Workbook and Competency Evaluation Review for

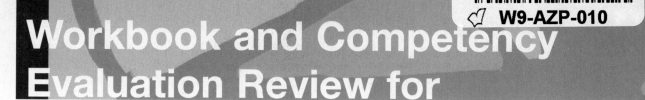

Mosby's Textbook
for
Long-Term Care Nursing Assistants

FIFTH EDITION

RELDA T. KELLY, RN, MSN

Professor Emeritus, Kankakee Community College
Kankakee, Illinois
Parish Nurse, Wesley United Methodist Church
Bradley, Illinois

Procedure Checklists by
HELEN CHIGAROS, RN, BS, MSN, CRRN, CNS

Professor Emeritus, Kankakee Community College
Kankakee, Illinois
Director, Azzarelli Outreach Clinic, St. Teresa Roman Catholic Church
Parish Nurse, St. Teresa Roman Catholic Church
Kankakee, Illinois

Competency Evaluation Review by
DIANN MUZYKA, PhD, RN

Clinical Associate Professor
Arizona State University
College of Nursing

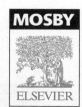

MOSBY

ELSEVIER

MOSBY
ELSEVIER

11830 Westline Industrial Drive
St. Louis, Missouri 63146

Notice

Nursing is an ever-changing field. Standard safety precautions must be followed, but as new
research and clinical experience broaden our knowledge, changes in treatment and drug therapy
may become necessary or appropriate. Readers are advised to check the most current product
information provided by the manufacturer. It is the responsibility of the licensed health care
provider, relying on experience and knowledge of the patient or resident, to determine the best
treatment for each individual patient or resident. Neither the publisher nor the authors assume
any liability for any injury and/or damage to persons or property arising from this publication.

The Publisher

ISBN-13: 978-0-323-04604-6
ISBN-10: 0-323-4604-5

Executive Editor: Susan R. Epstein
Senior Developmental Editor: Maria Broeker
Publishing Services Manager: John Rogers
Senior Project Manager: Doug Turner
Design Direction: Mark Oberkrom

Printed in the United States of America

Last digit is the print number: 9   8   7   6   5   4

This workbook is dedicated to my husband Earl who supported me as I worked on this edition. His encouragement and help in keeping my life in order kept me focused and on schedule!

Reviewers

Amy E. Green RN, BSN

Registered Nurse, Edward Hospital
and Health Services
Naperville, Illinois

Carolyn S. Leeder, RN

Inservice Coordinator
Georgia War Veterans Home
Milledgeville, Georgia

Preface

The *Workbook and Competency Evaluation Review for Mosby's Textbook for Long-Term Care Nursing Assistants*, fifth edition, is written to be used with the Sorrentino and Gorek textbook *Mosby's Textbook for Long-Term Care Nursing Assistants*, fifth edition. Students will not need other resources to complete the exercises in this Workbook. The answer key for the Workbook is found at the back of the Instructor's Resource Manual and includes page numbers on which the answers in the textbook are found.

The Workbook is designed to help students apply what they have learned in each chapter of the textbook. Students are encouraged to use this book as a study guide. Each chapter is thoroughly covered in the multiple-choice questions, which will give students practice to take the NAACEP test. In addition, other exercises such as fill-in-the-blank, matching, and crossword puzzles are used in many chapters. **Independent Learning Activities** at the end of each chapter may be used to apply the information learned in a practical setting. The section titled **Optional Learning Activities** may be used as an alternative exercise to give students more practice in studying the materials. Questions related to *Mosby's Nursing Assistant Skills Videos* have been added to the appropriate chapters. These questions will help students focus on the videos as they watch them.

In addition, **Procedure Checklists** that correspond with the procedures of the textbook are provided. These checklists are designed to help students become skilled at performing procedures that affect quality of care.

A brand-new **Competency Evaluation Review** includes a general review section and two practice exams with answers to help students prepare for the written certification exam. It also features a skills review guide that helps students practice procedures required for certification.

Assistive personnel are important members of the health team. Completing the exercises in this Workbook will increase the student's knowledge and skills. The goal is to prepare students to provide the best possible care and to encourage pride in a job well done.

Relda T. Kelly

Contents

1 Working in Long-Term Care

Key Terms

Acute illness	Hospice	Medicaid	Omnibus Budget
Alzheimer's disease	Independence	Medicare	Reconciliation Act of
(AD)	Interdisciplinary health	Nursing assistant	1987 (OBRA)
Assisted living facility	care team	Nursing center	Primary nursing
Board and care home	Involuntary seclusion	Nursing facility (NF)	Registered nurse (RN)
Case management	Licensed practical nurse	Nursing home	Residential care facility
Chronic illness	(LPN)	Nursing team	Skilled nursing
Deconditioning	Licensed vocational	Ombudsman	facility (SNF)
Functional nursing	nurse (LVN)		Team nursing

Fill in the Blanks: Key Terms

1. _____ is the process of becoming weak from illness or lack of exercise.

2. A person who has completed a 1-year nursing program and passed a licensing test is a _____.

3. Separating a person from others against his or her will is _____.

4. A _____ provides health care to persons who need regular or continuous care.

5. Another name for a nursing center or a nursing facility is a _____.

6. _____ means a person is not relying on or requiring care from others.

7. A sudden illness from which the person should recover is an _____.

8. A facility that provides nursing care for residents who have many or severe health problems or who need rehabilitation is called a _____ _____.

9. A _____ is an ongoing illness, slow or gradual in onset, that has no cure; the illness can be controlled and complications prevented with proper treatment.

10. An _____ provides housing, personal care, supportive services, health care, and social activities in a home-like setting.

11. In _____, a registered nurse is responsible for the person's total care.

12. RNs, LPNs/LVNs, and nursing assistants provide nursing care as part of the _____.

13. _____ is a disease that affects the brain tissue; there is increasing memory loss and confusion.

14. The nursing care pattern that focuses on tasks and jobs is _____.

15. _____ is a federal health insurance plan for persons 65 years of age or older and younger people with certain disabilities.

16. A _____ provides rooms, meals, laundry, and supervision to a few independent residents, often in a home setting.

17. A nursing center or nursing home may be called a _____.

18. _____ is a federal law concerned with the quality of life, health, and safety of residents.

19. In _____, a team of nursing staff is led by an RN who decides the amount and kind of care each person needs.

20. A person who has completed a 2-, 3-, or 4-year nursing program and who has passed a licensing test is a _____.

21. An _____ is someone who supports or promotes the needs and interests of another person.

22. Another name for a board and care home is a _____.

23. A nursing care pattern where an RN coordinates a person's care is _____.

24. A _____ gives basic nursing care under the supervision of a licensed nurse.

25. Another name for a licensed practical nurse is _____.

26. The many health care workers whose skills and knowledge focus on the person's total care is the _____.

27. _____ is a health care payment program sponsored by state and federal governments.

28. A health care agency or program for persons who are dying is a _____.

Circle the BEST Answer

29. Residents who live in a board and care home
    A. Receive care that meets the person's basic needs
    B. Stay there for a short time while recovering from an illness or surgery
    C. Are in a program for persons who are dying
    D. Are in a closed unit that provides a safer environment

30. Some assisted living facilities are part of
    A. A hospital
    B. Retirement communities or nursing centers
    C. A hospice
    D. A skilled care facility

31. Skilled nursing facilities provide
    A. Supportive care
    B. More complex care than nursing centers do
    C. A closed unit for residents who have Alzheimer's disease or other dementia
    D. Care for persons who are dying

32. Long-term care serves to
    A. Cure an acute illness
    B. Provide health care to persons who cannot care for themselves at home
    C. Help the person recover after surgery
    D. Cure a chronic illness

33. Colds and influenza can cause major health problems for older and disabled persons. These are called
    A. Chronic illnesses
    B. Communicable diseases
    C. Emotional illnesses
    D. Disabilities

34. What is the aim of rehabilitation or restorative care?
    A. A complete return of all functions
    B. Supportive care that meets basic physical needs
    C. To keep the person safe
    D. To help persons return to their highest possible level of physical and mental functioning

35. Children and pets usually can visit when a dying person is in
    A. An Alzheimer's unit   C. A hospice
    B. A hospital   D. A subacute care center

36. An Alzheimer's unit is a closed unit that provides
    A. A safer environment for the residents to wander freely
    B. A program for person who are dying
    C. A place for residents who are deconditioned after an acute illness
    D. A program for residents with a communicable disease

37. Which of these workers or areas in a health care center is not under the director of nursing in the organizational chart?
    A. Nursing assistant   C. Case managers
    B. Nurse managers   D. Social workers

38. The director of nursing is responsible for
    A. Coordinating resident care for a certain shift
    B. Planning and presenting educational programs
    C. The entire nursing staff
    D. All resident care and the actions of the nursing staff on a unit

39. Who coordinates care for a certain shift in the nursing center?
    A. Doctor   C. Shift manager
    B. Staff nurse   D. Director of nursing

40. Which of the following describes an RN?
    A. Completes 1-year nursing program and passes a licensing test
    B. Completes studies that qualifies the person to become the medical director of the nursing center
    C. Has formal training to give care and passes a competency examination
    D. Completes a 2-, 3-, or 4-year nursing program and has passed a licensing test

41. The nursing assistant gives basic nursing care under the supervision of
    A. The center administrator
    B. The director of nursing
    C. A licensed nurse
    D. Another nursing assistant

42. The nurse delegates care based on the person's needs and team member abilities in
    A. Functional nursing   C. Primary nursing
    B. Team nursing   D. Case management

43. Medicare is a federal health insurance plan that has benefits for
    A. Persons 65 years old and older
    B. Families with low incomes
    C. Individuals and families who buy the insurance
    D. Groups of individuals who buy the insurance

44. Part B of Medicare
    A. Pays for hospital costs and some SNF costs
    B. Benefits only persons 65 years of age and older
    C. Is administered by the Social Security Administration
    D. Helps pay for doctors' visits, outpatient hospital care, physical and occupational therapists, and some home care

45. Under a DRG (diagnosis-related group) plan
    A. Only persons 65 years of age and older receive care
    B. Payment is determined before the person receives care
    C. A decision is made about how much to pay for care in an SNF
    D. For a prepaid fee, persons receive all needed services offered

46. Under an RUG (resource utilization group) plan
    A. Only persons 65 years of age and older receive care
    B. Payment is determined before the person receives care
    C. A decision is made about how much to pay for care in an SNF
    D. For a prepaid fee, persons receive all needed services offered

47. If a person has managed care, the insured person will have costs covered based on
    A. Health care available in the community
    B. The age of the person
    C. His or her physical needs
    D. Pre-approval process used by his or her insurer

48. Under the Omnibus Budget Reconciliation Act of 1987 (OBRA), a resident has all of the following rights *except*
    A. The right to have a private room in which to live
    B. The right to have personal choice to choose what to wear and how to spend his or her time
    C. The right to personal privacy
    D. The right to refuse treatment
49. Under OBRA, if a resident is incompetent (not able) to exercise the rights, who can exercise these rights for the person?
    A. The doctor
    B. A responsible party such as a partner, spouse, or adult child
    C. The charge nurse
    D. A neighbor
50. If a resident refuses treatment, what should you do?
    A. Avoid giving any care to the person and go on to other duties
    B. Report the refusal to the nurse
    C. Tell the resident the treatment must be done and continue to carry out the treatment
    D. Tell his family so they can make him take the treatment
51. A student wants to observe a treatment, but the resident does not want her to be present. What is the correct action?
    A. The student cannot watch because this violates the resident's right to privacy
    B. The student may observe from the doorway where the resident cannot see her
    C. The staff nurse tells the resident he must allow the student to watch
    D. The nurse calls the resident's wife to get her permission
52. The resident should be given personal choice whenever it
    A. Is safely possible
    B. Does not interfere with scheduled activities
    C. Is approved by the director of nursing
    D. Is ordered by the doctor
53. If a resident voices concerns about care and the center promptly tries to correct the situation, this action meets the resident's right to
    A. Participate in a resident group
    B. Voice a dispute or grievance
    C. Personal choice
    D. Freedom from abuse, mistreatment, and neglect
54. A resident volunteers to take care of houseplants at the center. This is an acceptable part of the following *except*
    A. The care plan
    B. A requirement to receive care or care items
    C. The resident's regular activity
    D. Rehabilitation
55. When residents and their families plan activities together, this meets the residents' right to
    A. Privacy
    B. Freedom from restraint
    C. Freedom from mistreatment
    D. Participate in resident and family groups

56. The resident you are caring for has many old holiday decorations covering her nightstand. If you throw away these items without her permission you are denying her right to
    A. Privacy
    B. Work
    C. Care and security of personal possessions
    D. Freedom from abuse
57. A staff member tells a resident he cannot leave his room because he talks too much. This action denies the resident
    A. Freedom from abuse, mistreatment, and neglect
    B. Freedom from restraint
    C. Care and security of personal possessions
    D. Personal choice
58. When a resident is given certain drugs that affect his mood, behavior, or mental function, it may deny his right to
    A. Freedom from abuse, mistreatment, and neglect
    B. Personal choice
    C. Privacy
    D. Freedom from restraint
59. Which of these actions will promote dignity and privacy?
    A. Calling the resident by a nickname he does not choose
    B. Assist with dressing him in clothing appropriate to the time of day
    C. Changing the resident's hairstyle without her permission
    D. Leaving the bathroom door open so you can see the person
60. You ask a resident if you may touch him. This is an example of
    A. Courteous and dignified interactions
    B. Courteous and dignified care
    C. Providing privacy and self-determination
    D. Maintaining personal choice and independence
61. Assisting a resident to ambulate without interfering with his independence is an example of
    A. Courteous and dignified interaction
    B. Courteous and dignified care
    C. Providing privacy and self-determination
    D. Maintaining personal choice and independence
62. You provide privacy and self-determination for a resident when you
    A. Knock on the door before entering and wait to be asked in
    B. Allow the resident to smoke in designated areas
    C. Listen with interest to what the person is saying
    D. Groom his beard as he wishes
63. You allow the resident to maintain personal choice and independence when you
    A. Obtain her attention before interacting with her
    B. Provide extra clothing for warmth such as a sweater or lap robe
    C. Assist the resident to take part in activities according to his interests
    D. Use curtains or screens during personal care and procedures

64. Which of these activities would be carried out by an ombudsman?
    - A. Organize activities for a group of residents
    - B. Accompany residents to a religious service at a house of worship
    - C. Investigate and resolve complaints made by a resident
    - D. Assist the resident to choose friends
65. Nursing centers require certification to
    - A. Signal quality and excellence
    - B. Receive Medicare and Medicaid funds
    - C. Operate and provide care
    - D. Meet state and federal standards
66. A nursing assistant could prevent common nursing center deficiencies by
    - A. Protecting residents from abuse, mistreatment, and neglect when giving care
    - B. Hiring only people with no legal history of abusing, neglecting, or mistreating residents
    - C. Applying physical restraints to keep residents safe
    - D. Ignoring other caregivers who may be abusing or neglecting residents

Fill in the Blanks
Write out the meaning of each abbreviation.

67. RN _____
68. LPN or LVN _____
69. AD _____
70. NF _____
71. SNF _____
72. OBRA _____
73. DON _____
74. DRG _____
75. DRGs are for _____ costs
76. RUG _____
77. RUGs are for _____ payments
78. CMG _____
79. CMGs are used for _____ centers
80. HMO _____
81. PPO _____

Matching
Match the types of health care service with the correct example.

82. _____ Provides health care and nursing care for residents who have many or severe health problems or who need rehabilitation
83. _____ Provides rooms, meals, laundry, and supervision to a few independent residents
84. _____ Provides a unit closed off from the rest of the center. This provides a safe setting for residents to wander freely
85. _____ Health care agency or program for people who are dying
86. _____ Provides housing, personal care, supportive services, health care, and social activities in a home-like setting

A. Skilled care facility
B. Hospice unit
C. Board and care home
D. Alzheimer's unit
E. Assisted living facility

Match the types of nursing care pattern with the correct examples.

87. _____ RN leader delegates care of certain persons to other nurses. Nursing tasks and procedures are delegated to nursing assistants.
88. _____ The RN is responsible for the person's total care. The nursing team assists as needed.
89. _____ The RN coordinates a person's care from admission through discharge and into home setting.
90. _____ Each nursing team member has certain tasks or functions to do.

A. Functional nursing
B. Team nursing
C. Primary nursing
D. Case management

Nursing Assistant Skills Video Exercise
View the Basic Principles video to answer these questions.

91. To protect the right to confidentiality, you should _____.

92. You protect the right to personal choice by _____ _____.

93. Wherever you work, you must be familiar with the _____ and _____.

Optional Learning Exercises
Long-Term Care Centers Comparison

94. A board and care home provides _____ _____ in a home-like setting. What is the resident usually able to do with little help? _____ What happens if the person has an emergency in the middle of the night? _____

95. An assisted living facility provides _____ _____, _____ in a home-like setting. Help given includes _____. There is access to _____.

96. A nursing center provides health care to persons _____. The facility is required to employ _____ nurses on the staff.

97. A skilled nursing facility provides health and nursing care for residents who have _____.

98. What are the purposes and goals of long-term care centers?
A. Promote _____
B. Treat _____
C. Prevent _____
D. Provide _____

99. A hospice is an agency or program for _____ _____. What needs are met by a hospice? _____

100. An Alzheimer's unit is designed for persons with _____. An Alzheimer's unit is closed off from the rest of the center because these residents may _____.

101. Persons on a rehabilitation or subacute care unit often stay there for _____.

Health Team Members (Table 1-1)
Name the health team member who provides the service described.

102. Mr. Williams needs assistance to regain skills to dress, shave, and feed himself (ADL). He is assisted by the _____.

103. The nurse has concern about a drug action so calls the _____.

104. Mrs. Young needs the corns on her feet treated. The nurse notifies the _____.

105. Ms. Stewart has the responsibility of doing physical examinations, health assessments, and health educations for the center where she works. She is a _____.

106. Mr. Gomez keeps turning up the volume of his TV. His hearing is tested by the _____.

107. The _____ meets with a new resident and his family to discuss his nutritional needs.

108. Mr. Fox had a stroke and has weakness on his left side. The _____ assists him by developing a plan that focuses on restoring function and preventing disability from his illness.

109. The doctor orders x-rays after Mr. Jackson falls. The x-rays are done by the _____.

110. Mr. Ling has chronic lung disease and needs respiratory treatments. These are given by the _____.

111. Ms. Walker plans the recreational needs of a nursing center. She is an _____.

112. After a stroke, Mr. Stubbs has difficulty swallowing. He is evaluated by the _____.

113. When the doctor orders blood tests, the samples are collected by the _____.

OBRA Actions to Promote Dignity and Privacy (Box 1-2)
Match the action to promote dignity and privacy with the example.

114. _____ File fingernails and apply polish as resident requests
115. _____ Cover the resident with a blanket during a bath
116. _____ You gain the person's attention before giving care
117. _____ Show interest when a resident tells stories about his past
118. _____ Open containers and arrange food at mealtimes to assist the resident
119. _____ Close the door when the person asks for privacy
120. _____ Allow a resident to smoke in a designated area
121. _____ Make sure the resident is wearing his dentures when he goes to the dining room
122. _____ You take the resident to his weekly card game

A. Courteous and dignified interaction
B. Courteous and dignified care
C. Privacy and self-determination
D. Maintain personal choice and independence

Independent Learning Activities
Gather the following information about long-term centers in your area.
- How many board and care homes are located in your area? Choose one home and answer these questions:
  - Is this home attached to a nursing center, or is it a separate center?
  - What services are provided?
  - How many residents are in the home?
  - How many staff members work there? How many staff members are: RNs? LPNs/LVNs? Nursing assistants? What care is provided by nursing assistants?
- How many nursing centers are located in your area? Choose one center and answer these questions:
  - What types of residents are accepted in the center? (For example, does the center consider level of care needed, the resident's disease, or method of payment?)
  - How many residents live in the center?
  - How many staff members work there? How many staff members are: RNs? LPNs/LVNs? Nursing assistants? What care is provided by nursing assistants?
- How many nursing centers in your area provide skilled nursing care? Choose one center and answer these questions:
  - How many residents live in the center?
  - How many staff members work there? How many staff members are: RNs? LPNs/LVNs? Nursing assistants? What care is provided by nursing assistants?
- How many assisted living facilities are located in your area? Choose one center and answer these questions:
  - Is this facility independent or part of a long-term care center?
  - How many residents live in the facility?
  - What kind of living quarters do the residents have? (For example, does each resident have an apartment or studio? Do they share kitchen facilities, or does each person have a kitchen?)
  - How many staff members work there? How many staff members are: RNs? LPNs/LVNs? Nursing assistants? What care is provided by nursing assistants?
- Find a nursing center that has an Alzheimer's unit and answer these questions:
  - How is the unit identified? Is it a separate wing? Separate floor? Is the unit closed off?
  - How is the unit different from other units in the center?
  - Do the staff members who work on this unit receive special training? If so, what extra training are they given? What duties are assigned to nursing assistants on this unit?
- Does your area have a hospice program? If so, answer these questions about the program:
  - Is this program located within a center, or does it provide care in the person's facility or home?
  - What type of care is provided?
  - What special training is given to the staff? What duties can be performed by a nursing assistant?

2 The Nursing Assistant in Long-Term Care

Key Terms

Abuse
Accountable
Assault
Battery
Civil law
Crime
Criminal law

Defamation
Delegate
Elder abuse
Ethics
False imprisonment
Fraud
Invasion of privacy

Job description
Law
Libel
Malpractice
Neglect
Negligence
Responsibility

Slander
Standard of care
Tort
Will

Fill in the Blanks: Key Terms

1. _____ is negligence by a professional person.

2. Saying or doing something to trick, fool, or deceive another person is _____.

3. _____ is concerned with offenses against the public and society in general.

4. A _____ is a legal statement of how a person wishes to have property distributed after death.

5. Being responsible for one's actions and the actions of others who perform delegated tasks is called being _____.

6. A rule of conduct made by a government body is a _____.

7. _____ is the unauthorized touching of a person's body without the person's consent.

8. The intentional mistreatment or harm of another person is _____.

9. _____ is defamation through oral statements.

10. Injuring a person's name and reputation by making false statements to a third person is _____ _____.

11. _____ is knowledge of what is right conduct and wrong conduct.

12. Intentionally attempting or threatening to touch a person's body without the person's consent is _____.

13. A _____ is a wrong committed against a person or the person's property.

14. _____ is concerned with relationships between people.

15. A _____ is a list of responsibilities and functions the center expects you to perform.

16. The duty or obligation to perform some act or function is called _____.

17. Violating a person's right not to have his or her name, photograph, or private affairs exposed or made public without giving consent is _____ _____.

18. _____ is the skills, care, and judgment required by the health team member under similar circumstances.

19. To _____ means to authorize another person to perform a nursing task in a certain setting.

20. An act that violates a criminal law is a _____ _____.

21. _____ is the unlawful restraint or restriction of a person's movement.

22. Defamation through written statements is _____ _____.

23. _____ is an unintentional wrong in which a person does not act in a reasonable and careful manner and causes harm to a person or to the person's property.

24. Any knowing, intentional, or negligent act by a caregiver or any other person to an older adult is _____.

25. _____ is the failure to provide the person with goods or services needed to avoid physical harm, mental anguish, or mental illness.

Circle the BEST Answer

26. Until the 1980s, nursing assistants
    A. Attended nursing assistant classes approved by the state
    B. Were not used in giving basic nursing care
    C. Received on-the-job training from nurses
    D. Worked only in hospitals

27. What major political issues in the 1980s caused hospital closings, hospitals mergers, and changes in health care systems?
    A. Nursing shortages
    B. Changes made by OBRA
    C. Rising health care costs
    D. Changes in nurse practice acts

28. A staffing mix that includes nursing assistants are used in hospitals because of
    A. Nursing shortages
    B. An effort to reduce costs
    C. Changes in nurse practice acts
    D. Changes made in insurance payments
29. State laws that regulate nursing assistants' roles and functions are determined by
    A. OBRA
    B. The nurse practice act
    C. The state medical society
    D. Insurance companies
30. If you perform a task beyond the legal limits of your role, you could be
    A. Protected by the nurse practice act
    B. Practicing nursing without a license
    C. Protected by the nurse who supervises your work
    D. Accused of a criminal act
31. OBRA requires that the nursing assistant training and competency evaluation program have at least _____ hours of instruction
    A. 16
    B. 75
    C. 120
    D. 200
32. Which of these areas of study is *not* included in a training program for nursing assistants?
    A. Communication
    B. Elimination procedures
    C. Resident rights
    D. Phlebotomy (drawing blood)
33. The competency evaluation for nursing assistants has 2 parts. They are
    A. A written test and a skills test
    B. A multiple-choice test and a true-false test
    C. A skills test and a complete bed bath demonstration
    D. A written test and an oral question-and-answer test
34. If you fail the competency evaluation the first time you take it, you
    A. Can retest one more time
    B. Must repeat your training program
    C. Can retest two more times (for a total of three times)
    D. Can retest as often as necessary free of charge
35. All of the following information is contained in the nursing assistant registry information *except*
    A. Information about findings of abuse, neglect, or dishonest use of property
    B. Date of birth
    C. Number of dependents
    D. Date the competency examination was passed
36. OBRA requires that retraining and a new competency evaluation test must be taken if you have not worked as a certified nursing assistant for
    A. 24 months
    B. 5 years
    C. 1 consecutive year
    D. 6 months

37. Your work as a nursing assistant is supervised by
    A. An RN or LPN/LVN
    B. The doctor
    C. The director of nursing
    D. A nursing assistant with more experience
38. When in-service programs or training is scheduled, the nursing assistant
    A. Must attend those that are required
    B. Needs to attend only if the program is scheduled on a day he or she is scheduled to work
    C. Cannot attend if the program is scheduled during the work day
    D. Does not need to attend if it means he or she must come to work early or stay late
39. You are alone in the nurses' station and you answer the phone. Dr. Smith begins to give verbal orders to you. You should
    A. Hang up the phone
    B. Politely give him your name and title and ask him to wait while you get the nurse
    C. Quickly write down the orders and give them to the nurse
    D. Politely give him your name and title and ask him to call back later when the nurse is there
40. As a nursing assistant, you *never* give medications *unless*
    A. The nurse is busy and asks you to give them
    B. The resident is in the shower and the nurse leaves the medications at the bedside
    C. You have completed a state-required medication and training program about giving medications
    D. You are feeding the resident and the nurse asks you to mix the medications with the food
41. The nurse asks you to carry out a task that you do not know how to do. You should
    A. Ignore the order since it is something you cannot do
    B. Perform the task as well as you can
    C. Ask another nursing assistant to show you how to carry out the task
    D. Promptly explain to the nurse why you cannot carry out the task
42. The nurse asks you to assist him as he changes sterile dressings. You should
    A. Assist him as needed
    B. Tell him you cannot assist to perform any sterile procedures
    C. Tell him that this is something you cannot do
    D. Report his request to the supervisor
43. Who can tell the person or the family a diagnosis or prescribe treatments?
    A. The director of nursing
    B. The RN
    C. The doctor
    D. An experienced nursing assistant
44. When you read a job description, you should *not* take a job if it requires you to
    A. Carry out duties you do not like to do
    B. Maintain required certification
    C. Attend in-service training
    D. Function beyond your training limits

45. Which of the following is *not* acceptable?
    A. An RN delegates a task to an LPN/LVN
    B. An LPN/LVN delegates a task to a nursing assistant
    C. An RN delegates a task to a nursing assistant
    D. A nursing assistant delegates a task to another nursing assistant
46. When a nurse considers delegating tasks, the decision
    A. Should always result in the best care for the person
    B. Depends on whether the nurse likes the nursing assistant
    C. Depends on how busy the nurse is that day
    D. Depends on how well the nurse likes the person
47. You have been caring for Mr. Watson for several weeks. The nurse tells you that she will give his care today. Her delegation decision is based primarily on
    A. How well you performed his care yesterday
    B. Changes in Mr. Watson's condition
    C. Whether the nurse knows you or not
    D. How much supervision you need
48. Which of the following is *not* a right of delegation?
    A. The right task
    B. The right person
    C. The right time
    D. The right supervision
49. You agree to perform a task the nurse delegates to you. Which of these statements tells you it is the right circumstance for you to do this?
    A. You understand the purpose of the task for this person
    B. You are comfortable performing the task
    C. You have reviewed the task with the nurse
    D. You were trained to do the task
50. You may refuse to carry out a task for all of the following reasons *except*:
    A. The task is not in your job description
    B. You do not know how to use the supplies or equipment
    C. You are too busy
    D. The person could be harmed if you carry out the task
51. It is unethical if you
    A. Refuse to give care to a person with beliefs different from yours
    B. Refuse to carry out a task because you do not know how to do it
    C. Refuse to perform a task that is against your religious or moral beliefs
    D. Refuse to carry out a task beyond the legal limits of your role
52. Which of the following is *not* good conduct for a nursing assistant?
    A. Carry our any assignment given to you by the nurse
    B. Take only drugs that have been prescribed by your doctor
    C. Recognize limits of your role and your knowledge
    D. Consider the needs of the residents to be more important than your own needs

53. A nurse failed to do what a reasonable and careful nurse would have done. Legally, this is called
    A. A crime
    B. A tort
    C. Negligence
    D. Malpractice
54. If you fail to properly identify a person and perform a treatment on him intended for another, you are
    A. Committing a crime
    B. Legally responsible for your actions
    C. Not responsible legally, but are unethical
    D. Guilty of an intentional tort
55. A nursing assistant writes a note to a friend that injures the name and reputation of a person by making false statements. This is called
    A. Libel
    B. Slander
    C. Malpractice
    D. Negligence
56. The nursing assistant would violate the Health Insurance Portability and Accountability Act of 1996 (HIPAA) if he or she
    A. Says or does something that tricks or deceives a person
    B. Gives out information about the person's health care
    C. Signs a legal document for a resident
    D. Makes false statements about a resident to a third person
57. A nursing assistant tells a resident she is a nurse. She has committed
    A. Fraud
    B. Libel
    C. Slander
    D. Negligence
58. When a resident is confined to his room by a caregiver, he is a victim of
    A. Physical abuse
    B. False imprisonment
    C. Invasion of privacy
    D. Battery
59. If a resident tells you that he does not want you to dress him and you go ahead and touch him, you can be accused of
    A. Fraud
    B. Battery
    C. Assault
    D. False imprisonment
60. If you are asked to obtain a resident's signature on an informed consent, you should
    A. Make sure the resident is mentally competent
    B. Refuse. You are never responsible for obtaining a written consent
    C. Make sure the resident understands what he is signing
    D. Ask a family member to witness the signed consent

61. If a person is confused or unconscious, informed consent
    A. Is not necessary
    B. Cannot be obtained and so no treatments can be given
    C. Can be given by a husband, wife, son, daughter, or legal representative
    D. Can be given by the director of nursing

62. You can refuse to sign a will if
    A. You are named in the will
    B. You do not believe the person is of sound mind
    C. Your nursing center has policies that do not allow employees to witness wills
    D. All of the above

63. Which of the following is not an element of abuse?
    A. Willful causing of injury
    B. Intimidation
    C. Expecting a person to feed and dress himself within his abilities
    D. Depriving a person of food as punishment

64. What kind of abuse occurs when an elderly person is left to sit in urine or feces?
    A. Neglect
    B. Involuntary seclusion
    C. Mental
    D. Sexual

65. An example of verbal abuse can be
    A. Failing to answer a signal light
    B. Locking a person in a room
    C. Oral or written statements that speak badly of a person
    D. Making threats of being punished

66. Depriving a person of needs such as food, clothing, or a place to sleep is
    A. Verbal abuse
    B. Involuntary seclusion
    C. Physical or emotional abuse
    D. Sexual abuse

67. Which of the following may be a sign of elder abuse?
    A. The person answers questions openly
    B. The family makes sure the hearing aids have new batteries
    C. A caregiver is present during all conversations
    D. All medications are taken as scheduled

68. A sign of sexual abuse can be
    A. Small, circle-like burns on the body
    B. Bleeding or bruising in the genital area
    C. Weight loss and the person shows signs of poor nutrition
    D. Personal hygiene is lacking

69. If you suspect an elderly person is being abused, you should
    A. Call the police
    B. Discuss the situation and your observations with the nurse
    C. Discuss the situation with the family
    D. Notify community agencies that investigate elderly abuse

70. What happens to a nursing assistant who is found taking money from a resident's purse?
    A. The amount of money taken will be deducted from the next paycheck
    B. The nursing assistant can lose her job, and the state nursing assistant registry will be notified
    C. The nursing assistant will be transferred to another unit
    D. The nursing assistant will be expected to apologize to the resident

71. Which of these persons could be a child abuser?
    A. A person with little education
    B. A person with a high income
    C. A person who was abused as a child
    D. All of the above

72. Children who are deprived of food, clothing, shelter, and medical care are victims of
    A. Physical neglect
    B. Emotional neglect
    C. Physical abuse
    D. Sexual abuse

73. Children who are molested are victims of
    A. Physical neglect
    B. Emotional neglect
    C. Physical abuse
    D. Sexual abuse

74. If you suspect a child is being abused, you should
    A. Share your concerns with the nurse
    B. Talk with the child
    C. Inform the doctor
    D. Call a child protection agency

75. A husband does not allow his wife to use the car, to leave the home, or to visit with family and friends. This is a form of domestic violence called
    A. Verbal abuse
    B. Social abuse
    C. Physical abuse
    D. Economic abuse

Matching
Match the examples with the correct tort.

76. _____ While cleaning a resident's dentures, the nursing assistant drops and breaks them
77. _____ A nursing assistant opens a resident's mail and reads it without permission
78. _____ Instead of allowing the resident a choice, the nursing assistant tells him he will get a shower whether he wants one or not
79. _____ An individual touches a person's body without the person's consent
80. _____ An individual tricks or fools another person
81. _____ An individual restrains or restricts a resident's freedom of movement without a physician's order
82. _____ A nurse gives a treatment to the wrong person
83. _____ A nursing assistant injures the name and reputation of a resident by making false statements to a third person
84. _____ A nursing assistant writes notes falsely accusing another nursing assistant of stealing her purse

A. Negligence
B. Malpractice
C. Libel
D. Slander
E. False imprisonment
F. Assault
G. Battery
H. Fraud
I. Invasion of privacy

Nursing Assistant Skills Video Exercise
*View the **Basic Principles** video to answer these questions.*

85. As a nursing assistant, you are a member of the _____ that works together for the _____.
86. _____ and _____, and _____ define the roles and functions of each team member
87. Each member of the nursing team is concerned with the _____, _____, _____, and _____ needs of patients, residents, and their families.
88. The tasks you perform and the amount of supervision you need depend on
    A. _____
    B. _____
    C. _____
89. Never perform a function or task that _____ _____ or _____ _____.
90. When deciding to delegate, the nurse must protect the person's _____ and _____. The nurse can delegate only tasks that are _____ _____.
91. To ensure that tasks are delegated correctly and safely, nurses use the _____ _____.
92. Describe each of the "Five Rights of Delegation" listed.
    A. The "right task" means _____
    B. The "right circumstance" means _____
    C. The "right person" means _____
    D. The "right directions and communication" means _____
    E. The "right supervision" means _____
93. List four measures to protect the person's right to privacy.
    A. _____
    B. _____
    C. _____
    D. _____

Optional Learning Exercises
OBRA requirements related to the nursing assistant

94. The nursing assistant must meet federal and state training and competency requirements in order to work in _____ _____.
95. OBRA requires _____ hours of instruction. _____ hours must be supervised practical training. Where can the practical training take place? _____ or _____.
96. OBRA requires 15 areas of study. Write area of study where you learn the skill in each example.
    A. _____ You make a bed.
    B. _____ You close Mr. Smith's door to give him privacy.
    C. _____ You tell Mrs. Forbes the time of day and the day of week frequently during the day.
    D. _____ You apply lotion to a resident's dry skin.
    E. _____ You assist a resident to put on his shirt.
    F. _____ When assigned to a new unit, you check to find the location of the fire alarm.
    G. _____ You wash your hands before and after giving care.
    H. _____ You get help to move a resident from his bed to the chair.
    I. _____ When speaking to Mr. Jackson, you maintain good eye contact.
    J. _____ The nurse tells you to exercise a resident's extremities (limbs).
    K. _____ You shave Mr. Stewart.
    L. _____ You position a urinal for a resident in bed.
    M. _____ You assist Mrs. Young to walk in the hall.
    N. _____ You notice Mrs. Peck has an elevated temperature and her skin is warm.
    O. _____ You cut up the meat on Mr. Johnson's plate before helping him eat.

The National Nursing Assistant Assessment Program (NNAAP) (Appendix)

97. The NNAAP written test has _____ questions. List the percent of questions in each area.

    A. _____ Activities of Daily Living

    B. _____ Basic Nursing Skills

    C. _____ Restorative Skills

    D. _____ Emotional and Mental Health Needs

    E. _____ Spiritual and Cultural Needs

    F. _____ Communications

    G. _____ Client Rights

    H. _____ Legal and Ethical Behavior

    I. _____ Member of the Health Care Team

98. List the skills that are tested on the NNAAP.

    A. _____
    B. _____
    C. _____
    D. _____
    E. _____
    F. _____
    G. _____
    H. _____
    I. _____
    J. _____
    K. _____
    L. _____
    M. _____
    N. _____

O. _____
P. _____
Q. _____
R. _____
S. _____
T. _____
U. _____
V. _____
W. _____
X. _____
Y. _____

Position Description

99. During admission, transfer, and discharge procedures, the nursing assistant may be assigned to _____ and _____ the residents.

100. If the nursing assistant observes reddened areas or skin breakdown, the nursing assistant should _____.

101. When a nursing assistant tells the resident the date, day of the week, and time of day during daily care, he or she is meeting the job responsibility to provide _____.

102. When the nursing assistant attends in-service education programs as required, he or she will learn _____.

103. The nursing assistant is expected to attend at least _____ of staff meetings.

104. Current Basic Cardiac Life Support certification must be completed within _____ of hire date.

Independent Learning Activities
- Make a list of tasks that would conflict with your moral or religious beliefs.
  - How would you feel about performing these tasks in your job?
  - What would you say to you employer or co-workers?
- Role-play a situation in which you are asked to perform one of the tasks you identified in the previous activity. Have one student play the person asking you to perform the task. Have a second student observe and answer these questions:
  - What was your reaction when asked?
  - In what way did you communicate your discomfort?
  - What suggestions did you offer to make sure the task was done?
- Identify agencies in your community that help victims of abuse (elder, child, domestic). Visit one of the agencies and ask these questions:
  - How do you find out about the victim?
  - What services do you offer? What happens to the victim after you identify a problem? Do you have a place where they can be protected?

3 Work Ethics

Key Terms

Confidentiality	Gossip
Courtesy	Harassment

Preceptor	Stressor
Stress	Work ethics

Fill in the Blanks: Key Terms

1. A staff member who guides another staff member is a _____.

2. A _____ is the event or factor that causes stress.

3. Trusting others with personal and private information is _____.

4. _____ is behavior in the workplace.

5. _____ is to spread rumors or talk about the private matters of others.

6. The response or change in the body caused by any emotional, physical, social, or economic factor is _____.

7. _____ is a polite, considerate, or helpful comment or act.

8. _____ means to trouble, torment, offend, or worry a person by one's behavior or comments.

Circle the BEST Answer

9. Work ethics involve
   A. How well you do your skills
   B. What religion you practice
   C. How you treat and work with others
   D. Cultural beliefs and attitudes

10. Your diet will maintain your weight if
    A. You avoid salty and sweet foods
    B. You take in fewer calories than your energy needs require
    C. It includes foods with fats and oils
    D. The number of calories taken in equals your energy needs

11. Adults need about _____ hours of sleep daily
    A. 7
    B. 10
    C. 4
    D. 12

12. Exercise is needed for
    A. Rest and sleep
    B. Muscle tone and circulation
    C. Good body mechanics
    D. Good nutrition

13. Smoking odors
    A. Disappear quickly when the person finishes smoking
    B. Can be covered up by chewing gum
    C. Are noticed only by the smoker
    D. Stay on the person's breath, hands, clothing, and hair

14. The most important reason a person should not work under the influence of alcohol or drugs is it
    A. Affects the person's safety
    B. Causes the person to be disorganized
    C. Makes co-workers angry
    D. Is not allowed by your nursing center

15. Which of these is *not* part of good personal hygiene for work?
    A. Bathe daily and use a deodorant
    B. Practice good hand washing
    C. Cut toenails straight across
    D. Keep fingernails long and polished

16. Tattoos should be covered when working because they
    A. May offend residents, families, and co-workers
    B. Can become infected
    C. May confuse residents
    D. Increase the risk of skin injuries

17. When working, the nursing assistant may wear
    A. Jewelry in pierced eyebrow, nose, lips, or tongue
    B. Wedding and engagement rings
    C. Multiple earrings in each ear
    D. Nail polish

18. When working, the nursing assistant *should not* wear
    A. A beard or mustache that is clean and trimmed
    B. Hair that is off the collar and away from the face
    C. Perfume, cologne, or after-shave
    D. A wristwatch with a second hand

19. Displaying good work ethics at your clinical experience site may help you find a job because
    A. You will pass the course
    B. It will show you care
    C. You will get better grades
    D. The staff always looks at students as future employees

20. You should be well-groomed when looking for a job because it
    A. Shows you are cooperative
    B. Makes a good first impression
    C. Shows you are respectful
    D. Shows you have values and attitudes that fit with the center

21. How does an employer know you can perform required job skills?
    A. They will request proof of training and will check your record in the state nursing assistant registry
    B. They will have you give a demonstration of your skills
    C. You will be asked many questions about performing certain skills
    D. You will be required to take a written test

22. You can get a job application from
    A. The personnel office or the human relations office
    B. A friend who works at the center
    C. From the director of nursing
    D. The receptionist in the lobby of the center

23. You should take a dry run to a job interview to
    A. Show you follow directions well
    B. Show you listen well
    C. Make sure you will be on time for the interview
    D. Look over the center to see if you want to work there

24. When you are interviewing, it is correct to
    A. Have a glass of wine before going
    B. Look directly at the interviewer
    C. Wear a sweat suit and athletic shoes
    D. Shake hands very gently

25. What is a good way to share your list of skills with the interviewer?
    A. Tell the person verbally what you can do
    B. Ask for a list of skills and check the ones you know
    C. Bring a list of your skills and give it to the interviewer
    D. Tell the interviewer you will send a list as soon as possible

26. It is important to ask questions at the end of the interview because it
    A. Will show the interviewer you are interested in the job
    B. Will help you to decide if the job is right for you
    C. Shows you have good communication skills
    D. Shows you are dependable

27. If you are assigned a preceptor, the person may be
    A. An RN
    B. Another nursing assistant
    C. An LPN/LVN
    D. Any of the above

28. What is a common reason for losing a job?
    A. Not knowing how to perform a task
    B. Frequent absences or excessive tardiness
    C. Being disorganized
    D. Lacking self-confidence

29. If you are scheduled to begin work at 3 PM, you should arrive
    A. At 3 PM
    B. At 2:30 PM
    C. Early enough to be ready to work at 3 PM
    D. As close to 3 PM as you can

30. You can avoid being part of gossip by
    A. Remaining quiet when you are in a group where gossip is occurring
    B. Talking about residents and family members only to co-workers
    C. Repeating comments only in writing
    D. Removing yourself from a group or situation where gossip is occurring

31. Privacy and confidentiality for residents are rights protected by
    A. Your job description
    B. Resident rights under OBRA
    C. An agreement between the resident and the nurse
    D. Doctor's orders

32. When you are working, you should not wear
    A. Clothing that has not been washed and pressed
    B. A loose-fitting shirt
    C. A shirt with the top button open
    D. White socks

33. Slang or swearing should not be used at work because
    A. Words used with family and friends may offend residents and family members
    B. The resident may not understand you
    C. Resident may have difficulty hearing
    D. Co-workers may overhear it

34. You should say "please" and "thank you" to others because
    A. A courtesy means so much to people; it can brighten someone's day
    B. It shows respect to the person
    C. It is required by your job
    D. It shows you like the person

35. When you are working, it is acceptable to
    A. Take a pen to use at home
    B. Sell cookies for your child's school project
    C. Use a pay phone on your break to call your child
    D. Make a copy of a letter on the copier in the nurses' station

36. When you leave and return to the unit for breaks or lunch, you should
    A. Tell each resident
    B. Tell any family members present
    C. Tell the nurse
    D. All of the above

37. Safety practices are important to follow because
    A. They help you be more organized
    B. Negligent behavior affects the safety of others
    C. They save the center money
    D. You will get promoted more quickly

38. Care should be planned around
    A. Your break and lunch time
    B. Resident mealtimes, visiting hours, activities, and therapies
    C. Co-workers' schedules
    D. The time scheduled by the nurse

39. Stress occurs
    A. Only when you have unpleasant situations in your life
    B. Because you do not handle your problems well
    C. Because you are in the wrong job
    D. Every minute of every day and in everything you do

40. What physical effects of stress can be life-threatening?
    A. High blood pressure, heart attack, strokes, ulcers
    B. Increased heart rate, faster and deeper breathing
    C. Anxiety, fear, anger, depression
    D. Headaches, insomnia, muscle tension
41. Which of these actions is harassment?
    A. Offending others with gestures or remarks
    B. Offending others with jokes or pictures
    C. Making a sexual advance or requesting sexual favors
    D. All of the above

42. If you resign from a job, it is good practice to give
    A. One week's notice
    B. Two weeks' notice
    C. Four weeks' notice
    D. No notice
43. Good work ethics help residents
    A. Feel safe, secure, loved, and cared for
    B. Receive adequate care
    C. Recover from their illnesses
    D. Have more freedom to go to activities

Crossword
Use terms in Box 3-2 in the textbook to complete the crossword.

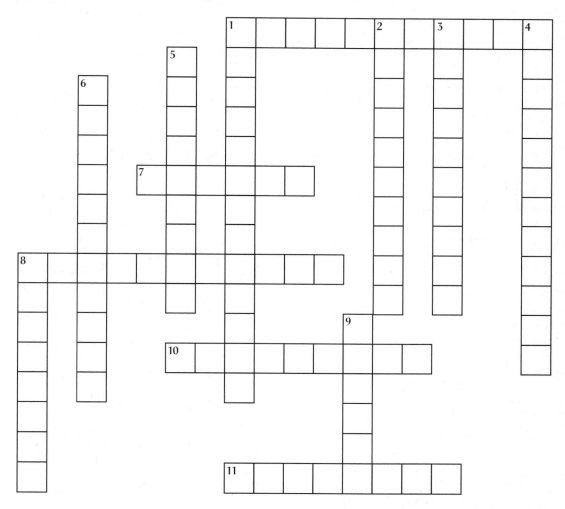

ACROSS
1. Respect the person's physical and emotional feelings
7. Have concern for the person
8. Willing to help and work with others
10. Be polite and courteous to residents, families, and visitors
11. See things from the person's point of view

DOWN
1. Be careful, alert, and exact in following directions
2. Report to work on time and when scheduled
3. Do not judge or condemn residents, and treat them with dignity and respect
4. Be eager, interested, and excited about your work
5. Know your feelings, strengths, and weaknesses
6. Residents and staff have confidence in you. They trust you will keep information confidential
8. Greet and talk to people in a pleasant manner
9. Accurately report the care given, your observations, and any errors

Nursing Assistant Skills Video Exercise

View the **Basic Principles** *video to answer these questions.*

44. Communication is oral and written. Information is also conveyed by

    A. _____

    B. _____

Optional Learning Exercises

45. List places you can find out about job openings.

    A. _____

    B. _____

    C. _____

    D. _____

    E. _____

    F. _____

    G. _____

    H. _____

Job Application (Box 3-3)

46. If a job application asks you to print in black ink, why is it a poor idea to use blue ink?

    _____

    _____

47. How can writing illegibly on a job application affect getting a job? _____

    _____

48. Why is it important to give information about employment gaps or leaving a job?

    _____

    _____

49. If you lie on a job application, it is _____. If you do this, what can happen?

    _____

Qualities and Characteristics of Good Work Ethics (Box 3-2)

Match the qualities and characteristics of good work ethics with the examples.

A. Caring   H. Courteous
B. Dependable   I. Conscientious
C. Considerate   J. Honest
D. Cheerful   K. Cooperative
E. Empathic   L. Enthusiastic
F. Trustworthy   M. Self-aware
G. Respectful

50. _____ While working with Mr. Smith, you try to understand and feel what it must be like to be paralyzed on one side.

51. _____ You realize you are very good at giving basic care. You know you need to improve your communication skills.

52. _____ When caring for elderly residents, you try to do small things to make them happy or to find ways to ease their pain.

53. _____ You thank co-workers when they help you, and remember to wish residents happy birthday as appropriate.

54. _____ When Mrs. Gibson is upset and angry, you remember to respect her feeling and to be kind.

55. _____ You report the blood pressure and temperature readings accurately to the nurse.

56. _____ You realize giving care to residents is important and you are excited about your work.

57. _____ Your supervisor tells you she knows she can count on you because you are always on time and perform delegated tasks as assigned.

58. _____ Even though Mr. Acevado's cultural and religious views are different from yours, you value his feelings and beliefs.

59. _____ Before you left home today you had an argument with your child. When you get to work, you make every effort to put that aside and be pleasant and happy.

60. _____ The nurse discusses a resident problem with you and states she knows you will keep the information confidential.

61. _____ When you are assigned to give care to a resident, you make sure his care is done thoroughly and exactly as instructed.

62. _____ Your co-worker says she needs help to turn her resident, and you cheerfully offer to help.

Independent Learning Activities

- How well do you take care of your own health? What can you do to improve your health practices?
  - Do you maintain a healthy weight by eating calories adequate for your energy needs? What can you do to improve your diet?
  - How much sleep do you get each night?
  - Do you practice good body mechanics at all times—not just at work?
  - How many hours do you exercise each week? What type of exercise do you do?
  - When did you last have your eyes checked? Do you wear glasses if they were prescribed?
  - Do you smoke? How much? Have you considered any smoking cessation programs?
  - Are you taking any drugs that affect your thinking, feeling, behavior, and function? Did a doctor prescribe them, or are you self-medicating? Have you talked with your doctor about the effect of any drugs you are taking?
  - Do you drink alcohol? How much? Have you been told it affects your behavior? Have you considered finding a program to help you quit drinking alcohol?

- Have you ever applied for a job? How did you feel when you were being interviewed? After reading this chapter, how would you handle a future interview?
- Role-play a job interview with a classmate. Take turns playing the interviewer and the job applicant. Use the lists in this chapter to ask questions. Practice answers that you can use in a real interview.
- Think of three people you could use as references when applying for a job. Ask their permission to use them as references. If they agree, make a list of the people and their titles, addresses, and telephone numbers to use when you apply for a job.

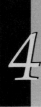

Communicating With the Health Team

Key Terms

Abbreviation
Chart
Communication
Conflict

Kardex
Medical record
Prefix

Progress note
Recording
Reporting

Root
Suffix
Word element

Fill in the Blanks: Key Terms

1. A _____ is a word element placed at the beginning of a word to change the meaning of the word.

2. An _____ is a shortened form of a word or phrase.

3. _____ is the exchange of information—a message sent is received and interpreted by the intended person.

4. A _____ is a clash between opposing interests and ideas.

5. A type of card file that summarizes information found in the medical record is a _____.

6. A part of a word is a _____.

7. The _____ is the medical record.

8. _____ is a verbal account of resident care and observations.

9. A written description of the care given and the person's response and progress is the

   _____.

10. A word element placed after a root; it changes the meaning of the word; it is a _____
    _____.

11. A word element containing the basic meaning of the word is the _____.

12. A _____ is a written account of a person's illness and response to the treatment and care given by the health team; chart.

13. Writing or charting resident care and observations is

   _____.

Circle the BEST Answer

14. For communication to be effective
    A. Use words that have the same meaning for the sender and the receiver
    B. Use terms that are unfamiliar to residents and families
    C. Add unrelated information to the message
    D. Answers should not be specific

15. The medical record will include all of the following *except*
    A. Physical examination results
    B. Graphic sheet
    C. Change-of-shift reports
    D. X-ray examination reports

16. To prevent errors and improper placement of records, the medical record is
    A. Kept in the resident's room
    B. Placed in a locked cabinet
    C. Stamped with the person's name, room number, and other identifying information on each page
    D. Printed on colored paper

17. Before a nursing assistant reads a resident's chart, he should
    A. Know the center's policy
    B. Ask the nurse for permission
    C. Ask the doctor's permission
    D. Sign a sheet to get permission

18. If a resident asks to see the chart, you should
    A. Give it to the resident because the person always has a right to see the chart
    B. Read the chart and tell the person what it says
    C. Report the request to your supervisor
    D. Tell the person that residents are not allowed to see the chart

19. The admission sheet is used to
    A. Find out the person's physical condition
    B. Help the person become familiar with the center
    C. Learn background information about a person
    D. Carry out a physical examination

20. Progress notes are usually written
    A. Every shift
    B. When there is a change in the person's condition
    C. Each day
    D. Once a year

21. OBRA requires that summaries of care be written
    A. Once a day
    B. Once every month
    C. At least every 3 months
    D. Once a year

22. What information is *not* included on the activities-of-daily-living flow sheet?
    A. Temperature, pulse, respirations
    B. Activity
    C. Bowel movements
    D. Amount of food taken in

23. If you make an error when recording, you should
   A. Erase it
   B. Use correction fluid to cover it
   C. Throw away the page and start over
   D. Draw a line through the incorrect part and date and initial the line

24. The resident and family can
   A. Attend the IDCP
   B. Attend problem-focused conferences
   C. Refuse actions suggested by the health team at a conference
   D. All of the above

Circle the word that is spelled correctly for each of the following definitions.

25. Slow heart rate
   A. Bradecardia   C. Bradacordia
   B. Bradycardia   D. Bradicardia

26. Difficulty in urinating
   A. Dysuria   C. Dysuira
   B. Dysurya   D. Disuria

27. Paralysis on one side of the body
   A. Hemyplegia   C. Hemoplega
   B. Hemaplegia   D. Hemiplegia

28. Opening into the ileum
   A. Ileostomie   C. Ileastoma
   B. Ileostomy   D. Illiostomy

29. Blue color or condition
   A. Cyonosis   C. Cyanosis
   B. Cyinosis   D. Cianosys

30. Opening into trachea
   A. Tracheastomy   C. Tracheostome
   B. Trachiostomy   D. Tracheostomy

31. Pain in a nerve
   A. Neuralgia   C. Nourealgia
   B. Neurolgia   D. Neurilegia

32. Examination of a joint with a scope
   A. Arthoscopie   C. Arethroscopy
   B. Arthroscopy   D. Artheroscope

33. Rapid breathing
   A. Tachepnea   C. Tachypnea
   B. Tachypinea   D. Tachypnia

34. Removal of gallbladder
   A. Cholecystectomy   C. Cholicystetomy
   B. Cholcystectomy   D. Cholecistectomy

Circle the BEST Answer

35. When you are given a computer password, you
   A. Must never change it
   B. Can share it with a coworker
   C. Should never tell anyone your password
   D. Can use another person's password when entering the computer

36. Computers should not be used to
   A. Send messages and reports to the nursing unit
   B. Store resident records and care plans
   C. Send e-mails that require immediate reporting
   D. Monitor blood pressure, temperatures, and heart rates

37. When you answer the telephone, do not put callers on hold if
   A. The person has an emergency
   B. It is a doctor
   C. The call needs to be transferred to another unit
   D. You are too busy to find the nurse

38. If you have a conflict with a co-worker, you should
   A. Ask the nurse in charge to schedule you at different times
   B. Ignore the person
   C. Identify the cause of the conflict and try to resolve it
   D. Talk to other co-workers to explain your side of the story

39. When a conflict occurs, what is the first step you should take?
   A. Talk with other co-workers to see if they have a conflict with the person also
   B. Confront the person and demand that the person meet with you
   C. Identify the real problem
   D. Assume the conflict will resolve itself if you ignore it

40. Why is it important to resolve a conflict at work?
   A. Unkind words or actions may occur
   B. The work environment becomes unpleasant
   C. Resident care is affected
   D. All of the above

Matching

Match the word with the correct definition.

41. _____ Neuralgia
42. _____ Gastrostomy
43. _____ Cholecystectomy
44. _____ Dysuria
45. _____ Gastritis
46. _____ Enteritis
47. _____ Bacteriogenic
48. _____ Glossitis
49. _____ Cyanotic
50. _____ Dermatology
51. _____ Oophorectomy
52. _____ Colostomy
53. _____ Nephritis
54. _____ Bronchoscope
55. _____ Proctoscopy

A. Difficulty urinating
B. Inflammation of kidneys
C. Pertaining to blue coloration
D. Caused by bacteria
E. Study of the skin
F. Incision into large intestine
G. Instrument used to examine bronchi
H. Inflammation of the tongue
I. Nerve pain
J. Examination of rectum with instrument
K. Excision of gallbladder
L. Excision of ovary
M. Incision into stomach
N. Inflammation of stomach
O. Inflammation of intestine

Fill in the Blanks

56. Next to each time, write the time using the 24-hour clock.

A. ____ 11:00 AM E. ____ 6:45 PM I. ____ 5:30 PM

B. ____ 8:00 AM   F. ____ 12 NOON J. ____ 10:45 PM

C. ____ 4:00 PM   G. ____ 3:00 AM K. ____ 11:55 PM

D. ____ 7:30 AM   H. ____ 4:50 AM L. ____ 9:15 PM

Write the definition of each prefix.

57. auto- _____

58. brady- _____

59. dys- _____

60. ecto- _____

61. leuk- _____

62. macro- _____

63. neo- _____

64. supra- _____

65. uni- _____

Write the definition of each root word.

66. adeno _____

67. angio _____

68. broncho _____

69. cranio _____

70. duodeno _____

71. entero _____

72. gyneco _____

73. masto _____

74. pyo _____

Write the definition of each suffix.

75. -asis _____

76. -genic _____

77. -oma _____

78. -phasia _____

79. -ptosis _____

80. -plegia _____

81. -megaly _____

82. -scopy _____

83. -stasis _____

Write the correct abbreviations.

84. Before meals _____

85. After meals _____

86. With _____

87. Cancer _____

88. Discontinued _____

89. Lower left quadrant _____

90. Every day _____

91. Range-of-motion _____

Convert the times in questions 92-101 from military to standard time and from standard to military time. Use figure as a guide.

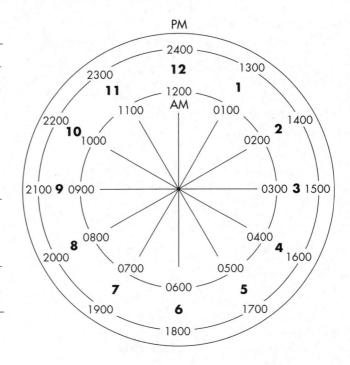

92. 2:00 AM = _____

93. 10:30 AM = _____

94. 5:00 AM = _____

95. 9:30 AM = _____

96. 5:45 PM = _____

97. 10:45 PM = _____

98. 0600 hrs = _____ AM/PM

99. 1145 hrs = _____ AM/PM

100. 1800 hrs = _____ AM/PM

101. 2200 hrs = _____ AM/PM

Labeling

102. Label the 4 abdominal regions. Use RUQ, LUQ, RLQ, LLQ to label.

    A. _____

    B. _____

    C. _____

    D. _____

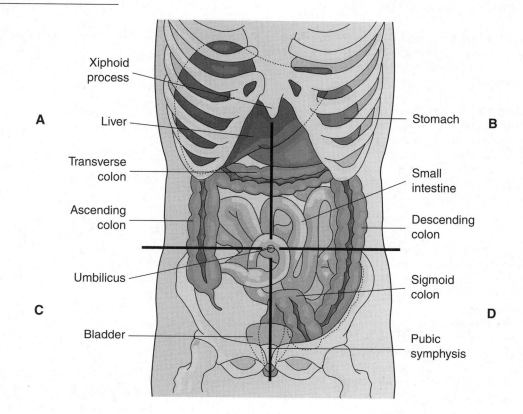

Nursing Assistant Skills Video Exercise
View the **Basic Principles** *video to answer these questions.*

103. After you finish a task, you must communicate with the nurse by reporting _____
_____
_____.

104. _____ is essential for coordinated and effective nursing care.

105. Knowing how to communicate effectively is essential for meeting _____, _____, and _____ requirements of your work.

106. For a message to be understood correctly, it must be _____, _____, and _____.

107. What should you do if someone uses a term you do not understand? _____

108. When charting, all entries must include

    A. _____

    B. _____

Optional Learning Exercise
Class Experiment

It is often difficult to describe fluids in a clear and precise manner. Set up the following examples that imitate situations where you need to describe intake, output, or drainage. Describe as accurately as possible what you see in terms of amounts, colors, and textures. Compare your notes with classmates to see if you are using words that all have the same meaning. What words were used that were clear to understand? What words were used that had more than one meaning?

- Bloody Drainage: Mix a teaspoon of ketchup and a teaspoon of water. Pour onto the center of a paper napkin.
- Urine: Pour a tablespoon of tea into the center of a paper towel.
- Bleeding: Smear a teaspoon of red jelly in the center of a paper towel.
- Broth: Pour 4 ounces of tea into a bowl.

Class Experiment

Substance	Observations
Bloody Drainage	
Urine	
Bleeding	
Broth	

Case Study

Mr. Larsen was admitted to a subacute care center after his abdominal surgery 1 week ago. This morning the nursing assistant gave Mr. Larsen a shower and assisted him to sit in a comfortable chair. The nursing assistant noticed that he sat there very still and held his arms across his abdomen. He asked for a pillow and held tightly against his abdomen.

Imagine you are the patient and answer these questions.
- What would you like the nursing assistant to ask you?
- How would you communicate your feelings to the nursing assistant?
- How could you let the nursing assistant know that you had pain without telling her?

Imagine you are the nursing assistant and answer these questions.
- As the nursing assistant, what observations would be important to make about Mr. Larsen?
- What questions could you ask Mr. Larsen?
- What nonverbal communication would give you information about Mr. Larsen?

Case Study

Mrs. Miller was admitted to the health care center since you worked 3 days ago. You have just started your shift and have been assigned to Mrs. Miller.
- What information would you need to know before giving care? Why?
- What information would be important to provide to the oncoming shift?
- What methods would you use to communicate this information?

Independent Learning Activities

1. Answer these questions about situations in which you may need to communicate with others.
   - When have you had a problem with communicating?
   - Why was it difficult?
   - How did you handle this?
2. Think about a situation in which you feel you communicated your point well.
   - What made the communication successful? How could you use a similar technique in caring for residents?
   - How would you communicate with a person who speaks a language that you do not speak or understand? What methods could you use to explain what you are going to do?
   - How would you communicate with a person from a different culture?
3. Make flash cards of the prefixes, suffixes, and root words in Chapter 4. Put the meaning of each one on the back of the appropriate card. Work alone or with a partner, and by looking at the cards, practice identifying the correct meaning of each term.
4. The next time you or a member of your family visits the doctor and is instructed to fill a prescription, look at what the doctor has written. Do you see any abbreviations that you learned in this chapter? What do they mean? How did this chapter help you understand what was written?

5 Assisting With the Nursing Process

Key Terms

Assessment
Comprehensive care plan
Evaluation
Goal

Implementation
Medical diagnosis
Nursing diagnosis
Nursing intervention

Nursing process
Objective data
Observation
Planning

Signs
Subjective data
Symptoms
Triggers

Fill in the Blanks: Key Terms

1. _____ are things a person tells you about that you cannot observe through your senses; symptoms.

2. _____ is to perform or carry out nursing measures in the care plan; a step in the nursing process.

3. The method RNs use to plan and deliver nursing care is the _____.

4. Another name for subjective data is _____.

5. A written guide about the care a person should receive is the _____

6. _____ is collecting information about the person; a step in the nursing process.

7. Another name for objective data is _____.

8. The _____ describes a health problem that can be treated by nursing measures; a step in the nursing process.

9. Information that is seen, heard, felt, or smelled is _____ or signs.

10. A step in the nursing process that is used to measure if goals in the planning step were met is called _____.

11. _____ is setting priorities and goals; a step in the nursing process.

12. A _____ is an action or measure taken by the nursing team to help the person reach a goal.

13. A _____ is that which is desired in or by the person as a result of nursing care.

14. Using the senses of sight, hearing, touch, and smell to collect information is _____.

15. The identification of a disease or condition by a doctor is a _____.

16. _____ are clues for the resident assessment protocols (RAPs).

Circle the BEST Answer

17. Which of these *is not* a step in the nursing process?
    A. Assessment   C. Planning
    B. Objective data   D. Evaluation

18. The nursing process focuses on
    A. The doctor's orders
    B. The person's nursing needs
    C. Tasks and procedures that are needed
    D. Reducing the cost of health care

19. The nursing process
    A. Stays the same from admission to discharge
    B. Helps all nursing team members do the same things for the person
    C. Cannot be used in home care
    D. Can be used only for adults

20. When you observe by using your senses, you assist the nurse to
    A. Assess the person
    B. Plan for care
    C. Implement care for the person
    D. Evaluate the person

21. Which of these is an example of objective data?
    A. Mrs. Hewitt complains of pain and nausea
    B. Mr. Stewart tells you he has a dull ache in his stomach
    C. You are taking Mrs. Jensen's blood pressure and you notice her skin is hot and moist
    D. Mrs. Murano tells you she is tired because she could not sleep last night

22. A minimum data set (MDS) is used
    A. For nursing center residents
    B. In all health care settings
    C. In acute care settings
    D. In home care

23. The MDS is updated
    A. Before each care conference
    B. Every month
    C. On discharge
    D. All of the above

24. A nursing diagnosis
    A. Identifies a disease or condition
    B. Helps identify drugs or therapies used by the doctor
    C. Describes a health problem that can be treated by nursing measures
    D. Identifies only physical problems

25. When a nurse uses the nursing process, the person is given
    A. Only one nursing diagnosis
    B. No more than five nursing diagnoses
    C. As many nursing diagnoses as are needed
    D. Nursing diagnoses that involve only physical needs
26. Planning involves
    A. Setting priorities and goals
    B. Choosing nursing interventions to help the person reach a goal
    C. Revising the care plan as a person's needs change
    D. All of the above
27. An interdisciplinary care planning conference is required
    A. For each person
    B. To meet agency guidelines
    C. To assess the person
    D. To implement the care plan
28. OBRA requires the use of resident assessment protocols (RAPs). They are
    A. Conferences held to update care plans
    B. Guidelines used to develop the person's care plan
    C. Conferences held when one problem affect a person's care
    D. Conferences attended by the person, family, and health team members
29. What part of the nursing process is being carried out when you give personal care to a person?
    A. Assessing
    B. Planning
    C. Implementation
    D. Evaluation
30. An assignment sheet will give information about
    A. Each person's care
    B. Evaluation of the goals for care
    C. An assessment of the person
    D. The nursing diagnoses for the person
31. Nurses will measure if goals in the planning steps are met during
    A. Assessing
    B. Planning
    C. Implementation
    D. Evaluation

Fill in the Blanks

32. When you make observations while you give care, what senses are used?
    A. _____
    B. _____
    C. _____
    D. _____

33. Each of the following is either subjective or objective data. In the blank next to each statement, place an "S" for subjective and an "O" for objective.
    A. _____Sleepy   F. _____Gas pain
    B. _____Chest pain   G. _____Pain when urinating
    C. _____Skin cool   H. _____Productive cough
    D. _____Cyanosis of   I. _____Breath has fruity odor
       nails   J. _____Pulse rapid
    E. _____Labored breathing

34. Name the body system or other area you are observing in each of these examples. *(from Box 5-1, Basic Observations)*
    A. Is the abdomen firm or soft? _____
    B. Is the person sensitive to bright lights? _____
    C. Are sores or reddened areas present? _____
    D. What is the frequency of the person's cough? _____
    E. Can the person bathe without help? _____
    F. Can the person swallow food and fluids? _____
    G. What is the position of comfort? _____
    H. Does the person answer questions correctly? _____
    I. Does the person complain of stiff or painful joints? _____

35. An assessment and screening tool completed when the person is admitted to a long-term care center is called _____.
    A. The form is updated before each _____.
    B. A new form is completed _____ and whenever _____.

36. When planning care, needs that are required for life and survival must be met before _____ _____.

37. A comprehensive care plan is
    A. Developed for _____
    B. Suggestions are welcomed from all _____
    C. It tells the health team members what care _____

38. The assignment sheet tells you about
    A. _____
    B. _____
    C. _____

Nursing Assistant Skills Video Exercise
*View the **Basic Principles** video to answer these questions about the Nursing Process*

39. The _____ is used to plan and provide nursing care in all health care agencies.

40. You assist with assessment by _____.
The nurse uses assessment information to make

_____.

41. The nursing care plan states _____ and identifies _____.

42. The nurse involves the entire nursing team in the nursing process.

    A. True

    B. False

Optional Learning Exercises
List at least three nursing interventions for each of these nursing diagnoses and goals:

43.

Nursing Diagnosis: Feeding self-care deficit: Related to weakness in right arm

Goal: Patient will eat 75% of each meal by 2/1.

Nursing Interventions:

    A. _____

    B. _____

    C. _____

44.

Nursing Diagnosis: Hygiene self-care deficit: Related to forgetfulness

Goal: Patient will be assisted to maintain good hygiene throughout hospital stay.

Nursing Interventions:

    A. _____

    B. _____

    C. _____

Independent Learning Activities

- Ask permission to look at the nursing care plans used at the agency where you have your clinical experience. Answer these questions about the nursing care plans:
- How do the nurses develop the plans? What resources do they use?
- How often are the plans reviewed and revised?
- How are the plans used by the nursing assistants?
- How do nursing assistants help develop and revise the interventions?
- How do the nurses communicate the information on the nursing care plan?

6 Understanding the Resident

Key Terms
Body language
Comatose
Culture
Disability

Esteem
Holism
Need
Nonverbal communication

Optimal level of function
Paraphrasing
Religion

Self-actualization
Self-esteem
Verbal communication

Fill in the Blanks: Key Terms

1. Experiencing one's potential is called _____.

2. _____ is thinking well of oneself, seeing oneself as useful, and being well thought of by others.

3. A person's highest potential for mental and physical performance is the _____.

4. A _____ is that which is necessary or desirable for maintaining life and mental well-being.

5. Communication that uses the written or spoken word is called _____.

6. _____ is lost, absent, or impaired physical or mental function.

7. _____ is communication that does not involve words.

8. The characteristics of a group of people—language, values, beliefs, habits, likes, dislikes, customs—passed from one generation to the next is called _____.

9. The worth, value, or opinion one has of a person is _____.

10. _____ is spiritual beliefs, needs, and practices.

11. A person who is _____ has an inability to respond to verbal stimuli.

12. Restating the person's message in your own words is called _____.

13. _____ sends messages through facial expressions, gestures, posture, and body movements.

14. _____ is a concept that considers the whole person.

Circle the BEST Answer

15. Who is the most important person in the nursing center?
    A. The director of nursing
    B. The resident
    C. The doctor
    D. The nurse

16. Which of these losses may have happened to an older resident?
    A. Loss of home, family members
    B. Loss of the person's role in the family or community
    C. Loss of body functions
    D. All of the above

17. When speaking about the resident, which of these statements is best?
    A. "Mrs. Jones in 135 needs a pain pill."
    B. "Granny Jones needs something for pain."
    C. "135 needs a pain pill."
    D. "Janie is complaining of pain."

18. What is the main reason you call a resident by a title such as Mr., Mrs., or Miss?
    A. It best identifies the person
    B. It gives the person dignity and respect
    C. It is polite
    D. It shows the person you are in charge

19. When is it acceptable to call a person by his or her first name or another name?
    A. You have cared for the person for several months
    B. The person is confused
    C. The person asks you to use the name
    D. The person has difficulty hearing

20. Which of these needs is affected when the person is ill or elderly?
    A. Physical   C. Psychological
    B. Social   D. All are affected

21. What needs are most important for survival?
    A. Physical   C. Love and belonging
    B. Safety and security D. Self-esteem

22. It is important for the person to know what to expect when care is given because the person will
    A. Be combative
    B. Feel safer and more secure
    C. Have a more meaningful relationship
    D. Experience his potential

23. What need is rarely, if ever, totally met?
    A. Physiological   C. Self-esteem
    B. Safety and security D. Self-actualization

24. Mrs. Young is a new resident. All of the following will help her feel more secure *except*
    A. Give her explanations of routines and procedures only one time
    B. Treat her with kindness and patience
    C. Make sure she understands how a procedure is to be done
    D. Listen to her concerns, and explain all routines and procedures as often as needed

26

25. Mrs. Peck never has visitors and is becoming weaker and unable to care for herself. What need is not being met?
    A. Physiological
    B. Safety and security
    C. Love and belonging
    D. Self-esteem
26. Which of these practices may relate to both religion and culture?
    A. Language
    B. Hygiene habits
    C. Days of worship
    D. Beliefs about causes and cures of illness
27. When you are caring for a person of a different culture, you should
    A. Expect all people in the culture to follow the same practices
    B. Judge the person by your standards
    C. Remember that each person is unique
    D. Ignore the cultural practices
28. A person who is ill and disabled is often very angry because
    A. The care he is receiving is poor
    B. The person is angry at the situation
    C. The person does not like you
    D. The person has a bad temper
29. How can you help Mr. Clay maintain his optimal level of functioning?
    A. Give him complete care
    B. Encourage him to be as independent as possible
    C. Avoid staying with him to visit
    D. Do not respond promptly when he asks for help
30. Mrs. Nelson is alert and oriented. Why would she require care in a nursing center?
    A. She has trouble remembering where she is
    B. She cannot tell you what she needs or wants
    C. She has physical problems so she requires help
    D. She does not know who she is
31. Which of these is a reason confusion and disorientation may be temporary?
    A. The person has a disabling disease
    B. The person has recently been admitted to the nursing center
    C. The person needs complete help with all activities of daily living (ADL)
    D. The person is terminally ill
32. Mrs. Smithers is admitted to the nursing center. The nurse tells you she will be here only short-term. You know the reason for most short-term admissions is to
    A. Provide quality care to dying residents
    B. Give complete care to the resident
    C. Help the resident recover from fractures, acute illness, or surgery
    D. Prevent injury of the resident
33. Respite care provides
    A. Time to recover from surgery or acute illness
    B. Time to recover from temporary confusion
    C. Care for a dying person
    D. The caregiver a chance to take a vacation, tend to business, or rest

34. A person who needs life-long care has a disability that occurs
    A. Because of birth defects or childhood illnesses or injuries
    B. Because of mental illness
    C. Because of the aging process
    D. Because the person is dying
35. If a resident is comatose, how would you know the person is in pain?
    A. The person cries and lies very still
    B. The person asks for pain medications
    C. Pain is shown by grimacing and groaning
    D. You cannot tell if the person is in pain
36. Which of these ways to deal with a person with behavior issues would *not* be helpful?
    A. Argue with the person to show him he is wrong
    B. Explain reasons for long waits
    C. Answer the person's questions clearly and thoroughly
    D. Stay calm and professional if the anger and hostility is directed at you
37. Which of these would *not* help effective communication?
    A. Use words that have the same meaning to both you and the person
    B. Communicate in a logical and orderly manner
    C. Give facts and be specific
    D. Use medical terminology when talking to the person
38. Mrs. Stevens cannot speak. How does she use verbal communication?
    A. She may use touch
    B. Her body language sends messages
    C. She can use gestures to communicate
    D. She may write messages on a paper pad
39. When you go to Mrs. Hart's room, you can tell she is not happy or not feeling well because
    A. Her hair is well groomed
    B. She has a slumped posture
    C. She smiles when you come in the room
    D. She protects an affected body part
40. All of these would show you listen effectively *except*
    A. You face the person and have good eye contact
    B. You lean back and cross your arms
    C. You ask the person questions
    D. You use words the person can understand
41. Which of these is paraphrasing?
    A. "You don't know how long you will be here."
    B. "Do you want to take a tub bath or a shower?"
    C. "Tell me about living on a farm."
    D. "Can you explain what you mean?"
42. When you say, "Mr. Davis, have you taken a shower this morning?," you are
    A. Paraphrasing his thoughts
    B. Asking a direct question
    C. Focusing his thoughts
    D. Asking an open-ended question

43. Responses to open-ended questions generally are
    A. Longer and give more information than direct questions
    B. Yes or no answers
    C. Able to make sure you understand the message
    D. Focused on dealing with a certain topic
44. Mr. Parker often rambles and tells long stories in which his thoughts wander. You need to know if he had a bowel movement today, so you will
    A. Make a clarifying statement
    B. Ask an open-ended question
    C. Ask a focusing question
    D. Paraphrase his thoughts
45. What is best if the person takes long pauses between statements?
    A. You do not need to talk. Just being there helps
    B. Try to cheer the person up by talking
    C. Leave the room
    D. Find another resident to talk with him
46. Mrs. Duke has visitors and you need to give care. What would you do?
    A. Give the care while visitors are present
    B. Politely ask the visitors to leave the room
    C. Tell the visitors to give the care
    D. Tell the visitors that they must leave the nursing center

Basic Needs Exercise
47. List the basic needs for life as described by Maslow from the lowest level to the highest level.
    A. _____
    B. _____
    C. _____
    D. _____
    E. _____

Optional Learning Exercises
Basic Needs
Physical needs
48. What are the six physical needs required for survival?
    _____
49. The physical needs must be met before the _____ needs.
Safety and security
50. Safety and security needs relate to feeling safe from _____, _____, and _____.
51. Why do many people feel a loss of safety and security when admitted to a nursing center?
    A. _____
    B. _____
    C. _____
Love and belonging
52. The need for love and belonging relates to _____, _____, and _____. These needs also involve _____.
53. How can you help a resident feel loved and accepted?
    _____

Self-Esteem
54. What does self-esteem relate to?
    A. _____
    B. _____
    C. _____
55. Why is it important to encourage residents to do as much as possible for themselves?
    _____

Self-Actualization
56. What does self-actualization involve? _____, _____, and _____
57. What happens if self-actualization is postponed?
    _____

Cultural Practices
Religion
58. How can you help a resident observe religious practices if services are held in the nursing center?
    _____
59. If the resident wants to have a visit from a spiritual leader, you should tell _____.
60. If the resident wants a spiritual leader or advisor to visit in the room, you should _____, _____, and _____.
Cultural health care beliefs
Mexican Americans
61. If hot causes the illness, _____ is used for the cure.
62. Hot and cold are found in _____, _____, and _____.
Vietnamese Americans
63. Hot is given to balance _____ illnesses.
64. Cold is given to balance _____ illnesses.
Cultural sick practices
65. How do Vietnamese-American folk practices treat these illnesses?
    A. Common cold _____
    B. Headache and sore throat _____
66. What illnesses do these Russian-American folk practices treat?
    A. _____ An ointment is placed behind the ears and temples and also on the back of the neck.
    B. _____ A dough made of dark rye flour and honey is placed on the spinal column.
Cultural touch practices
67. Why is touch important in Mexico and the Philippine cultures? _____
68. Men who are from India or Vietnam may not wish to shake hands with a _____.
69. Residents from some countries might not like to be touched. Two examples of these countries are _____ and _____.

Cultural eye contact practices

70. Why would you avoid making direct eye contact with a person from an Asian or American-Indian culture?
_____

71. If a resident from Vietnam blinks when you explain a procedure, it probably means that the message _____.

72. Direct eye contact is practiced among people from _____ and _____.

Cultural family roles in sick care

73. You are caring for a resident from China. You might expect the family members to _____, _____, and _____ the person.

74. A man from Mexico is a resident, and his daughter says she cannot care for him when he goes home. This may be because in Mexico women cannot give care if _____.

Case Study

You have completed your duties for the morning and have some free time. Mr. Harry Donal is a resident in the nursing center. He rarely has visitors, and you try to spend time with him when you can. Answer the following questions about communication techniques you use when you visit with Mr. Donal.

75. You sit in a chair next to Mr. Donal so you can see each other. This position will help you to have better_____.

76. You should lean _____ Mr. Donal to show interest.

77. Mr. Donal says, "I know this is the best place for me, but I miss my flower garden at home." You respond, "You miss your home." This is an example of _____.

78. You ask Mr. Donal, "You told me you did not sleep well last night. Can you tell me why?" He replies, "There was a lot of noise in the hall." This is an example of a _____.

79. You say to Mr. Donal, "Tell me about your flower garden at home." This is an _____ question.

80. When you say, "Can you explain what that means," you are asking a person to _____.

81. Mr. Donal says he "hurts all over" and then begins to talk about the weather. You say, "Tell me more about where you hurt. You said you hurt all over." This statement helps in _____ the topic.

82. Mr. Donal begins to cry when he talks about his flower garden. How can you show caring and respect for his situation and feelings?
_____

83. When Mr. Donal begins to cry, you quickly begin to talk about the activities planned this morning. Changing the subject is a _____

Independent Learning Activities

- Use the section of Chapter 6 that discusses needs to think about how well you are meeting your own needs:
  - Do you smoke? What need may be affected by smoking?
  - What kinds of foods and fluids do you eat? Is your diet meeting your basic needs for food and water?
  - How much rest and sleep do you get each day? How much do you need to feel well rested?
  - How safe do you feel at home? At school? In your community? How do your feelings affect your ability to hold a job or attend school?
  - Who are the people who make you feel loved? Who helps you when you have problems?
  - What are you doing that helps you meet the need for self-actualization?
- Answer these questions about your personal health care practices:
  - What health care practices are followed in your family? How are these practices related to your cultural or religious beliefs?
  - How often do you go to the doctor? For regular checkups? Only when ill?
  - When do you go to the dentist? Once or twice a year for cleaning and checkups? Only when you have a toothache?
  - When a family member is in a health care center, how does your family respond? Does someone stay with the person and do all of the care" Or do family members visit for brief periods and let health care workers provide all care? Is the family response related to any cultural or religious practices?
- Look at your answers to both sets of questions above:
  - How well are you meeting your basic needs? How could you improve in meeting needs? What changes would be the most beneficial?
  - How much influence on your practices comes from cultural or religious traditions in your family? Are these influences helping you or hindering you to meet needs?

7 Body Structure and Function

Key Terms

Artery
Capillary
Cell
Digestion

Hemoglobin
Hormone
Immunity
Menstruation

Metabolism
Organ
Peristalsis
Respiration

System
Tissue
Vein

Fill in the Blanks: Key Terms

1. The substance in red blood cells that carries oxygen and gives blood its color is _____.

2. _____ is protection against a disease or condition.

3. The process of supplying the cells with oxygen and removing carbon dioxide from them is _____.

4. The process of physically and chemically breaking down food so that it can be absorbed for use by the cells is _____.

5. _____ is the burning of food for heat and energy by the cells.

6. A blood vessel that carries blood away from the heart is an _____.

7. _____ is the involuntary muscle contractions in the digestive system that move food down the esophagus through the alimentary canal.

8. Organs that work together to perform special functions form a _____.

9. The basic unit of body structure is a _____.

10. Groups of tissues with the same function form an _____.

11. A _____ is a tiny blood vessel.

12. A group of cells with similar function is _____.

13. _____ is the process in which the lining of the uterus breaks up and is discharged from the body through the vagina.

14. A chemical substance secreted by the glands into the bloodstream is a _____.

15. A _____ is a blood vessel that returns blood to the heart.

Circle the BEST answer

16. A cell is
    A. Found only in muscles
    B. The basic unit of body structure
    C. Can live without oxygen
    D. A group of tissues

17. The control center of a cell is the
    A. Membrane   C. Cytoplasm
    B. Protoplasm   D. Nucleus

18. Genes control
    A. Cell division
    B. Tissues
    C. Physical and chemical traits inherited by children
    D. Organs

19. Connective tissue
    A. Covers internal and external body surface
    B. Receives and carries impulses to the brain and back to body parts
    C. Anchors, connects, and supports other body tissues
    D. Allows the body to move by stretching and contracting

20. Living cells of the epidermis contain
    A. Blood vessels and many nerves
    B. Sweat and oil glands
    C. Pigment that gives skin color
    D. Hair roots

21. Sweat glands help
    A. The body regulate temperature
    B. Keep the hair and skin soft and shiny
    C. Protect the nose from dust, insects, and other foreign objects
    D. The skin sense pleasant and unpleasant sensations

22. Long bones
    A. Allow skill and ease in movement
    B. Bear the weight of the body
    C. Protect organs
    D. Allow various degrees of movement and flexion

23. Blood cells are manufactured in
    A. The heart   C. Blood vessels
    B. The liver   D. Bone marrow

24. Joints move smoothly because of
    A. Cartilage   C. Muscle
    B. Synovial fluid   D. Ligaments

25. A joint that moves in all directions is a
    A. Ball and socket   C. Pivot
    B. Hinge   D. All of the above

26. Voluntary muscles are
    A. Found in the stomach and intestines
    B. Attached to bones
    C. Cardiac muscle
    D. Tendons

27. Muscles produce heat by
    A. Contracting   C. Maintaining posture
    B. Relaxing   D. Working automatically

30

28. The central nervous system consists of
    A. A myelin sheath
    B. Nerves throughout the body
    C. The brain and spinal column
    D. Cranial nerves
29. The medulla controls
    A. Muscle contraction and relaxation
    B. Heart rate, breathing, blood vessel size, and swallowing
    C. Reasoning, memory, and consciousness
    D. Hearing and vision
30. Cerebrospinal fluid
    A. Cushions shocks that could injure structure of the brain and spinal cord
    B. Controls voluntary muscles
    C. Lubricates movement
    D. Controls involuntary muscles
31. Cranial nerves conduct impulses between the
    A. Brain and the head, neck, chest, and abdomen
    B. Brain and the skin and extremities
    C. Brain and internal body structure
    D. Spinal cord and lower extremities
32. When you are frightened, the _____ nervous system is stimulated
    A. Sympathetic   C. Central
    B. Parasympathetic   D. Cranial
33. Receptors for vision and nerve fibers of the optic nerve are found in the
    A. Sclera   C. Retina
    B. Choroids   D. Cornea
34. What structure of the ear is involved in balance?
    A. Malleus   C. Tympanic membranes
    B. Auditory canal   D. Semicircular canals
35. Hemoglobin in red blood cells gives blood its red color and carries
    A. Oxygen   C. Waste products
    B. Food to cells   D. Water
36. Red blood cells live for
    A. About 9 days   C. 4 days
    B. 3 or 4 months   D. A year
37. White blood cells or leukocytes
    A. Protect the body against infection
    B. Are necessary for blood clotting
    C. Carry food, hormones, chemicals, and waste products
    D. Pick up carbon dioxide
38. The left atrium of the heart
    A. Receives blood from the lungs
    B. Receives blood from the body tissues
    C. Pumps blood to the lungs
    D. Pumps blood to all parts of the body
39. Arteries
    A. Return blood to the heart
    B. Pass food, oxygen, and other substances into the cells
    C. Pick up waste products including carbon dioxide from the cells
    D. Carry blood away from the heart
40. In the lungs, oxygen and carbon dioxide are exchanged
    A. In the epiglottis
    B. Between the right bronchus and the left bronchus
    C. By the bronchioles
    D. Between the alveoli and capillaries

41. The lungs are protected by
    A. The diaphragm
    B. The pleura
    C. A bony framework of the ribs, sternum, and vertebrae
    D. The lobes
42. Food is moved through the alimentary canal (GI tract) by
    A. Chyme   C. Swallowing
    B. Peristalsis   D. Bile
43. Water is absorbed from chyme in the
    A. Small intestine C. Esophagus
    B. Stomach   D. Large intestine
44. Digested food is absorbed through tiny projections called
    A. Jejunum   C. Villi
    B. Ileum   D. Colon
45. A function of the urinary system is to
    A. Remove waste products from the blood
    B. Rid the body of solid waste
    C. Rid the body of carbon dioxide
    D. Burn food for energy
46. A person feels the need to urinate when the bladder contains about
    A. 1000 ml of urine C. 250 ml of urine
    B. 500 ml of urine   D. 125 ml of urine
47. Testosterone is needed for
    A. Male secondary sex characteristics
    B. Female secondary sex characteristics
    C. Sperm to be produced
    D. Ova to be produced
48. The prostate gland lies
    A. In the scrotum   C. Just below the bladder
    B. In the testes   D. In the penis
49. The ovaries secrete progesterone and
    A. Estrogen   C. Ova
    B. Testosterone   D. Semen
50. When an ovum is released from an ovary, it travels first through the
    A. Uterus   C. Endometrium
    B. Fallopian tubes   D. Vagina
51. Menstruation occurs when
    A. The hymen is ruptured
    B. An ovum is released by the ovary
    C. The endometrium breaks up
    D. Fertilization occurs
52. A fertilized cell implants in the
    A. Ovary   C. Endometrium
    B. Fallopian tubes   D. Vagina
53. The master gland is the
    A. Thyroid gland
    B. Parathyroid gland
    C. Adrenal gland
    D. Pituitary gland
54. Thyroid hormone regulates
    A. Growth
    B. Metabolism
    C. Proper functioning of nerves and muscles
    D. Energy produced during energy

55. If too little insulin is produced by the pancreas, the person has
   A. Tetany   C. Diabetes mellitus
   B. Slow growth   D. Slowed metabolism
56. When antigens enter the body, they are attacked and destroyed by
   A. Antibodies   C. B cells
   B. Lymphocytes   D. T cells

Matching
Match the descriptions on the left with the correct term on the right.

Musculoskeletal

57. _____ Connective tissue at end of long bones		A. Periosteum
58. _____ Skeletal muscle		B. Joint
59. _____ Membrane that covers bone		C. Cartilage
60. _____ Connects muscle to bone		D. Synovial fluid
61. _____ Point at which two or more bones meet		E. Striated muscle
62. _____ Heart muscle		F. Smooth muscle
63. _____ Involuntary muscle		G. Cardiac muscle
64. _____ Acts as a lubricant so the joint can move smoothly		H. Tendons

Nervous system

65. _____ Contains eustachian tubes and ossicles	A. Sclera
66. _____ Has 12 pairs of cranial nerves and 31 pairs of spinal nerves	B. Cornea
67. _____ White of the eye	C. Retina
68. _____ Outside of cerebrum; controls highest function of brain	D. Cerumen
69. _____ Inner layer of eye; receptors for vision are contained here	E. Middle ear
70. _____ Controls involuntary muscles, heart beat, blood pressure, and other functions	F. Inner ear
71. _____ Light enters eye through this structure	G. Brainstem
72. _____ Contains midbrain, pons, and medulla	H. Cerebral cortex
73. _____ Waxy substance secreted in auditory canal	I. Autonomic nervous system
74. _____ Contains semicircular canal and cochlea	J. Peripheral nervous system

Circulatory system

75. _____ Liquid part of blood	A. Plasma
76. _____ Thin sac covering heart	B. Erythrocytes
77. _____ Very tiny blood vessels	C. Hemoglobin
78. _____ Substance in blood that picks up oxygen	D. Leukocytes
79. _____ Carry blood away from heart	E. Thrombocytes
80. _____ White blood cells	F. Pericardium
81. _____ Carry blood toward heart	G. Myocardium
82. _____ Red blood cells	H. Endocardium
83. _____ Thick, muscular portion of heart	I. Arteries
84. _____ Platelets; necessary for clotting	J. Veins
85. _____ Membrane lining inner surface of heart	K. Capillaries

Respiratory system

86. _____ Air passes from larynx into this structure	A. Epiglottis
87. _____ A two-layered sac that covers the lungs	B. Larynx
88. _____ Piece of cartilage that acts like a lid over larynx	C. Bronchiole
89. _____ Separates lungs from the abdominal cavity	D. Trachea
90. _____ The voice box	E. Alveoli
91. _____ Several small branches that divide from the bronchus	F. Diaphragm
92. _____ Tiny one-celled air sacs	G. Pleura

Digestive system

93. _____ Structure that adds more digestive juices to chyme	A. Liver
94. _____ Semiliquid food mixture formed in stomach	B. Chyme
95. _____ Portion of GI tract that absorbs food	C. Colon
96. _____ Stores bile	D. Duodenum
97. _____ Portion of GI tract that absorbs water	E. Jejunum
98. _____ Produces bile	F. Saliva
99. _____ Moistens food particles in the mouth	G. Pancreas
100. _____ Produces digestive juices	H. Gallbladder

Urinary system

101. _____ Basic working unit of the kidney
102. _____ Bean-shaped structure that produces urine
103. _____ A cluster of capillaries in Bowman's capsule
104. _____ Structure that allows urine to pass from the bladder
105. _____ A tube attached to the renal pelvis of the kidney
106. _____ Hollow, muscular sac that stores urine
107. _____ Opening at the end of the urethra
108. _____ Fluid and waste products form urine in this structure

A. Bladder
B. Glomerulus
C. Kidney
D. Meatus
E. Nephrons
F. Tubules
G. Ureter
H. Urethra

Reproductive system

109. _____ Male or female sex organs
110. _____ Two folds of tissue on each side of the vagina
111. _____ Sac between thighs that contains testes
112. _____ External genitalia of female
113. _____ Testicles; sperm produced here
114. _____ Attached to uterus; ovum travels through this structure
115. _____ Stores sperm and produces semen
116. _____ Tissue lining the uterus

A. Scrotum
B. Testes
C. Seminal vesicle
D. Gonads
E. Fallopian tubes
F. Endometrium
G. Labia
H. Vulva

Endocrine system

117. _____ Released by pancreas; regulates sugar in blood
118. _____ Sex hormone secreted by testes
119. _____ Sex hormone secreted by ovaries
120. _____ Regulates metabolism
121. _____ Regulates calcium levels in the body
122. _____ Stimulates to produce energy during emergencies

A. Epinephrine
B. Estrogen
C. Insulin
D. Parathormone
E. Testosterone
F. Thyroxine

Immune system

123. _____ Normal body substances that recognize abnormal or unwanted substances
124. _____ Type of cell that destroys invading cells
125. _____ Type of white blood cell that digests and destroys microorganisms
126. _____ Type of cell that causes production of antibodies
127. _____ An abnormal or unwanted substance
128. _____ Types of white blood cells that produce antibodies

A. Antibodies
B. Antigens
C. Phagocytes
D. Lymphocytes
E. B cells
F. T cells

Labeling

129. Name the parts of the cell.

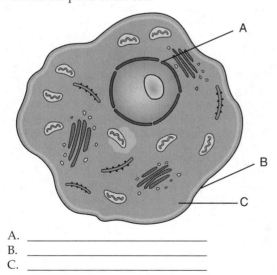

A. _____
B. _____
C. _____

130. Name each type of joint.

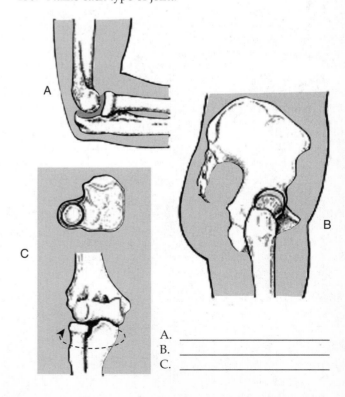

A. _____
B. _____
C. _____

131. Name the parts of the brain.

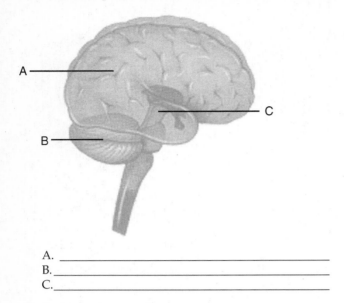

A. _____

B. _____

C. _____

132. Name the four chambers of the heart.

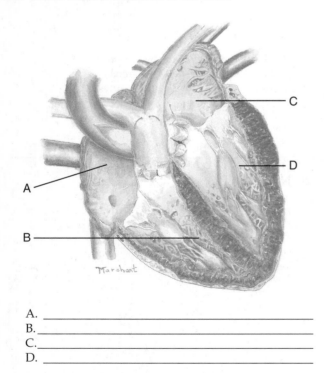

A. _____

B. _____

C. _____

D. _____

133. Name the structures of the respiratory system.

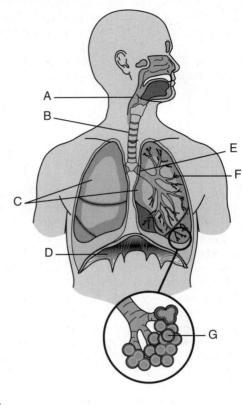

A. _____

B. _____

C. _____

D. _____

E. _____

F. _____

G. _____

134. Name the structures of the digestive system.

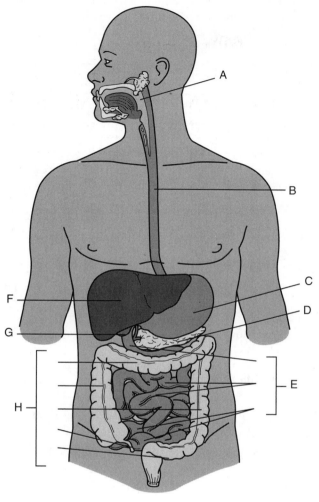

A. _____
B. _____
C. _____
D. _____
E. _____
F. _____
G. _____
H. _____

135. Name the structures of the urinary system.

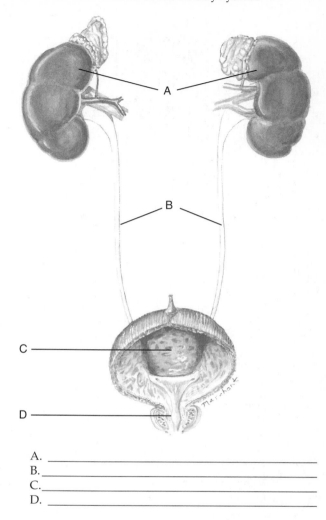

A. _____
B. _____
C. _____
D. _____

136. Name the structures of the male reproductive system.

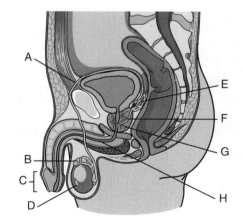

A. _____
B. _____
C. _____
D. _____
E. _____
F. _____
G. _____
H. _____

137. Name the external female genitalia.

Marchant

A. _____
B. _____
C. _____
D. _____
E. _____
F. _____

Optional Learning Exercises

138. Explain the function of each part of the cell.
    A. Cell membrane _____
    B. Nucleus _____
    C. Cytoplasm _____
    D. Protoplasm _____
    E. Chromosomes _____
    F. Genes _____

139. List what structures are contained in the two skin layers.
    A. Epidermis_____
    B. Dermis _____

140. Explain the function of the types of bone.
    A. Long bones _____
    B. Short bones _____
    C. Flat bones _____
    D. Irregular bones _____

141. Describe how each type of joint moves, and give an example of each type.
    A. Ball and socket _____
    Ex: _____
    B. Hinge _____
    Ex: _____
    C. Pivot _____
    Ex: _____

142. Explain what happens when muscles contract.
    _____
    _____
    _____

143. Explain the function of the three main parts of the brain. Include the function of the cerebral cortex and the midbrain, pons, and medulla.
    A. Cerebrum _____
    Cerebral cortex _____
    B. Cerebellum _____
    _____
    C. Brainstem _____
    Midbrain and Pons _____
    _____
    Medulla _____
    _____

144. Explain how the sympathetic and parasympathetic nervous systems balance each other.
    _____
    _____

145. Explain what happens to each of these structures when light enters the eye.
    A. Choroid _____
    B. Cornea _____
    C. Lens _____
    D. Retina _____

146. Explain how each of these structures helps carry sound in the ear.
    A. Ossicles _____
    B. Cochlea _____
    C. Auditory nerve _____

147. Where are red blood cells destroyed as they wear out?
    _____

148. When an infection occurs, what do white blood cells do?
    _____

149. Explain the function of the four atria of the heart.
    A. Right atrium _____
    B. Left atrium _____
    C. Right ventricle _____
    D. Left ventricle _____

150. Explain where each of these veins carries blood.
    A. Inferior vena cava _____
    B. Superior vena cava _____

151. Explain what happens in the alveoli. _____
    _____
    _____

152. After food is swallowed, explain what happens in each of these parts of the digestive tract.
    A. Stomach _____
    B. Duodenum _____
    C. Jejunum and ileum _____
    D. Colon _____
    E. Rectum _____
    F. Anus _____

153. Explain what happens in these structures of the kidney.
   A. Glomerulus _____
   B. Collecting tubules _____
   C. Ureters _____
   D. Urethra _____
   E. Meatus _____

154. Sperm is produced in the testicles. What happens to the sperm in each of these structures?
   A. Testes _____
   B. Vas deferens _____
   C. Seminal vesicle _____
   D. Ejaculatory duct _____
   E. Prostate gland _____
   F. Urethra _____

155. What is the function of the endometrium? _____
_____

156. Menstruation occurs about every _____ days. Ovulation usually occurs on or about day _____ of the cycle.

157. What is the function of each of these pituitary hormones?
   A. Growth hormone _____
   B. Thyroid-stimulating hormone _____
   C. Adrenocorticotropic hormone _____
   D. Antidiuretic hormone _____
   E. Oxytocin _____

158. What is the function of insulin? _____
_____
What happens if too little insulin is produced? _____
_____

159. What happens when the body senses an antigen? ____
_____

Independent Learning Activities

- Using your own body, move joints of each type to see how they move.
  - What joint is a ball and socket? How many ways were you able to move it?
  - What joint moves like a hinge? How does it work differently from the ball and socket?
  - What joint is a pivot joint? Compare its movement with the other two joint.
- Listen to a friend's chest with a stethoscope.
  - What sounds do you hear?
  - What body systems are making the sounds?
  - Are you able to count any of the sounds you hear? What are you counting?
- Listen to your lower abdomen with a stethoscope.
  - What sounds can you hear?
  - What causes sound in the abdomen? What body system is involved in this activity?
  - What is occurring when you hear your "stomach growl"? What is the term for this activity that you learned in this chapter?
- Look at a friend's eyes in a dimly lit area and observe the size of the pupils.
  - What size are the pupils? Are they both the same?
  - Shine a flashlight in the eye. What happens to the pupil?
  - What happens when you move the light away? If you see a change, how quickly does it occur?

8 The Older Person

Key Terms

Development
Developmental task
Dysphagia
Dyspnea
Geriatrics
Gerontology
Growth
Menopause
Old
Old-old
Presbyopia
Young-old

Fill in the Blanks: Key Terms

1. When menstruation stops, it is called _____.

2. _____ is a skill that must be completed during a stage of development.

3. Difficult, labored, or painful breathing is _____.

4. Persons age 85 and older are considered _____.

5. _____ is difficulty swallowing.

6. Persons between the ages of 65 and 74 are considered
   _____.

7. The care of aging people is _____.

8. Persons between the ages of 75 and 84 are considered
   _____.

9. The study of the aging process is _____.

10. _____ is age-related farsightedness.

11. Changes in mental, emotional, and social function is _____.

12. Physical changes that are measured and that occur in a steady, orderly manner is _____.

Circle the BEST Answer

13. In 2003, how many people were 65 and older?
    A. 4,200,000   C. 36,000,000
    B. 14,400,000   D. 100,000

14. Most older people live
    A. In a nursing center   C. In a family setting
    B. Alone   D. With non-relatives

15. A stage of growth and development in late adulthood is
    A. Adjusting to aging parents
    B. Developing new friends and relationships
    C. Developing a satisfactory sex life
    D. Developing leisure-time activities

16. A person would be in the old-old age range when
    A. 65-74 years   C. 60-65 years
    B. 75-84 years   D. Over 85 years

17. As aging occurs
    A. Illness and disability always result
    B. Changes are slow
    C. The person is lonely and isolated
    D. Most persons live in nursing centers

18. Psychological and social changes include
    A. Mental function declines
    B. Physical disabilities
    C. Retirees need activities to replace work
    D. Decreased physical strength

19. It may be difficult to meet all self-esteem needs when retired because:
    A. The person can do whatever he wants
    B. Work helps meet love, belonging, and self-esteem needs
    C. A retired person develops new relationships
    D. Physical strength decreases

20. Retired people may feel fulfilled and useful when they
    A. Travel
    B. Work part-time or do volunteer work
    C. Live alone
    D. Live with adult children

21. Money problems can result with retirement because
    A. Income is reduced
    B. The person lives alone
    C. The person is unable to work
    D. The person plans for retirement with savings and investments

22. Loneliness may be a bigger problem for foreign-born persons because
    A. Families from other cultures do not care about older persons
    B. They are not accepted by native-born persons
    C. They may not have anyone to talk to in their native language
    D. They have more chronic illnesses

23. An older person can adjust to social relationship changes by doing all of these *except*
    A. Finding new friends
    B. Developing hobbies, church and community activities
    C. Having regular contact with family
    D. Staying at home alone to save money

24. When children care for older parents
    A. The older person may feel unwanted and useless
    B. The older person may feel more secure
    C. Tension may develop among the children and the family
    D. All of the above

25. What causes wrinkles to appear on an older person?
    A. Decreases in oil and sweat gland secretions
    B. Fewer nerve endings
    C. Loss of elasticity, strength, and fatty tissue layer
    D. Poor circulation

26. Skin breakdown may heal slowly in older people because
    A. Older people eat a poor diet
    B. Blood vessels decrease in number
    C. The skin has more nerve endings
    D. Secretions from oil and sweat glands decrease
27. Bones may break easily because
    A. Joints become stiff and painful
    B. Joints become slightly flexed
    C. Bones lose strength and become brittle
    D. Vertebrae shorten
28. Older persons can prevent bone loss and loss of muscle strength by
    A. Activity, exercise, and diet
    B. Taking hormones
    C. Resting with feet elevated
    D. Taking vitamins
29. Dizziness may increase in older people because
    A. They have difficulty sleeping
    B. Blood flow to the brain is decreased
    C. Nerve cells are lost
    D. Brain cells are lost
30. Painful injuries and disease may go unnoticed because
    A. The person is confused
    B. Touch and sensitivity to pain are reduced
    C. Memory is shorter
    D. The blood flow is reduced
31. Eyes are irritated easily because
    A. The lens yellows
    B. The eye takes longer to adjust to changes in light
    C. Tear secretion is less
    D. The person becomes farsighted
32. If circulatory changes occur, the person
    A. May be encouraged to walk long distances
    B. May need to rest during the day
    C. May not do any kind of exercise
    D. Should exercise only once a week
33. A person with dyspnea can breathe easier when
    A. Lying flat in bed
    B. Covered with heavy bed linens
    C. Allowed to stay in one position on bedrest
    D. Resting in the semi-Fowler's position
34. Dulled taste and smell decrease
    A. Peristalsis   C. Saliva
    B. Appetite   D. Swallowing
35. Older persons need
    A. Fewer calories   C. More calories
    B. Less fluids   D. Low-protein diets
36. Many older persons have to urinate several times during the night because
    A. Bladder infections are common
    B. Urine is more concentrated
    C. Bladder muscles weaken and bladder size decreases
    D. Urinary incontinence may occur
37. Sexual activity in older persons changes because
    A. Orgasms for men and women are less intense or forceful
    B. The vaginal secretions increase
    C. An erection lasts longer
    D. Sex hormones increase

38. All of these are advantages of an older person living with family except
    A. It provides companionship
    B. The family can provide care during illness or disability
    C. They can share living expenses
    D. Sleep arrangements may change
39. Adult day-care centers
    A. Provide meals, supervision, and activities for older persons
    B. Accept only self-care persons and those who can walk without help
    C. Provide complete care
    D. Provide respite care
40. A common dining room or meals are usually not provided when the person lives in
    A. An apartment   C. A board and care home
    B. Congregate housing D. A residential hotel
41. Assisted living residences provide the following except
    A. Nursing care
    B. Help with daily living
    C. Health care and 24-hour oversight
    D. Social contact with other residents
42. Continuing care retirement communities (CCRC) may have
    A. Independent living units
    B. Food service and help nearby
    C. Added services as the person's needs change
    D. All of the above
43. Nursing centers are housing options for older persons who
    A. Need only companionship
    B. Cannot care for themselves
    C. Need care during the daytime while family works
    D. Are developmentally disabled
44. Moving to a nursing center
    A. Is an exciting change for the older person
    B. Can cause a loss of identity
    C. Is always a permanent move
    D. Allows the person to have more personal freedom
45. A quality nursing center is certified
    A. By the medical society
    B. For Medicare and Medicaid
    C. By the state board of nursing
    D. By the local health department
46. A quality nursing center would not be required to have
    A. An activity area for residents' use
    B. Halls wide enough for two wheelchairs to pass with ease
    C. Toilet facilities that can be accessed wheelchairs
    D. Private rooms for each resident
47. Sufficient space and equipment requirements by OBRA include
    A. Halls with hand rails and other safety needs
    B. A private bathroom for each resident
    C. Expecting residents to provide furniture for their rooms
    D. Using tablecloths and cloth napkins in dining room

Matching

Match physical changes during the aging process with the body system affected.

48. _____ Reduced blood flow to kidneys
49. _____ Arteries narrow and are less elastic
50. _____ Forgetfulness
51. _____ Gradual loss of height
52. _____ Decreased strength for coughing
53. _____ Decreased secretion of oil and sweat glands
54. _____ Difficulty digesting fried and fatty foods
55. _____ Heart pumps with less force
56. _____ Bladder muscles weaken
57. _____ Difficulty seeing green and blue colors
58. _____ Difficulty swallowing
59. _____ Lung tissue less elastic
60. _____ Bone mass decreases
61. _____ Testosterone level decreases
62. _____ Facial hair in some women

A. Integumentary
B. Musculoskeletal
C. Nervous
D. Circulatory
E. Respiratory
F. Digestive
G. Urinary
H. Reproductive

Optional Learning Exercises

Nursing concerns with physical changes.

63. When bathing an older person, what kind of soap should be used? _____. Often no soap is used on the _____.

64. What can happen if a nick or cut occurs on the feet? _ _____ Why can this happen? _____ _____

65. What types of skin growths are common in older persons?
    A. _____
    B. _____

66. Why are these skin growths dangerous if untreated? _____

67. When bone mass decreases, why is it important to turn an older person carefully? _____ _____

68. Why does an older person often have a gradual loss of height? _____

69. What types of exercise help prevent bone loss and loss of muscle strength? _____ _____

70. Older people have changes in the nervous system. When the changes listed below happen, what physical problems occur?

    A. Nerve conduction and reflexes are slower. _____ _____

    B. Blood flow to brain is reduced. _____ _____

    C. Progressive loss of brain cells occurs. _____ _____

71. When you are eating with an older person, you notice she puts salt on vegetables that taste fine to you? What may be a reason she does this? _____

72. A female nurse has a high-pitched voice, and several residents seem to have difficulty hearing her. They do not complain about hearing the male charge nurse. What may be a reason for the difference? _____ _____

73. How can you help the circulation of persons confined to bed? _____ What other body system will be helped by this activity? _____

74. What can the nursing assistant do to prevent respiratory complications from bedrest? _____

75. The stomach and colon empty slower and flatulence and constipation are common in the older person. What causes all of these problems? _____ _____

76. How do good oral hygiene and denture care improve food intake? _____

77. Why should you plan to give most fluids to the older person before 1700 (5:00 PM)? _____

Independent Learning Activities

- Interview an older person who lives independently. Use these questions to find what concerns the person has about remaining independent.
  - What physical problems does the person have, if any?
  - What activities are more difficult than they were when the person was younger?
  - What does the person use to provide safety? (Walkers, canes, alarms, daily phone calls, etc.)
  - What comfort measures are needed to decrease pain or help the person sleep?

- ○ What are transportation needs? Does the person drive? How does the person grocery shop? Visit with family, friends? Attend social functions?
  - ○ How are social needs met? How often does the person go to socialize? How often does the person have visitors?
- Interview an older person and talk about life when the person was young.
  - ○ Observe facial expression and tone of voice when the person talks about events remembered. What changes do you see?
  - ○ Compare how well the person remembers events of long ago with those that happened recently.
  - ○ How do you feel differently about the person after hearing about the person's youth?

9 Sexuality

Key Terms

Bisexual
Erectile dysfunction
Heterosexual

Homosexual
Impotence
Sex

Sexuality
Transgender

Transsexual
Transvestite

Fill in the Blanks: Key Terms

1. _____ is a broad term to describe people who express their sexuality or gender in other than the expected way.

2. Another name for impotence is _____.

3. _____ is the physical, psychological, social, cultural, and spiritual factors that affect a person's feelings and attitudes about his or her sex.

4. A _____ is a person who becomes sexually excited by dressing in the clothes of the other sex.

5. A person attracted to both sexes is _____.

6. A _____ is a person who believes that he or she is really a member of the other sex.

7. A _____ is a person who is attracted to members of the same sex.

8. The physical activities involving the organs of reproduction, is _____.

9. A person who is attracted to members of the other sex is _____.

10. The inability of the male to have an erection is erectile dysfunction, or _____.

Circle the BEST Answer

11. Sexuality
    A. Involves the personality and the body
    B. Is the physical activities involving reproductive organs
    C. Is unimportant in old age
    D. Is done for pleasure or to have children

12. A woman who is attracted to men is
    A. Homosexual   C. Lesbian
    B. Heterosexual   D. Bisexual

13. Transvestites are often
    A. Homosexual   C. Married and heterosexual
    B. Transsexual   D. Bisexual

14. Diabetes, spinal cord injuries, and multiple sclerosis may cause
    A. Impotence   C. Sexual aggression
    B. Menopause   D. Heterosexuality

15. Which of these are *not* true about sexuality and older persons?
    A. An orgasm is less forceful than in younger persons
    B. Arousal takes longer
    C. Older persons lose sexual needs and desires
    D. Love, affection, and intimacy are needed throughout life

16. When older adult couples live in a nursing center, OBRA requires that they
    A. Are allowed to share the same room
    B. Are placed in separate rooms
    C. Are not encouraged to be intimate
    D. Cannot share a bed

17. When a person in a nursing center is sexually aggressive, it may be the result of
    A. Confusion
    B. Using a way to gain your attention
    C. Genital soreness or itching
    D. All of the above

18. If a person touches you in the wrong way, you should
    A. Ignore it and realize the person is not responsible
    B. Tell the person you do not like him or her
    C. Tell the person that those behaviors make you uncomfortable
    D. Refuse to give care to the person

19. If you do not share a person's sexual attitudes, values, practices, or standards, you should
    A. Not judge or gossip about the person
    B. Avoid the person
    C. Tell him or her your feelings
    D. Discuss the person's relationships with other staff members

Fill in the Blanks

20. Sexuality develops when the baby's _____.

21. Children know their own sex at age _____.

22. Bisexuals often _____ and have _____.

23. Sexual function may be affected by chronic illnesses such as
    A. _____
    B. _____
    C. _____

24. What reproductive surgeries may affect sexuality?
    A. Men _____
    B. Women _____

25. Some older people do not have intercourse. They may express their sexual needs or desires by _____ _____.

26. When you are assisting persons, what grooming practices will promote sexuality for residents?
    A. Men _____
    B. Women _____

42

Copyright © 2007, 2003 by Mosby, Inc., an affiliate of Elsevier Inc. All rights reserved.

27. What can you do to allow privacy for a person and a partner?
   A. Close _____
   B. Remind the person about _____
   C. Tell other _____
   D. Knock _____

28. Masturbation is a normal _____.

29. What health-related problems may cause a person to touch his or her genitals?
   A. _____ or _____ system disorders
   B. Poor _____
   C. Being _____ or _____ from urine and feces

Optional Learning Exercises

Mr. and Mrs. Davis are 78-year-old residents in a nursing center, where they share a room. They need assistance with ADL but are mentally alert. They are an affectionate couple who care deeply for each other. Answer these questions about meeting their sexuality needs.

30. Mr. Davis has diabetes and high blood pressure. What effect can these disorders have on sexuality?

   _____

31. What do you think would be an important thing you could do when they ask for privacy?

   _____

Independent Learning Activities

1. Consider this situation about a sexually aggressive person, and answer the questions about how you would respond.

   SITUATION: John James is 72 and has paraplegia because of an accident several years ago. His caregivers report that recently he has begun to make sexually suggestive remarks. While you are giving his morning care, he touches you several times in private areas and makes frequent sexually suggestive remarks. The other nursing assistants tell you they just ignore him or joke around with him about the actions.

   ○ What would you say to Mr. James when he touched you in private areas?
   ○ How would you respond to his suggestive remarks?
   ○ What would you say to your colleagues who suggest you ignore or joke with Mr. James?
   ○ Has this type of situation ever occurred to you? How did you handle it then? What would you do differently after studying this chapter?

2. Consider this situation about caring for a person who is gay. Answer the questions about how you would respond.

   SITUATION: Bobbie Freeman is 45 and has had gallbladder surgery. While assisting her to ambulate, she begins to talk about her friend Judy. She tells you that they have been lovers for 15 years.

   ○ What would you say to a person who tells you she is homosexual?
   ○ What effect would this information have on the care you provide for the person?
   ○ Has this type of situation ever occurred when you were caring for a person? How did you respond? How would you respond after studying this chapter?

10 Safety

Key Terms

Coma	Electrical shock	Hemiplegia	Quadriplegia
Dementia	Ground	Incident	Suffocation
Disaster	Hazardous substance	Paraplegia	Workplace violence

Fill in the Blanks: Key Terms

1. The loss of cognitive and social function caused by changes in the brain is _____.

2. Paralysis from the neck down is _____.

3. _____ is any chemical in the workplace that can cause harm.

4. A _____ is a sudden catastrophic event in which many people are injured and killed and property is destroyed.

5. _____ occurs when breathing stops from the lack of oxygen.

6. Paralysis on one side of the body is _____.

7. A _____ is a state of being unaware of one's surroundings and being unable to react or respond to people, places, or things.

8. That which carries leaking electricity to the earth and away from an electrical appliance is a _____.

9. _____ is paralysis from the waist down.

10. _____ occurs when electrical current passes through the body.

11. Violent acts directed toward persons at work or while on duty is _____.

12. An _____ is any event that has harmed or could harm a resident, staff member, or visitor.

Circle the BEST Answer

13. To protect the person from harm, you need to
    A. Use restraints
    B. Follow the person's care plan
    C. Limit mobility
    D. Lock all doors

14. Age can increase a person's risk of accidents because of all of these except
    A. Balance is affected and they fall easily
    B. They may have poor vision or hearing problems
    C. They are less sensitive to heat and cold
    D. They are more sensitive to hazardous materials

15. People with dementia are at risk of injury because they
    A. No longer know what is safe and what is dangerous
    B. Are in a coma
    C. Have problems sensing heat and cold
    D. Have poor vision

16. Drugs can be a risk factor for accidents because side effects can
    A. Affect hearing
    B. Reduce ability to sense heat and cold
    C. Cause loss of balance or lack of coordination
    D. Cause hemiplegia

17. Identifying the person is most important because
    A. You must give the right care to the right person
    B. Visitors may ask your help to find someone
    C. You need to call the person by the right name
    D. You will have to give care to two people if you give it to the wrong person first

18. Which of these is not a reliable way to identify the person?
    A. Check the identification bracelet
    B. Use the person's picture to compare with the person
    C. If resident is alert and oriented, follow the center policy to identify
    D. Call the person by name

19. Burns can be prevented if
    A. Smoking is allowed when the person is in bed
    B. Residents are allowed to smoke only in smoking areas
    C. No smoking is allowed
    D. Smoking materials are kept at each person's bedside

20. Which of these personal care items can cause poisoning?
    A. Soap and shampoo
    B. Mouthwash
    C. Lotion and deodorant
    D. All of the above

21. Suffocation can be caused by
    A. Cutting food into small, bite-size pieces
    B. Making sure dentures fit properly and are in place
    C. Giving oral food and fluids to a person with a feeding tube
    D. Checking the care plan for swallowing problems

22. If a person clutches the throat and is unable to speak, he or she has a
    A. Sore throat
    B. Dangerous level of carbon monoxide
    C. Severe airway obstruction
    D. Mild airway obstruction

23. When a severe foreign body airway obstruction occurs and the person is conscious, you should first
    A. Place the person in bed and go for help
    B. Perform the Heimlich maneuver until the object is expelled
    C. Do a finger sweep to remove the object
    D. Ask the person to cough to expel the object

24. An electrical appliance cannot be used if
    A. It has a three-pronged plug
    B. It is connected directly to a wall outlet
    C. It has not been checked by the maintenance staff
    D. The cord is in good repair
25. An electrical shock is especially dangerous because it can
    A. Start a fire
    B. Damage equipment
    C. Affect the heart and cause death
    D. Violate OBRA regulations
26. If you are shocked by electric equipment, you should
    A. Take the item to the nurse
    B. Try to see what is wrong with the equipment
    C. Make sure it has a ground prong
    D. Test the equipment in a different outlet
27. Wheelchair brakes are locked when
    A. Transporting the person
    B. Taking a wheelchair up or down stairs
    C. A person is moving to or from the wheelchair
    D. Storing the wheelchair
28. When moving a person on a stretcher, all of these practices are correct *except*
    A. Safety straps or side rails are used only when the person is confused
    B. Lock the stretcher before transferring the person
    C. Do not leave the person alone
    D. Stand at the head of the stretcher. Your co-worker stands at the foot
29. Which of these is *not* a health hazard caused by chemicals?
    A. A burn from an explosion
    B. Damage to the kidneys, nervous system, lungs, skin, eyes, or mucous membranes
    C. Blood cell formation and function affected by chemicals
    D. Birth defects, miscarriages, and fertility problems
30. What should be done if a label is missing from a hazardous substance?
    A. Take the container to the nurse
    B. Return the container to the cupboard or shelf
    C. Use the substance as usual
    D. Leave the container where you found it, and go for help
31. All of this information is found in the Material Safety Data Sheet (MSDS) *except*
    A. How to clean up a spill or leak
    B. Conditions that could cause a chemical reaction
    C. How to use the substance
    D. Explosion information and fire-fighting measures
32. When you are cleaning up a hazardous substance, you should
    A. Work from clean areas to dirty areas using circular motions
    B. Wear personal protective equipment listed on the MSDS
    C. Dispose of hazardous waste in sealed bags or containers
    D. All of the above

33. _____ requires a hazard communication program so that employees know how to handle hazardous substances.
    A. Omnibus Budget Reconciliation of 1987 (OBRA)
    B. Occupational Safety and Health Administration (OSHA)
    C. Joint Commission on Accreditation of Healthcare Organizations (JCAHO)
    D. Material Safety Data Sheet (MSDS)
34. Where would you find the Material Safety Data Sheets (MSDS) for hazardous materials?
    A. Attached to the substance
    B. In the administrator's office
    C. In a binder at a certain place on each nursing unit
    D. On the Internet
35. If a resident is receiving oxygen, he is at special risk for
    A. Burns   C. Poisoning
    B. Suffocation   D. Electrical shock
36. All of these things are needed for a fire *except*
    A. Spark or flame
    B. Electrical equipment
    C. Materials that will burn
    D. Oxygen
37. If a fire occurs, what should you do first?
    A. Rescue people in immediate danger
    B. Sound the nearest fire alarm and call the switchboard operator
    C. Close doors and windows to confine the fire
    D. Use a fire extinguisher on a small fire that has not spread to a larger area
38. When using a fire extinguisher, the "P" in the word PASS means
    A. Pull the fire alarm
    B. Pull the safety pin
    C. Rescue person in immediate danger
    D. Push the handle or lever down
39. If evacuating is necessary, residents who are
    A. Closest to the outside door are rescued first
    B. Able to walk are rescued last
    C. Closest to the fire are taken out first
    D. Helpless are rescued last
40. If there is a disaster, you
    A. Are expected to go to your nursing center immediately
    B. May be called into work if you are off duty
    C. Should stay away or leave to get out of the way
    D. May go home to check on your family
41. Why is workplace violence a big concern in health care?
    A. According to OSHA, more assaults occur in health care settings than in other industries
    B. Acutely disturbed and violent persons may seek health care
    C. Agency pharmacies are a source of drugs and therefore a target for robberies
    D. All of the above

42. Which of these would *not* be effective to prevent or control workplace violence?
    A. Stand away from the person
    B. Know where to find panic buttons, call bells, and alarms
    C. Sit quietly with the person in his room. Hold his hand to calm him
    D. Tell the person you will get a nurse to speak to him or her

43. Which of these could *not* be used as a weapon by an aggressive person?
    A. Your jewelry or scarf
    B. Long hair that is worn up and off the collar
    C. Keys, scissors, or other items
    D. Tools or items left by maintenance staff

44. Risk management involves
    A. Training the staff to understand MSDS
    B. Identifying and controlling risks and safety hazards
    C. Firing employees who have accidents
    D. Hiring security staff to prevent injuries

45. When you are filling out a valuables list or envelope, which of these would be the best description?
    A. "A diamond in a gold setting"
    B. "A one-carat diamond in a 14K gold setting"
    C. "A white stone in a yellow setting"
    D. "A white diamond-like stone in a gold-like setting"

46. Which of these would *not* be reported as an accident or error?
    A. Forgetting to give care
    B. Giving the wrong care
    C. Assisting a co-worker to give care
    D. Losing a resident's dentures

Matching
Match each safety measure with the risk of injury it prevents.

47. _____ Do not let person use electric blanket
48. _____ Keep soap and shampoo in safe place
49. _____ Be sure residents smoke only in smoking areas
50. _____ Keep electrical items away from water
51. _____ Make sure casters face forward
52. _____ Do not leave the person alone
53. _____ Do not give resident shower or tub bath when there is an electrical storm
54. _____ Keep matches away from confused and disoriented persons
55. _____ Report loose teeth or dentures to the nurse
56. _____ Do not let the person stand on the footplates
57. _____ Do not touch a person who is experiencing an electrical shock
58. _____ Move all residents from the area if you smell gas or smoke
59. _____ Do not allow smoking near oxygen tanks or concentrators
60. _____ Fasten safety straps when the person is properly positioned

A. Burns
B. Suffocation
C. Poisoning
D. Fire
E. Electrical
F. Wheelchair
G. Stretcher

Fill in the Blanks

61. Before giving care, use the _____ to identify the person.

62. _____ is a gas produced by the burning of fuel.

63. Forceful _____ can remove the object causing a mild airway obstruction.

64. The Heimlich maneuver is not used for very _____ persons or _____ women.

65. If a ground (three-pronged) plug is not used, it can cause _____ and possible _____.

66. Before using a hazardous substance, you check the _____ for safety information.

67. If a person is receiving oxygen therapy, _____ signs are placed on the door and near the bed.

68. If an incident occurs that has harmed a person, you should _____ at once.

Optional Learning Exercises

69. What factors related to age make older persons more at risk for accidents?
    A. Decreased _____
    B. Poor balance makes it hard to avoid _____
    C. Less sensitive to _____ and _____

70. How do impaired smell and touch increase accident risks?
    A. Person may not detect _____ or _____ odors
    B. Person has problems sensing _____ and _____
    C. Decreased _____ sense

71. Warning labels on hazardous substances identify
    A. _____
    B. _____
    C. _____
    D. _____
    E. _____

72. If a person is receiving oxygen therapy, why are wool blankets and synthetic fabrics removed from the room? _____

73. What does RACE mean when a fire occurs?
    A. R _____
    B. A _____
    C. C _____
    D. E _____

74. When using a fire extinguisher, what does the word PASS stand for?
    A. P _____
    B. A _____
    C. S _____
    D. S _____

75. What kinds of threats are considered workplace violence?
    A. _____
    B. _____
    C. _____

76. What information is required on an incident report?
    A. _____
    B. _____
    C. _____
    D. _____
    E. _____
    F. _____

Read the following examples, and write the related guideline from Boxes 10-4 and 10-5 in the textbook.
77. The nursing assistant tells the resident his shower will be delayed until the storm passes. _____

78. The nursing assistant tells the nurse she has never used the portable footbath before. _____

79. The nursing assistant dries her hands carefully before plugging in a razor. _____

80. An electric fan will not work, and the staff member follows the correct procedure to have it repaired.
_____

81. The nursing assistant moves an electrical cord that is lying across a heat vent. _____

82. The nursing assistant makes sure the person has both feet on the wheelchair footrests. _____

83. The nursing assistant notices one wheel is flat on a wheelchair and reports it to the nurse. _____

84. The nursing assistant locks the wheelchair when the person is sitting in it next to his bed. _____

When handling hazardous materials, what should you do in these situations? (Box 10-6)
85. When cleaning up a hazardous material, how do you know what equipment to wear? _____

86. When a spill occurs, what is the correct way to wipe it up? _____

87. The nurse tells the nursing assistant the resident is having an x-ray done in her room. _____

88. The staff opens the windows when cleaning up a hazardous material. _____

What fire prevention measure is being practiced in each example? (Box 10-7)
89. The resident is taken to the smoking area in his wheelchair. _____

90. When cleaning the smoking area, the staff member uses a metal can partially filled with sand. _____

91. When heating food for a resident, the nursing assistant remains in the kitchen. _____

What measures to prevent or control workplace violence are being used or should be used in these examples? (Box 10-8)
92. How can jewelry serve as a weapon? _____

93. Why is long hair worn up? _____

94. Why are few pictures, vases, and other items kept in some areas? _____

95. What type of glass protects nurses' stations, reception areas, and admitting areas? _____

96. What clothing items should be worn by staff to assist the ability to run? _____

List personal safety practices that apply in these situations. (Box 10-9)

97. Parking your car in a parking garage. _____

98. What items should you keep in the car for safety? ___

99. Why is a "dry run" important? _____

100. If you think someone is following you, what should you do? _____

101. If someone wants your wallet or purse, what should you do? _____

102. How can you use your car keys as a weapon? _____

103. How can you use your thumbs as a weapon? _____

104. What part of the body can you attack on either a man or a woman? _____

Independent Learning Activities

- Safety is important to everyone and needs to be practiced at all times. Check the following items or areas in your own home to determine whether it is safe:
  - What areas are adequately lighted for safety? What areas need improved lighting?
  - Check electrical cords and plugs on appliances and lamps. How many have frayed cords? Ungrounded plugs? Other problems that make them unsafe to use?
  - How many smoke detectors do you have in your home? When were the batteries last replaced? How can you check the smoke detector to make sure it is working correctly?
  - How many scatter rugs are used on slippery surfaces? How many have some type of backing to prevent slipping?
  - Where are hazardous materials (medications, cleaning solutions, painting supplies, etc.) stored? Which of these could be reached by children? What could be done to store them more safely?
  - Make a list of good safety practices in your home. Make a list of safety practices that could be improved.
- Develop a plan for your home and family that helps everyone know how to escape if a fire occurs:
  - Make sure every person knows at least two escape routes form the sleeping area.
  - Practice how to check a door for heat before opening.
  - Arrange a place to meet once you are outside the building.

11 Preventing Falls

Key Terms
Bedrail   Gait belt   Transfer belt

Fill in the Blanks: Key Terms
1. A device used to support a person who is unsteady or disabled is a _____.

2. A _____ is a device that serves as a guard or barrier along the side of the bed.

3. Another name for a transfer belt is a _____ _____.

Circle the BEST Answer
4. Most falls occur in
   A. Hallways
   B. Resident rooms and bathrooms
   C. Outside
   D. Dining areas
5. Falls are more likely to occur
   A. After midnight
   B. During shift changes
   C. At mealtime
   D. In the morning after breakfast
6. Which of these would help prevent falls?
   A. Answer call light promptly
   B. Take the person to the bathroom once a shift
   C. Always keep side rails up
   D. Have the person wear socks to walk in room
7. Which of these physical problems can cause falls?
   A. Low blood pressure
   B. Joint pain and stiffness
   C. Incontinence
   D. All of the above
8. Bed rails
   A. Are used for all older persons
   B. Are considered restraints by OBRA
   C. Prevent falls
   D. Are never used when giving care
9. When giving care, the bed wheels are
   A. Unlocked
   B. Locked
   C. Unlocked on the side of the bed where you are working
   D. Locked when moving the bed
10. A transfer belt is
    A. Always applied over clothing
    B. Applied with the buckle over the spine
    C. Applied very loosely
    D. Always applied next to the skin
11. If a person begins to fall, you should
    A. Try to prevent the fall
    B. Call for help and hold the person up
    C. Ease the person to the floor
    D. Stand back and let the person fall

Fill in the Blanks
12. Most falls occur between _____ and _____.

13. You may calm an agitated person by giving the person a _____, _____, or a _____.

14. Tubs and showers may be made safer if they have _____ surfaces.

15. The need for bed rails is noted in the person's _____ and _____.

16. You raise the bed to give care. If the person uses bed rails and you are working alone, what do you do with the side rails?
    A. _____
    B. _____

17. After you are done giving care, how is the bed positioned? _____

18. Hand rails in hallways and stairways give support to persons who are _____ _____.

19. When a transfer belt is applied, you should be able to slide _____ fingers under the belt.

20. When a person starts to fall, you should protect the person's _____ as you ease the person to the floor.

21. What information is recorded on an incident report when a person falls?
    A. _____
    B. _____
    C. _____
    D. _____
    E. _____

Optional Learning Exercises
22. Why are falls more likely to happen during shift changes? Staff _____.
    Confusion _____ _____

23. What kinds of equipment help make bathrooms and showers safer?
    A. _____
    B. _____
    C. _____
    D. _____

24. Why should floor coverings be one color in areas where older persons are living? _____
    _____

25. Why are falls prevented when the person's phone, lamp, and personal belongings are at the bedside?
    _____

26. What kind of footwear and clothing will help prevent falls?
    A. Footwear_____
    B. Clothing_____

27. Why is it important to answer signal lights promptly?
    _____
    _____

28. If a person needs bed rails, keep them up at all times except _____.

29. For a person who uses bed rails, always raise the far bed rail if you _____
    _____.

30. If a person does not use bed rails and you are giving care, how do you protect him or her from falling?
    _____

31. Wheels are locked at all times except when _____
    _____.

32. If a person starts to fall, you _____.
    This lets you control _____.

Independent Learning Activities

- Look at the nursing center where you are assigned to answer these questions about safety.
  - How quickly are signal lights answered? How does the staff know who should answer each light?
  - If you are there during shift change, how does the staff make sure residents do not fall?
  - What safety measures do you see being used? (Use Box 11-2 as a guide to check for these measures.)
  - How many residents use bed rails? What are the reasons these residents need bed rails?
- Practice easing a falling person to the floor with a classmate.
  - How did you support the person?
  - How did using the transfer/gait belt help control the fall?
  - What was easy and what was difficult about this practice?
  - How did this practice help you to feel more confident about helping a falling person?

12 Restraint Alternatives and Safe Restraint Use

Key Terms
Active physical restraint   Passive physical restraint   Restraint

Fill in the Blanks: Key Terms

1. Any item, object, device, garment, material, or chemical that limits or restricts a person's freedom of movement or access to one's body is a _restraint_.

2. An _____ is a restraint attached to the person's body and to a stationary (non-movable) object.

3. A _____ is a restraint near but not directly attached to the person's body; it does not totally restrict freedom of movement and allows access to certain body parts.

Circle the BEST Answer

4. Restraints are used
   A. Whenever the nurse feels they are necessary
   B. Only as a last resort to protect residents from harming themselves or others
   C. To make sure the person does not fall
   D. To decrease work for the staff

5. The decision to find ways to meet the person's safety needs is made by
   A. The doctor
   B. The nurse and family
   C. The health team at a resident care conference
   D. The nursing assistants giving care

6. Research shows that restraints
   A. Prevent falls
   B. Cause falls
   C. Are used whenever the nurse decides
   D. Are necessary protective devices

7. A person's harmful behaviors may be caused by
   A. Being afraid of a new setting
   B. Being too hot or too cold
   C. Being hungry or thirsty
   D. All of the above

8. Guidelines about using restraints are part of
   A. FDA regulations
   B. State laws
   C. OBRA and CMS regulations
   D. All of the above

9. Restraints are *not* used to
   A. Prevent harm to the person
   B. Discipline or punish the person
   C. Prevent a person from pulling at a wound or dressing
   D. Keep an IV from being pulled out

10. Which of these can be a type of restraint?
   A. A soft chair with a footstool to elevate the feet
   B. A bed without rails
   C. A geriatric (geri) chair
   D. A drug that helps a person function at his or her highest level

11. The most serious risk from restraints is
   A. Cuts, bruises, and fractures
   B. Death from strangulation
   C. Falls
   D. Depression, anger, and agitation

12. After receiving instructions about the correct use of a restraint, you should
   A. Ask for help to apply it to a resident
   B. Demonstrate correct application to the nurse before using it on a person
   C. Watch someone else apply it to a resident
   D. Apply it to the resident independently

13. Which of these is *not* a physical restraint?
   A. A vest restraint
   B. A chair with an attached tray
   C. A drug that affects the person's mental function
   D. Sheets tucked in so tightly they restrict movement

14. To use a restraint, the nurse must
   A. Get permission from the family
   B. Have a written doctor's order
   C. Get permission from the health care team
   D. Receive OBRA permission

15. Which of these is an active physical restraint?
   A. Vest   C. Wedge cushion
   B. Bed rail   D. Pillow

16. OBRA requires informed consent. This consent is obtained by
   A. The resident's legal representative
   B. The doctor or nurse
   C. The resident
   D. The nursing assistant

17. When restraining a combative and agitated person, it should be done
   A. Slowly by only one person
   B. Only after explaining to the person what will be done
   C. With enough help to protect the person and staff from injury
   D. In a public area so the person is distracted

18. The person who is restrained must be observed every
   A. 5 minutes   C. Hour
   B. 15 minutes   D. 2 hours

19. Wrist restraints are used when a person
   A. Tries to get out of bed
   B. Moves his wheelchair without permission
   C. Pulls at tubes used in medical treatments
   D. Slides out of a chair easily

20. A belt restraint
   A. Is more restrictive than other restraints
   B. Allow the person to turn from side to side
   C. Must be released by the staff
   D. Can be used only in bed

21. A vest restraint
    A. Always crosses in the front
    B. Is applied next to the skin under clothing
    C. Must be secured very tightly to be safe
    D. Crosses in the back
22. When applying wrist restraints
    A. Tie the straps to the bed rail
    B. Tie firm knots in the straps
    C. Place the restraints over clothing
    D. Place the soft part toward the skin
23. When you apply mitts restraints
    A. Make sure the person's hand is clean and dry
    B. Pad the mitt with soft material
    C. Make sure the mitt is securely tied so the hand
       cannot move
    D. Make sure you can slide 3 or 4 fingers between the
       wrist and the restraint
24. When using a vest restraint in bed
    A. The straps are secured at waist level out of the
       person's reach
    B. The straps are secured to the bed rail
    C. The vest crosses in the back
    D. The person can turn over
25. How can you improve the quality of life for a person
    with restraints?
    A. Provide water or other fluids frequently
    B. Check often to make sure breathing and circulation
       are normal
    C. Treat the person with kindness, caring, respect,
       and dignity
    D. All of the above

Matching
Match the safety guidelines with the correct example.

26. _____ Injuries and deaths have occurred from improper restraint and poor observation.
27. _____ A restraint is used only when it is the best safety precaution for the person.
28. _____ The nurse gives you the printed instructions about applying and securing the restraint safely.
29. _____ Restrained persons need repeated explanations and reassurance.
30. _____ The doctor gives the reason for the restraint, what to use, and how long to use the restraint.
31. _____ Residents in immediate danger of harming themselves or others are restrained quickly.
32. _____ Because they are the least restrictive, passive physical restraints should be used when possible.
33. _____ The goal of this guideline is to meet person's needs using as little restraint as possible.
34. _____ If told to apply a restraint, you must clearly understand the need.
35. _____ When the restraint is removed, range-of-motion exercises are done or the person is ambulated.
36. _____ The care plan must include measures to protect the resident and to prevent the person from harming others.
37. _____ The resident must understand the reason for the restraints.
38. _____ The person must be comfortable and able to move the restrained part to a limited and safe extent. Food, fluid, comfort, safety, exercise, and elimination needs must be met.

A. Restraints are used to protect the person. OBRA and CMS do not allow restraints for staff convenience or to discipline a person
B. Restraints require a doctor's order.
C. OBRA and CMS require using the least-restrictive method.
D. Restraints are used only after trying other methods to protect the person.
E. Unnecessary restraint is false imprisonment.
F. OBRA requires informed consent for restraint use.
G. The manufacturer's instructions are followed.
H. The health team meets the restrained person's basic needs.
I. Restraints are applied with enough help to protect the person and staff from injury.
J. Restraints can increase a person's confusion and agitation.
K. OBRA requires that the resident's quality of life be protected.
L. The resident is observed at least every 15 minutes or more often as required by the care plan.
M. The restraint is removed, the person repositioned, and basic needs met at least every 2 hours.

Fill in the Blanks

39. When using restraints, what information is reported and recorded?
    A. _____
    B. _____
    C. _____
    D. _____
    E. _____
    F. _____
    G. _____
    H. _____
    I. _____
    J. _____
    K. _____

40. Persons restrained in a supine position must be monitored constantly because they are a great risk for
    _____.

41. You should carry scissors with you because in an emergency _____
    _____.

42. At what angle should a belt restraint be applied?
    _____

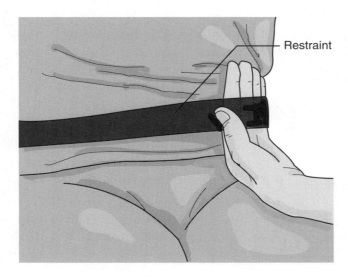

Restraint

Labeling

43. Explain what is being done in the figure._____
    _____

Nursing Assistant Skills Video Exercise
View the **Safety** *and* **Restraints** *video to answer these questions.*

44. Being in an unfamiliar environment increases the risk of accidents.
    A. True
    B. False

45. As a member of the nursing team, you are responsible for the following:
    A. _____
    B. _____
    C. _____
    D. _____
    E. _____
    F. _____

46. List the safety measures practiced when assisting Mr. Rydell to the bathroom.
    A. _____
    B. _____
    C. _____
    D. _____
    E. _____
    F. _____
    G. _____
    H. _____
    I. _____
    J. _____
    K. _____

47. What safety measures were practiced after assisting Mr. Rydell back to bed?
    A. _____
    B. _____
    C. _____

48. Restraints are used only as a last resort, when other measures have failed to do one or all of the following:
    A. _____
    B. _____
    C. _____

49. Explain what "the least restrictive device" means.
    _____

50. For which persons are vest or jacket restraints ordered? _____
    _____

51. For which person are mitt restraints ordered?_____
    _____

52. The person with a _____, _____, or _____ restraint is at great risk for strangulation and suffocation if he or she gets caught in the restraint or if the restraint is too tight.

53. If a person with a vest, jacket, or belt restraint is having difficulty breathing or is not breathing, you must _____.

54. _____, _____, and _____
    may prevent accidents, injury, and restraint use.

Optional Learning Exercises

55. How is a drug considered a restraint?
    A. _____
    B. _____
    C. _____

56. How does a restraint increase incontinence?

_____

_____

57. What life-long habits and routines could be included in the nursing care plan as alternatives to restraints?

_____

_____

58. Why would a person in restraints be at risk for dehydration?

_____

_____

59. Why would video tapes of family and friends or visiting with family be good alternatives to restraints?

_____

_____

Independent Learning Activities

Role play: One person is a nursing assistant, and one is a person who is restrained. An active physical restraint is applied as the person sits in a chair or wheelchair. When the restraint is in place, the nursing assistant leaves and does not return for 15 minutes. Discuss the following questions with each other after the experiment:

- How did the person feel when the restraints were applied? What did the nursing assistant tell the person about the restraints?
- Did the nursing assistant ask the person if toileting was needed? If the person was thirsty?
- Was the chair comfortable? Was there any padding? Did the nursing assistant check for wrinkles? Could the person move around to reposition the body for comfort?
- How was the person able to get help during the 15 minutes of being alone?
- What diversions were offered while the person was restrained? TV or radio? Reading materials? A window with a pleasant view? If any of these were provided, who chose the channel, station, book, or view?
- Was the person told someone would return in 15 minutes? Was a clock or watch available to see the time? How long did it seem?
- What was learned from this experience by both people?

136. If you are asked to assist with a sterile procedure,
what information do you need before beginning?
A. _____
B. _____
C. _____
D. _____
E. _____

Independent Learning Activities

Hand-washing practices are important to use whenever you are to prevent the spread of infection. Use this exercise to make yourself aware of your own habits.

- Make a list of when you washed your hands for one day.
  - How did you wash your hands? Did you use the method taught in this chapter?
  - How many times did you wash your hands at work? At home?
  - How many times did you realize you had forgotten to wash your hands? What were the reasons you forgot?
- How can you improve your hand-washing practices? What will you change after studying this chapter?

14 Body Mechanics

Key Terms
Base of support
Body alignment
Body mechanics
Dorsal recumbent position

Ergonomics
Fowler's position
Lateral position

Posture
Prone position
Semi-prone position

Side-lying position
Sims' position
Supine position

Fill in the Blanks: Key Terms

1. Another name for the lateral position is _____.

2. The way in which the head, trunk, arms, and legs are aligned with one another is _____ or posture.

3. The _____ is also called the side-lying position.

4. The _____ is the same as the back-lying or supine position.

5. The area on which an object rests is the _____.

6. _____ is a left side-lying position in which the upper leg is sharply flexed so that it is not on the lower leg and the lower arm is behind the person.

7. A semi-sitting position with the head of the bed elevated 45 to 90 degrees is _____.

8. Lying on the abdomen with the head turned to one side is _____.

9. _____ is using the body in an efficient and careful way.

10. The back-lying or dorsal recumbent position is also called the _____.

11. _____ or body alignment is the way in which body parts are aligned with one another.

12. _____ is the science of designing the job to fit the worker.

13. Another name for the Sims' position is _____.

Circle the BEST Answer

14. Using good body mechanics will
    A. Prevent good posture
    B. Cause back injuries
    C. Reduce the risk of injury
    D. Cause muscle injury

15. For a wider base of support
    A. Keep your feet close together
    B. The head, trunk, arms, and legs are aligned with one another
    C. Stand with your feet apart
    D. Make sure you are in good physical condition

16. When you bend your knees and squat to lift a heavy object, you are
    A. Using good body alignment
    B. In danger of injury
    C. Likely to strain your back
    D. Using good body mechanics

17. If you need to move a heavy object
    A. Push, slide, or pull the object
    B. Get help from a co-worker
    C. Bend your hips and knees to lift from the floor
    D. All of the above

18. Work-related musculoskeletal disorders (WMSDs) are a risk
    A. When the worker does not exercise regularly
    B. When the worker is small and weak
    C. When force or repeating action is used when moving persons
    D. Only when the staff member is using poor body mechanics

19. If you have pain when standing or rising from a seated position. you
    A. May have a back injury
    B. Are using poor body mechanics
    C. Have worked too many hours
    D. Should exercise more

20. According to the Occupational Safety and Health Administration (OSHA), which of these is *not* a factor that can lead to back disorders?
    A. Reaching while lifting
    B. Getting help when lifting or moving heavy objects
    C. Bending while lifting
    D. Lifting with forceful movement

21. Which of these activities will help prevent back injury?
    A. Reach across the bed to give care
    B. Bend at the waist to pick up an object from the floor
    C. Lift an object above your shoulder
    D. Have a co-worker help you move heavy objects

22. Regular position changes and good alignment
    A. Cause pressure ulcers and contractures
    B. Promote comfort and well-being
    C. Interrupt rest and sleep
    D. Decrease circulation

23. A resident who depends on the nursing team for position changes needs to be positioned
    A. At least every 2 hours   C. Every 15 minutes
    B. Once an hour   D. Once a shift

24. Linens need to be clean, dry, and wrinkle-free to help prevent
    A. Pressure ulcers   C. Breathing problems
    B. Contractures   D. Frequent repositioning

25. Persons with heart and respiratory disorders usually can breathe more easily in the
    A. Fowler's position   C. Supine position
    B. Semi-Fowler's position   D. Prone position

26. Most older persons have limited range of motion in their necks and so do not tolerate
    A. Lateral position   C. Fowler's position
    B. Sims' position   D. Prone position

27. When positioning a person in the supine position, the nurse may ask you to place a pillow under the person's lower legs to
    A. Improve the circulation
    B. Assist the person to breathe easier
    C. Lift the heels off of the bed
    D. Prevent swelling of the legs and feet

28. A small pillow is positioned against the person's back in the
    A. Lateral position   C. Supine position
    B. Prone position   D. Semi-Fowler's position

29. Older persons usually are not comfortable in
    A. Lateral position   C. Supine position
    B. Sims' position   D. Chair position

30. In the chair position, a pillow is not used
    A. To position paralyzed arms
    B. To support the feet
    C. Under the upper arm and hand
    D. Behind the back if restraints are used

Fill in the Blanks

31. Where are strong, large muscles located that are used to handle and move heavy objects?
    A. _____
    B. _____
    C. _____
    D. _____

32. Back injuries are a major risk when lifting. For good body mechanics, you should:
    A. _____
    B. _____

33. Describe these risk factors for musculoskeletal disorders (WMSDs) in nursing centers:
    A. Force _____
    B. Repeating action _____
    C. Awkward postures _____

34. Early signs and symptoms of WMSDs are _____
    _____.

35. What nursing tasks are known to be high risk for WMSDs?
    A. _____
    B. _____
    C. _____
    D. _____
    E. _____
    F. _____
    G. _____
    H. _____
    I. _____
    J. _____

36. Instructions to reposition a person are received from the _____ and the _____.

37. If you are delegated the task of positioning the person, what information do you need?
    A. _____
    B. _____
    C. _____
    D. _____
    E. _____
    F. _____
    G. _____
    H. _____
    I. _____
    J. _____
    K. _____

38. What measures are needed for good alignment when the person is in Fowler's position?
    A. _____
    B. _____
    C. _____

39. In supine position?
    A. _____
    B. _____
    C. _____

40. In prone position?
    A. _____
    B. _____
    C. _____

41. In lateral position?
    A. _____
    B. _____
    C. _____
    D. _____
    E. _____
    F. _____

42. In Sims' position?
    A. _____
    B. _____
    C. _____
    D. _____

43. In chair position?
    A. _____
    B. _____
    C. _____

Labeling
44. Label the positions in each of the drawings.

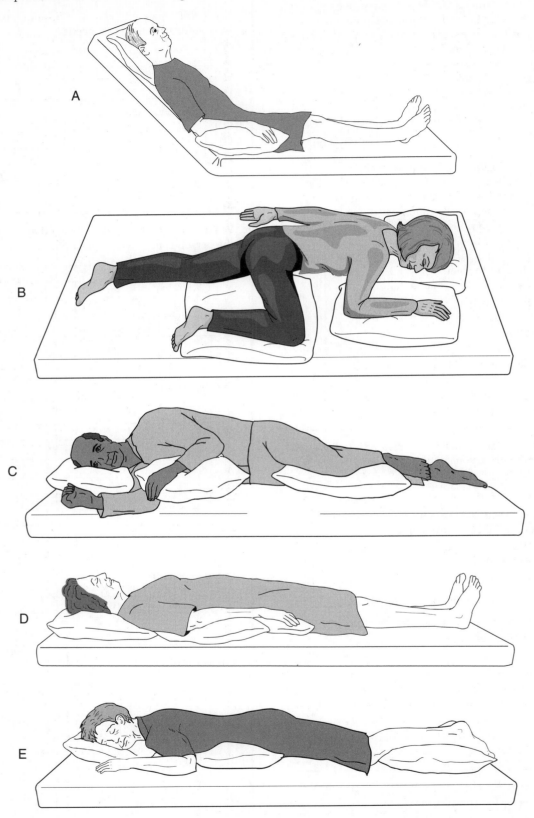

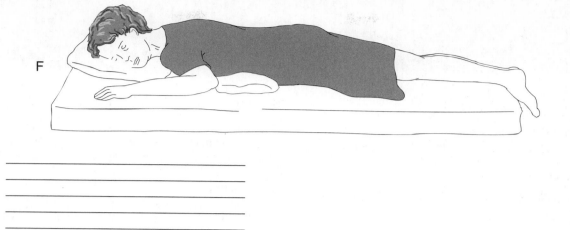

F

A. _____

B. _____

C. _____

D. _____

E. _____

F. _____

Nursing Assistant Skills Video Exercise
View the **Body Mechanics and Exercise** *video to answer these questions.*

45. How you perform your tasks as a nursing assistant affects:

    A. _____

    B. _____

46. The principles of body mechanics involve:

    A. _____

    B. _____

    C. _____

Optional Learning Exercises

47. According to OSHA, certain factors can lead to back injuries. Read the examples and list the factor that could cause a back injury in each one. *(listed in textbook)*

    A. The nursing assistant does not raise the level of the bed when changing linens.

    _____

    B. While you are walking with Mr. Smith, he slips and starts to fall.

    _____

    C. Mrs. Tippett slides down in bed and looks uncomfortable. _____

    _____

D. You assist Mrs. Miller to use the toilet in her small bathroom.

   _____

E. Water is spilled on the hallway floor. _____

   _____

F. You lean across the bed to hold the person in position while the nurse changes a dressing. _____

   _____

48. Regular position changes and good alignment promote:

    A. _____

    B. _____

    C. _____

    D. _____

    It prevents:

    E. _____

    F. _____

49. _____, _____, and _____ help prevent contractures.

Independent Learning Activities
After learning about using good body mechanics in this chapter, think about how well you practice body mechanics in your daily life and answer these questions:

- How much do the books you carry with you each day weigh? How do you carry them? When carrying them, where is your base of support? Is your body in good alignment?
- Do you have small children that you pick up? How do you lift them? What methods listed in the chapter do you use?
- When carrying groceries into the house, do you carry them held close to the body? How well are you using good body mechanics?
- At the end of the day, how do you feel? How could using good body mechanics help you avoid any discomfort?

15 Safe Resident Handling, Moving, and Transfers

Key Terms
Friction   Logrolling   Shearing   Transfer

Fill in the Blanks: Key Terms
1. _____occurs when skin sticks to a surface and muscles slide in the direction the body is moving.

2. Moving a person from one place to another is a _____.

3. The rubbing of one surface against another is _____.

4. Turning the person as a unit, in alignment, with one motion is _____.

Circle the BEST Answer
5. To prevent injuries when moving older persons
   A. Move the person without help
   B. Grab the person under the arms
   C. Allow the person to move himself or herself
   D. Move the person carefully to prevent injury or pain

6. When moving a person up in bed, prevent hitting the headboard with the head by
   A. Keeping the person in good body alignment
   B. Placing the pillow upright against the headboard
   C. Placing your hand on the person's head
   D. Asking the person to bend his or her neck forward

7. When moving residents, it is best if you move the person
   A. By yourself
   B. With at least 2 or 3 staff members
   C. Using a mechanical lift
   D. Only with staff members that you like

8. To prevent work-related injuries, OSHA recommends that
   A. Manual lifting be minimized or eliminated when possible
   B. Manual lifting be used at all times
   C. Any person or object is never lifted alone
   D. Mechanical lifts are always used for any lifting

9. Which of these would *not* be correct when you are using manual lifting?
   A. Try to keep what you are moving close to you
   B. Stand with your feet close together
   C. Lift on the "count of 3" when working with others
   D. Move the person toward you, not away from you

10. To make lateral transfers safe for the staff members
    A. Make sure bed rails are up
    B. Never use drawsheets, turning pads, or other devices to assist in the move
    C. Adjust surfaces so they are at about waist height
    D. Reach across the bed or stretcher to transfer the person

11. When the person can bear some weight, can sit up with help, and may be able to pivot to transfer, you know that the person's level of dependence is
    A. Code 4   C. Code 2
    B. Code 3   D. Code 1

12. Why are beds raised to move persons in bed?
    A. It prevents the person from falling out of bed
    B. It reduces friction and shearing
    C. It prevents pulling on drainage tubes
    D. It reduces bending and reaching for the staff

13. How can you reduce friction and shearing?
    A. Raise the head of the bed to a sitting position before moving the person
    B. Roll or lift the person to reposition
    C. Pull the person up in bed by grasping under the arms
    D. Massage the skin

14. If a person with dementia resists being moved, you should
    A. Move the person by yourself
    B. Proceed slowly and use a calm, pleasant voice
    C. Let the person alone and do not reposition him
    D. Tell the person firmly that he must cooperate to be moved

15. When you are delegated to move a person in bed, you need to know all of these *except*
    A. What equipment is needed
    B. Whether the person is awake
    C. How many workers are needed to safely move the person
    D. Any limits in the person's ability to move or be repositioned

16. When raising a person's head and shoulders
    A. It is best to have help with an older person to prevent pain and injury
    B. A mechanical lift should be used
    C. You can always do this alone
    D. A transfer belt will be needed

17. To correctly raise the head and shoulders
    A. Both of your hands are placed under the person's back
    B. The person puts his near arm under your near arm and behind your shoulder
    C. Use a lift sheet to raise the person up
    D. Your free arm rests on the edge of the bed

18. You may move a person up in bed alone if the
    A. Person can push against the mattress with his or her feet
    B. Rest of the staff is busy and cannot help
    C. Nurse tells you to use a lift sheet or slide sheet
    D. Nurse says you have to move the person alone

68

19. What is the position of the bed when you are moving a person up in bed?
    A. Fowler's
    B. Flat
    C. As flat as possible for the person's condition
    D. Semi-Fowler's
20. The person is moved
    A. On the "count of 3"
    B. On the "count of 2"
    C. When the person says he is ready
    D. As soon as the workers are all in position
21. An assist device such as a lift sheet is used for
    A. A person who weighs less than 200 pounds
    B. A person who weighs more than 200 pounds
    C. A person with a dependence level of Code 4: Total Dependence
    D. All of the above
22. Where is the lift sheet positioned?
    A. Under the head and shoulders
    B. Under the buttocks
    C. From the head to above the knees or lower
    D. From the hips to below the knees
23. When using a lift sheet as an assist device, the workers should
    A. Roll the sheet up close to the person
    B. Grasp the sheet at the edges
    C. Move one side of the sheet at a time
    D. Grasp the sheet only at the top edge
24. A person is moved to the side of the bed before turning because
    A. Otherwise, after turning, the person lies on the side of the bed
    B. It makes it easier to turn the person
    C. It prevents injury to the person
    D. It prevents friction and shearing
25. When you move a person in segments, which of these is *incorrect*?
    A. First place your arms under the person's neck and shoulders and grasp the far shoulder
    B. First move the hips and legs
    C. Move the center part of the body by placing one arm under the waist and one under the thighs
    D. Rock backward and shift your weight to your rear leg when moving the upper part of the body
26. When using a drawsheet to move a person to the side of the bed, support the
    A. Back   C. Head
    B. Knees   D. Hips
27. After the person is turned
    A. Give the person good personal care
    B. Position him or her in good body alignment
    C. Elevate the head of the bed
    D. Elevate the bed to its highest position
28. When delegated to turn a person, you need all of this information from the nurse and care plan *except*
    A. How much help the person needs
    B. Which procedure to use
    C. Whether the doctor has ordered turning
    D. What supportive devices are needed for positioning

29. When you have completed turning a person in bed, he or she should
    A. Have the back against the bed rail
    B. Have his or her face near the bed rail
    C. Be positioned in good body alignment near the middle of the bed
    D. Lie flat on the mattress without any supportive pillows
30. When a person is turned, musculoskeletal injuries, skin breakdown, and pressure ulcers could occur if a person is not in
    A. A special bed   C. Good body mechanics
    B. Good body alignment D. The middle of the bed
31. How do you decide whether to turn the person toward you or away from you?
    A. Check the doctor's order
    B. It depends on the person's condition and the situation
    C. Use the method you like best
    D. Ask the person which way is best
32. Why do you need 2 or 3 staff members to logroll a person?
    A. A person who is being logrolled is usually in pain
    B. It is important to keep the spine straight and in alignment
    C. The person is probably a Code 4 level of dependence and needs extra help
    D. No assistive devices are used when you logroll
33. When preparing to logroll a person, place a pillow
    A. At the head of the bed   C. Under the head
    B. Between the knees   D. Under the shoulders
34. What information do you need before dangling a person?
    A. The person's diagnosis
    B. When the person ate last
    C. The person's dependence level
    D. Whether the person likes to dangle
35. What should you do if a person who is dangling becomes faint or dizzy?
    A. Lay the person down
    B. Go and report this to the nurse
    C. Tell the person to take deep breaths
    D. Have the person move his or her legs back and forth in circles
36. When preparing to dangle a person, the head of the bed should be
    A. Flat
    B. Slightly raised
    C. In a sitting position
    D. At a comfortable height for the person
37. When preparing to transfer a person, you should
    A. Arrange the room so there is enough space for a safe transfer
    B. Keep furniture in the position the resident likes
    C. Remove all furniture from the room
    D. Ask the person how to arrange the furniture

38. The person being transferred should wear non-skid footwear to
    A. Protect the person from falls
    B. Allow the person to bend the feet more easily
    C. Promote comfort for the person
    D. Keep the feet warm
39. Lock the bed, wheelchair, or assist device wheels when transferring to
    A. Help the staff use good body mechanics
    B. Prevent damage to the equipment being used
    C. Prevent the bed and the device from moving during the transfer
    D. Make sure the person is kept in good body alignment
40. When a person is transferring from a chair or wheelchair, help the person of out of bed on
    A. The right side of the bed
    B. His or her strong side
    C. His or her weak side
    D. The side of the bed that is most convenient for the staff
41. Which of these is the preferred method for chair or wheelchair transfers?
    A. Use a gait/transfer belt
    B. Have the person put his or her arms around your neck
    C. Put your arms around the person and the grasp the shoulder blades
    D. Use a mechanical lift
42. When a person is seated in a wheelchair, you can increase the person's comfort by
    A. Placing pillows around the person
    B. Making sure nothing covers the vinyl seat and back
    C. Covering the back and seat with a folded bath blanket
    D. Removing any cushions or positioning devices
43. When you transfer a person, the nurse may ask you to take and report the _____ before and after the transfer.
    A. Blood pressure   C. Respirations
    B. Pulse rate   D. Temperature
44. When using a transfer belt, you can prevent the person from sliding or falling by
    A. Bracing your knees against the person's knees
    B. Using the knee and foot of one leg to block the person's weak leg or foot
    C. Straddling your legs around the person's weak leg
    D. All of the above
45. A transfer belt must be used for a transfer unless
    A. The doctor has written an order that states no belt is needed
    B. You are directed by the nurse and care plan to transfer without a belt
    C. The person asks you not to use the belt
    D. You feel safer moving the person without the belt
46. When you are transferring a person back to bed from a chair or wheelchair, the person should be positioned
    A. With the weak side near the bed
    B. With the strong side near the bed
    C. With the chair in the same position as it was when the person got out of bed
    D. Where you have the most space to work

47. A mechanical sling is used
    A. For all persons regardless of the level of dependence
    B. For persons who are too heavy for the staff to transfer
    C. When staff members prefer to use them instead of manually lifting
    D. Only when ordered by the doctor
48. When you are delegated to use a mechanical lift, you need to know
    A. The person's dependency level
    B. What sling to use
    C. How many staff members are needed to perform the task safely
    D. All of the above
49. As a person is lifted in the sling of the mechanical lift, the person
    A. May hold the swivel bar
    B. May hold the straps or chains
    C. Must keep the arms folded across the chest
    D. Should keep the legs outstretched
50. When transferring a person from a wheelchair to the toilet
    A. The toilet should have a raised seat
    B. The toilet seat should be removed
    C. Always position the wheelchair next to the toilet
    D. Unlock the wheelchair to allow movement during the transfer
51. A slide board may be used to transfer a person from a wheel chair to a toilet if
    A. The person can stand and pivot
    B. There is enough room to position the wheelchair next to the toilet
    C. The staff member does not want to use a transfer belt
    D. The person has lower body strength
52. When moving a person who weighs more than 200 pounds to a stretcher, OSHA recommends
    A. Use a lateral sliding aid and 2 staff members
    B. Use a lateral sliding aid and 3 staff members
    C. Use a lateral sliding aid or a friction-reducing device and 2 staff members
    D. Use a drawsheet, a turning pad, or a large incontinence underpad
53. During transport on the stretcher, the person is moved feet first so
    A. The staff member at the foot can clear the pathway
    B. The staff member at the head can watch the person's breathing and color
    C. The person can see where he or she is going
    D. The person does not become disoriented
54. It is important to reposition a person sitting in a chair or wheelchair
    A. For good alignment and safety
    B. To make sure the back and buttocks are against the back of the chair
    C. Because some persons cannot move and reposition themselves
    D. All of the above

Fill in the Blanks

55. To prevent injuries in older persons with fragile bones and joints, what safety measures need to be used?
   A. _____
   B. _____
   C. _____
   D. _____
   E. _____

56. To promote mental comfort when handling, moving, or transferring the person, you should:
   A. _____
   B. _____

57. To promote physical comfort when handling, moving, or transferring the person, you should:
   A. _____
   B. _____
   C. _____
   D. _____

58. When manual lifting, you use good body mechanics when you:
   A. _____
   B. _____
   C. _____
   D. _____
   E. _____

59. To prevent work-related injuries when handling, moving, and transfers, the nurse and health team determine:
   A. _____
   B. _____
   C. _____
   D. _____

60. Explain how a person is lifted and transferred for each level of dependence:
   A. Code 4: Total Dependence _____
   _____
   B. Code 3: Extensive Assistance _____
   _____
   C. Code 2: Limited Assistance _____
   _____
   D. Code 1: Supervision _____
   _____
   E. Code 0: Independent _____
   _____

61. When you move a person in bed, report and record:
   A. _____
   B. _____
   C. _____
   D. _____
   E. _____

62. Friction and shearing can be reduced when moving a person in bed by:
   A. _____
   B. _____
   C. _____

63. You can sometimes move a person up in bed alone if the person can use a _____.

64. When moving a person up in bed and the person can assist, ask the person to:
   A. Flex _____
   B. Grasp the _____
   C. Move on the count of _____

65. An assist device is used to move persons:
   A. With a dependence level of _____
   B. With a dependence level of _____
   C. Who are recovering from _____

66. What assist devices, other than mechanical lifts, are used to move persons to the side of the bed?
   _____

67. Why are assist devices used when moving a person to the side of the bed?
   A. Prevent _____ and _____ damage
   B. Prevent injury to the _____

68. Before turning and repositioning a person, what information do you need from the nurse and care plan?
   A. _____
   B. _____
   C. _____
   D. _____
   E. _____
   F. _____
   G. _____
   H. _____
   I. _____
      i. _____
      ii. _____
      iii. _____
      iv. _____
      v. _____

69. After turning and repositioning a person, it is common to place a small pillow under the _____
   _____.

70. When a person is logrolled, the spine is _____.

71. Logrolling is used to turn these persons:
   A. _____
   B. _____
   C. _____
   D. _____

72. When a person is dangling, the circulation can be stimulated by having the person move _____
   _____.

73. What observations should be reported and recorded after dangling a person?
    A. _____
    B. _____
    C. _____
    D. _____
    E. _____
    F. _____
    G. _____

74. While a person is dangling, check the person's condition by:
    A. Asking _____
    B. Checking _____
    C. Checking _____
    D. Noting _____

75. A person can transfer from the bed to the chair with a stand-and-pivot transfer if the:
    A. _____
    B. _____
    C. _____

76. During a chair or wheelchair transfer, the person must not put his or her arms around your neck because _____.

77. Locked wheelchairs may be considered to be restraints if the person _____.

78. When using a transfer belt to transfer a person to a chair or wheelchair, grasp the belt at _____ and from _____.

79. If you transfer a person to a chair without a transfer belt, place your hands _____ and around the person's _____.

80. For what reasons would you use the slings listed?
    A. Standard full sling _____
    B. Extended length sling _____
    C. Bathing sling _____
    D. Amputee sling _____

81. What information do you need when you are delegated to use a mechanical lift?
    A. _____
    B. _____
    C. _____
    D. _____
    E. _____

82. To promote mental comfort when using a mechanical lift, you should explain _____ and show the person _____.

83. A slide board can be used when transferring a person to and from a toilet if:
    A. _____
    B. _____
    C. _____
    D. _____

84. If a person weighs more than 200 pounds and is being moved to a stretcher, OSHA recommends the use of one of the following:
    A. _____
    B. _____
    C. _____

Nursing Assistant Skills Video Exercises
View the Body Mechanics and Exercise video to answer these questions.

85. When you are delegated lifting, moving, positioning, and transfer activities, you need to:
    A. _____
    B. _____
    C. _____
    D. _____
    E. _____
    F. _____
    G. _____

86. You are preparing to transfer Mr. Anderson. How will you know how much help he needs?
    _____

87. When transferring a person from the bed to the wheelchair, where is the wheelchair positioned?
    _____

88. The transfer belt was placed just below Mr. Anderson's rib cage with the buckle centered in the front.
    A. True
    B. False

89. Where did the nursing assistant place her hands to transfer Mr. Anderson when not using the transfer belt?
    _____

90. After transferring a person, where should the wheelchair be positioned? _____

Optional Learning Exercises

91. Why is it important to know the person's height and weight, dependence level, physical abilities, and medical condition? _____

92. What decisions need to be made before moving a person that will help prevent work-related injuries?
    A. _____
    B. _____
    C. _____

93. If you need to move a person with dementia, he or she may resist because he or she may not _____. What measures in the care plan will help you give safe care?
    A. _____
    B. _____
    C. _____

94. It is safe to move a person up in bed alone only if:
    A. _____
    B. _____
    C. _____
    D. _____
    E. _____
    F. _____
    G. _____

95. What type of pad is not strong enough to be used during a lift? _____

    _____
    For a safe lift, the underpad must:
    A. _____
    B. _____
    C. _____

96. How does moving a person to the side of the bed avoid work-related injuries for you?

    _____

97. When you are delegated to turn a person, how will you know whether to turn him or her alone, with help, or by using logrolling? _____

98. When you turn a person and reposition him or her, what must be done to the bed level before you leave the room?

    _____

99. When two staff members are logrolling a person without a turning sheet, where does each person place the hands?
    A. Staff at head _____
    B. Staff at legs _____

100. Why should a person dangle for 1 to 5 minutes before walking or transferring?

    _____

101. What simple hygiene measures can be performed while the person is dangling? _____
    In addition to refreshing the person, what is another benefit this activity will provide? _____

102. After you are finished using a mechanical lift, what should do with it that will help teamwork and time management?
    A. _____
    B. _____

103. If a person cannot bear some or all of his or her weight and cannot assist with the transfer, what method would be safe to use in a bed-to-chair transfer? _____

    _____

104. Why should you know the person's weight before using a mechanical lift? _____

    _____

105. What should you do if the mechanical lift available is different from one you have used before?

    _____

106. When you are moving or transferring a person, how can you protect these rights?
    A. Privacy:
       i. _____
       ii. _____
       iii. _____
    B. Personal choice:
       i. _____
       ii. _____
       iii. _____
    C. Freedom from restraint:
       i. _____

Independent Learning Activities
Work with classmates and practice the following activities. Each of you should take a turn as the resident.
- Practice moving a person up in bed with and without assist devices. Answer these questions after you have completed this exercise:
  ○ Which method was easier for the worker? For the person being moved?
  ○ How did you feel when you were being moved? Did anyone explain what was being done?
- Practice transferring a person who is weak on one side to a chair from the bed and then return the person to the bed. Answer these questions after you complete the exercise:
  ○ *As the worker:* How did you position the chair? How did the chair position change when you returned the person to bed?
  ○ *As the person:* How safe did you feel during the transfer? What could the worker have done to help you feel safe? What else could the staff have done to make you more comfortable?
- Practice logrolling a person with and without a turning sheet. Answer these questions after you have completed the exercise:
  ○ *As the worker:* How many workers were used to logroll the person? Which method was easier—with or without the turning sheet? How well do you think the workers did with the turns? Did the spine stay straight?
  ○ *As the person:* How did you feel—did you understand what was being done? Was the turn smooth, or did you feel as if your spine twisted?

- Ask your instructor if you can use a mechanical lift to practice with each other. If the instructor approves this exercise, answer these questions:
  - *As the worker:* What did you do before beginning the lift? What questions did you ask? What other information should you have gathered before starting?
  - *As the person:* How did you feel when you were lifted? Did you feel as if you understood what was happening? What other information would have helped make you more comfortable?
- Overall, how will these practices help you as you move residents? What would do differently, now that you have practiced these exercises?

16 The Resident's Unit

Key Terms

Fowler's position
Full visual privacy
Resident unit
Reverse Trendelenburg's position
Semi-Fowler's position
Trendelenburg's position

Fill in the Blanks: Key Terms

1. The personal space, furniture, and equipment provided for the individual by the nursing center is the

   _____.

2. In _____, the head of the bed is raised 30 degrees; or the head of the bed is raised 30 degrees, and the knee portion is raised 15 degrees.

3. _____ is a semi-sitting position; the head of the bed is raised 45 to 60 degrees.

4. The head of the bed is raised, and the foot of the bed is lowered in _____.

5. In _____, the head the bed is lowered, and the foot of the bed is raised.

6. The person has the means to be completely free from public view while in bed when they have

   _____.

Circle the BEST Answer

7. When residents share a room
   A. You may rearrange items and furniture in the room as needed
   B. Each person has a private area of the room
   C. Residents may use each other's belongings
   D. They generally share furniture such as a dresser

8. OBRA requires that nursing centers maintain a temperature range of
   A. 68° to 74° F
   B. 61° to 71° F
   C. 71° to 81° F
   D. 78° to 85° F

9. Persons who are older and chronically ill
   A. May need cooler room temperatures
   B. May need warmer room temperatures
   C. Are insensitive to room temperature changes
   D. Will need a warmer room at night

10. Which of these factors that affect comfort cannot be controlled by the nursing staff?
    A. Illness
    B. Temperature
    C. Noise
    D. Odors

11. If an older person complains of a draft
    A. Have the person go to bed
    B. Give the person a hot shower
    C. Offer a lap robe or a warm sweater to wear
    D. Pull the privacy curtain around the person

12. If unpleasant odors occur, do all of these except
    A. Use spray deodorizers around all residents
    B. Provide good personal hygiene for residents
    C. Change and dispose of soiled linens and clothing
    D. Empty and clean bedpans, commodes, urinals, and kidney basins promptly

13. Noises in a strange setting, such as a nursing center, may keep a resident from meeting the need for
    A. Love and belonging
    B. Self-esteem
    C. Rest
    D. Safety and security

14. Which of these measures will not reduce noises in a nursing center?
    A. Have drapes in rooms
    B. Use only metal equipment
    C. Answer telephone promptly
    D. Oil wheels on equipment to keep it in good working order

15. Soft, non-glare lighting is helpful for all except
    A. Helping residents relax
    B. Decreasing agitation in residents with dementia
    C. Improving orientation in residents with dementia
    D. Helping residents rest

16. Cranks on manual beds are kept down when not in use to
    A. Prevent residents from operating the bed
    B. Prevent anyone walking past the crank from bumping into it
    C. Keep the bed in the correct position
    D. Make sure they are ready to use at all times

17. How can the staff prevent a person from adjusting an electric bed to unsafe positions?
    A. Lock the bed into a position
    B. Unplug the bed
    C. Put the person in a bed that cannot be repositioned
    D. Keep reminding the person not to change the position

18. What bed position may adjust the head of the bed and the knee portion to prevent sliding down in bed?
    A. Fowler's
    B. Semi-Fowler's
    C. Trendelenburg's
    D. Reverse Trendelenburg's

19. If a person becomes trapped in the hospital bed system, you should
    A. Immediately go for help
    B. Call 911
    C. Try to release the person
    D. Lower the bed rails

20. What items should not be placed on the overbed table?
    A. Meals
    B. Personal care items
    C. Writing and reading materials
    D. Bedpans, urinals, and soiled linens

21. Where are the bedpan and urinal kept in the bedside table?
    A. Wherever the person wants
    B. The top shelf or drawer
    C. The bottom shelf or drawer
    D. The middle shelf or drawer

22. OBRA requires that the resident unit always has
    A. Two chairs
    B. A straight-back chair
    C. A reclining chair
    D. At least one chair for personal and visitor use
23. Privacy curtains
    A. Are sometimes used in rooms with more than one bed
    B. Are always pulled completely around the bed when care is given
    C. Can block sounds and conversations
    D. May be open when giving personal care
24. Personal care items
    A. Are usually supplied by the nursing center
    B. Must be provided by the resident
    C. Must be ordered by the doctor
    D. Are required by OBRA
25. When the resident is weak on the left side, the signal light
    A. Is placed on the left side
    B. Is removed from the room
    C. Is placed on the right side
    D. Is replaced by an intercom
26. If a confused person cannot use a signal light
    A. Explain often how to use the signal light
    B. Use an intercom instead
    C. Remove the signal light
    D. Check the person often
27. Elevated toilet seats
    A. Help residents with joints problems
    B. Make wheelchair transfers more difficult
    C. Are required by OBRA
    D. Are used on all toilets in a nursing center
28. When a person uses a bathroom signal light
    A. It flashes above the room door and at the nurses' station
    B. It makes the same sound as the room signal light
    C. It activates the intercom
    D. The signal sounds and flashes only above the bathroom door
29. Closet and drawer space
    A. Is shared by persons in a room with more than one person
    B. Can be opened and searched by a staff member at any time
    C. Cannot be searched without the resident's permission
    D. Is not required in a nursing center
30. What equipment may be in rehabilitation and subacute rooms that usually is not found in long-term care centers?
    A. Televisions
    B. Commode chairs
    C. Blood pressure equipment or wall outlets for oxygen and suctioning
    D. Electric beds

31. Residents can bring some furniture and personal items to use in the room as long as the choices
    A. Do not interfere with the rights of others
    B. Match the color and decoration in the room
    C. Can be cared for by the resident or the family
    D. Do not need to be attached to the wall

Labeling

32. In this figure:

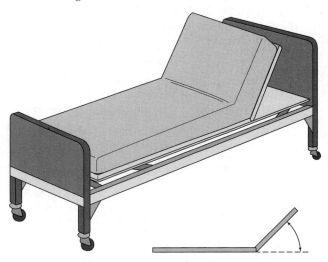

    A. What is the bed position called? _____
    B. What is the angle of the head of the bed? _____
    C. Why is this position used? _____

33. In this figure:

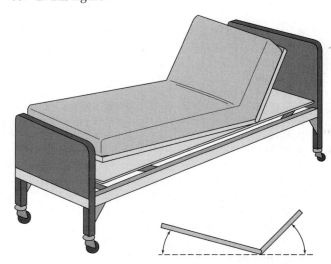

    A. What is the bed position called? _____
    B. What is the angle of the head of the bed? _____
    C. The angle of the knee portion? _____
    D. Raising the knee portion can _____

34. In this figure:

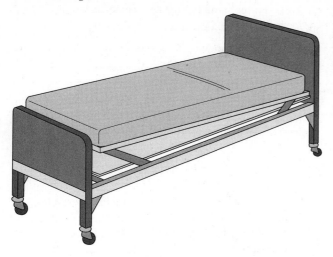

    A. What is the bed position called? _____
    B. What is the position of the head of the bed and the foot of the bed? _____
    C. This position requires a _____

35. In this figure:

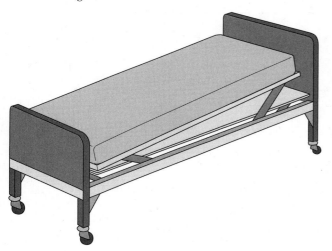

    A. What is the bed position called? _____
    B. What is the position of the head of the bed and the foot of the bed? _____
    C. This position requires a _____

Optional Learning Exercises

36. What are three factors that affect comfort that usually cannot be controlled?
    A. _____
    B. _____
    C. _____

37. What factors that affect comfort can be controlled?
    A. _____
    B. _____
    C. _____
    D. _____.

38. In these situations, how would help protect a resident from drafts?
    A. The person is dressing for the day. _____
    _____

    B. The person is sitting in a wheelchair. _____
    _____

    C. You are assisting a resident who is going to bed for the night._____
    _____

    D. You are giving personal care to the resident. ____
    _____

39. How can you help eliminate odors in these situations?
    A. You are caring for a person who is frequently incontinent. _____
    _____

    B. The person is vomiting and has wound drainage.
    _____

    C. The person uses the bathroom by herself. _____
    _____

    D. The person keeps a urinal at his bedside and uses it himself during the day. _____

40. When the staff talks loudly and laughs in hallways, some persons may think that _____
    _____.

41. Why do persons with dementia react more to loud noises at night?_____
    _____

42. How can the staff reduce noises and increase resident comfort?
    A. Control_____
    B. Handle _____
    C. Keep _____
    D. Answer _____

43. What are 2 situations when bright lights are helpful for a resident with poor vision? _____ and
    _____

44. In dementia units, how does adjusting lighting help the residents?
    A. Soft, non-glare _____
    B. Brighter _____

45. The bed in the flat position is used for:
    A. _____
    B. _____

46. Fowler's position is used for persons with _____
    _____.

47. Semi-Fowler's has 2 definitions. They are:
    A. _____
    B. _____

48. How do you know which of the ways in #47 to position the bed when semi-Fowler's position is ordered?
    _____

49. To raise the foot of the bed with Trendelenburg's position, you may put _____.

50. Describe the entrapment zones that can occur in a hospital bed system:
   A. Zone 1 _____
   B. Zone 2 _____
   C. Zone 3 _____
   D. Zone 4 _____
   E. Zone 5 _____
   F. Zone 6 _____
   G. Zone 7 _____

51. When the nursing team uses the overbed table as a work area, what are the only items that can be placed on it? _____

52. What are your responsibilities in these situations regarding the signal light?
   A. The resident is sitting in a chair next to the bed.
   _____

   B. The person is weak on the right side. _____

   C. The person calls out instead of using the signal light. _____

D. The resident is embarrassed because she soiled the bed after signaling for assistance. _____

E. The emergency light in a room rings while you are busy in another room. _____

53. The resident is allowed to bring personal items to make his space as home-like as possible. The health team must make sure the resident's choices:
   A. _____
   B. _____
   C. _____

54. List the OBRA requirement that relates to each of these items in the resident unit:
   A. Number of residents in a room _____
   B. Windows _____
   C. Closets _____
   D. Call system _____
   E. Odors, noise, lighting _____
   F. Handrails, bedrails _____

Independent Learning Activities

When you are in the health care center as a student, find an empty resident room and practice using the equipment. Answer these questions about the equipment.
- Where are the controls for the bed?
  - How do you operate the head of the bed?
  - How do you operate the knee control of the bed?
  - How do you adjust the height of the bed?
- Where is the signal light located?
- Where are controls for the television and radio?
- Does the center have an intercom system? How is it used?

Ask the staff these questions about the signal lights.
- How does the staff know when a resident turns on the signal light?
- When a resident uses a bathroom signal light, how does the staff know the difference?

Think about what temperature is comfortable for you and answer these questions. This exercise will help you understand the importance of individual preferences for residents in the health care center.
- What is the usual temperature of your home?
- Who decides what the temperature will be in your home? Partner, spouse, roommate, children?
- Would the temperature you prefer be comfortable for an infant? An older person? Why or why not?

Think about the noises in your home and how they affect you. This exercise will help you understand why noise levels in the nursing center can affect the residents.
- When you study, do you turn on the TV or radio? Listen to music? Prefer complete silence?
- What noises do you like when going to sleep? TV? Radio? Soft music?
- Does everyone in your household agree on how loud or soft to play a radio or TV? How are conflicts about noise levels resolved?
- If noisy surroundings are unacceptable to you, how do you react? How does it affect your ability to think? To rest? To study? How does it affect your relationship with others?

17 Bedmaking

Key Terms

Cotton drawsheet　　　　Drawsheet　　　　Plastic drawsheet

Fill in the Blanks: Key Terms

1. A waterproof drawsheet made of plastic placed between the bottom sheet and the cotton drawsheet to protect the mattress and bottom linens from dampness and soiling is the _____.

2. A _____ is a small sheet placed over the middle of the bottom sheet.

3. A drawsheet made of cotton that helps keep the mattress and bottom linens clean and dry is a _____ _____.

Circle the BEST Answer

4. In nursing centers, bed linens are changed
   A. Only when the linens are wet or soiled
   B. Every day after baths
   C. On the person's bath or shower day
   D. Once a week on a scheduled day

5. Follow Standard Precautions and the Bloodborne Pathogen Standard when you
   A. Handle any bed linens
   B. Make the bed every morning
   C. May have contact with wet, soiled, or damp linens soiled with the person's blood, body fluids, secretions, or excretions
   D. Place clean linens on the bed

6. All of these statements about a closed bed are true *except*
   A. A closed bed is made after a person is discharged
   B. The top linens are fan-folded back to make it easier for the person to get into bed with ease
   C. Closed beds are made for persons who are out of bed most of the day
   D. If a bedspread is used, it covers the pillow and is tucked under the pillow

7. When making a bed, you use good body mechanics when you
   A. Bend from the waist when removing and replacing the linens
   B. Stretch across the bed to smooth the linens
   C. Raise the bed to a comfortable height
   D. Lock the wheels

8. If extra clean linens are brought to a person's room, you should
   A. Return the unused linens to the linen room
   B. Store the extra linens in the person's closet
   C. Put the unused linens in the dirty laundry
   D. Use the linens for a person in the next room

9. An open bed is
   A. Made with the person in it
   B. In use. The top linens are folded back so that the person can get into bed
   C. Not in use until bedtime. The top linens are not folded back
   D. Made to transfer a person from a stretcher to the bed

10. When handling linens and making beds, all of these actions follow the rules of medical asepsis *except*
    A. Put the dirty linens on the floor
    B. Hold the linens away from your body and uniform
    C. Never shake linens in the air
    D. Place clean linens on a clean surface

11. Which of these linens will be collected first?
    A. Bath towel　　　　C. Mattress pad
    B. Bath blanket　　　 D. Top sheet

12. When you remove dirty linens, which of these actions is *incorrect*?
    A. Gather all the linens in one large roll
    B. Roll each piece away from you
    C. Top and bottom sheets, drawsheets, and pillowcases are always changed
    D. The blanket and bedspread may be reused for the same person

13. A plastic drawsheet can
    A. Cause discomfort and skin breakdown
    B. Be hard to keep tight and wrinkle-free
    C. Keep the mattress and bottom linens clean and dry
    D. All of the above

14. When you are delegated to make a bed, why do you need to know the person's schedule for treatments, therapies, and activities?
    A. You need to make sure the bed is flat
    B. It is best to change linens after the treatment or when the person is out of the room
    C. You need to unlock beds that have been locked in a certain position
    D. You will know what type of bed to make

15. When assigned to make a bed, which of these is *not* information you need from the nurse or care plan?
    A. What type of bed to make
    B. If the person uses bed rails
    C. When the bed was changed last
    D. How to position the person and positioning devices needed

16. When a person is discharged from a hospital or nursing center, what is done in addition to changing the bed?
    A. New pillows are placed on the bed
    B. The bed frame and mattress are cleaned and disinfected
    C. The bed is sterilized
    D. The bedspread and blanket may be reused

17. When making a bed, position the bottom sheet with
    A. The lower edge even with the top of the mattress
    B. The hem-stitching facing downward
    C. The large hem at the bottom and the small hem at the top
    D. The center crease across the bed
18. When the top sheet, blanket, and bedspread are in place on the bed
    A. Each one is tucked under the mattress separately
    B. The sheet and blanket are tucked together and the bedspread is allowed to hang loose over them
    C. All three are tucked together under the foot of the bed and the corners are mitered
    D. All three are allowed to hang loose over the foot of the bed
19. The pillow is placed on the bed
    A. So the open end of the pillowcase is away from the door
    B. The seam of the pillowcase is toward the foot of the bed
    C. Leaning against the head of the bed
    D. So the open end of the pillowcase is toward the door
20. If you are making an occupied bed for a person who is comatose, it is important to
    A. Keep the bed in the low position
    B. Unlock the wheels
    C. Use special linens
    D. Explain each step of the procedure to the person before it is done
21. A bath blanket is used when making an occupied bed to
    A. Protect the person from injury
    B. Provide warmth and privacy for the person
    C. Protect the bed linens
    D. Protect the person from dirty linens
22. To provide safety when making an occupied bed for a person who does not use bed rails, you should
    A. Have a co-worker work on the opposite side of the bed
    B. Push the bed against the wall
    C. Always keep one hand on the person while you are making the bed
    D. Only change linens when the person is out of the bed for tests or therapies
23. When making an occupied bed, how is privacy provided?
    A. Close the door
    B. Cover the person with a bath blanket when linens are removed
    C. Pull the curtain around the bed in a semi-private room
    D. All of the above
24. Which of these steps is *not* done when making a surgical bed?
    A. Tuck all top linens under the mattress together and make a mitered corner
    B. Remove all linens from the bed
    C. Put the mattress pad on the mattress
    D. Place the bottom sheet with the lower edge even with the bottom of the mattress

25. You allow the person the right of personal choice when you
    A. Allow the person to use bed linens from home
    B. Decide which linens will look best in the room
    C. Tell the person you will make the bed at 9 AM
    D. Choose the pillows and blanket the person needs for comfort

Fill in the Blanks
26. Number this list from 1-13 in the order you would collect the linens to make a bed.
    _____ Pillowcase(s)
    _____ Top sheet
    _____ Gown or pajamas
    _____ Bottom sheet (flat or fitted)
    _____ Mattress pad
    _____ Bedspread
    _____ Plastic drawsheet
    _____ Bath blanket
    _____ Hand towel
    _____ Cotton drawsheet
    _____ Bath towel(s)
    _____ Blanket
    _____ Washcloth

Nursing Assistant Skills Video Exercise
View the **Bedmaking** *video to answer these questions.*
27. Linens are always changed when _____.
28. Follow these procedure guidelines when making a bed:
    A. _____
    B. _____
    C. _____
    D. _____
29. Wash your hands _____ handling clean linens and _____ handling dirty linens.
30. Your uniform is considered _____. Linens must be held _____
31. You must never place clean or soiled linens _____ _____.
32. Never shake linens because _____.
33. How should you fold the bedspread and blanket if they will be reused?
34. Which piece of linen is used to cover the person before the top sheet is removed?
35. When fan-folding used bottom linens, you need to keep the side that touched the person
36. Before putting on clean linens, you need to

37. Place the clean bottom sheet on the bed with the hem-stitching _____
_____.

38. The cotton drawsheet must cover the entire plastic drawsheet.
   A. True
   B. False

39. Top linens must be loose enough to allow _____
_____.

40. All top linens are tucked under the mattress together.
   A. True
   B. False

41. After making the bed, you need to:
   A. _____
   B. _____
   C. _____
   D. _____
   E. _____
   F. _____
   G. _____

Optional Learning Exercise
42. When is a complete linen change made in a nursing center? _____
_____

43. Clean, dry, and wrinkle-free linens are important to promote _____ and to prevent _____ and
_____.

44. What should you do to keep beds neat and clean?
   A. _____
   B. _____
   C. _____
   D. _____
   E. _____
   F. _____

45. When handling linens, practice medical asepsis. Explain why each of the following actions would be *poor* medical asepsis:
   A. Holding the linens close to your body and uniform. _____
_____
   B. Shaking the linens to straighten them. _____
_____
   C. Placing the dirty linens on the floor. _____
_____

46. Family and visitors may question the quality _____ and the quality_____ if the bed is unmade, messy, or dirty.

Independent Learning Activities
- When you make beds at home this week, practice the methods you learned in this chapter.
  - What linens did you collect? What was the order of the linens?
  - Did you remember to make as much of one side of the bed as possible before moving to the other side?
  - What step could *not* be carried out at home that would have helped you use good body mechanics?
  - Think about the methods you used to change your bed before reading this chapter. How did you change your bedmaking practices now that you studied this chapter?
- Practice with a classmate and take turns as a resident who must have an occupied bed made. Ask these questions about your feelings:
  - In what ways was your privacy protected?
  - Did the caregiver offer you any choices before making your bed? What were these choices?
  - Did you feel safe at all times? If not, what made you feel unsafe?
  - What was uncomfortable during the bed change?
  - How were you positioned after the bed was made?
- It is sometimes difficult for a new nursing assistant to remember the order in which to collect linens. If you have difficulty with this, make a list in a pocket notebook or on a 3 × 5 index card so you can carry it with you when you are working.

18 Hygiene

Key Terms

AM care
Aspiration
Denture

Early morning care
Evening care
Morning care

Oral hygiene
Pericare
Perineal care

Plaque
PM care
Tartar

Fill in the Blanks: Key Terms

1. Another name for PM care is _____.

2. _____ is cleansing the genital and anal areas; pericare.

3. Sometimes evening care is called _____ _____.

4. Routine care performed before breakfast or early morning care is called _____.

5. _____ is mouth care or measures that keep the mouth and teeth clean.

6. Hardened plaque on teeth is _____.

7. _____ occurs when breathing fluid or an object into the lungs.

8. Care given after breakfast when cleanliness and skin care are more thorough is called _____.

9. Another name for perineal care is _____.

10. _____ is a thin film that sticks to the teeth. It contains saliva, microorganisms, and other substances.

11. Another name for AM care is _____.

12. An artificial tooth or a set of artificial teeth is a _____.

Circle the BEST Answer

13. If a person needs help with personal hygiene, you can find out what needs they have by
    A. Following the nurse's directions and the care plan
    B. Asking the family
    C. Asking other staff members
    D. Making your own decisions

14. You should assist a person with personal hygiene
    A. Only when the person asks
    B. Only in the morning
    C. Whenever help is needed
    D. Only when it is your assignment

15. When giving personal hygiene, you need to remember to protect the person's right to
    A. Privacy and personal choice
    B. Care and security of personal possessions
    C. Activities
    D. Environment

16. Which of these hygiene measures is *not* done before breakfast?
    A. Assisting with elimination
    B. Straightening resident units, including making beds
    C. Changing wet or soiled linens and garments
    D. Assisting with oral hygiene

17. Which of these is done every time you assist with hygiene measures throughout the day?
    A. Assist with dressing and hair care
    B. Face and hand washing
    C. Assist with activity
    D. Help person change into sleepwear

18. If good oral hygiene is not done regularly, the person may develop tartar, which will lead to
    A. A dry mouth
    B. Periodontal disease
    C. A bad taste in the mouth
    D. Plaque

19. All of these health team members may assess the person's need for mouth care *except* the
    A. Speech/language pathologist
    B. Physical therapist
    C. Nurse
    D. Dietitian

20. Teeth are flossed to
    A. Remove plaque from the teeth
    B. Remove tartar from the teeth
    C. Remove food from between the teeth
    D. All of the above

21. Which of these steps is *incorrect* to do when flossing the teeth?
    A. Start at the lower back tooth on the right side
    B. Hold the floss between the middle fingers
    C. Move the floss gently up and down between the teeth
    D. Move to a new section of floss after every second tooth

22. Sponge swabs are used for
    A. Persons with sore, tender mouths and for unconscious persons
    B. Cleaning dentures
    C. Oral care on children
    D. Oral care on all residents

23. You follow Standard Precautions and the Bloodborne Pathogen Standard when giving oral hygiene because
    A. You will not spread bacteria to the person
    B. It will help you avoid bad breath odors from the person
    C. Gums may bleed during mouth care
    D. You will avoid any loose teeth or rough dentures

24. When the person is able to perform oral hygiene in bed, you arrange the items on
    A. The overbed table   C. The sink counter
    B. The bedside table   D. The bed
25. When you are brushing the person's teeth, which of these steps would be *incorrect*?
    A. Let the person rinse the mouth with water
    B. Only use a sponge swab to clean the teeth
    C. Brush the person's tongue gently, if needed
    D. Floss the person's teeth
26. When providing mouth care for an unconscious person, position the person on one side with the head turned well to the side to
    A. Make it easier to brush the teeth
    B. Make the person more comfortable
    C. Prevent or reduce the risk of aspiration
    D. Make is easier for the person to breathe
27. When giving oral hygiene to an unconscious person who wears dentures, you should
    A. Remove the dentures, clean them, and replace them in the mouth
    B. Dentures are not worn when the person is unconscious
    C. Clean the dentures in the mouth without removing them
    D. Place a padded tongue blade in the mouth to prevent biting
28. Mouth care is given to an unconscious person
    A. After each meal
    B. When AM and PM care are given
    C. At least every 2 hours
    D. Once a day
29. A padded tongue blade is used when giving oral hygiene to an unconscious person to
    A. Keep the mouth open   C. Clean the tongue
    B. Clean the teeth   D. Prevent aspiration
30. When cleaning dentures at a sink, line the sink with a towel to
    A. Prevent infections
    B. Prevent damage to the dentures if they are dropped
    C. Dry the dentures
    D. Clean the dentures
31. If dentures are not worn after cleaning, store them in
    A. Cool water   C. A soft towel
    B. Hot water   D. Soft tissues or a napkin
32. If the person cannot remove the dentures, you can use _____ to get a good grip on the slippery dentures.
    A. Gloves   C. Gauze squares
    B. Washcloth   D. Bare hands
33. Older persons usually need a complete bath or shower twice a week because
    A. They are less active
    B. They are often ill
    C. They have increased perspiration
    D. Dry skin often occurs with aging

34. If a person has dry skin, which of these will help keep it soft?
    A. Soaps
    B. Lotions and oils
    C. Powders
    D. Deodorants and antiperspirants
35. If a person with dementia resists bathing, you should
    A. Hurry through the bath
    B. Speak firmly in a loud voice
    C. Try giving a partial bath or try the bath later
    D. Use restraints so the person will not harm you
36. For skin care products for bathing, you should choose
    A. Soap
    B. Products the person prefers
    C. Bath oils
    D. Creams and lotions
37. The water temperature for a complete bed bath is usually between 110° and 115° F (43.3° to 46.1° C) for adults. For older persons, the temperature
    A. Should be between 110° and 115° F (43.3° to 46.1° C)
    B. May need to be lower
    C. Should be whatever you feel is comfortable
    D. May need to be warmer
38. When applying powder
    A. Shake or sprinkle the powder directly on the person
    B. Sprinkle a small amount of powder onto your hands or a cloth
    C. Apply a thick layer of powder
    D. You should never use powder on any older person
39. A complete bed bath is given to persons who
    A. Cannot bathe themselves
    B. Are unconscious or paralyzed
    C. Are weak from illness or surgery
    D. All of the above
40. When you are giving a complete bed bath, the bed linens are changed
    A. Only if needed
    B. Before the bath begins
    C. After the bath is completed
    D. After the person gets out of bed
41. Using the bedpan, urinal, commode, or bathroom is
    A. Offered before the bath begins
    B. Offered after the bath ends
    C. Not important in giving a bath
    D. Not offered at all during the bath procedure
42. During the bath, the bath blanket is placed
    A. Over the top linens
    B. Under the top linens
    C. Over the person as the top linens are removed
    D. Under the person
43. Do not use soap when washing
    A. The face, ears, and neck
    B. Around the eyes
    C. The abdomen
    D. The perineal area

44. How do you avoid exposing the person when washing the chest?
    A. Keep the bath blanket over the area
    B. Keep the top linens over the chest
    C. Place a bath towel over the chest crosswise
    D. Make sure the curtains are closed

45. Bath water is changed
    A. Every 5 minutes during the bath
    B. Only when it becomes cool and soapy
    C. Before giving perineal care
    D. After washing the face, ears, and neck

46. A person _____ may respond well to a towel bath.
    A. With dementia
    B. Who has been incontinent
    C. With breaks in the skin
    D. Who needs a partial bath

47. A partial bath involves bathing
    A. Areas the person cannot reach
    B. The face, hands, axillae (underarms), back, buttocks, and perineal area
    C. The arms, legs, and feet
    D. The chest, abdomen, and underarms

48. When giving any type of bath, you should
    A. Wash from the dirtiest to cleanest areas
    B. Allow the skin to air dry to avoid rubbing
    C. Provide for privacy
    D. Decide what is best for the person

49. A tub bath should not last longer than
    A. 10 minutes   C. 20 minutes
    B. 15 minutes   D. 30 minutes

50. If a person is weak or unsteady, a _____ should be used when the person showers.
    A. Shower chair   C. Wheelchair
    B. Transfer belt   D. Stretcher

51. Which of these would be good time management when giving a tub bath or shower?
    A. Take the person to the shower room and then collect your equipment
    B. Ask a co-worker to give the shower for you
    C. Ask a co-worker to make the person's bed while you give the bath
    D. Clean and disinfect the tub or shower before returning the person to his or her room

52. When assisting with a tub bath or shower, which of these steps is first?
    A. Help the person undress and remove footwear
    B. Assist or transport the person to the tub or shower room
    C. Put the *Occupied* sign on the door
    D. Place a rubber bathmat in the tub or on the shower floor

53. The best position for a back massage is
    A. Prone position   C. Side-lying position
    B. Supine position   D. Semi-Fowler's position

54. Back massages are dangerous for persons with all of these problems *except*
    A. Certain heart diseases
    B. Lung disorders
    C. Arthritis
    D. Back injuries or surgeries

55. When giving a back massage, the strokes
    A. Start at the shoulders and go down to the buttocks
    B. Should be light and gentle
    C. Start at the buttocks and go up to the shoulders
    D. Are continued for at least 10 minutes

56. When cleaning the perineal area
    A. You do not need to wear gloves
    B. Work from the anal area to the urethra
    C. Work from the urethra to the anal area
    D. Work from the dirtiest area to the cleanest

57. When gathering equipment for perineal care, you will need
    A. One washcloth   C. At least 3 washcloths
    B. Two washcloths   D. At least 4 washcloths

58. When giving perineal care to a male, you
    A. Retract the foreskin if he is uncircumcised
    B. Wash from the scrotum to the tip of the penis
    C. Use one washcloth for the entire procedure
    D. Leave the foreskin retracted after finishing the care

59. If a family member or friend offers to help provide hygiene to a person
    A. You should check the center policy
    B. The person must consent to this
    C. Accept the offer and allow him or her to give the care
    D. Tell the family or friend this is not allowed

Matching

Match the skin care product with the benefits or the problem that may occur if you use the product.

60. _____ Absorbs moisture and prevents friction
61. _____ Makes showers and tubs slippery
62. _____ Protects skin from the drying effect of air and evaporation
63. _____ Excessive amounts can cause caking and crusts that can irritate the skin
64. _____ Masks and controls body odors
65. _____ Tends to dry and irritate skin
66. _____ Keeps skin soft and prevents drying of skin
67. _____ Removes dirt, dead skin, skin oil, some microbes, and perspiration

A. Soaps
B. Bath oils
C. Creams and lotions
D. Powders
E. Deodorants and antiperspirants

Fill in the Blanks

68. The _____ and _____ must be intact to prevent microbes from entering the body and causing an _____.

69. The religion of East Indian Hindus requires at least _____ a day.

70. Some Hindus believe that bathing after _____ causes injury.

71. What are times when you would give oral hygiene to a person? _____

72. When you are delegated to give oral hygiene, what observations should you report?
    A. _____
    B. _____
    C. _____
    D. _____
    E. _____
    F. _____

73. If flossing is done only once a day, the best time to floss is at _____.

74. When giving oral care to an unconscious person, explain what you are doing, because you always assume _____ _____.

75. When following the rules for bathing in Box 18-1, you protect the skin by following these rules:
    A. Rinse _____
    B. Pat _____
    C. Dry _____

76. What methods can be used to measure the water temperature used for a bed bath?
    A. _____
    B. _____

77. When you place a person's hand in the basin during the bed bath, you may have the person _____ the hands and fingers.

78. When the person takes a partial bath, you may need to wash and dry _____.

79. A tub bath can cause a person to feel _____ _____, especially if the person was on bedrest.

80. When the shower room has more than one stall or cabinet, you must protect the person's right _____. What can you do to protect this right?
    A. _____
    B. _____

81. When giving a tub bath or shower, you use safety measures to protect the person from _____, _____, and _____.

82. When giving a back massage, what is the effect of
    A. Fast movements? _____
    B. Slow movements? _____

83. When you are delegated to give a back massage, what observations should you report and record?
    A. _____
    B. _____
    C. _____
    D. _____

84. When you are assisting a person with perineal care, what terms may help the person understand what you are going to do? _____ _____

85. What observations made while assisting with hygiene should be reported at once?
    A. _____
    B. _____
    C. _____

Labeling

86. Look at the figure and answer these questions:

    A. Why is the person positioned on his side? _____ _____
    B. What is the purpose of the padded tongue blade? _____

87. In this figure, what is the staff member using to remove the upper denture?_____ Why? _____

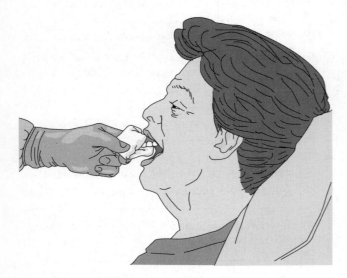

88. In this figure, explain what the staff member is doing. _____ Why is the towel positioned vertically on the person? _____

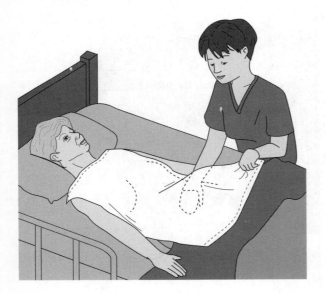

Nursing Assistant Skills Video Exercise
View the **Bathing** *video to answer these questions.*

89. Bathing is necessary to clean the skin of
   _____, _____,
   _____, and
   _____.

90. When you are delegated a person's bath or shower, you must follow procedure guidelines. The nurse's directions and the care plan tell you:
   A. _____
   B. _____
   C. _____

91. When giving a bath or shower, you provide for the person's warmth, privacy, and safety by:
   A. _____
   B. _____
   C. _____
   D. _____

92. You must give explanations about the procedure in the language the person understands.
   A. True
   B. False

93. Explain why you need to use proper positioning and body mechanics.
   _____

94. Before starting the bed bath, you need to ask for help if_____
   _____.

95. Before starting the bed bath, adjust the bed height to promote _____
   _____.

96. You do not have a bath thermometer. How should you test the water temperature for a bed bath? _____
   _____

97. You need to wear gloves if there is the potential for contact with _____
   _____.

98. How did the nursing assistant protect Mr. Bennett's privacy while removing his gown?

99. Soaking the feet is avoided when the person has _____ or _____.

100. Before washing the person's back and buttocks, you need to _____.

101. You need to provide for _____ any time you are giving personal care.

102. Report reddened areas to the nurse immediately.
   A. True
   B. False

103. Explain why you should not massage reddened areas.
   _____

104. You should always encourage the person to let you do his or her perineal care.
   A. True
   B. False

105. Before beginning perineal care, you need to _____ _____ and _____.

106. When washing the scrotum, you need to observe for
   _____.

107. When giving female perineal care, wash from the anus to the vagina.
   A. True
   B. False

View the **Personal Hygiene and Grooming** *video to answer these questions.*

108. By giving skillful and considerate care, you:
    A. _____
    B. _____

109. Oral hygiene is important for the following reasons:
    A. _____
    B. _____

110. When delegated oral hygiene, you need to follow these procedure guidelines:
    A. Follow the nurse's direction and the care plan for:
        i. _____
        ii. _____
        iii. _____
    B. Follow Standard Precautions and the Bloodborne Pathogen Standard because of:
        _____
        _____
    C. Provide for the person's privacy, comfort, and safety, taking special care to prevent
        _____
    D. Give explanations of each procedure and your actions when you give care. This is especially important when caring for the unconscious person because _____

111. Mrs. Callahan was able to assist with her oral hygiene. List the supplies provided for Mrs. Callahan:
    A. _____
    B. _____
    C. _____
    D. _____
    E. _____
    F. _____

112. Aspiration can cause _____ and _____.

113. List supplies needed when giving oral care to the unconscious person:
    A. _____
    B. _____
    C. _____
    D. _____
    E. _____
    F. _____
    G. _____
    H. _____

114. How was Mr. Harris positioned for oral care? _____
    _____

115. To clean dentures, you need these supplies:
    A. _____
    B. _____
    C. _____
    D. _____
    E. _____
    F. _____
    G. _____
    H. _____
    I. _____

116. Explain why the sink is lined with a towel and filled with water when cleaning dentures.
    _____

117. As you clean dentures, you need to note:
    A. _____
    B. _____
    C. _____

118. Dentures are stored in the denture cup filled with cool water because _____

Optional Learning Exercises

119. Hygiene promotes comfort, safety, and health. Answer these questions about hygiene:
    A. Intact skin prevents _____
    B. What other areas must be clean to maintain intact skin? _____
    C. Besides cleansing, what are the other benefits of good hygiene?
        _____
    D. What are 2 other reasons hygiene is important? It is _____ and _____.

120. What factors cause mouth dryness for an unconscious person?
    A. _____
    B. _____
    C. _____

121. The factors listed above cause crusting on the _____ and _____.

122. Oral hygiene keeps the mouth _____ and _____. It also prevents _____.

123. What are the benefits of bathing?
    A. Cleans _____
    B. Also cleans _____
    C. Removes _____
    D. Bath is _____ and _____
    E. Stimulates _____
    F. Exercises _____
    G. You can make _____
    H. You have time _____

124. When you are bathing a person with dementia, what measures are important to help the person through the bath?
    A. _____
    B. _____
    C. _____
    D. _____
    E. _____
    F. _____
    G. _____
    H. _____
    I. _____
    J. _____
    K. _____
    L. _____
    M. _____
    N. _____

125. You are delegated to give Mrs. Johnson a bath. Before beginning, what information do you need?
    A. _____
    B. _____
    C. _____
    D. _____
    E. _____
    F. _____

126. As you are bathing Mrs. Johnson, what observations should you make to report and record?
    A. _____
    B. _____
    C. _____
    D. _____
    E. _____
    F. _____
    G. _____
    H. _____
    I. _____
    J. _____

127. You are preparing to give perineal care to Mrs. Johnson. How many washcloths should you gather? _____
    Why?_____
    _____

Independent Learning Exercises

- Discuss the following questions with several classmates to understand personal preferences about personal hygiene:
  - Do you prefer a shower or tub bath?
  - What time of day do you usually bathe?
  - What skin care products do you use to keep your skin healthy?
  - What special measures do you use when brushing your teeth? Special brush? Toothpaste? Do you floss? How often?
- As part of your preparation for caring for residents, you may give a classmate a back massage and receive a back massage. Answer these questions about how you felt when you were the "resident":
  - How did the lotion feel on your back? Was it warm or cold?
  - Which strokes were relaxing? Which were more stimulating?
  - How long do you think the back massage lasted? Did you look at the clock to see the actual time?
  - What would you like to tell the person giving the back massage that would improve the back massage?
  - How will this practice help you when you give a back massage to another person?
- As part of your preparation for caring for residents, you may give a classmate oral hygiene. Answer these questions about how you felt when you were the "resident":
  - What did the "nursing assistant" tell you before beginning the oral hygiene?
  - What choices were offered? Position? Equipment? Products?
  - How did it feel to have someone else give you oral hygiene? Floss your teeth?
  - How clean did your teeth feel when the oral hygiene was completed?
  - What would you like to tell the person who gave the oral hygiene that would help improve the procedure?
  - How will this experience help you when you give oral hygiene to a resident?

19 Grooming

Key Terms

Alopecia   Dandruff   Pediculosis (lice)   Pediculosis corporis
Anticoagulant   Hirsutism   Pediculosis capitis   Pediculosis pubis

Fill in the Blanks: Key Terms

1. The infestation with lice is _____.

2. _____ is an excessive amount of dry, white flakes from the scalp.

3. The infestation of the body with lice is _____.

4. Hair loss is _____.

5. _____ is the infestation of the pubic hair with lice.

6. Excessive body hair in women and children is _____ _____.

7. The infestation of the scalp with wingless insects is _____.

8. A drug that prevents or slows blood-clotting time is an _____.

Circle the BEST Answer

9. Hair care, shaving, and nail and foot care are important to residents because they affect the needs for
   A. Safety and security
   B. Love and belonging and self-esteem needs
   C. Physical needs
   D. Self-actualization needs

10. If you see any sign of lice, you should report it to the nurse because
   A. Lice bites can cause severe infections
   B. Lice are easily spread to other persons through clothing, furniture, bed linens, and sexual contact
   C. It can cause the person's hair to fall out
   D. The lice will cause the hair to mat and tangle

11. Who chooses how you will brush, comb, and style a person's hair?
   A. The person
   B. You decide
   C. The nurse tells you
   D. It is written in the care plan

12. If long hair becomes matted or tangled, you should
   A. Braid the hair
   B. Cut the hair to remove the tangles and matting
   C. Talk to the nurse and ask for directions
   D. Get the family's permission to change the hairstyle

13. If hair is curly, coarse, and dry, which of these would *not* be done?
   A. Braid or cut the hair
   B. Use a wide-toothed comb
   C. Work upward, lifting and fluffing hair outward
   D. Apply a conditioner or petroleum jelly to make combing easier

14. When shampooing the person who has small braids
   A. Undo the hair and rebraid each time it is shampooed
   B. The braids are left intact for shampooing
   C. Undo the braids only at night
   D. Comb out the braids once a week

15. If a woman's hair is done by the beautician
   A. Wash her hair only once a week
   B. Shampoo her hair on the day she goes to the beautician
   C. Make sure she wears a shower cap during the tub bath or shower
   D. Wash her hair each time she gets a shower or tub bath

16. If a person has limited range of motion in the neck, he or she is *not* shampooed
   A. At the sink or on a stretcher
   B. In the shower
   C. During a tub bath
   D. In bed

17. Which of these is *not* an observation that is made when shampooing?
   A. Scalp sores
   B. The presence of nits or lice
   C. The amount of hair on the head
   D. Matted or tangled hair

18. If a person receives anticoagulants and needs shaving
   A. Use only an electric razor
   B. Use disposable safety razors
   C. It must be done by the nurse or barber
   D. It should be done only during the shower or bath

19. When using safety razors (blade razors)
   A. The same razor can be used for several persons until it becomes dull
   B. Use the resident's own razor several times
   C. Use a new disposable razor each time
   D. Be careful when shaving a person who takes anticoagulants

20. Why is an electric razor used when shaving a person with dementia?
   A. The person usually bleeds easily
   B. The person may resist care and move suddenly
   C. It is faster than using a safety razor
   D. The skin is tender and sensitive

21. When shaving a person with a safety razor, wear gloves
   A. To protect the person from infections
   B. To prevent contact with blood
   C. When applying shaving cream
   D. To maintain sterile technique

22. When caring for a mustache and beard, all of these are done *except*
    A. Wash the mustache or beard daily
    B. Combing daily is usually needed
    C. Ask the person how to groom his beard or mustache
    D. Trim a beard or mustache when needed
23. Nursing assistants can trim nails
    A. Whenever they have time
    B. On all persons
    C. If center policy allows them to trim nails
    D. If the person agrees to the care
24. When caring for the fingernails or toenails, which of these is *wrong*?
    A. Cut the nails with small scissors
    B. Clean under the nails with an orange stick
    C. Clip the nails straight across with nail clippers
    D. Shape the nails with an emery board or nail file
25. When changing clothing, remove the clothing from
    A. The weak side first
    B. The lower limbs first
    C. The right side last
    D. The strong or "good" side first
26. When you are undressing a person, it is usually done
    A. With the person in the bed in the supine position
    B. With the person sitting in a chair
    C. By having the person stand at the bedside
    D. In the bathroom
27. When you are changing the person's clothes, you use good body mechanics by
    A. Having a good base of support
    B. Holding objects close to your body
    C. Raising the bed to a good working level
    D. Lifting with the large muscles
28. To provide warmth and privacy when changing clothes, you
    A. Keep the top sheets in place
    B. Cover the person with a bath blanket
    C. Close the curtains
    D. Close the door
29. When changing the gown of a person with an IV
    A. Turn off the IV
    B. Lay the IV bag on the bed and remove the gown
    C. Slide the gathered sleeve over the tubing, hand, arm, and IV site
    D. Disconnect the IV
30. When you have finished changing the gown of a person with an IV, you should
    A. Restart the pump
    B. Reconnect the IV
    C. Ask the nurse to check the flow rate
    D. Check the flow rate

Fill in the Blanks

31. When you are giving care, report these signs and symptoms of lice to the nurse at once:
    A. _____
    B. _____
    C. _____
    D. _____
    E. _____

32. When you brush and comb the hair, you should report and record:
    A. _____
    B. _____
    C. _____
    D. _____
    E. _____
    F. _____
    G. _____
33. If you give hair care to a person in bed after a linen change, collect falling hair by _____.
34. It may help to prevent tangled and matted hair when you brush and comb, starting at the _____.
35. If hair has become matted and tangled, brush and comb near the _____ and work up to the _____ _____.
36. You can protect the person's eyes during shampooing by asking the person to hold a _____.
37. What delegation guidelines do you need when shaving a person?
    A. _____
    B. _____
    C. _____
    D. _____
    E. _____
38. What should be reported at once when you are shaving a person?
    A. _____
    B. _____
    C. _____
39. When you are shaving the face and underarms with a safety razor, shave in the direction of the _____.
40. When shaving legs with a safety razor, shave _____ _____.
41. When using an electric shaver, shave _____.
42. When you are delegated to give nail and foot care, report and record:
    A. _____
    B. _____
    C. _____
    D. _____
    E. _____
43. Foot care for persons with diabetes or poor circulation is provided by _____ or _____.

44. When undressing the person who cannot raise the head and shoulders:
    A. _____
    B. _____
    C. _____
    D. _____
    E. _____

45. When dressing the person who cannot raise the hips and buttocks:
    A. _____
    B. _____
    C. _____
    D. _____
    E. _____

46. Before changing a person's hospital gown, what information do you need from the nurse and the care plan?
    A. _____
    B. _____

Nursing Assistant Skills Video
View the **Personal Hygiene and Grooming** *video to answer these questions.*

47. When you are delegated hair care, you need to follow the nurse's directions and the care plan for:
    A. _____
    B. _____
    C. _____
    D. _____

48. When shampooing Mr. Steele's hair in bed, the nursing assistant started from the _____ and worked toward the _____.

49. When shaving with a blade razor, you need to:
    A. Follow _____ and the _____
    B. Shave in the direction of _____
    C. Apply _____ to nicks and cuts

50. The nails and feet need special attention to:
    A. _____
    B. _____

51. The _____ and the _____ will tell you when to give nail and foot care.

52. When giving nail and foot care, you need to check the water temperature to prevent _____.

53. When are clean clothes needed?
    A. _____
    B. _____

54. Assistance with dressing is needed when the person has _____, _____, _____, or _____.

55. Why is clothing removed from the strong or unaffected side first? _____

Optional Learning Exercises

56. You are caring for a person who is receiving cancer treatments. What effect could this treatment have on the person's hair? _____

57. Dandruff not only occurs on the scalp, but it may involve the _____.

58. Brushing the hair increases _____ to the scalp. It also brings _____ along the hair shaft.

59. Why do older persons usually have dry hair? _____

60. What water temperature is usually used when shampooing the hair? _____

61. How can the beard be softened before shaving? _____

62. After shaving, why do some people apply after-shave or lotion?
    A. Lotion _____
    B. After-shave _____

63. Injuries to the feet of a person with poor circulation are serious because poor circulation _____.

64. When changing clothing or hospital gowns, what rules should be followed?
    A. _____
    B. _____
    C. _____
    D. _____
    E. _____
    F. _____

65. How does grooming improve quality of life?
    A. Promotes _____
    B. Helps person's _____ and _____
    C. Whenever possible, it allows for _____
    D. Treats personal _____ and _____

Independent Learning Exercises
- Ask another person if you may shave him or her with a safety razor. (Some instructors may be concerned about the liability of this exercise. Make sure that the instructor approves this exercise, especially if you are using a classmate as a partner.) Ask the person you shaved to help you answer these questions.
  - What did you use for lubricating the skin? Shaving cream? Soap? Water only? How did it feel to the person? What worked best?
  - Which technique worked best? When you applied more pressure? Less pressure?
  - Shave one side of face with hair growth and one side against the hair growth. Which way was better? Why?

- What way can the person help you shave the face better?
  - What area was the most difficult to shave? How did you deal with this area?
  - Ask the person you shaved for any tips on how to improve your shaving skills.
- Role-play this situation with a classmate. Take turns being the resident and the nursing assistant. Remember to keep your left arm and leg limp when you are the resident.

Situation: Mr. Olsen is a 58-year-old resident who has weakness on the left side. You are assigned to take off his sleepwear and dress him for the day. You need to remove his pajamas and dress him in a shirt, a pullover sweater, slacks, socks, and shoes.

  - How did you provide privacy?
  - How was Mr. Olsen positioned for the clothing change?
  - What difficulties did you have when you removed his pajamas?
  - Which arm did you redress first? What difficulty did you have getting his arms into the shirt?
  - How did you put on the sweater? What was most difficult about this?
  - What was the most difficult part of putting on the slacks?
  - How did you put on the socks and shoes?
  - What did you learn from this role-play situation? Did you follow the procedure in the chapter to assist you?
  - Discuss with each other how it felt to have someone dress you when you were "Mr. Olsen."

20 Urinary Elimination

Key Terms

Catheter
Catheterization
Dysuria
Foley catheter
Functional incontinence
Hematuria
Indwelling catheter

Micturition
Mixed incontinence
Nocturia
Oliguria
Ostomy
Overflow incontinence
Polyuria

Reflex incontinence
Retention catheter
Stoma
Straight catheter
Stress incontinence
Urge incontinence

Urinary frequency
Urinary incontinence
Urinary urgency
Urination
Urostomy
Voiding

Fill in the Blanks: Key Terms

1. The production of abnormally large amounts of urine is _____.

2. _____ is having more than one type of incontinence.

3. A Foley or indwelling catheter is also called a _____.

4. The process of inserting a catheter is _____ _____.

5. _____ is the inability to control the loss of urine from the bladder.

6. Frequent urination at night is _____.

7. A catheter left in the bladder so urine drains constantly into a drainage bag is called a retention, Foley, or _____.

8. A _____ is a diversion of urine away from the bladder through a surgically created opening in the skin.

9. The loss of urine when the bladder is too full is _____ _____.

10. The process of emptying the bladder is called urination, voiding, or _____ _____.

11. _____ is the involuntary, unpredicted loss of urine from the bladder.

12. An artificial opening to the outside of the body is a _____.

13. Another name for micturition or voiding, which is the process of emptying urine from the bladder, is _____.

14. A _____ is a tube used to drain or inject fluid through a body opening.

15. Blood in the urine is _____.

16. A catheter that drains the bladder and then is removed is a _____.

17. Voiding at frequent intervals is _____.

18. An indwelling or retention catheter is also called a _____.

19. The loss of small amounts of urine with exercise and certain movements is _____.

20. Another word for urination or micturition is _____.

21. _____ is the need to void at once.

22. An artificial opening is a _____.

23. The loss of urine in response to a sudden, urgent need to void is _____.

24. Painful or difficult urination is _____.

25. The loss of urine at predictable intervals when the bladder is full is _____.

26. A scant amount of urine, usually less than 500 ml in 24 hours, is _____.

Circle the BEST Answer

27. Solid wastes are removed from the body by the
    A. Digestive system   C. Blood
    B. Urinary system   D. Integumentary system

28. A healthy adult excretes about _____ of urine a day.
    A. 500 ml   C. 1500 ml
    B. 1000 ml   D. 2000 ml

29. You can provide privacy when the person is voiding by doing all of these *except*
    A. Pull drapes or window shades
    B. Always stay in room to give assistance
    C. Pull the curtain around the bed
    D. Close room and bathroom doors

30. If the person has difficulty starting the urine stream, you can
    A. Play music on the TV
    B. Provide perineal care
    C. Use a stainless steel bedpan
    D. Run water in a nearby sink

31. The urine may be bright yellow if the person eats
    A. Asparagus
    B. Carrots and sweet potatoes
    C. Beets and blackberries
    D. Rhubarb

32. When using a steel bedpan, you should
    A. Keep the pan in the utility room
    B. Warm the pan with water and dry it before use
    C. Sterilize the pan after each use
    D. Cool the pan with water and dry it before use
33. When you are getting ready to give a person the bedpan, you should
    A. Raise the head of the bed slightly
    B. Position the person in the Fowler's position
    C. Wash the person's hands
    D. Place the bed in a flat position
34. Urinals are usually placed at the bedside on
    A. Bed rails   C. Bedside stands
    B. Overbed tables   D. The floor
35. If a man is unable place a urinal to void, you should
    A. Tell the nurse
    B. Ask a male co-worker to help the man
    C. Place the penis in the urinal
    D. Pad the bed with incontinent pads
36. A commode chair is used when the person
    A. Is unable to walk to the bathroom
    B. Cannot sit up unsupported on the toilet
    C. Needs to be in the normal position for elimination
    D. All of the above
37. When you place a commode over the toilet
    A. Restrain the person
    B. Stay in the room with the person
    C. Lock the wheels
    D. Make sure the container is in place
38. Dribbling of urine that occurs with laughing, sneezing, coughing, lifting, or other activities means the person has
    A. Urge incontinence   C. Overflow incontinence
    B. Stress incontinence   D. Functional incontinence
39. When you do not answer lights quickly or do not position the signal light within the person's reach, it can cause
    A. Overflow incontinence
    B. Mixed incontinence
    C. Reflex incontinence
    D. Functional incontinence
40. All of these will help prevent urinary tract infections *except*
    A. Promote fluid intake as the nurse directs
    B. Decrease fluid intake at bedtime
    C. Encourage the person to wear cotton underwear
    D. Keep perineal area clean and dry
41. When providing perineal care, all of these would be correct steps *except*
    A. Provide perineal care once a day
    B. Wash, rinse, and dry the perineal area and buttocks
    C. Remove wet incontinence products, garments, and linens
    D. Use a safe and comfortable water temperature
42. A catheter that is inserted and is then removed is
    A. An indwelling catheter
    B. A straight catheter
    C. A condom catheter
    D. A Foley catheter

43. A catheter is used for all of these *except*
    A. To keep the bladder empty before, during, and after surgery
    B. When a person is dying
    C. For all persons with incontinence
    D. To protect wounds and pressure ulcers from contact with urine
44. A last resort for incontinence is
    A. Bladder training
    B. Answering signal lights promptly
    C. An indwelling catheter
    D. Adequate fluid intake
45. When cleaning a catheter, you should
    A. Wipe 4 inches up the catheter to the meatus
    B. Disconnect the tubing from the drainage bag
    C. Clean the catheter from the meatus down the catheter about 4 inches
    D. Wash and rinse the catheter by washing up and down the tubing
46. The drainage bag from a catheter should *not* be attached to the
    A. Bed frame   C. Lower part of an IV pole
    B. Back of a chair   D. Bed rail
47. If a catheter is accidentally disconnected from the drainage bag, you should tell the nurse at once and then
    A. Quickly reconnect the drainage system
    B. Clamp the catheter to prevent leakage
    C. Wipe the end of the tube and end of the catheter with antiseptic wipes
    D. Discard the drainage bag and get a new bag
48. If a person uses a leg drainage bag, it
    A. Is switched to a drainage bag when the person is in bed
    B. Is attached to the clothing with tape or safety pins
    C. Is attached to the bed rail when the person is in bed
    D. Can be worn 24 hours a day
49. A leg bag needs to be emptied more often than a drainage bag because
    A. It holds less than 1000 ml and the drainage bag holds about 2000 ml
    B. It is more likely to leak than the drainage bag
    C. It holds about 250 ml and the drainage bag holds 1000 ml
    D. It interferes with walking if it is full
50. When you empty a drainage bag, you
    A. Disconnect the bag from the tubing
    B. Clamp the catheter to prevent leakage
    C. Open the clamp on the drain and drain into a graduate
    D. Take the bag into the bathroom to empty it
51. When applying a condom catheter
    A. Apply elastic tape in a spiral around the penis
    B. Make sure the catheter tip is touching the head of the penis
    C. Apply tape securely in a circle entirely around the penis
    D. Remove and reapply every shift

52. The goal of bladder training is
    A. To keep the person dry and clean
    B. To control urination
    C. To prevent skin breakdown
    D. To prevent infection
53. When you are assisting the person with bladder training to have normal elimination
    A. Help the person to the bathroom every 15 to 20 minutes
    B. Give the person 15 to 20 minutes to start voiding
    C. Make sure the person drinks at least 1000 ml each shift
    D. Tell the person he or she can void only once a shift
54. When you assist with bladder training for a person with an indwelling catheter
    A. Empty the drainage bag every hour
    B. At first, clamp the catheter for 1 hour
    C. At first, clamp the catheter for 3 to 4 hours
    D. Give the person 15 to 20 minutes to start voiding
55. A person with a urostomy
    A. Has an indwelling catheter from the bladder to a drainage bag
    B. Will be able to void normally
    C. Has had the bladder removed and has a urinary diversion
    D. Has no urine output
56. When changing a urostomy pouch
    A. It is best to change it after a meal or at bedtime
    B. Make sure it is changed at least once a day
    C. You know that the stoma does not have sensation
    D. Skin irritation around the stoma is normal
57. When a person needs dialysis, it means that the
    A. Person has urinary incontinence
    B. Urine contains sugar or blood
    C. Person has nocturia
    D. Kidneys are producing little or no urine
58. When you care for a person who has dialysis done, you know the person
    A. Is transported to the hospital or dialysis centers 2 or 3 times a week
    B. Will void large amounts of urine
    C. Will drink a large amount of fluids
    D. Eats a regular diet

Fill in the Blanks
59. What substances increase urine production?
    A. _____
    B. _____
    C. _____
    D. _____

60. A normal position for voiding for women is _____
    _____. For men, a normal position is _____.

61. What can you do to mask urination sounds?
    A. _____
    B. _____
    C. _____

62. Fracture pans are used for persons:
    A. _____
    B. _____
    C. _____
    D. _____
    E. _____
    F. _____

63. When a person voids in a bedpan or urinal, what observations about the urine are important?
    A. _____
    B. _____
    C. _____
    D. _____

64. When you are handling bedpans, urinals, and commodes and their contents, you should follow _____ and _____.

65. When you are delegated to provide a urinal, what guidelines should you follow?
    A. _____
    B. _____
    C. _____
    D. _____
    E. _____
    F. _____

66. When you transfer a person to a commode from bed, you must practice safe transfer practices and use a _____.

67. Name five causes of urge incontinence.
    A. _____
    B. _____
    C. _____
    D. _____
    E. _____

68. Stress incontinence is common in women because the pelvic muscles weaken from _____ and with _____.

69. Overflow incontinence may occur in men because of a _____.

70. _____ incontinence occurs with nervous system disorders and injuries.

71. When a catheter is inserted after a person voids, it is measuring how _____ _____.

72. When you provide perineal care after a person is incontinent, remember to:
    A. _____
    B. _____
    C. _____
    D. _____
    E. _____
    F. _____

73. A catheter is secured to the inner thigh or the man's abdomen to prevent _____ _____.

74. When a person has a catheter, what observations should you report and record?
    A. _____
    B. _____
    C. _____
    D. _____
    E. _____

75. When you give catheter care, clean the catheter about _____ inches. Clean _____ from the meatus with _____ stroke.

76. Is the urinary system sterile or nonsterile?
    _____

77. What happens if a drainage bag is higher than the bladder? _____ This can cause _____.

78. If a drainage system is disconnected accidentally, what should you do?
    A. Tell _____
    B. Do not _____
    C. Practice _____
    D. Wipe _____
    E. Wipe _____
    F. Do not _____
    G. Connect _____
    H. Discard _____
    I. Remove _____

79. Before applying a condom catheter, you should provide _____ and observe the penis for _____.

80. The catheter is clamped for 1 hour at first, and eventually for 3 to 4 hours when _____ is being done.

Labeling

81. Mark the places you would secure the catheter.

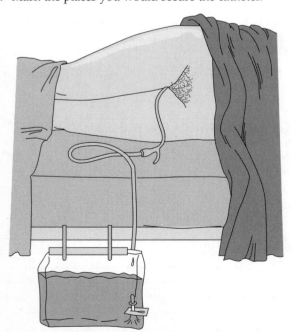

Explain why the catheter is secured this way. _____
_____

82. Mark the places you would secure the catheter.

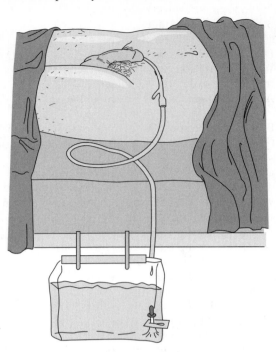

Explain why the catheter is secured this way. _____
_____

Crossword

Fill in the crossword by answering the clues below with the words from this list:

Dysuria   Nocturia
Frequency   Oliguria
Hematuria   Polyuria
Incontinence   Urgency

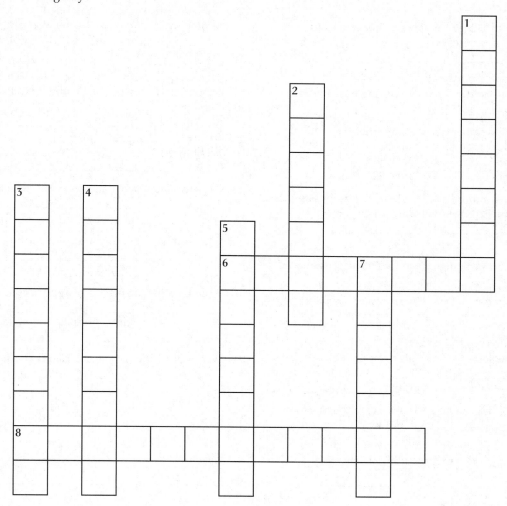

ACROSS

6. Scant amount of urine, usually less than 500 ml in 24 hours
7. Inability to control loss of urine from bladder.

DOWN

1. Production of abnormally large amount of urine.
2. Painful or difficult urination.
3. Blood in the urine.
4. Voiding at frequent intervals.
5. Frequent urination at night.
7. Need to void immediately.

Nursing Assistant Skills Video Exercise

*View the **Normal Elimination** video to answer these questions.*

83. The passageway for the urine to leave the body is the
    A. Bladder   C. Kidney
    B. Urethra   D. Ureter

84. Do not place the urinal on the bedside stand because
    _____
    _____ .

85. Before handling the urinal, you need to put on gloves.
    A. True   B. False

86. _____ are used for urinary and bowel elimination when the person cannot get out of bed.

87. Before you assist the person off the bedpan, you need to:
    A. _____
    B. _____
    C. _____

88. Catheter care is required to reduce the potential for

_____.

89. When delegated catheter care, the nurse and the care plan tell you:
    A. _____
    B. _____

90. Providing catheter care offers an important opportunity to observe _____ and make sure _____

_____.

91. You need to hold the catheter during washing to prevent _____ or _____.

92. When giving catheter care, clean from the urethral opening down the catheter about
    A. 2 inches   C. 8 inches
    B. 4 inches   D. 12 inches

93. Wear gloves and follow Standard Precautions and the Bloodborne Pathogen Standard when _____, _____, or _____ condom catheters.

94. Every time you change a condom catheter, you need to:
    A. _____
    B. _____

Optional Learning Exercises

95. When a person eats a diet high in salt, it causes the body _____. When this happens, how does it affect urine output? _____

96. You would ask the nurse to observe urine that looks or _____. You would also report complaints of _____

_____.

97. A fracture pan can be used with older persons who have _____ or _____.

98. Covering the lap and legs of a person using a commode provides _____ and promotes

_____.

99. If you are caring for an incontinent person and you become short-tempered and impatient, _____ _____. What right are you protecting when you do this? _____

100. Even though catheters are a last resort for incontinent persons, they may be used with weak, disabled, or dying persons to:
    A. Promote _____
    B. Prevent _____
    C. Protect _____ and _____
    D. Allow _____

101. Catheters may have diagnostic reasons for use such as:
    A. _____
    B. _____

102. What can happen if microbes enter a closed drainage system? _____

_____

103. What type of tape is used to apply a condom catheter? _____ Why? _____
What can happen if you use the wrong tape?

_____

104. Why is a urostomy pouch replaced anytime it leaks?

_____

Independent Learning Activities

• Role-play the following situation with a classmate. Take turns playing the person using the bedpan and the nursing assistant. Answer the questions about the activity.
   Situation: Mrs. Donnelly is a 70-year-old who must use the bedpan. She finds it difficult to move easily and usually does not have enough strength to raise her hips to get on the bedpan. She tells you she will try to help as much as she can.
   As Mrs. Donnelly:
   ○ When you tried to assist, how easy was it to raise your hips? How did the nursing assistant help you get on the pan?
   ○ When you were rolled onto the bedpan, how did it feel? How well was the pan positioned under you?
   ○ How did you feel about sitting on the pan in bed? Did you feel as if this would be an easy or difficult way to void? Explain your feelings.
   ○ How could the nursing assistant made this procedure better?
   As the nursing assistant:
   ○ How did you position the bedpan to get ready to slide it under Mrs. Donnelly? Did this method work? How could you improve this?
   ○ When you rolled Mrs. Donnelly onto the pan, how well positioned was she? What adjustments were necessary?
   ○ When you rolled her off the pan, what happened? If urine had been in the pan, what would have occurred?
   ○ How could you change some of your steps to make this procedure better?

21 Bowel Elimination

Key Terms
Colostomy
Constipation
Defecation
Dehydration
Diarrhea

Enema
Fecal impaction
Fecal incontinence
Feces

Flatulence
Flatus
Ileostomy
Ostomy

Peristalsis
Stoma
Stool
Suppository

Fill in the Blanks: Key Terms
1. A surgically created opening is a _____.

2. The process of excreting feces from the rectum through the anus is a bowel movement or _____.

3. The excessive formation of gas in the stomach and intestines is _____.

4. A _____ is a cone-shaped solid medication that is inserted into a body opening.

5. The frequent passage of liquid stools is _____.

6. _____ is the prolonged retention and buildup of feces in the rectum.

7. _____ is the excessive loss of water from tissues.

8. Gas or air passed through the anus is _____.

9. The introduction of fluid into the rectum and lower colon is an _____.

10. Excreted feces is _____.

11. An artificial opening between the colon and abdominal wall is a _____.

12. _____ is the alternating contraction and relaxation of intestinal muscles.

13. The passage of a hard, dry stool is _____.

14. _____ is the inability to control the passage of feces and gas through the anus.

15. An opening is a _____.

16. The semisolid mass of waste products in the colon is _____.

17. An artificial opening between the ileum and the abdominal wall is an _____.

Circle the BEST Answer
18. People normally have a bowel movement
    A. Every day
    B. Every 2 to 3 days
    C. 2 or 3 times a day
    D. All of these can be normal
19. Bleeding in the stomach and small intestines causes stool to be
    A. Brown   C. Red
    B. Black   D. Clay-colored

20. The characteristic odor of stool is caused by
    A. Poor personal hygiene
    B. Poor nutrition
    C. Bacterial action in the intestines
    D. Adequate fluid intake
21. When you observe stool that is abnormal
    A. Ask the nurse to observe the stool
    B. Report your observation and discard the stool
    C. Ask the person if the stool is normal for him
    D. Record your observation when you finish his care
22. Which of these could interfere with defecation?
    A. Being able to relax by reading a book or newspaper
    B. Eating a diet with high-fiber foods
    C. Using a bedpan or commode in a semiprivate room
    D. Drinking 6 to 8 glasses of water daily
23. A person who must stay in bed most of the time may have irregular elimination and constipation because of
    A. Poor diet   C. Lack of activity
    B. Poor fluid intake   D. Lack of privacy
24. Which of these would provide safety for the person during bowel elimination?
    A. Make sure the bedpan is warm
    B. Place the signal light and toilet tissue within the person's reach
    C. Provide perineal care
    D. Allow enough time for defecation
25. Constipation can be relieved by
    A. Giving the person a low-fiber diet
    B. Increasing activity
    C. Decreasing fluids
    D. Ignoring the urge to defecate
26. A person tries several times to have a bowel movement and cannot. Liquid feces seep from the anus. This probably means he has
    A. Diarrhea   C. A fecal impaction
    B. Constipation   D. Fecal incontinence
27. When the nurse finds a fecal impaction is present, he or she sometimes tries to relieve it by
    A. Changing the person's diet
    B. Telling the nursing assistant to give more fluids
    C. Removing the fecal mass with a gloved finger
    D. Increasing the activity of the person
28. Good skin care is important when a person has diarrhea because
    A. This prevents odors
    B. Skin breakdown and pressure ulcers are risks
    C. It prevents the spread of microbes
    D. It prevents fluid loss

29. Why is diarrhea very serious in older persons?
   A. It causes skin breakdown
   B. It causes odors
   C. It can cause dehydration
   D. It increases activity
30. When fecal incontinence occurs, the person may need all of these *except*
   A. Increased fluid intake
   B. Bowel training
   C. Help with elimination after meals
   D. Incontinent products to keep garments and linens clean
31. If flatus is not expelled, the person may complain of
   A. Abdominal cramping or pain
   B. Diarrhea
   C. Fecal incontinence
   D. Nausea
32. Which of these *is not* a goal of bowel training?
   A. To give laxatives daily to maintain regular bowel movements
   B. To gain control of bowel movements
   C. To develop a regular pattern of elimination
   D. To prevent fecal impaction, constipation, and fecal incontinence
33. When bowel training is planned, which of these is included in the care plan?
   A. The amount of stool the person expels
   B. How many bowel movements the person has each day
   C. The usual time of day the person has a bowel movement
   D. The foods that cause flatus
34. When the nurse delegates you to prepare a soapsuds enema, mix
   A. 2 teaspoons of salt in 500–1000 ml of tap water
   B. 3-5 ml of castile soap in 500–1000 ml of tap water
   C. 2 ml of castile soap in 500 ml of tap water
   D. Mineral oil with sterile water
35. When you give a cleansing enema, it should be given to the person
   A. Within 5 minutes
   B. Over about 30 minutes
   C. In about 10-15 minutes
   D. Over about 15-20 minutes
36. The person receiving an enema is usually placed in a
   A. Supine position   C. Semi-Fowler's position
   B. Prone position   D. Side-lying or Sims' position
37. When you prepare and give an enema, you will do all of these *except*
   A. Prepare the solution at 110° F
   B. Insert the tubing 3 to 4 inches into the rectum
   C. Hold the solution container about 12 inches above the bed
   D. Lubricate the enema tip before inserting it into the rectum
38. When the doctor orders enemas until clear
   A. Give one enema
   B. Give as many enemas as necessary to return a clear fluid
   C. Ask the nurse how many enemas to give
   D. Give only tap water enemas

39. If you are giving an enema and the person complains of cramping
   A. Tell the person that is normal and continue to give the enema
   B. Clamp the tube until the cramping subsides
   C. Discontinue the enema immediately and tell the nurse
   D. Lower the bag below the level of the bed
40. When giving a small volume enema, do not release pressure on the bottle because
   A. It will cause cramping if pressure is released
   B. The fluid will leak from the rectum
   C. Solution will be drawn back into the bottle
   D. It will cause flatulence
41. When giving a small-volume enema
   A. Place the person in the prone position
   B. Insert the enema tip 2 inches into the rectum
   C. Heat the solution to 105° F
   D. Clamp the tubing if cramping occurs
42. An oil-retention enema is given to
   A. Cleanse the bowel to prepare for surgery
   B. Regulate the person who is receiving bowel training
   C. Relieve flatulence
   D. Soften the feces and lubricate the rectum
43. If you feel resistance when you are giving an enema
   A. Lubricate the tube more thoroughly
   B. Push more firmly to insert the tube
   C. Stop and call the nurse
   D. Ask the person to take a deep breath and relax
44. When you are caring for a person with an ostomy
   A. All of the stools are solid and formed
   B. Stomas do not have nerve endings and are not painful
   C. An ostomy is always temporary and is reconnected after healing
   D. A pouch is worn to protect the stoma
45. Which of these statements is true about an ileostomy?
   A. The stool is solid and formed
   B. The stoma is an opening into the colon
   C. The pouch is changed daily
   D. The skin around the ileostomy can be irritated by the digestive juices in the stool
46. When carrying for a person with a stoma, the pouch is
   A. Changed daily
   B. Changed every 3 to 7 days and when it leaks
   C. Worn only when the person thinks he or she will have a bowel movement
   D. Changed every time the person has a bowel movement
47. The best time to change the ostomy bag is before breakfast because
   A. The stoma is less likely to expel stool at this time
   B. The person has more time in the morning
   C. It should be changed before morning care
   D. The person tolerates the procedure better before eating

48. When cleaning the skin around the stoma, you use
    A. Sterile water and sterile gauze squares
    B. Alcohol and sterile cotton
    C. Gauze squares or washcloths and water or soap and other cleansing agent as directed by the nurse
    D. Adhesive remover and sterile cotton balls

49. You give the person with an ostomy the right of personal choice when you
    A. Allow the person to manage the care when able
    B. Choose the time when care is done
    C. Choose the care measures and equipment used
    D. Ask the nurse to determine the care to be done

Fill in the Blanks

50. When observing stool, what should be reported to the nurse?
    A. _____
    B. _____
    C. _____
    D. _____
    E. _____
    F. _____
    G. _____
    H. _____

51. What three food groups are high in fiber?
    A. _____
    B. _____
    C. _____

52. Name six gas-forming foods:
    A. _____
    B. _____
    C. _____
    D. _____
    E. _____
    F. _____

53. Drinking warm fluids such as coffee, tea, hot cider, and warm water will increase _____.

54. How will dehydration affect these?
    A. Skin is _____
    B. Urine is _____
    C. Blood pressure _____
    D. Pulse and respirations _____

55. Flatulence may be caused when the person _____ while eating and drinking.

56. When a nurse inserts a suppository for bowel training, how soon would you expect the person to defecate?
    _____

57. Before giving an enema, make sure that:
    A. _____
    B. _____
    C. _____
    D. _____
    E. _____

58. After giving an enema, what should be reported and recorded?
    A. _____
    B. _____
    C. _____
    D. _____
    E. _____
    F. _____

59. Because you will likely contact stool while giving an enema, you should follow _____ and _____.

60. How can cramping be prevented during an enema?
    A. _____
    B. _____

61. How long does it usually take for a tap-water, saline, or soapsuds enema to take effect? _____

62. A small-volume enema irritates and distends the _____.

63. A person should retain a small volume enema for _____.

64. When you start to insert the tube to give an enema, ask the person to _____.

65. What can you place in the ostomy pouch to prevent odors? _____

66. Showers and baths are delayed 1 to 2 hours after applying a new pouch to allow _____.

Labeling
Answer questions 67 through 70 using the following illustrations.

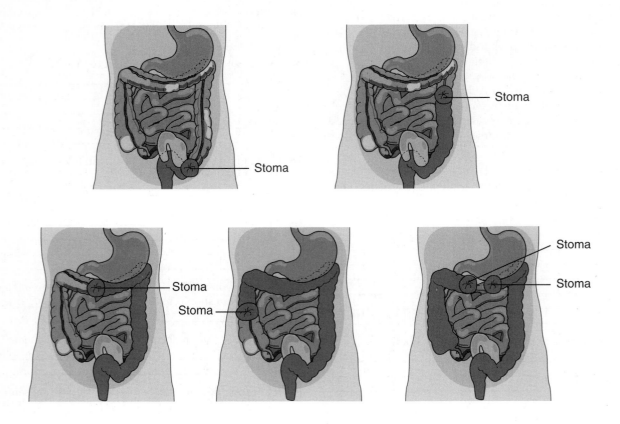

67. Name the five types of colostomies shown.
    A. _____
    B. _____
    C. _____
    D. _____
    E. _____

68. Which colostomy will have the most solid and formed stool? _____

69. Which colostomy will have the most liquid stool? _____

70. Which colostomy is a temporary colostomy? _____

Answer questions 71 through 73 using the following illustration.

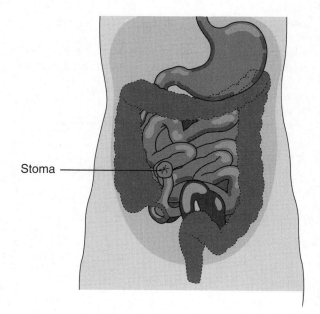

Stoma —

71. What type of ostomy is shown? _____

72. What part of the bowel has been removed? _____

73. Will the stool from the ostomy be liquid or formed?
_____

Nursing Assistant Skills Video Exercise
View the **Normal Elimination** *video to answer these questions.*

74. Enemas are ordered to _____ and
_____. An enema may also be
used to _____.

75. When you are preparing to administer an enema, you need to follow the nurse's directions and the care plan for:
   A. _____
   B. _____
   C. _____
   D. _____
   E. _____

76. Why is the Sims' or left side-lying position used to administer an enema?
_____

77. Why should you ask the person to take a few deep breaths before inserting the lubricated enema tube?
_____
_____

78. The enema tube is *never* inserted more than 6 inches into the rectum.
   A. True   B. False

79. When administering an enema solution, you should clamp the tube if the person:
   A. _____
   B. _____
   C. _____

80. Clamp the tube before the solution bag is empty to prevent_____
_____.

Optional Learning Exercises

81. You are caring for Mr. Evans, who is in a semi-private room. His roommate has a large family and many visitors. Mr. Evans has not had a bowel movement in 3 days, even though he is eating well and taking medications to assist elimination. What could be a reason he has not had a bowel movement?
_____

82. Mrs. Weller usually has a bowel movement after breakfast. What are some activities that may assist her to defecate more easily? _____
_____

83. The nurse tells you to make sure Mr. Johnson eats the high-fiber foods in his diet to assist in his elimination. What foods are high in fiber?
_____

84. Mrs. Shaffer tells you she cannot digest fruits and vegetables and she refuses to eat them. What may be added to her cereal and prune juice to provide fiber?
_____

85. You offer Mr. Murphy _____ of water each day to promote normal bowel elimination.

86. Mr. Hernandez has been taking an antibiotic, which is a drug to treat his pneumonia, and he has developed diarrhea. You think he may have diarrhea because
_____.

87. You are caring for 83-year-old Mrs. Chen, and you helped her to the bathroom 30 minutes ago, where she had a bowel movement. When you enter her room to make her bed, she tells you she needs to use the bathroom for a bowel movement. You know that older people _____.

88. The two goals of bowel training are _____ and _____.

89. Why are tap-water enemas dangerous? _____ How many tap-water enemas can be given? _____ Why? _____

90. Compare small-volume enemas and oil-retention enemas.
   A. Small-volume enemas are given to _____.
      Oil-retention enemas are given to _____.
   B. Small-volume enemas take effect in about _____ minutes. Oil-retention enemas should be retained for at least _____ minutes.
   C. The nurse may want an oil-retention enema retained for _____ hours.

Independent Learning Activities

- Think about times when you have had a problem with bowel irregularity. Answer these questions about how you handled the problems:
  - What causes you to have irregularity? Foods? Illness? Stress? Inactivity?
  - What methods have you used to treat irregularity? Diet? Medication?
  - How does irregularity affect you physically? Your appetite? Energy level? Sleep and rest?
  - How does irregularity affect your mood? Your daily activities?
- Interview a person who has a colostomy or an ileostomy. You may know someone who has an ostomy. Or you may care for someone who has one. Your community may have an ostomy support group that you can contact. Talk to the person and ask these questions:
  - How long has the person had the ostomy? Is it permanent or temporary?
  - What was the hardest part of learning to live with an ostomy? What was the easiest part?
  - How has living with an ostomy affected the person's life? Has the person's work been affected? Were leisure activities affected?
  - How has the ostomy affected the person's family? What changes have occurred?
  - What equipment works best for the person? How expensive is the equipment? How much time is required each day to care for the ostomy?

22 Nutrition and Fluids

Key Terms
Anorexia	Daily Value (DV)	Edema	Nutrient
Aspiration	Dehydration	Graduate	Nutrition
Calorie	Dysphagia	Intake	Output

Fill in the Blanks: Key Terms

1. _____ is the amount of fluid taken in.

2. The _____ is how a serving fits into the daily diet. It is expressed in a percent based on a daily diet of 2000 calories..

3. The loss of appetite is _____.

4. The amount of fluid lost is _____.

5. A substance that is ingested, digested, absorbed, and used by the body is a _____.

6. _____ is difficulty or discomfort in swallowing.

7. The breathing of fluid or an object into the lungs is _____.

8. The many processes involved in the ingestion, digestion, absorption, and use of food and fluids by the body is _____.

9. The amount of energy produced from the burning of food by the body is a _____.

10. A decrease in the amount of water in body tissues is _____.

11. A _____ is a calibrated container used to measure fluid.

12. _____ is the swelling of body tissues with water.

Circle the BEST Answer

13. Which of these occurs when the person has a poor diet and poor eating habits?
    A. Decreased risk for infection and chronic diseases
    B. Wounds heal well
    C. Affects physical and mental well-being
    D. Decreased risk of acute and chronic infections

14. Body fuel for energy is found in
    A. Vitamins
    B. Minerals
    C. Fats, proteins, and carbohydrates
    D. Water

15. A healthy diet as described in the *Dietary Guidelines for Americans 2005* should
    A. Be high in fruits, vegetables, and whole grains
    B. Be high in fats and cholesterol
    C. Include all types of meats, poultry, and fish
    D. Aim to include 2500 mg of sodium each day

16. *Dietary Guidelines for Americans 2005* states that you should *not* eat
    A. Any sodium or added sugar
    B. Raw or undercooked fish or shellfish
    C. Hardboiled eggs
    D. Certain deli meats that have been reheated to steaming hot

17. What percent of calories should come from total fat intake according to the *Dietary Guidelines for Americans 2005*?
    A. 20 to 30   C. 40 to 50
    B. 5 to 10   D. 0 to 10

18. How much sodium should be consumed each day according to the *Dietary Guidelines for Americans 2005*?
    A. No more 1000 mg a day
    B. No more than 3500 mg a day
    C. Less than 2300 mg a day
    D. Up to 5000 mg a day

19. In the *Dietary Guidelines for Americans 2005*, the risk of chronic illness can be reduced if you engage in
    A. Cardiovascular conditioning
    B. Stretching exercises
    C. Resistance exercises
    D. 30 minutes of moderate to vigorous activity most days

20. The kind and amounts of food to eat daily in MyPyramid depend on
    A. The ethnic and cultural background of the person
    B. The person's age, gender, and activity level
    C. The person's weight
    D. Religious dietary restrictions

21. The color bands on MyPyramid stand for
    A. The number of calories eaten daily
    B. The amount of physical activity daily
    C. The amount of food eaten in each group
    D. The five food groups and oils

22. Foods lower in the color bands of MyPyramid
    A. Are cheaper
    B. Should be chosen less often for the daily intake
    C. Are foods that most people like
    D. Should be chosen more often than those higher in the band

23. Which of these statements is *not* true?
    A. A person needs at least 3 ounces of whole-grain cereals
    B. Vegetables can be fresh, frozen, canned, or dried
    C. Fruits contain potassium, dietary fiber, vitamin C, and folate
    D. Oils are solid at room temperature

24. An example of moderate physical activity in MyPyramid would be
    A. Bicycling at less than 10 miles per hour
    B. Freestyle swimming laps
    C. Chopping wood
    D. Competitive basketball
25. Which nutrient is needed for tissue growth and repair?
    A. Carbohydrates   C. Vitamins
    B. Fats   D. Protein
26. Which vitamin is needed for the formation of substances that hold tissue together?
    A. Vitamin K   C. Vitamin A
    B. Vitamin C   D. Vitamin B_{12}
27. Food labels have all of this information *except*
    A. The serving size
    B. All vitamins and minerals in the food
    C. Total amount of fat and amount of saturated and trans fats
    D. Amount of cholesterol and sodium
28. A cultural group that eats a diet low in fat and high in sodium is in
    A. The Philippines   C. Poland
    B. China   D. Mexico
29. All pork and pork products are forbidden by
    A. Seventh Day Adventists
    B. Muslim or Islam
    C. Church of Jesus Christ of Latter Day Saints
    D. Roman Catholic
30. People with limited incomes often buy
    A. More protein foods
    B. Carbohydrate foods
    C. Foods high in vitamins and minerals
    D. Fatty foods
31. When people buy cheaper foods, the diet may lack
    A. Fats
    B. Starchy foods
    C. Protein and certain vitamins and minerals
    D. Sugars
32. Appetite can be stimulated by
    A. Illness and medications
    B. Decreased senses of taste and smell
    C. Aromas and thoughts of food
    D. Anxiety, pain, and depression
33. Personal choice of foods is influenced by
    A. Foods served at home
    B. Age and social experience
    C. Allergies
    D. All of the above
34. During illness
    A. Appetite increases
    B. Fewer nutrients are needed
    C. Nutritional needs increase to fight infection and heal tissue
    D. The person will prefer protein foods
35. All of these may occur with aging *except*
    A. Increases in taste and smell
    B. Secretion of digestive juices decreases
    C. Difficulty in swallowing
    D. A need for fewer calories than younger people

36. Requirements for food served in long-term care centers are made by
    A. MyPyramid
    B. OBRA
    C. The nursing center
    D. The public health department
37. All of these are requirements for food served in long-term care centers *except*
    A. The center provides needed adaptive equipment and utensils
    B. The person's diet is well-balanced, nourishing, and tastes good
    C. All food is served at room temperature
    D. Each person must receive at least three meals a day and be offered a bedtime snack
38. A general diet
    A. Is ordered for person with difficulty swallowing
    B. Has no dietary limits or restrictions
    C. May have restricted amounts of sodium
    D. Has an increased amount of sugar
39. The body needs no more than _____ of sodium each day.
    A. 2400 mg   C. 5000 mg
    B. 3000 mg   D. 1000 mg
40. When the body tissues swell with water, what organ has to work harder?
    A. Kidneys   C. Heart
    B. Liver   D. Lungs
41. When you are caring for a person with diabetes, you should do all of these *except*
    A. Serve the person's meals and snacks on time
    B. Tell the nurse what the person did and did not eat
    C. Give the person extra food and snacks whenever it is requested
    D. Provide a between-meal nourishment if all the food was not eaten
42. A person may be given a mechanical soft diet because
    A. Nausea and vomiting have occurred
    B. The person has chewing problems
    C. The person has been advanced from a clear-liquid diet
    D. The person has constipation
43. If you are serving a meal to a person on a fiber- and residue-restricted diet, the meal would *not* include
    A. Raw fruits and vegetables
    B. Strained fruit juices
    C. Canned or cooked fruit without skin or seeds
    D. Plain pasta
44. A person who has serious burns would receive a
    A. Sodium-controlled diet   C. High-calorie diet
    B. Fat-controlled diet   D. High-protein diet
45. When a person has dysphagia, the thickness of the food served is chosen by the
    A. Person
    B. Nursing assistant
    C. Family
    D. Speech/language pathologist, dietitian, and doctor or nurse

46. Food on a dysphagia diet that is a thickened liquid is served
    A. From a cup
    B. In a bowl
    C. By stirring right before serving
    D. With a spoon
47. Which of these may be a sign of a swallowing problem (dysphagia)?
    A. Person complains that food will not go down or that food is stuck
    B. Foods that need chewing are avoided
    C. There is excessive drooling of saliva
    D. All of the above
48. When assisting a person with meals, you can help prevent aspiration while the person is eating by placing him in
    A. A semi-Fowler's position
    B. A Fowler's position
    C. The side-lying position
    D. The supine position
49. If fluid intake exceeds fluid output, the person will
    A. Have edema in the tissues
    B. Be dehydrated
    C. Have vomiting and diarrhea
    D. Have increased urinary output
50. How much fluid is needed every day for normal fluid balance?
    A. 1500 ml   C. 2000-2500 ml
    B. 1000-1500 ml   D. 3000-4000 ml
51. If the person you are caring for has an order for restricted fluids, which of these should you do?
    A. Offer a variety of liquids
    B. Thicken all fluids
    C. Keep the water pitcher out of sight
    D. Do not allow the person to swallow any liquids during oral hygiene
52. When you are keeping I&O records, you should measure all of these except
    A. Milk, water, coffee, and tea
    B. Mashed potatoes and creamed vegetables
    C. Creamed cereals and gelatin
    D. Ice cream, custard, and pudding
53. When you are measuring I&O, you need to know that 1 ounce equals
    A. 10 ml   C. 100 ml
    B. 500 ml   D. 30 ml
54. When you are using the graduate to measure output, you read the amount by
    A. Holding the graduate at waist level and reading the amount
    B. Looking at the graduate while it is held above eye level
    C. Keeping the container at eye level
    D. Setting the graduate on the floor and reading it
55. When I&O is ordered, which of the following is not included in the measurement?
    A. Urine   C. Drainage from suction
    B. Solid stool   D. Vomitus

56. What is the advantage for residents when they receive their meals in assistive dining?
    A. The person is with others at mealtime
    B. The food is served in bowls and on platters
    C. This prevents distractions during meals
    D. Food is served as in a restaurant
57. Which of the following needs to be done before the person is served a meal?
    A. Give complete personal care
    B. Change all linens
    C. Make sure the person is clean and dry
    D. Make sure the person has been shaved or has makeup applied
58. You can provide comfort during meals by
    A. Making sure unpleasant sights, sounds, and sounds are removed
    B. Making sure dentures, eyeglasses, or hearing aids are in place
    C. Giving the person good oral care before and after meals
    D. All of the above
59. What should you do if a food tray has not been served within 15 minutes?
    A. Recheck the food temperatures
    B. Serve the tray immediately
    C. Throw the food away
    D. Serve only the cold items on the tray
60. How can you make sure the food tray is complete?
    A. Ask the person being served
    B. Ask the nurse
    C. Call the dietary department
    D. Check items on the tray with the dietary card
61. If you become impatient while feeding a resident with dementia, you should
    A. Refuse to continue caring for the person
    B. Return the person to his or her room
    C. Talk to the nurse
    D. Make the person eat his or her food
62. When you are feeding a person, you should
    A. Not allow the person to assist
    B. Give the person a fork and knife to assist with cutting the food
    C. Feed the person in a private area to maintain confidentiality
    D. Use a spoon because it is less likely to cause injury
63. When feeding a person, liquids are given
    A. Only at the start of feeding
    B. During the meal alternating with solid foods
    C. At the end of the meal when all solid food have been eaten
    D. Only if the person has difficulty swallowing
64. When providing fresh water to residents, you would not
    A. Give fresh water when the pitcher is empty
    B. Put ice in all pitchers
    C. Practice the rules of medical sepsis
    D. Ask the nurse about any special orders
65. When you keep track of calorie intake, you include
    A. What time the person ate
    B. Only the liquids that the person drinks
    C. All of the food that was served to the person
    D. What the person ate and how much

66. When residents are included in deciding what foods they eat, the person's right to _____ is being met.
   A. Personal choice   C. Confidentiality
   B. Privacy   D. Good nutrition

Fill in the Blanks
67. How many calories are in each of these?
   A. 1 gram of fat _____
   B. 1 gram of protein _____
   C. 1 gram of carbohydrate _____

Questions 68 through 73 relate to the **Dietary Guidelines for Americans 2005.**
68. What is included in a healthy diet?
   A. _____
   B. _____
   C. _____

69. Nutrient-dense foods have little or _____
   _____.

70. What recommendations are made for older persons for each of these?
   A. Vitamin D _____
   B. Sodium intake _____
   C. Potassium requirement _____

71. What recommendations are made for weight management?
   A. _____
   B. _____

72. What foods are high in each of these fats?
   A. Saturated fats _____
   B. Trans fats _____
   C. Cholesterol _____

73. The diet should include at least _____ of whole-grain products each day. At least _____ of the daily grain requirement should come from whole grains.

Questions 74 through 77 relate to MyPyramid.
74. What are the five food groups that the color bands stand for?
   A. _____
   B. _____
   C. _____
   D. _____
   E. _____

75. Foods near the base of MyPyramid have the most _____ and the _____.

76. Some of the bands are wider than others. What does this mean? _____

77. Which food group or groups have the following health benefits?
   A. May reduce the risk of osteoporosis _____
   B. Good source of protein and iron _____
   C. May prevent constipation _____
   D. May reduce risk of kidney stones _____
   E. May prevent birth defects _____
   F. May help lower calorie intake _____
   G. Rich sources of vitamin E (list food group and the specific foods) _____

78. What is the most important nutrient? _____

79. If dietary fat is not needed by the body, it is stored as _____.

80. What is the function of each of these nutrients?
   A. Protein _____
   B. Carbohydrates _____
   C. Fats _____
   D. Vitamins _____
   E. Minerals _____
   F. Water _____

81. Which vitamins can be stored by the body? _____

82. Which vitamins must be ingested daily? _____

83. What vitamin is important for these functions: *formation of substances that hold tissues together; healthy blood vessels, skin, gums, bones, and teeth; wound healing; prevention of bleeding; resistance to infection?*
   _____

84. Milk and milk products, liver, green leafy vegetables, eggs, breads, and cereals are good sources of which vitamin? _____

85. What mineral allows red blood cells to carry oxygen? _____

86. When the diet does not have enough _____, it may affect nerve function, muscle contraction, and heart function.

87. Calcium is needed for _____.

88. What information is found on food labels?
   A. _____
   B. _____
   C. _____

89. Those who practice _____ as their religion eat only fish with scales and fins.

90. Alcohol and coffee are not allowed by these religious groups (4).
   _____

91. What religious group may have members that fast from meats on certain Fridays of the year?
   _____

92. Nutritional needs increase during illness when the body must _____.

93. Older persons need _____ than younger people do.

94. Why do the diets of some older people lack protein?
   _____

95. What OBRA requirement relates to the temperature of foods served in long-term care centers? _____

96. What foods are included in a clear-liquid diet? _____
   _____
   _____

97. When the person receives a full-liquid diet, it will include all of the foods on the clear-liquid diet as well as these foods. _____
_____

98. If a person has poorly fitted dentures and has chewing difficulties, the doctor may order a _____ diet.

99. A person who is constipated and has other GI disorders may receive a _____ diet. The foods in this diet increase the _____ to stimulate _____.

100. If a person is receiving a high-calorie diet, the calorie intake is _____
_____.

101. What vegetables juices are high in sodium? _____

102. When a person is receiving a diabetic diet, the same amount of _____ are eaten each day.

103. If you are feeding a person a dysphagia diet, what observations should be reported to the nurse immediately?
A. _____, _____, or _____ during or after meal
B. _____ or _____

104. Why is it important to offer water often to older persons?_____
_____

105. When you give oral hygiene to a person who is receiving nothing by mouth, the person must not _____.

106. List the amount of milliliters in the following:
A. 1 ounce equals _____ ml
B. 1 pint equals about _____ ml
C. 1 quart equals about _____ ml

107. What information do you need when you are delegated to measure intake and output?
A. _____
B. _____
C. _____
D. _____
E. _____

108. What two types of dining programs may be used with persons who are oriented or are quietly confused? _____

109. What can be done to promote comfort when preparing residents for meals?
A. _____
B. _____
C. _____
D. _____
E. _____

110. If a food tray is not served within 15 minutes, what should be checked? _____

111. When you are delegated to serve meal trays, what information do you need from the nurse or care plan?
A. _____
B. _____
C. _____
D. _____

112. When you are serving meal trays, you make sure the right person gets the right tray by checking _____
_____.

113. When you are feeding a person, the spoon should be filled _____.

114. Why is it important to sit facing the person when you feed him or her?
A. _____
B. _____
C. _____

115. What should be reported after you have fed a person?
A. _____
B. _____
C. _____
D. _____

Labeling
Use the chart below to answer question 116.

OSF SM
ST. JOSEPH MEDICAL CENTER
Bloomington, Illinois

FLUID BALANCE CHART

Water Glass	250cc	Ice Cream	120cc
Styrofoam Cup	180cc	Ice Chips	1/2 amt. of
Cup (coffee)	250cc		cc's in cup
Milk Carton	240cc		
Pop (1 can)	360cc	Pitcher	
Broth-Soup	175cc	(Yellow)	1000cc
Juice Carton	120cc		
Juice Glass	120cc		
Jello	120cc		

DATE _____

	INTAKE			OUTPUT					
				URINE		OTHER		CONT. IRRIGATION	
TIME	ORAL	Parenteral	Amt. cc Absbd.	Method Collected	Amt. (cc)	Method Collected	Amt. (cc)	In	Out
2400-0100		cc from previous shift							
0100-0200									
0200-0300									
0300-0400									
0400-0500									
0500-0600									
0600-0700									
0700-0800									
		8 - hour Sub-total		8-hr T		8-hr T			
0800-0900		cc from previous shift							
0900-1000									
1000-1100									
1100-1200									
1200-1300									
1300-1400									
1400-1500									
1500-1600									
		8 - hour Sub-total		8-hr T		8-hr T			
1600-1700		cc from previous shift							
1700-1800									
1800-1900									
1900-2000									
2000-2100									
2100-2200									
2200-2300									
2300-2400									
		8 - hour Sub-total		8-hr T		8-hr T			
		24 - hour Sub-total		24-hr T		24-hr T			

310' Marie Mills

Source Key:

URINE

V	- Voided
C	- Catheter
INC	- Incontinent
U.C.	- Ureteral Catheter

Source Key:

OTHER

G.I.T.	- Gastric Intestinal Tube
T.T.	- T. Tube
Vom.	- Vomitus
Liq S.	- Liquid Stool
H.V.	- Hemovac

Form No. MF36722 (Rev. 5/97) **MFI**

Modified from OSF St. Joseph Medical Center, Bloomington, Ill.

116. Enter this information on the intake and output record. Total amounts for the 8-hour and 24-hour periods. Amounts in parentheses indicate how much the person ate or drank. (Use 2400-0800, 0800-1600, and 1600-2400 as 8-hour periods.)

0200 *Voided 300 ml*
0600 *Voided 500 ml*
0730 **Breakfast**
    Orange juice (whole glass)
    Milk (1/2 carton)
    Coffee (1 cup)
0700 *Voided 300 ml*
1000 *Water pitcher filled*
1130 **Lunch**
    Soup (whole bowl)
    Milk (1/2 carton)
    Tea (1 cup)
    Jell-O (1 serving)
1330 *Voided 450 ml*
1400 *Pop (1 can)*
1430 *Water pitcher 500 ml*
    (refilled)
1530 *Vomited 50 ml*
1730 **Dinner**
    Soup (whole bowl)
    Tea (1 cup)
    Juice (whole glass)
    Ice cream (all)
1730 *Voided 250 ml*
1830 *Vomited 100 ml*
1915 *Voided 500 ml*
2000 *Milk (1 carton)*
2015 *Voided 300 ml*
2330 *Voided 200 ml*

117. Label the plate with numbers so that you can describe the location of food to a blind person. How would tell a visually impaired person who asks you where to find the food items on the plate?

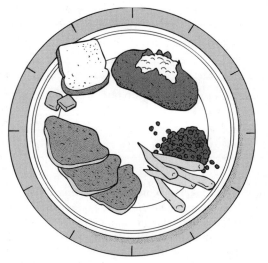

A. Bread _____
B. Baked potato _____
C. Vegetables _____
D. Meat _____

Nursing Assistant Skills Video Exercise
View the **Nutrition and Fluids** *video to answer these questions.*

118. List four factors that can interfere with meeting nutritional needs of patients and residents.
    A. _____
    B. _____
    C. _____
    D. _____

119. Always provide _____ and _____ care when assisting patients and residents with meals.

120. _____ are the most common causes of dysphagia in adults.

121. Dysphagia should be suspected when the person:
    A. _____
    B. _____
    C. _____

122. _____ are the most difficult foods for a person with dysphagia to swallow.

123. Before helping a person with dysphagia with food and fluids, you need to _____
_____.

124. When assisting a person with dysphagia with food and fluids, you need to report signs of difficulty to the nurse immediately.
    A. True   B. False

125. List four factors that may affect a person's appetite and ability to eat.
    A. _____
    B. _____
    C. _____
    D. _____

126. You need to assist the person with hand washing before and after meals.
    A. True   B. False

127. To prepare Mrs. Burger for meals, the nursing assistant did the following:
    A. _____
    B. _____
    C. _____
    D. _____
    E. _____

128. Serving food promptly ensures that _____.

129. Make sure the tray is complete by _____.

130. The _____ and the _____ tell you what observations and measurements are needed.

131. To make sure the tray is complete, ask the patient or resident if the correct food and needed items are present.
    A. True   B. False

132. Always explain what foods are on the tray and where
they are located.
A. True   B. False

133. _____ can help
relieve feelings of helplessness and loss of control.

134. Letting the person help to the extent possible is
important for_____
_____.

135. Before feeding a person, you need to review:
A. _____
B. _____

136. You need to report signs and symptoms of dysphagia
to the nurse when you finish feeding the person.
A. True   B. False

137. Food is served in the order preferred by the person.
A. True   B. False

138. Checking for food that becomes pocketed in the
mouth helps prevent _____ and
_____.

139. When a person has finished eating, you need to:
A. _____
B. _____
C. _____
D. _____
E. _____
F. _____
G. _____
H. _____
I. _____
J. _____

View the **Measurements** *video to answer these questions.*
140. Calibrated containers are used to measure intake and
output. They are measured at eye level.
A. True   B. False

141. If you are careful, there is no need to wear gloves
when measuring output.
A. True   B. False

142. When measuring intake, you need to follow these steps:
A. _____
B. _____
C. _____
D. _____

143. Intake and output have been ordered for Mr.
Bernardo. Why is it important to remind him to use
the signal light when the specimen container or urinal
needs emptying? _____
_____

Optional Learning Exercises

144. This is a person's food intake for 1 day. Place the foods
in the correct food group on MyPyramid.

Breakfast	Lunch	Dinner
3/4 cup orange juice	1 cup tomato soup	2 pork chops (4 oz)
1 cup oatmeal	Grilled cheese sandwich	Baked potato/butter
2 slices toast	1/2 cup applesauce	1/4 cup green beans
1/4 cup milk	Can of regular soda	2 brownies
2 cups black coffee	Candy bar	2 cups black coffee

Snacks
1 apple
1 bag potato chips (4 oz)
1/3 cup nuts
Can of regular soda
1/2 cup ice cream

A. Grains _____
_____

B. Vegetables _____
_____

C. Fruits _____
_____

D. Milk _____

E. Meat and beans _____
_____

F. Oils _____
_____

G. Other _____
_____

145. Which group or groups meet the needs for daily
servings? _____
_____

146. Which group or groups do not meet the needs for
daily servings? _____
_____

Independent Learning Activities
Now that you have learned about good nutrition, use this exercise to find out whether you eat a nutritious diet.
List your intake for 1 day. Be sure to include the amount of each item. Remember, the portion size is important.
Group the foods and liquids you eat according to the parts of MyPyramid. If you wish, you may go to
www.MyPyramid.gov and follow the directions there to group the foods. Answer the following questions:
○ How many servings did you eat of grains? How many of these servings were whole grain?
○ How many servings of fruit did you eat? How many were fresh fruit? Canned fruit? Fruit juice? Had added sugars?
○ How many vegetable servings did you eat? How many were raw? Cooked? How much sodium was contained in
prepared vegetables?
○ How many servings of milk and milk products did you eat? How many were low-fat or fat-free?
○ How many servings of meat and beans did you eat? How many were high in fat? Low in fat? High in sodium?

- How many foods did you eat that count as oils?
- In which food groups are you meeting your daily needs?
- In which groups do you need to increase your intake? Decrease your intake?
- How much physical activity did you include in your daily plan?
- After completing this exercise, what changes in your diet and activity level will you consider?

- **Role-play with a classmate and take turns feeding each other as you would a resident. You may choose any spoon-fed foods you wish. (Pudding, gelatin, and soup are suggestions.) You should also give a beverage to the person.** *After you have fed each other, answer these questions:*
  - How were your physical needs met before you were fed (toileting, hand washing, oral hygiene)?
  - Where were you fed (bed, chair, at a table)? Who made the decision about your location?
  - Which food was offered first? Who made the choice of how food was offered? Were you offered a variety of foods?
  - When was a beverage offered? Between food items? Only at the end of feeding? How did the person feeding you decide the order of foods and beverages? The temperature of these items?
  - When you were being fed, how was the nursing assistant positioned? Sitting? Standing? How did the person's position make you feel?
  - What kind of conversation was carried on while you were eating? What chances were offered to rest while you were eating? Did you feel relaxed or rushed?
  - After this exercise, what will you do differently when you feed a resident?

23 Nutritional Support and IV Therapy

Key Terms
Aspiration
Enteral nutrition
Flow rate
Gastrostomy tube

Gavage
Intravenous (IV) therapy
Jejunostomy tube
Nasoduodenal tube

Nasogastric (NG) tube
Nasointestinal tube
Nasojejunal tube
Parenteral nutrition

Percutaneous endoscopic
  gastrostomy (PEG) tube
Regurgitation

Fill in the Blanks: Key Terms

1. Giving nutrients into the gastrointestinal (GI) tract through a feeding tube is _____ _____ .

2. A _____ is a tube inserted through a surgically created opening in the stomach.

3. A feeding tube inserted through the nose into the jejunum of the small intestine is a _____ _____ .

4. _____ is the backward flow of stomach contents into the mouth.

5. A _____ is a feeding tube inserted into a surgically created opening in the jejunum of the small intestine.

6. The process of giving a tube feeding is called _____ .

7. The _____ is the number of drops per minute.

8. A feeding tube inserted through the nose into the small intestine is a _____ _____ .

9. _____ is breathing fluid or an object into the lungs.

10. Giving nutrients through a catheter inserted into a vein is _____ .

11. A feeding tube inserted through the nose into the small intestine is a _____ _____ .

12. _____ is giving fluids through a needle or catheter inserted into a vein.

13. A feeding tube inserted through the nose into the stomach is a _____ _____ .

14. A _____ is a feeding tube into the stomach through a small incision made through the skin.

Circle the BEST Answer

15. The doctor may order nutritional support for a person who
    A. Cannot eat enough to meet his or her nutritional needs
    B. Has a problem swallowing
    C. Refuses to eat or drink
    D. All of the above

16. Which of these tubes are used for short-term nutritional support?
    A. Nasogastric tubes   C. Jejunostomy tubes
    B. Gastrostomy tubes   D. PEG tubes

17. Opened formula for a gavage feeding can remain at room temperature for
    A. 1 hour   C. About 4 hours
    B. An 8-hour shift   D. Overnight

18. If a person is receiving intermittent (scheduled) feedings, the nurse will
    A. Attach the feeding to a pump
    B. Give feeding four or more times each day
    C. Give the feedings over a 24-hour period
    D. Give the feeding directly from the refrigerator

19. A major risk with tube feedings is
    A. Nausea
    B. Complaints of flatulence
    C. Aspiration
    D. Elevated temperature

20. If a person is receiving a continuous feeding, you should report
    A. Elevated blood pressure
    B. Signs and symptoms of respiratory distress
    C. A normal pulse rate
    D. The person is sleeping

21. You can help prevent regurgitation when a person is receiving gavage when you
    A. Position the person in a left side-lying position
    B. Maintain Fowler's or semi-Fowler's position after the feeding
    C. Position the person in a supine position
    D. Position the person in a prone position

22. When a person is receiving nutrition through a tube, frequent mouth care is needed because
    A. It stimulates peristalsis to aid digestion
    B. It prevents discomfort from dry mouth, dry lips, and sore throat
    C. It provides additional fluid intake
    D. It provides additional nutrition

23. Which of these are *never* done by nursing assistants?
    A. Insert a feeding tube
    B. Remove a feeding tube
    C. Give tube feedings
    D. Clean area around a feeding tube

24. When a person is receiving TPN, the nursing assistant would assist by
    A. Removing the tube
    B. Inserting the tube
    C. Providing frequent oral hygiene and other basic needs
    D. Giving the feedings

25. When caring for a person receiving IV therapy, the nursing assistant can
    A. Adjust the flow rate if it is too fast or too slow
    B. Report to the nurse if no fluid is dripping
    C. Disconnect the IV to give basic care
    D. Change the IV bag when it is empty

26. You may change a dressing on a peripheral IV if
    A. The nurse asks you to do this
    B. You observe that it is loose and soiled
    C. Your state lets nursing assistants perform the procedure
    D. You think you know how to do this procedure

Fill in the Blanks

27. Nasogastric and nasointestinal tubes are in place for short-term nutritional support, usually for less than

    _____.

28. Gastrostomy, jejunostomy, and PEG tubes are used for long-term support, usually longer than _____

    _____.

29. Formula given through a feeding tube is given at room temperature because cold fluids cause

    _____.

30. Coughing, sneezing, vomiting, suctioning, and poor positioning are common causes of _____

    _____.

31. What can the nursing assistant do to assist the nurse in preventing regurgitation and aspiration?
    A. _____
    B. _____
    C. _____

32. What comfort measures will help a person with a feeding tube who has a dry mouth?
    A. _____
    B. _____
    C. _____

33. The nose and nostrils are cleaned every 4 to 8 hours because a feeding tube can _____ and

    _____.

34. If you are delegated to give a tube feeding, what should the nurse check first?
    A. _____
    B. _____

35. How much flushing solution is used before giving a tube feeding to an adult?

    _____

36. When caring for a person receiving IV therapy, what complications would you observe at the IV site?
    A. _____
    B. _____
    C. _____
    D. _____
    E. _____

Crossword

Fill in the crossword by answering the clues below with the words from this list:

Enteral	Nasoduodenal
Gastrostomy	Nasointestinal
Gavage	Nasojejunal
Jejunostomy	PEG
Nasogastric	

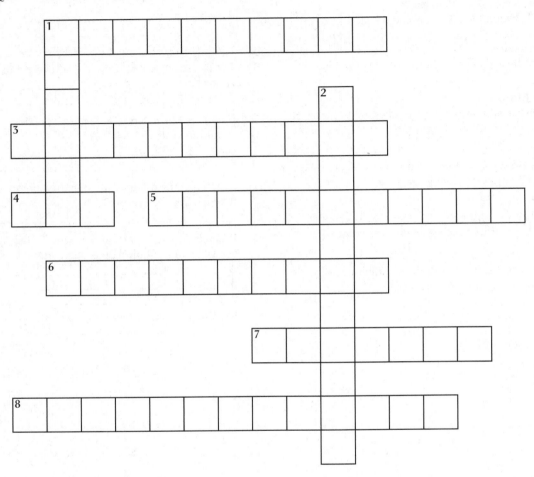

ACROSS

1. A tube inserted through a surgically created opening into the stomach
3. A feeding tube inserted through the nose into the duodenum of the small intestine
4. A feeding tube inserted into the stomach through a small incision made through the skin
5. A feeding tube inserted into a surgically created opening in the jejunum of the small intestine
6. A feeding tube inserted through the nose into the jejunum of the small intestine
7. Giving nutrition into the gastrointestinal tract through a feeding tube
8. A feeding tube inserted through the nose into the small intestine

DOWN

1. The process of giving a tube feeding
2. A feeding tube inserted through the nose into the stomach

Optional Learning Exercises

37. What type of feeding tube would each of these persons probably have in place?

A. The nurse tells you Mr. S. is expected to have a feeding tube to his stomach for 2-3 weeks.

_____

B. Mrs. G. has had a feeding tube in her stomach for 9 months. _____ or
_____

C. The nurse tells you to observe Mr. H. for irritation of his nose and nostril when you give care.
_____ or _____

D. The nurse tells you that Mrs. K. is at great risk for regurgitation from her feeding tube.
_____ or _____

38. Why is formula sometimes warmed to room temperature and at other times, ice chips are used to cool it?

A. Warmed when _____

B. Kept cool when _____

39. Why are older persons more at risk for regurgitation and aspiration?

A. _____

B. _____

40. What would you do if a person with a feeding tube asks you for something to eat or drink?
_____ Why? _____
_____

41. Mrs. H. has a feeding tube in her nose. Answer these questions about caring for her nose and nostrils:

A. How often should the nose and nostrils be cleaned? _____

B. How is the tube secured to the nose? _____

C. Why is the tube secured to the person's garment at the shoulder? _____
_____

D. What are two ways the tube can be secured at the shoulder?

i. _____

ii. _____

42. When giving tube feedings, what answers would you likely get if you asked the nurse these questions?

A. What feeding method is used? _____

B. What size syringe is used? _____

C. How is the person positioned for the feeding?
_____

D. How is the person positioned after the feeding?
_____

E. How high is the syringe raised or the feeding bag hung? _____

F. How much fluid is used to flush the tubing?
_____

G. How fast is the feeding given if using a syringe?
_____

43. If a person is receiving TPN, how will you assist the nurse?

A. _____

B. _____

C. _____

44. How can you check the flow rate of an IV?
_____

45. What would you tell the RN at once when you check the flow rate?

A. _____

B. _____

C. _____

46. When you assist the person with an IV in turning and repositioning, how should the IV bag be handled?

A. _____

B. _____

Independent Learning Activities

- Have you or anyone you know ever needed enteral nutrition? Either answer these questions or ask the person you know to answer them:
  - How long was the tube in place? What type of tube was used?
  - What discomfort or pain was felt?
  - How did having a feeding tube affect your activity? Your personal care and grooming?
- Have you ever had an IV? Answer these questions about the experience:
  - What type of IV did you have? Where was it inserted?
  - How long was the IV in place?
  - How did the IV interfere with your care, grooming, or activity?
- You may care for a person who is not receiving any nutritional support or IV therapy. Answer these questions about how you handle this situation:
  - How would you feel about caring for a person who is not receiving any nutritional support?
  - How would your religious or cultural values affect you in this situation?
  - If the situation made you uncomfortable, what would you do?

24 Exercise and Activity

Key Terms

Abduction
Adduction
Ambulation
Atrophy
Contracture
Deconditioning

Dorsiflexion
Extension
External rotation
Flexion
Footdrop

Hyperextension
Internal rotation
Orthostatic hypotension
Plantar flexion
Postural hypotension

Pronation
Range of motion (ROM)
Rotation
Supination
Syncope

Fill in the Blanks: Key Terms

1. If _____ is present, the foot is bent down at the ankle.

2. A brief loss of consciousness or fainting is _____ _____.

3. Bending a body part is _____.

4. Moving a body part away from the midline of the body is _____.

5. _____ is the movement of a joint to the extent possible without causing pain.

6. Turning the joint outward is _____.

7. A drop in blood pressure when the person stands is postural hypotension or _____.

8. _____ occurs when moving a body part toward the midline of the body.

9. Turning the joint upward is called _____.

10. Bending the toes and foot up at the ankle is _____.

11. Excessive straightening of a body part is _____.

12. A decrease in size or the wasting away of tissue is _____.

13. Turning the joint is _____.

14. _____ is straightening of a body part.

15. _____ is another name for orthostatic hypotension.

16. _____ is permanent plantar flexion; the foot falls down at the ankle.

17. The act of walking is _____.

18. _____ is turning the joint downward.

19. The loss of muscle strength from inactivity is _____.

20. _____ is turning the joint inward.

21. The lack of joint mobility caused by abnormal shortening of a muscle is a _____.

Circle the BEST Answer

22. If a person is on bedrest, he or she
    A. May be allowed to perform some activities of daily living (ADL)
    B. May use the bedside commode for elimination needs
    C. May not perform any activities of daily living
    D. May use the bathroom for elimination needs

23. Complications of bedrest include all of these *except*
    A. Contractures in fingers, wrists, knees, and hips
    B. Muscle atrophy
    C. Increased appetite and improved muscle strength
    D. Orthostatic hypotension and syncope

24. If a contracture develops
    A. It will require extra range-of-motion exercises to correct it
    B. You need to position the person in good body alignment
    C. The person is permanently deformed and disabled
    D. It will be relieved as soon as the person is able to walk and exercise

25. When you are caring for a person who has orthostatic hypotension, you should
    A. Raise the head of the bed slowly to Fowler's position
    B. Have the person get out of bed quickly to prevent weakness
    C. Keep the bed flat when getting the person out of bed
    D. Have the person walk around to decrease weakness and dizziness

26. Nursing care that prevents complications from bedrest includes all of these *except*
    A. Positioning in good body alignment
    B. Range-of-motion exercises
    C. Frequent position changes
    D. Deconditioning

27. If a person sitting on the edge of the bed complains of weakness, dizziness, or spots before the eyes, you should
    A. Assist the person to stand
    B. Help the person to sit in a chair or walk around
    C. Help the person to Fowler's position
    D. Tell the person that is a normal response and continue to get the person up

28. Bed boards are used to
    A. Keep the person in alignment by preventing the mattress from sagging
    B. Prevent plantar flexion that can lead to footdrop
    C. Keep the hips abducted
    D. Keep the weight of top linens off the feet

29. Plantar flexion must be prevented to
    A. Keep the feet from bending down at the ankle (footdrop)
    B. Keep the hips from rotating outward
    C. Keep the wrist, thumb, and fingers in normal position
    D. Maintain good body alignment
30. To prevent the hips and legs from turning outward, you can use
    A. Bed cradles   C. Trochanter rolls
    B. Hip abduction wedges   D. Splints
31. Exercise occurs when
    A. Activities of daily living (ADL) are done
    B. The person turns and moves in bed without help
    C. The person uses a trapeze to lift the trunk off the bed
    D. All of the above
32. When another person moves the joints through their range of motion, it is called
    A. Active range-of-motion
    B. Activities of daily living
    C. Active-assistive range-of-motion
    D. Passive range-of-motion
33. A nursing assistant can perform range-of-motion exercises on the _____ only if allowed by center policy.
    A. Shoulder   C. Hip
    B. Neck   D. Knee
34. A goal in rehabilitation is to
    A. Have the person recover all functions
    B. Improve the person's independence so he or she can go home
    C. Give complete care and meet all of the person's needs
    D. Perform only passive range-of-motion
35. When exercising the wrist, you will perform all of these motions *except*
    A. Abduction   C. Flexion
    B. Hyperextension   D. Extension
36. Which joint is adducted and abducted?
    A. Neck   C. Forearm
    B. Hip   D. Knee
37. When you help a person walk, you should
    A. Apply a gait (transfer) belt
    B. Help the person lean on furniture to walk around room
    C. Put soft socks on the feet without shoes
    D. Let the person walk without any help
38. When the person is walking with crutches, the person should wear
    A. Soft slippers on the feet
    B. Clothes that fit well
    C. Clothes that are loose
    D. A gait belt
39. When walking with a cane, it is held
    A. On the strong side of the body
    B. On the weak side of the body
    C. In the right hand
    D. On the left side of the body

40. When a person is using a walker, it is
    A. Picked up and moved 3 to 4 inches in front of the person
    B. Moved forward with a rocking motion
    C. Moved first on the left side and then on the right
    D. Picked up and moved 6 to 8 inches in front of the person
41. When you are caring for a person who wears a brace, it is important to report at once
    A. How far the person walks
    B. What care the person can do alone
    C. The amount of mobility in joints when doing range-of-motion exercises
    D. Any redness or signs of skin breakdown when you remove a brace
42. Recreational activity is important for all of these reasons *except*
    A. It forces the person to find new interests
    B. Joints and muscles are exercised
    C. Circulation is stimulated
    D. Activities are mentally stimulating

Fill in the Blanks

43. To prevent deconditioning, is it important to promote _____ and _____ in all persons to the extent possible.

44. Bedrest is ordered to:
    A. _____
    B. _____
    C. _____
    D. _____
    E. _____

45. The nurse tells you the resident is on bedrest but can use the bathroom for elimination. This means the resident is ordered _____.

46. When a person has a contracture, the person is _____ deformed and disabled.

47. When a person is moved from lying or sitting to a standing position, the blood pressure may _____. This is called _____.

48. Supportive devices such as bed boards are used to _____ and _____ the person in a certain position.

49. When you use a foot board, the soles of the feet are _____ against it to prevent _____.

50. A trochanter roll is placed along the body to prevent the hips and legs from _____.

51. Handrolls or handgrips prevent _____ of the thumb, fingers, and wrists.

52. A device used to keep the wrist, thumb, and fingers in normal position is a _____.

53. Bed cradles are used because the weight of top linens can cause _____ and _____.

54. A trapeze bar allows the person to lift the _____ off the bed. It also allows the person to _____ and _____ in bed.

55. When a person does exercises with some help, the person is doing _____ range-of-motion exercises.

56. When range-of-motion exercises are done, what should be reported or recorded?
    A. _____
    B. _____
    C. _____
    D. _____
    E. _____

57. When performing range-of-motion, each movement should be repeated _____ times or the _____.

58. List the rules to follow when performing range-of-motion.
    A. _____
    B. _____
    C. _____
    D. _____
    E. _____
    F. _____
    G. _____
    H. _____

59. When you help a person walk, you should walk to the _____ and _____ the person. Provide support with the _____, or have_____ _____.

60. Many people prefer a walker because it gives more support than a _____.

61. When recreational activities are offered, it protects the person's right to _____.

Labeling

62. ROM exercises for the _____ joint are shown in these drawings. Name the movements shown in each drawing.
    A. _____
    B. _____
    C. _____

63. ROM exercises for the _____ are shown in these drawings. Name the movements shown in each drawing.
    A. _____
    B. _____

64. ROM exercises for the _____ are shown in these drawings. Name the movements shown in each drawing.
    A. _____
    B. _____
    C. _____
    D. _____

Crossword

Fill in the crossword by answering the clues below with the words from this list:

Abduction   Rotation
Adduction   Internal rotation
Extension   External rotation
Flexion   Plantar flexion
Hyperextension   Pronation
Dorsiflexion   Supination

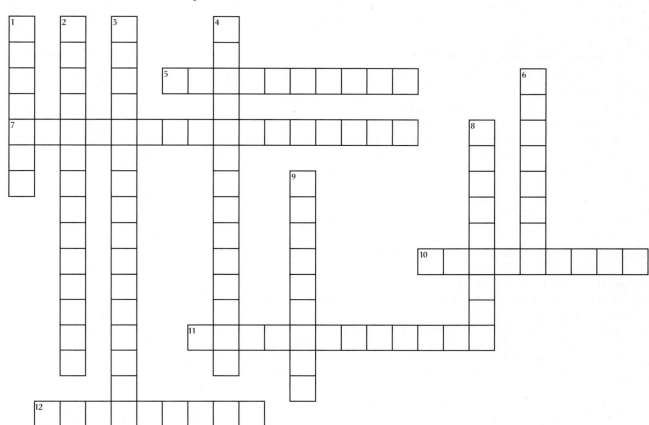

ACROSS
  5. Turning the joint upward
  7. Turning the joint inward
10. Straightening a body part
11. Bending the toes and foot up at the ankle
12. Turning the joint downward

DOWN
  1. Bending a body part
  2. Bending the foot down at the ankle
  3. Turning the joint outward
  4. Excessive straightening of a body part
  6. Turning the joint
  8. Moving a body part from the midline of the body
  9. Moving a body part toward the midline of the body

Nursing Assistant Skills Video
View the related portions of the **Body Mechanics and Exercise** *video to answer these questions.*

65. Being active is important for _____ and _____ well-being.

66. Inactivity affects normal function of every body system and the person's mental well-being.
    A. True
    B. False

67. You are performing range-of-motion exercises on a patient. How many times do you need to repeat ROM to each joint? _____ or _____
_____

68. Signs and symptoms of orthostatic hypotension include:
    A. _____
    B. _____
    C. _____
    D. _____

Optional Learning Exercises

69. What kind of range of motion would be used with each of these residents?
A. The resident needs complete care for bathing, grooming, and feeding.

    _____

B. The resident takes part in many activities in the center. She walks to most activities independently.

    _____

C. The resident has weakness on his left side. He is able to feed himself but needs help with bathing and dressing.

    _____

70. As you plan to help a person out of bed, you are concerned about orthostatic hypotension. To make sure the person is able to stand and get up safely, you plan to take the blood pressure, pulse, and respirations several times. When would you take the blood pressure?
A. _____
B. _____
C. _____
D. _____
E. _____

71. When doing range-of-motion exercises, you should ask the person if he or she:
A. _____
B. _____

72. When you ambulate a person, what observations are reported and recorded?
A. _____
B. _____
C. _____
D. _____
E. _____

73. How does the person use a standard walker?
A. _____
B. _____
C. _____

74. Why does the nurse assess the skin under braces every shift? _____

Independent Learning Activities

- Role-play with a classmate and take turns acting as the nursing assistant and a person with left-sided weakness. Perform range-of-motion exercises on the person. Answer these questions about how you felt after this activity:
  ○ What did the nursing assistant explain to you before performing the exercises?
  ○ How were you positioned for exercising? What did the nursing assistant ask about your comfort and personal wishes in the position used?
  ○ How was your privacy maintained? Was there anything that made you feel exposed or embarrassed?
  ○ How were your joints supported during the exercises? Did you feel any discomfort or pain during the exercises?
  ○ What exercises were you encouraged to carry out independently? With some assistance?
  ○ Which exercises were done first? Were the exercises carried out in an organized pattern? How did you know what exercise would be done next?
  ○ After this activity, what will you do differently when giving range-of-motion exercises to a person?
- With a classmate, role-play assisting a weak, older person to ambulate. Take turns acting as the person and the nursing assistant. Answer these questions about how you felt and what you learned:
  ○ What did the nursing assistant tell you before preparing to walk with you? What choices were offered about the time you were to ambulate, what clothing to wear, and where you were going to walk?
  ○ What safety devices were used? What did the nursing assistant tell you about the devices or equipment used?
  ○ What assessments were made before you sat up? When you dangled? After walking?
  ○ How did the nursing assistant make you feel secure during ambulation? How did the nursing assistant hold you?
  ○ What did you learn from this activity that will help you when you ambulate a person?

25 Comfort, Rest, and Sleep

Key Terms

Acute pain
Chronic pain
Circadian rhythm
Comfort
Discomfort

Distraction
Enuresis
Guided imagery
Insomnia

NREM sleep
Pain
Phantom pain
Radiating pain

Relaxation
REM sleep
Rest
Sleep

Fill in the Blanks: Key Terms

1. Another name for discomfort is _____.

2. _____ is pain that is felt suddenly from injury, disease, trauma, or surgery; it generally lasts less than 6 months.

3. _____ is a way to change a person's center of attraction.

4. A state of unconsciousness, reduced voluntary muscle activity, and lowered metabolism is _____.

5. Pain lasting longer than 6 months is _____. It may be constant or occur off and on.

6. _____ is to be free from mental or physical stress.

7. _____ is a state of well-being. The person has no physical or emotional pain and is calm and at peace.

8. To be calm, at ease, and relaxed is to _____. The person is free of anxiety and stress.

9. Creating and focusing on an image is _____.

10. The stage of sleep when there is rapid eye movement is _____.

11. _____ is a chronic condition in which the person cannot sleep or stay asleep throughout the night.

12. The day-night cycle or body rhythm is also called _____. This daily rhythm is based on a 24-hour cycle.

13. _____ is pain felt at the site of tissue damage and in nearby areas.

14. To ache, hurt, or be sore is _____. It is also called pain.

15. _____ is the phase of deep sleep when there is no rapid eye movement.

16. Pain felt in a body part that is no longer there is _____.

17. Urinary incontinence in bed at night is _____.

Circle the BEST Answer

18. Rest and sleep are needed
    A. For well-being and energy
    B. To decrease function and quality of life
    C. To increase muscle strength
    D. All of the above

19. OBRA requirements related to comfort, rest, and sleep include
    A. Only two people in a room
    B. Bright lighting in all areas
    C. Room temperature between 65° and 71° F
    D. Adequate ventilation and room humidity

20. When a person complains of pain
    A. The person has pain
    B. It must be carefully measured to see if the person really has pain
    C. You can easily measure to find out how much pain is present
    D. You can tell if the person really has pain by the way he or she acts

21. When a person complains of pain that is nearby an area of tissue damage, this is _____ pain.
    A. Acute   C. Radiating
    B. Chronic   D. Phantom

22. If pain is ignored or denied, it may be because the person thinks pain is a sign of weakness. Which factor that affects pain would this be?
    A. Attention
    B. Past experience
    C. Value or meaning of pain
    D. Support from others

23. A person from Mexico may react to pain by
    A. Showing a strong emotional response
    B. Appearing very stoic
    C. Accepting pain quietly
    D. Viewing it as the will of God

24. When a person has anxiety, the person
    A. Will usually feel increased pain
    B. Will usually feel less pain
    C. May deny having pain
    D. May be stoic and show no reaction to pain

25. When you ask a person "Where is the pain?," you are asking the person to
    A. Describe the pain
    B. Explain the intensity of the pain
    C. Tell you the onset and duration of the pain
    D. Tell you the location of the pain

26. When a person tells you he has pain when coughing or deep breathing, this is
    A. A factor causing pain
    B. A measurement of the onset of pain
    C. Words used to describe the pain
    D. The location of the pain

27. A distraction measure to promote comfort and relieve pain may be
    A. Focusing on an image
    B. Learning to breathe deeply and slowly
    C. Listening to music or playing games
    D. Contracting and relaxing muscle groups

28. If the nurse has given a person pain medication, it is best if you
    A. Give the person a bath
    B. Walk the person according to the care plan
    C. Wait one-half hour before giving care
    D. Give care before the medication makes the person sleepy

29. You may help promote comfort and relieve pain by doing all of these *except*
    A. Allow family members and friends at the bedside as requested by the person
    B. Keep the room brightly lit and play loud music
    C. Provide blankets for warmth and to prevent chilling
    D. Use touch to provide comfort

30. You can help promote rest by doing all of these *except*
    A. Meeting physical needs such as thirst, hunger, and elimination needs
    B. Making sure the person feels safe
    C. Allowing the person to practice rituals or routines before resting
    D. Giving care at a time most convenient to you

31. When caring for an ill or injured person, you know the person may need more rest. You can help the person get rest by making sure you
    A. Provide plenty of exercise to prevent weakness
    B. Provide rest periods during or after a procedure
    C. Give complete hygiene and grooming measures quickly
    D. Spend time talking with the person to distract him or her

32. Which of these does *not* occur during sleep?
    A. The person is unaware of the environment
    B. Metabolism is reduced
    C. Vital signs (blood pressure, temperature, pulse, respirations) increase
    D. There are no voluntary arm or leg movements

33. Some people function better in the morning because of
    A. The circadian rhythm
    B. Getting enough sleep
    C. Interference with the body rhythm
    D. Changes in the work schedule

34. During REM sleep, the person
    A. Is hard to arouse
    B. Has a gradual fall in vital signs
    C. Is easily aroused
    D. Has tension in voluntary muscles

35. Which stage of sleep is usually not repeated during the cycles of sleep?
    A. REM
    B. Stage 1: NREM
    C. Stage 2: NREM
    D. Stage 3: NREM

36. Which age-group requires the least amount of sleep?
    A. Toddlers
    B. Young adults
    C. Adolescents
    D. Older adults

37. Which of these factors increases the need for sleep?
    A. Illness
    B. Weight loss
    C. Emotional problems
    D. Drugs and other substances

38. When a person takes sleeping pills, sleep may not restore the person mentally because
    A. Caffeine prevents sleep
    B. Some have difficulty falling asleep
    C. The length of REM sleep is reduced
    D. It upsets the usual sleep routines

39. Exercise should be avoided for 2 hours before sleep because
    A. It requires energy
    B. People usually feel good after exercise
    C. It causes the release of substances in the bloodstream that stimulate the body
    D. The person tires after exercise

40. Persons who are ill or in intensive care units are at great risk for
    A. Sleep deprivation
    B. Sleepwalking
    C. Insomnia
    D. Increased sleep times

41. If a person has decreased reasoning, red and puffy eyes, and coordination problems, report this to the nurse because the person
    A. Is having a reaction to sleeping medications
    B. Has signs and symptoms of sleep disorders
    C. Needs more exercise before bedtime
    D. May need an increase in sleeping pills

42. Which of these measures *would not* help promote sleep?
    A. Provide blankets or socks for those who tend to be cold
    B. Have the person void or make sure incontinent persons are clean and dry
    C. Follow bedtime rituals
    D. Offer the person a cup of coffee or tea at bedtime

Fill in the Blanks

43. OBRA has requirements about the person's room. List the requirements that relate to each of these:
    A. Suspended curtain _____
    B. Linens _____
    C. Bed _____
    D. Room temperature _____
    E. Persons in room _____

44. Name the type of pain described:
    A. A person with an amputated leg may still sense leg pain. _____
    B. There is tissue damage. The pain decreases with healing. _____
    C. Pain from a heart attack is often felt in the left chest, left jaw, left shoulder, and left arm. _____
    D. The pain remains long after healing. Common causes are arthritis and cancer. _____

45. What is the reason persons from the Philippines may appear stoic in reaction to pain? _____

46. Older persons may ignore or deny new pain because:
    A. _____
    B. _____

47. Persons with dementia may signal pain by changes _____.

48. When gathering information about a person in pain, you can use a scale of 0 to 10. Which end of the scale is the most severe pain? _____

49. What happens to vital signs when the person has acute pain? _____

50. When the person uses words to describe pain such as aching, knifelike, or sore, what do you report to the nurse? _____

51. What body responses may be signs or symptoms that the person has pain?
    A. _____
    B. _____
    C. _____
    D. _____
    E. _____

52. What changes in these behaviors may be symptoms of pain?
    A. Speech _____
    B. Affected body part _____
    C. Body position _____

53. List nursing measures to promote comfort and relieve pain related to these clues:
    A. Position of the person _____
    B. Linens _____
    C. Blankets _____
    D. Pain medications _____
    E. Family members _____

54. If a person is receiving strong pain medication or sedatives, what safety measures are important?
    A. _____
    B. _____
    C. _____
    D. _____

55. When you explain the procedure before performing it, you may help a person rest better because you met the need for _____.

56. A clean, neat, and uncluttered room can promote rest by meeting _____ needs.

57. The mind and body rest, the body saves energy, and body functions slow during _____.

58. Mental restoration occurs during a phase of sleep called _____.

59. The deepest stage of sleep occurs during _____.

60. If work hours change, it can affect the normal _____ cycle or _____ rhythm.

61. Alcohol tends to cause drowsiness and sleep, but it interferes with _____.

62. Insomnia may be caused by:
    A. Fear of _____
    B. Afraid of not _____
    C. Fear of not being able _____
    D. Physical and emotional _____

63. When a person has dementia and wanders at night, the best approach for some persons is to allow _____.

Optional Learning Exercises

64. You are caring for two residents who both have arthritis. Mr. Forman tells you this is the first time he has had any health problems. Mrs. Wegman tells you she has had several surgeries and has had three children. Which of these two persons is likely to be more anxious about the pain and to be unable to handle the pain well? _____ Why? _____

65. Mr. Forman tells you his pain seems much worse at night. What could be the reason for this reaction? _____

66. You are caring for Mrs. Reynolds. She tells you she misses her children who have moved to another state. Today, Mrs. Reynolds is complaining of pain in her abdomen. In spite of providing nursing comfort measures, she still rates her pain at a 7. What is a possible reason Mrs. Reynolds is not getting relief of her pain? _____

67. When a person is ill, how do these affect sleep?
    A. Treatments and therapies _____
    B. Care devices such as traction or a cast _____
    C. Emotions that affect sleep include _____

68. Certain foods affect sleep. Tell how these foods affect sleep, and list foods that contain the substances.
    A. Caffeine _____ sleep. It is found in _____.
    B. L-tryptophan _____ sleep. It is found in _____.

Independent Learning Activities

- Form a group with several classmates and share your personal experiences with pain. Discuss these questions to understand the different ways you respond to pain and treat the pain:
  - What experiences have you had with pain? Accidents? Illnesses? Childbirth? Surgery?
  - What type of pain have you had? Acute? Chronic? Other types?
  - How would you rate your pain on a scale of 0 to 10? How long did it last?
  - How did your family and friends respond to your pain? How much support did you receive from them? How did the support (or lack of it) affect the pain?
  - What measures were used to treat the pain? What was the most effective? The least effective?
  - What did you learn from this discussion with others about their pain? How will this help you as you care for others with pain?
- Form a group with several classmates to talk about differences in sleep habits. Answer these questions to understand differences in personal practices concerning rest and sleep:
  - How many hours do you sleep each day? How many hours of sleep do you think you *should* get each day?
  - If you did not have to follow a schedule (work, school, etc), when would you go to bed and wake up?
  - What rituals do you perform before going to bed? How is your sleep affected if you cannot perform these rituals?
  - What factors interfere with your sleep? What do you do to avoid these factors?
  - When do you feel most alert? Morning? Afternoon? Night?
  - How do you feel when you wake up? Alert? Pleasant? Grouchy? Tired?
  - How often do you take naps? What time of day do you like to nap? How do you feel when you wake from a nap?
  - How will this discussion help you understand differences in sleep patterns when you are caring for others? How will it affect how you help the persons you care for to get the rest and sleep they need?

26 Oxygen Needs

Key Terms

Allergy	Hemothorax	Kussmaul respirations	Pneumothorax
Apnea	Hyperventilation	Mechanical ventilation	Pollutant
Biot's respirations	Hypoventilation	Orthopnea	Respiratory arrest
Bradypnea	Hypoxemia	Orthopneic position	Respiratory depression
Cheyne-Stokes	Hypoxia	Oxygen concentration	Suction
Dyspnea	Intubation	Pleural effusion	Tachypnea
Hemoptysis			

Fill in the Blanks: Key Terms

1. _____ are respirations that are rapid and deep followed by 10 to 30 seconds of apnea.

2. Bloody sputum is called _____.

3. _____ is inserting an artificial airway.

4. Air in the pleural space is _____.

5. Rapid breathing in which respirations are usually more than 24 per minute is called _____.

6. An _____ is a sensitivity to a substance that causes the body to react with signs and symptoms.

7. Difficult, labored, or painful breathing is _____.

8. _____ is blood in the pleural space.

9. Being able to breathe deeply and comfortably only while sitting is _____.

10. Respirations that are fewer than 12 per minute is slow breathing or _____.

11. A reduced amount of oxygen in the blood is _____.

12. _____ describes slow, weak respirations that occur at a rate of fewer than 12 per minute.

13. The lack or absence of breathing is_____.

14. _____ is a pattern of respirations that is rapid and deeper than normal.

15. Using a machine to move air into and out of the lungs is _____.

16. A harmful chemical or substance in the air or water is a _____.

17. The process of withdrawing or sucking up fluid is _____.

18. _____ are respirations that gradually increase in rate and depth and then become shallow and slow. Breathing may stop for 10 to 20 seconds.

19. The _____ is sitting up and leaning over a table to breathe.

20. The escape and collection of fluid in the pleural space is _____.

21. When breathing stops, it is _____.

22. Very deep and rapid respirations are _____.

23. _____ is the amount of hemoglobin containing oxygen.

24. When cells do not have enough oxygen, it is called _____.

25. Respirations that are slow, shallow, and sometimes irregular is _____.

Circle the BEST Answer

26. Capillaries and cells must exchange O_2 and CO_2 in the
    A. Respiratory system   C. Nervous system
    B. Cardiovascular system D. Red blood cells

27. Oxygen needs increase when
    A. The person is aging
    B. Drugs are taken
    C. The person has fever or pain
    D. The person is well-nourished

28. Respiratory depression can occur when
    A. The person exercises
    B. Allergies are present
    C. Narcotic drugs are taken in large doses
    D. The person smokes

29. Restlessness is an early sign of
    A. Hypoxia   C. Hyperventilation
    B. Apnea   D. Bradypnea

30. Which of these would not be a sign of hypoxia?
    A. Disorientation and confusion
    B. Decrease in pulse rate and respirations
    C. Apprehension and anxiety
    D. Cyanosis of the skin, mucous membranes, and nail beds

31. When you prepare a person for a chest x-ray, you
    A. Make sure the person does not eat for several hours before the test
    B. Help the person to remove all clothing and jewelry from the waist to the neck
    C. Tell the person not drink any fluids before the x-ray
    D. Keep the person on bedrest for at least 1 hour before the x-ray

32. If you are caring for a person who just had a pulmonary function test, you would expect the person to
    A. Tell you he has chest pain
    B. Be very tired
    C. Have hemoptysis
    D. Complain of nausea and vomiting
33. If a pulse oximeter is being used on a person with tremors or poor circulation, which of these sites would be best to use?
    A. A toe on a foot that is swollen
    B. A finger that has nail polish on the nail
    C. A toe with an open wound
    D. An earlobe
34. When you are delegated to place a pulse oximeter on a person, report to the nurse if
    A. The person is sleeping
    B. The person's pulse does not equal the pulse on the display
    C. You remove nail polish on the nail before attaching the pulse oximeter
    D. You tape the oximeter in place
35. When a person has breathing difficulties, it is usually easier for the person to breathe
    A. In the supine position
    B. Lying on one side for long periods
    C. In the semi-Fowler's or Fowler's position
    D. In the prone position
36. Deep-breathing and coughing exercises
    A. Help prevent pneumonia and atelectasis
    B. Decrease pain after surgery or injury
    C. Are done once a day
    D. Cause mucus to form in the lungs
37. When assisting with coughing and deep breathing, you tell the person to
    A. Inhale through the mouth
    B. Hold the breath for 30 seconds
    C. Exhale slowly through pursed lips
    D. Repeat the exercise 1 or 2 times
38. When a person uses an incentive spirometer, it allows the person to
    A. Take shallow breaths
    B. See air movement when inhaling
    C. See air movement with exhaling
    D. Exhale quickly
39. If a person is receiving oxygen, you may
    A. Set the flow rate
    B. Apply the oxygen device to the person
    C. Set up the system
    D. Turn on the oxygen
40. If you are caring for a person with oxygen therapy, you may *not*
    A. Start and maintain oxygen therapy
    B. Remove the mask for meals
    C. Tell the nurse if the rate is too high or too low
    D. Check for irritation from the device
41. If a person receives oxygen through a nasal cannula, it is important to look for irritation
    A. On the nose, ears, and cheekbones
    B. Under the mask
    C. In the throat
    D. In the oral cavity

42. If you are delegated to set up for oxygen administration, you will do all of these *except*
    A. Collect the device with connecting tubing
    B. Attach the flow meter to the wall outlet or tank
    C. Apply the oxygen administration device to the person
    D. Fill the humidifier with distilled water
43. If you are near a person receiving oxygen, which of these should you report?
    A. The humidifier is bubbling
    B. The humidifier has enough water
    C. The humidifier is not bubbling
    D. The person is in a semi-Fowler's position
44. If you are caring for a person with an artificial airway, your care should always include
    A. Removing the device to clean it
    B. Comforting and reassuring the person that the airway helps breathing
    C. Suctioning to maintain the airway
    D. Making sure the person never takes a tub bath
45. The person with an ET tube can communicate by
    A. Whispering or speaking quietly
    B. Speaking in a normal voice
    C. Using paper and pencil, Magic Slate, or communication boards
    D. Having a family member ask and answer questions
46. When suctioning is done, the nurse
    A. Uses sterile technique and follows Standards Precautions
    B. Makes sure a suction cycle is no more than 20 to 30 seconds
    C. Waits about 5 seconds between each suction cycle
    D. Suctions as many times as needed to clear the airway
47. When you are caring for a person with an artificial airway, tell the nurse at once if
    A. The person needs frequent oral hygiene
    B. If the person feels as if he or she is gagging or choking
    C. If the airway comes out or is dislodged
    D. If the person cannot speak
48. When a person has a tracheostomy, the stoma is
    A. Uncovered when the person is outdoors
    B. Covered with plastic when outdoors to prevent dust from entering
    C. Covered when shaving
    D. Covered with a loose gauze dressing
49. If you are caring for a person with a mechanical ventilator and the alarm sounds, you should first
    A. Get the nurse
    B. Reset the alarms
    C. Reassure the person
    D. Check to see if the person's tube is attached to the ventilator
50. If a person has chest tubes, petrolatum gauze is kept at the bedside to
    A. Cover the insertion site if the chest tube comes out
    B. Lubricate the site of the chest tube
    C. Cleanse the skin around the chest tube
    D. Cover the site of the chest tube insertion

51. To provide safe care to a person with oxygen needs, you do all of these *except*
    A. Make sure a nurse supervises you if you are doing complex tasks
    B. Have necessary training to perform or assist in care
    C. Give oxygen when you understand oxygen therapy and its safety rules
    D. Provide care that will protect the right to privacy

Fill in the Blanks

52. As a person ages, what factors affect the person's oxygen needs?
    A. Respiratory muscles _____
    B. Lung tissue _____
    C. Strength for coughing _____
    D. Risk for respiratory _____

53. Three diseases are caused by or related to smoking. They are:
    A. _____
    B. _____
    C. _____

54. How does alcohol increase the risk of aspiration? It depresses the _____ and reduces the _____ and increases _____.

55. What terms can be used to describe sputum when reporting and recording?
    A. Color: _____
    B. Odor: _____
    C. Consistency: _____
    D. Hemoptysis: _____

56. If you are caring for a person with a pulse oximeter, how is the reading recorded and what do the letters mean?
    A. Recorded as _____
    B. S = _____
    C. P = _____
    D. O$_2$ = _____

57. If a person has difficulty breathing, he or she may prefer a position where the person is sitting
    _____.
    This position is called _____.

58. If a person has a productive cough, what respiratory hygiene and cough etiquette should be taught?
    A. _____
    B. _____
    C. _____
    D. _____

59. If a person is using an incentive spirometer, how long is the breath held to keep the balls floating?
    _____

60. What observations should be reported after a person uses an incentive spirometer?
    A. _____
    B. _____
    C. _____
    D. _____

61. When a person wears a mask to receive oxygen, what should you do when the person needs to eat? _____ How will the person receive oxygen during the meal? _____

62. Oxygen is humidified because it will _____.

63. If you are caring for a person with a tracheostomy, you call the nurse if:
    A. You note signs and symptoms _____
    B. If the outer _____

64. When giving care to a person with a tracheostomy, it is important to cover the stoma because _____.

65. If a person has mechanical ventilation, where do you find a plan for communication? _____ Why is it important for everyone to use the same signals for communication? _____

66. When a person has chest tubes, why is it important to prevent kinks in the tubing?
    _____

Crossword

Fill in the crossword by answering the clues below with the words from this list:

Abnormal respirations   Hyperventilation
Apnea   Hypoventilation
Biot's   Kussmaul
Bradypnea   Orthopnea
Cheyne-Stokes   Tachypnea
Dyspnea

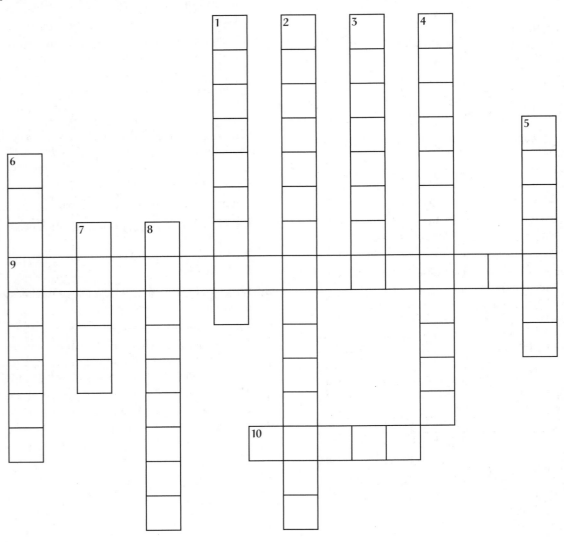

ACROSS

9. Respirations are rapid and deeper than normal
10. Rapid and deep respirations followed by 10 to 30 seconds of apnea; occur with nervous disorders

DOWN

1. Respirations are 24 or more per minute
2. Respirations are slow, shallow, and sometimes irregular
3. Very deep and rapid respirations; signal diabetic coma
4. Respirations gradually increase in rate and depth; common when death is near
5. Difficult, labored, or painful breathing
6. Breathing deeply and comfortably only when sitting
7. Lack or absence of breathing
8. Respirations are fewer than 12 per minute

Optional Learning Exercises

SITUATION: *You are caring for Mr. R., age 84, who has chronic obstructive pulmonary disease. Answer questions 67 and 68 about caring for Mr. R.*

67. What position would make it easier for Mr. R. to breathe when he is in bed?

_____

68. How can you increase his comfort when he sitting up? _____ What is this position called? _____

SITUATION: *Mrs. F. is receiving oxygen through a nasal cannula at 2 L/min. Her respirations are unlabored at 16 per minute unless she is walking about or doing personal care. Then her respirations are 28 and dyspneic. Answer questions 69 through 72 about her care.*

69. Why is there no humidifier with the oxygen set-up for Mrs. F? _____

70. Where should you check for signs of irritation from the cannula? _____ _____

71. You should make sure there are _____ in the tubing and that Mrs. F. does not _____ of the tubing.

72. What are the abnormal respirations called that Mrs. F. has with activity? _____

Independent Learning Activities

Work with a classmate and carry out these exercises. They will help you understand how it feels to be a person with breathing problems.

- Have your partner count your respirations while you are at rest. Then exercise by running or jogging in place for at least 2 minutes. Now have your partner check your respirations again. How have they changed? Rate? Rhythm or pattern? Easy or labored?
- While you exercise, try first to breathe only through your nose. Then try breathing through your mouth. Which way makes you feel you are getting enough air?
- Place a drinking straw in your mouth, and close your lips tightly around it. Now breathe only through the straw while at rest and during exercise. When you are at rest, how comfortable does this feel? Are you getting enough air? How is your air supply during exercise?
- Take a drinking straw and place small pieces of paper in one end so that it is fairly tight. Now try breathing through the straw at rest and exercise. What is the difference between the open and blocked straw? Imagine if every breath you take feels like it does with the blocked straw. This is how many people with breathing problems feel all the time.

Key Terms

Assisted living residence   Medication reminder   Service plan
(ALR)

Fill in the Blanks: Key Terms

1. A _____ is reminding the person to take drugs, observing that they were taken as prescribed, and charting that they were taken.

2. A written plan that lists the services needed by the person and who provides them is a _____.

3. An _____ provides housing, support services, and health care to persons needing help with activities of daily living.

Circle the BEST Answer

4. Which of these persons *would not* be living in an ALR?
   A. Someone who needs help taking drugs at certain times
   B. A person who has problems with thinking, reasoning, and judgment
   C. A person who needs complete care with all ADL
   D. Someone who is lonely and wants to live with people

5. When a person lives in an ALR, one requirement is
   A. At least two rooms and a bath
   B. Both a bathtub and a shower
   C. A door that locks and the person keeps the key
   D. A double or queen-size bed

6. Environmental requirements in an ALR include
   A. Common bathrooms have toilet paper, soap, and cloth towels or a dryer
   B. Pets or animals must be kept in kennels
   C. Hot water temperatures are between 110° F and 130° F
   D. Garbage is stored in covered containers lined with plastic bags that are removed at least once day

7. Which of these is *not* included in the Assisted Living Resident's Rights?
   A. May participate in religious, social, community, and other activities
   B. May communicate privately and freely with any person
   C. Has a doctor or pharmacist assigned by the facility
   D. Must be given information on how residents and others can file complaints

8. An Alzheimer's Special Care Unit provides
   A. Programs that rehabilitate the person to normal function
   B. Activities that provide stimulation and promote the highest level of function
   C. Each person with a private room that locks
   D. A private apartment with cooking facilities

9. A staff member in an ALR would be expected to have training in all of these areas *except*
   A. Assisting with drugs
   B. Early signs of illness and the need for health care
   C. Food preparation, service, and storage
   D. Measuring and giving medications

10. Which of these is a requirement of a resident in an ALR?
    A. The person must be able to leave the building in an emergency
    B. The person may require skilled nursing services
    C. The person has complex nursing problems
    D. The person must not be paralyzed or be chronically ill

11. A service plan for a person in an ALR
    A. Is reviewed every 90 days
    B. Lists the services needed by the person and who provides them
    C. States the medications that the person takes each day
    D. Is reviewed and revised only when needs change

12. Which of these is a service offered in an ALR?
    A. Daily housekeeping
    B. A garage for cars owned by residents
    C. A 24-hour emergency communication system
    D. A bank in the facility

13. Meals in an ALR
    A. Are always served in the person's room
    B. Include the noon meal only
    C. Are posted in a weekly menu
    D. Cannot meet special dietary needs

14. When you assist with housekeeping, you will be expected to
    A. Clean the tub or shower after each use
    B. Put out clean towels and washcloths every week
    C. Use a disinfectant or water and detergent to clean bathroom surfaces once a week
    D. Dust furniture every day

15. A measure you should follow when handling, preparing, or storing foods is
    A. Use leftover food within 4 or 5 days
    B. Wash all pots and pans in a dishwasher
    C. Date and refrigerate containers of leftovers and refrigerate as soon as possible
    D. Clean kitchen appliances, counters, tables, and other surfaces once a day

16. When practicing food safety, which of these is *incorrect*?
    A. Use a garbage disposer for food and liquid garbage
    B. Place leftover food in refrigerator as soon as possible
    C. Wash meat and poultry
    D. Place washed eating and cooling items in a drainer to dry

17. When assisting with laundry, a guideline to follow is
    A. Sort items according to the amount of soil on the items
    B. Wear gloves when handling soiled laundry
    C. Use hot water to wash all items
    D. Use the highest setting on the dryer to sanitize the items
18. When you assist a person with medication, it may involve
    A. Opening containers for person who cannot do so
    B. Measuring the medications for the person
    C. Explaining to a person the action of the medication
    D. Preparing a pill organizer for the person each week
19. If a drug error occurs, you should
    A. Tell the person not to do it again
    B. Make sure the person takes the correct medication at the next scheduled time
    C. Report the error to the nurse
    D. Take all medications away from the person immediately
20. An attendant is needed in an ALR 24 hours a day to
    A. Give care to those who need it
    B. Make sure medications are dispensed when ordered
    C. Assist those who need assistance if an emergency occurs
    D. Provide activities for the residents
21. A resident can be transferred, discharged, or evicted from the ALR if
    A. The facility closes
    B. The person is a threat to the health and safety of self or others
    C. The person fails to pay for services as agreed upon
    D. All of the above
22. Which of these is *not* a right of a resident in assisted living?
    A. The right to confidentiality of the medical record
    B. The right to have overnight guests whenever the resident wishes
    C. The right to refuse to work for the facility
    D. The right to request to relocate or refuse to relocate within the facility

Fill in the Blanks
23. When working in an assisted living setting, you should follow _____ when contact with blood, body fluids, secretions, excretions, or potentially contaminated items is likely.
24. According to the American Association of Retired Persons (AARP), most persons in assisted living settings need help with:
    A. _____
    B. _____
    C. _____
    D. _____
    E. _____
    F. _____
25. Almost half of persons in an ALR are _____.

26. A bathroom in an ALR must provide privacy and:
    A. _____
    B. _____
    C. _____
    D. _____
    E. _____
27. If you are assigned to work on an Alzheimer's unit, you know the staff must have training about _____. Many states require _____.
28. The ALR cannot employ a person with a _____ _____.
29. The service plan lists:
    A. _____
    B. _____
30. The service plan also relates to:
    A. _____
    B. _____
    C. _____
    D. _____
    E. _____
    F. _____
31. A 24-hour emergency communication system is provided to be used for _____ or to _____.
32. The time between the evening meal and breakfast usually is no more than _____. It can be longer if _____.
33. When you wash eating and cooking items by hand, what is the order in which they are washed?
    _____
34. If you are assisting the person with taking medications, you should know the six rights of drug administration. They are:
    A. _____
    B. _____
    C. _____
    D. _____
    E. _____
    F. _____
35. If a person is taking his or her drugs and states that a pill looks different, what should you do?
    _____
36. If a person needs a medication reminder, it means reminding _____, observing _____, and charting _____.
37. If you are assisting in drug administration, you should report any drug error to the RN. Errors would include:
    A. _____
    B. _____
    C. _____
    D. _____
    E. _____
    F. _____

Optional Learning Exercise

You are working in an assisted living facility. What would you do in these situations?

38. You are providing housekeeping assistance to Mrs. Miller, who lives alone. The stove is on, and a pan has burning food in it. Mrs. Miller tells you she did not put the pan on the stove. What should you do? _____
What is a likely reason for her behavior? _____ _____

39. A resident in the facility has lived there for 2 years and has needed little assistance. He recently had a stroke and now needs care for all of his ADL. Why is he being moved to a nursing facility? _____ _____

40. Mrs. Jenkins tells you she is expecting an important phone call and wants to eat her lunch in her room. What should you do? _____ _____

41. Mr. Shante asks you to get his medicines ready for him to take. What assistance are you allowed to give when the nurse has trained you?
    A. _____
    B. _____
    C. _____
    D. _____
    E. _____
    F. _____
    G. _____
    H. _____

42. When you are assisting Mrs. Clyde with her medicines, you notice two of the labels have an expired date. What should you do? _____ _____

43. Mrs. Johnson asks you when the next meeting of the quilting group will be held. She also asks what days the community crafts fair is planned. Where would you direct her to find this information? _____ _____

Independent Learning Activities

- Find out if your community has any assisted living facilities. They may be part of another facility or may be an independent facility. Visit the facility to answer these questions:
  - What services are offered in the facility? Who provides the services? Nursing assistants? Other assistants? What training is required?
  - What kinds of living quarters are provided? What belongings can the person bring from home?
  - What activities are scheduled? How are residents given information about these activities?
  - How do the residents act? Happy? Withdrawn? Sad? How do the staff members act?
- Find out what laws in your state apply to assisted living facilities. Answer these questions about the laws:
  - What type of license is required for an assisted living facility? Do the laws apply to independent facilities as well as those attached to other facilities?
  - What laws apply to staff training for these facilities? Does the state require workers to be nursing assistants with special training?
  - What does the state law state about assisting with medications? What non-licensed persons can assist with medications? What training is required?

28 Measuring Vital Signs

Key Terms

Apical-radial pulse
Blood pressure
Body temperature
Bradycardia
Diastole

Diastolic pressure
Fever
Hypertension
Hypotension
Pulse

Pulse deficit
Pulse rate
Respiration
Sphygmomanometer
Stethoscope

Systole
Systolic pressure
Tachycardia
Vital signs

Fill in the Blanks: Key Terms

1. A rapid heart rate is _____. The heart rate is over 100 beats per minute.

2. The _____ is taking the apical and radial pulse at the same time.

3. An instrument used to listen to the sounds produced by the heart, lungs, and other body organs is a

   _____.

4. A condition in which the systolic blood pressure is below 90 mm Hg and the diastolic pressure is below 60 mm Hg is _____.

5. The _____ is the number of heartbeats or pulses felt in 1 minute.

6. The amount of heat in the body that is a balance between the amount of heat produced and amount lost by the body is the _____.

7. _____ is the period of heart muscle contraction.

8. _____ is the persistent blood pressure measurements above the normal systolic (140 mm Hg) or diastolic (90 mm Hg) pressures.

9. The instrument used to measure blood pressure is a _____.

10. The beat of the heart felt at an artery as a wave of blood passes through the artery is the _____.

11. Temperature, pulse, respirations, and blood pressure are _____.

12. _____ is a slow heart rate, the rate less than 60 beats per minute.

13. The amount of force it takes to pump blood out of the heart into the arterial circulation is the

    _____.

14. The period of heart muscle relaxation is _____.

15. The difference between the apical and radial pulse rates is the _____.

16. _____ is the amount of force exerted against the walls of an artery by the blood.

17. The act of breathing air into and out of the lungs is _____.

18. _____ is the pressure in the arteries when the heart is at rest.

19. Elevated body temperature is _____.

Circle the Best Answer

20. Residents usually have vital signs measured
    A. Once a shift
    B. Every 4 hours
    C. Once a month
    D. Daily or weekly

21. Unless otherwise ordered, take vital signs when the person
    A. Is lying or sitting
    B. Has been walking or exercising
    C. Has just finished eating
    D. Is getting ready to take a shower or tub bath

22. Body temperature is lower in the
    A. Afternoon
    B. Morning
    C. Evening
    D. Night

23. If you are taking vital signs on a person with dementia, it may be better if
    A. You have 2 or 3 co-workers help you
    B. The vital signs are taken when the person is asleep
    C. You take the pulse and respirations at one time and the temperature and blood pressure at another time
    D. You ask the nurse to take the vital signs

24. What should you do if a resident asks his or her vital sign measurements?
    A. You can tell the person the measurements if center policy allows
    B. Tell the nurse that the person wants to know the measurements
    C. Tell the person you cannot tell him or her this information
    D. This information is private and cannot be shared

25. If you take a rectal temperature, the normal range of the temperature would be
    A. 96.6° to 98.6° F (35.9° to 37.0° C)
    B. 97.6° to 99.6° F (36.5° to 37.5° C)
    C. 98.6° to 100.6° F (37.0° to 38.1° C)
    D. 98.6° F (37° C)

26. If you are taking the temperature of an older person, you would expect the temperature to be
    A. Lower than the normal range
    B. Higher than the normal range
    C. About in the middle of the normal range
    D. The same as for a younger adult

27. A glass rectal thermometer has
  A. A stubby tip color-coded in red
  B. A long or slender tip
  C. A pear-shaped tip
  D. A blue color-coded end
28. To read a glass thermometer, you should hold it at the
  A. Stem above eye level and look up to read it
  B. Bulb end and bring it to eye level
  C. Stem and bring it to eye level to read it
  D. Bulb at waist level and look down to read it
29. An oral temperature may be taken with a glass thermometer for a person who
  A. Is receiving oxygen
  B. Has a history of convulsive disorders
  C. Breathes through the mouth
  D. Is alert and needs a routine temperature taken
30. If you are preparing to take an oral temperature, ask the person not to
  A. Eat, drink, or smoke for at least 15 to 20 minutes
  B. Shower or bathe right before the temperature is taken
  C. Exercise for 30 minutes before
  D. Eat, drink, or smoke for at least 5 to 10 minutes
31. A glass thermometer is inserted into the rectum
  A. 1 inch   C. 1/2 inch
  B. 2 inch   D. 3 inches
32. When recording an axillary temperature of 97.6° F, it is written
  A. 97.6°   C. 97.6° A
  B. 97.6° R   D. 97.6° axillary
33. When using an electronic thermometer, you can prevent the spread of infection by
  A. Discarding the thermometer after each use
  B. Discarding the probe cover after each use
  C. Keeping a thermometer for each person at the bedside
  D. Sterilizing the thermometer after each use
34. When taking a temperature on a resident with dementia, the best choice would be to
  A. Take a rectal temperature
  B. Use a glass oral thermometer
  C. Take an axillary temperature
  D. Use an electronic thermometer
35. Which pulse is most commonly used?
  A. Carotid   C. Radial
  B. Brachial   D. Popliteal
36. A _____ pulse is taken during cardiopulmonary resuscitation (CPR).
  A. Carotid   C. Femoral
  B. Temporal   D. Radial
37. When using a stethoscope, you can help prevent infection by
  A. Warming the diaphragm in your hand
  B. Wiping the earpieces and diaphragm with alcohol before and after use
  C. Placing the diaphragm over the artery
  D. Placing the earpieces in your ears so the bend of the tips points forward

38. When a pulse rate is 120 beats per minute, you
  A. Report that the person has bradycardia
  B. Know that this is a normal pulse rate
  C. Report that the person has tachycardia
  D. Report that the pulse is irregular
39. The pulse rate is the number of heartbeats or pulses felt in
  A. 30 seconds   C. 1 minute
  B. 15 seconds   D. 5 minutes
40. You cannot get information about pulse _____ with electronic blood pressure equipment.
  A. Rhythm and force   C. Tachycardia
  B. Rate   D. Bradycardia
41. When taking the radial pulse, place
  A. The thumb over the pulse site
  B. Two or three fingers on the middle of the wrist
  C. Two or three fingers on the thumb side of the wrist
  D. The stethoscope on the chest wall
42. The apical pulse is counted for 1 minute if
  A. It is irregular
  B. Required by the center policy
  C. Directed by the nurse
  D. All of the above
43. An apical pulse of 72 is recorded as
  A. Pulse 72   C. 72Ap
  B. 72 – Apical pulse   D. P 72
44. An apical-radial pulse is taken by
  A. Taking the radial pulse for 1 minute and then taking the apical pulse for 1 minute
  B. Subtracting the apical pulse from the radial pulse
  C. Having two staff members take the pulses at the same time
  D. Having two persons take the apical pulse at the same time
45. When counting respirations, the best way is to
  A. Stand quietly next to the person and watch the chest rise and fall
  B. Keep your fingers or stethoscope over the pulse site so the person thinks you are still counting the pulse
  C. Tell the person to breathe normally so you can count the respirations
  D. Use the stethoscope to hear the respirations clearly and count for 1 full minute
46. Each respiration involves
  A. One inhalation
  B. One exhalation
  C. One inhalation and one exhalation
  D. Counting for 30 seconds and multiplying by two
47. The blood pressure may be higher in older persons because
  A. They have orthostatic hypotension
  B. The diet is higher in sodium
  C. Arteries narrow and are less elastic
  D. They are usually overweight
48. The blood pressure should not be taken on an arm
  A. If the person has had breast surgery on that side
  B. With a cast
  C. That has a dialysis access site
  D. All of the above

49. You will find out the size of blood pressure cuff needed
    A. By asking the nurse
    B. By measuring the person's arm
    C. In the doctor's orders .
    D. By asking the person
50. When taking the blood pressure, you place the stethoscope diaphragm
    A. Over the radial artery on the thumb side of the wrist
    B. Over the brachial artery at the inner aspect of the elbow
    C. Lightly against the skin
    D. Over the apical pulse site
51. When getting ready to take the blood pressure, position the person's arm
    A. Above the level of the heart
    B. Level with the heart
    C. Below the level of the heart
    D. Abducted from the body
52. The blood pressure cuff is inflated _____ beyond the point where you last felt the radial pulse.
    A. 10 mm Hg   C. 30 mm Hg
    B. 20 mm Hg   D. 40 mm Hg

Fill in the Blanks
53. Vital signs are taken when drugs are taken that affect
    _____.

54. When vital signs are taken, immediately report to the nurse if:
    A. _____
    B. _____
    C. _____

55. Sites for measuring temperature are the:
    A. _____
    B. _____
    C. _____
    D. _____
    E. _____

56. Which site has the highest baseline temperature?
    _____

57. Which site has the lowest baseline temperature?
    _____

58. If a mercury-glass thermometer breaks, _____ immediately because mercury _____.

59. When you read a Fahrenheit thermometer, the short lines mean _____.

60. List how long the glass thermometer remains in place for these sites:
    A. Oral _____ or as required by center policy
    B. Rectal _____ or as required by center policy
    C. Axillary _____ or as required by center policy

61. When taking an oral temperature, place the bulb end of the thermometer _____.

62. When taking an axillary temperature, the axilla must be _____.

63. Tympanic membrane and temporal artery thermometers are used for confused persons because they are
    _____.

64. When using an electronic thermometer, what does the color of the probe mean?
    A. Blue: _____
    B. Red: _____

65. When you take a rectal temperature, _____ the tip of the thermometer or the end of the covered probe.

66. When taking a tympanic membrane temperature, pull back on the ear to _____.

67. The adult pulse rate is between _____ and _____ per minute.

68. List words used to describe:
    A. Forceful pulse: _____
    B. Hard-to-feel pulse: _____

69. If a pulse is irregular, count the pulse for _____.

70. When you take a pulse, what observations should be reported and recorded?
    A. _____
    B. _____
    C. _____
    D. _____
    E. _____

71. Do not use your thumb to take a pulse because
    _____.

72. When taking an apical pulse, each *lub-dub* sound is counted as _____.

73. The apical pulse rate is never less than the
    _____.

74. A healthy adult has _____ respirations per minutes.

75. What observations should be reported and recorded when counting respirations?
    A. _____
    B. _____
    C. _____
    D. _____
    E. _____
    F. _____

76. One respiration is counted for each _____.

77. Respirations are counted for _____ if they are abnormal or irregular.

78. Blood pressure is controlled by:
    A. _____
    B. _____
    C. _____

79. Normal ranges for blood pressures are:
    A. Systolic _____
    B. Diastolic _____

80. If a person has been exercising, let the person rest for _____ before taking the blood pressure.

81. In what positions is the person placed to take the blood pressure? _____ Sometimes the doctor orders blood pressure in the _____ position.

82. When listening to the blood pressure, the first sound you hear is the _____ pressure and the point where the sound disappears is the _____ pressure.

Labeling

83. Name the thermometers shown.

A. _____

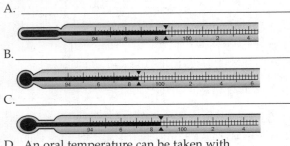

B. _____

C. _____

D. An oral temperature can be taken with

_____.

E. A rectal temperature is taken with

_____.

84. Fill in the drawings so that the thermometers read correctly.

A. 95.8° F   F. 35.5° C
B. 98.4° F   G. 36.5° C
C. 100.2° F   H. 37° C
D. 101° F   I. 38.5° C
E. 102.6° F   J. 39.5° C

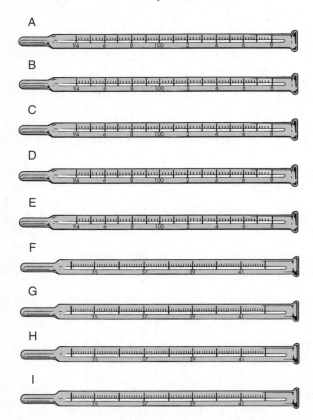

85. Name the pulse sites shown for A through H.

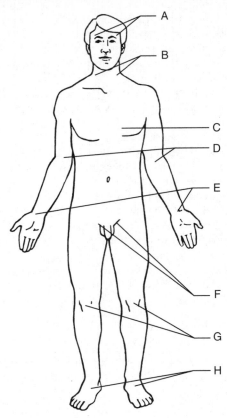

A. _____
B. _____
C. _____
D. _____
E. _____
F. _____
G. _____
H. _____

I. Which pulse is used during cardiopulmonary resuscitation (CPR)? _____

J. Which pulse is most commonly taken? _____

K. Which pulse is used when taking the blood pressure? _____

L. Which pulse is found with a stethoscope?

_____

86. Fill in the drawings so that the dials show the correct blood pressures.
    A. 168/102
    B. 104/68

A 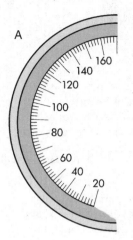 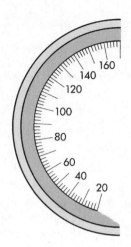 B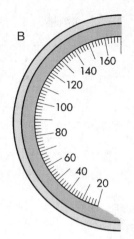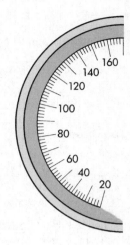

87. Fill in the drawings so that the mercury columns show the correct blood pressures.
    A. 152/86
    B. 198/110

A 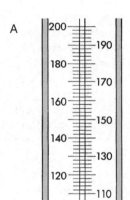 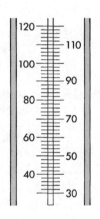 B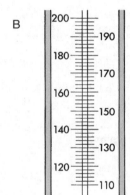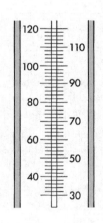

88. Record the readings on the thermometers shown.

A

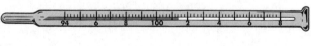

B

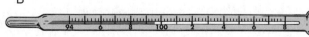

C

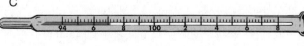

    A. _____
    B. _____
    C. _____

Nursing Assistant Skills Video Exercise
View the parts of the **Measurements** *video that apply to this chapter to answer these questions.*

89. What procedure guidelines are followed for these measurements?
   A. Body temperature: _____
   _____
   B. Pulse: _____
   _____
   C. Respirations: _____
   _____
   D. Blood pressure: _____
   _____

90. Body temperature range is the same for all temperature sites.
   A. True   B. False

91. When using an electronic thermometer, you need to use a new probe cover each time.
   A. True   B. False

92. A rectal temperature must be performed skillfully and with attention to _____, _____, and _____.

93. Note the pulse _____, _____, and _____ before you count the pulse rate.

94. You need to clean the _____ and the _____ of the stethoscope with alcohol wipes before and after measuring the apical pulse.

95. Count each rise of the chest as one respiration and each fall of the chest as one respiration.
   A. True   B. False

Optional Learning Exercises
Taking temperatures
96. You prepare to take Mr. Harrison's temperature with a glass thermometer. When you take the thermometer from the container, it reads 97.8° F. What should you do? _____

97. If the thermometer registers between 2 short lines, record the temperature to the _____.

98. How would you record these temperature readings?
   A. An oral temperature of 97.4° F _____ 36.5° C _____
   B. A rectal temperature of 99.8° F _____ 38.1° C _____
   C. An axillary temperature of 96.2° F _____ 36.1° C _____

Taking pulses and respirations
99. You are assigned to take Mrs. Sanchez' pulse and respirations. You note that the pulse rate and respirations are regular, so you take each one for _____. When you complete counting the pulse, you keep your _____ and count _____. This is done so that Mrs. Sanchez will _____.

100. When you finish counting Mrs. Sanchez' pulse and respirations, your numbers are pulse 36 and respirations 9. What numbers should be recorded?
   Pulse: _____. Respirations: _____.
   Why? _____

101. The nurse tells you to take an apical-radial pulse on Mrs. Hellman. Why do you ask a co-worker to help you? _____

102. How long is an apical-radial pulse counted? _____ After you have taken the apical-radial pulse, how do you find the pulse deficit? _____
   _____

Taking blood pressures
103. You are assigned to take Mr. Hardaway's blood pressure. You know that he goes for dialysis 3 times a week. What do need to know before you take his blood pressure? _____ Why?
   _____

104. When you inflate the cuff, you cannot feel the pulse after you pump the cuff to 130 mm Hg. How high will you inflate the cuff to take his blood pressure? _____

105. You should deflate the cuff at an even rate of _____ per second.

Independent Learning Activities

- Take turns measuring vital signs on 3 or 4 classmates. If possible, use glass, electronic, and tympanic thermometers for each person to see if they give similar results. Use this table to record the results.

Person	Temperature	Pulse	Respiration	Blood Pressure
#1	Glass	Radial	Rate	
	Electronic	Apical	Rhythm	
	Tympanic		Depth	
#2	Glass	Radial	Rate	
	Electronic	Apical	Rhythm	
	Tympanic		Depth	
#3	Glass	Radial	Rate	
	Electronic	Apical	Rhythm	
	Tympanic		Depth	
#4	Glass	Radial	Rate	
	Electronic	Apical	Rhythm	
	Tympanic		Depth	

- Answer these questions about this exercise:
  - If you used different thermometers, how did the results compare?
  - What differences did you find in finding the radial pulses among your classmates?
  - What differences did you find in the rates and rhythms?
  - How were you able to measure respirations so that the person did not know you were watching?
  - What differences in rhythm and depth of respirations did you find among your classmates?
  - What differences did you find in locating the brachial artery in different people?
  - How did the sounds of the blood pressure differ among your classmates?
  - What difficulties did you have with any of the measurements taken?
  - What will you change about measuring vital signs on a resident after this practice?
- Practice taking an apical-radial pulse with classmates. Take turns acting as the staff members and the person having the pulses taken. Answer these questions after the exercise is completed:
  - How was privacy maintained for the person having the pulse measured?
  - How did the "staff members" decide who would begin and end the count?
  - What problems did you have in counting for a minute?
  - How did the apical and radial counts compare?
  - What will you change about measuring the apical-radial pulses on a resident after this experience?

29 Assisting With the Physical Examination

Key Terms

Dorsal recumbent position
Horizontal recumbent
  position

Knee-chest position
Laryngeal mirror
Lithotomy position

Nasal speculum
Ophthalmoscope
Otoscope

Percussion hammer
Tuning fork
Vaginal speculum

Fill in the Blanks: Key Terms

1. An instrument vibrated to test hearing is a _____ _____.

2. In the _____, the woman lies on the back with the hips at the edge of the exam table, the knees are flexed, the hips are externally rotated, and the feet are in stirrups.

3. The supine position with the legs together is called the _____.

4. An _____ is a lighted instrument used to examine the external ear and the eardrum (tympanic membrane).

5. A _____ is an instrument used to open the vagina so it and the cervix can be examined.

6. When a person kneels and rests the body on the knees and chest, and the head is turned to one side, the arms are above the head or flexed at the elbows, the back is straight, and the body is flexed about 90 degrees at the hip, the person is in the _____.

7. A _____ is an instrument used to tap body parts to test reflexes.

8. An instrument used to examine the mouth, teeth, and throat is called a _____.

9. An instrument used to examine the inside of the nose is a _____.

10. The dorsal recumbent position is also called the _____.

11. An _____ is a lighted instrument used to examine the internal structures of the eye.

Circle the BEST Answer

12. In nursing centers, residents have a physical examination
    A. Only when the person is admitted
    B. Once a month
    C. At least once a year
    D. Only when the person is ill

13. If a resident is having a physical examination, you may be asked to do all of these *except*
    A. Measure vital signs, height, and weight
    B. Assist the doctor or nurse with an examination
    C. Explain why the examination is being done and what to expect
    D. Position and drape the person

14. When the doctor is examining the person's mouth, teeth, and throat, you may be asked to hand him or her the
    A. Ophthalmoscope   C. Tuning fork
    B. Percussion hammer   D. Laryngeal mirror

15. Which of these *would not* protect the right to personal choice for a person having a physical examination?
    A. Having the person urinate before the exam begins
    B. Telling the person who will do the exam and when it will be done
    C. Explaining the procedure
    D. Allowing a family member to be present if the person requests

16. The right to privacy is protected by
    A. Removing all clothes for a complete examination
    B. Explaining the reasons for the examination
    C. Exposing only the body part being examined
    D. Explaining the exam results with a family member present

17. It is important to have a person empty the bladder before an examination because
    A. An empty bladder allows the examiner to feel the abdominal organs
    B. A full bladder can change the normal position and shape of organs
    C. A full bladder can cause discomfort when the abdominal organs are felt
    D. All of the above

18. Which of these steps *would not* promote safety and comfort during an exam?
    A. Expose only the body part being examined
    B. Have an extra bath blanket nearby
    C. Prevent drafts to protect the person from chilling
    D. Do not leave the person unattended

19. After you have taken the person to the exam room and placed the person in position, you should
    A. Put the signal light on for the nurse or examiner
    B. Leave the room
    C. Go to the nurse or examiner to report the person is ready
    D. Open the door, so the nurse or examiner knows you are ready

20. When the abdomen, chest, and breasts are to be examined, you will place the person in the
    A. Lithotomy position
    B. Sims' position
    C. Dorsal recumbent (horizontal recumbent) position
    D. Knee-chest position

142

21. If a person is asked to stand on the floor during an exam, you should
    A. Assist the person to put on shoes or slippers
    B. Place paper or paper towels on the floor
    C. Place a sheet on the floor
    D. Wipe the floor carefully with an antiseptic cleaner before the person stands on it

Fill in the Blanks

22. List the equipment you need to collect when the ears are being examined.
    A. _____
    B. _____

23. What equipment is needed to examine the eyes?
    A. _____
    B. _____

24. When the nose, mouth, and throat are being examined, you should collect:
    A. _____
    B. _____
    C. _____
    D. _____

25. What are common fears the person may have when a physical examination is done?
    A. _____
    B. _____

26. To maintain the person's right to privacy, who are the only persons who have a right to see the person's body during the exam?
    _____

27. Who are the only persons who need to know the reason for the exam and its results?
    _____

Labeling
Use this figure to answer questions 28–31.

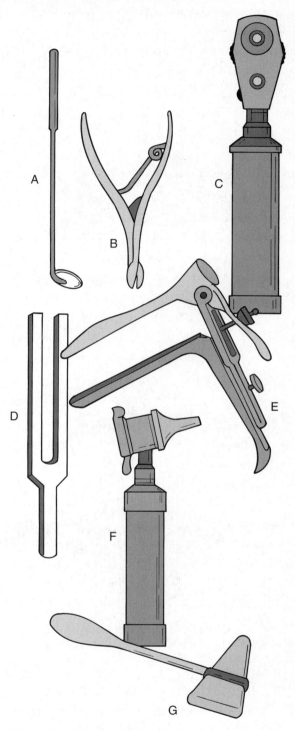

28. Name the instruments.
    A. _____
    B. _____
    C. _____
    D. _____
    E. _____
    F. _____
    G. _____

29. Which instrument is used to examine the nose? _____

30. When the eye is examined, the examiner uses the _____.

31. If a person has a sore throat, the examiner will look at the throat with the _____.

32. The reflexes are examined by using the _____.

A

B

C

D

33. Name the positions.
    A. _____
    B. _____
    C. _____
    D. _____

34. Which positions may be used when a rectal examination is done?
    A. _____
    B. _____

35. When the abdomen, chest, and breasts are examined, the person is placed in _____.

36. The _____ is used for a vaginal exam.

Optional Learning Exercises

37. When you are delegated the job of preparing a person for an exam, why do you need the following information?
    A. The time the examination is to be done.

    B. The two reasons it would helpful to know which examinations will be done.

    C. What equipment will be needed if you are assigned to take vital signs.

38. You are a female nursing assistant assisting a male examiner with an examination of a female resident. The nurse tells you to stay in the exam room during the entire procedure. Why is this important to the examiner and to the woman?_____

Independent Learning Activities
- You probably have had a physical examination at some time. Perhaps you needed one to be a student in this class. Answer these questions about your experience when you had the physical done to you:
  - Who explained what to expect during the exam? What were you told about any discomfort?
  - What steps were taken to give you privacy? While you changed clothes? During the exam?
  - Who was present during the exam? Were you given a choice of having another person in the room with you and the examiner? How did you feel about having (or not having) another person in the room?
  - How did you know what was being done? How much information were you given about procedures? Positions? Tests?
  - What positions were used during the exam? Which positions shown in this chapter were used? How comfortable did you feel? How did the examiner and assistant help to make you more comfortable with the positions?
  - What questions did you have during the exam? Who was able to answer these? How well were they answered to make you understand what was being done?
  - How comfortable did you feel about the exam? What could have been done to make you more comfortable physically and psychologically?
  - How did this experience help you understand the feelings of persons you may assist during an exam?

30 Collecting and Testing Specimens

Key Terms
Acetone
Glucosuria
Glycosuria

Hematuria
Hemoptysis

Ketone
Ketone body

Melena
Sputum

Fill in the Blanks: Key Terms

1. Bloody sputum is _____.

2. A ketone or acetone is also called _____.

3. A black, tarry stool is _____.

4. _____ is glucosuria or sugar in the urine.

5. _____ is mucus from the respiratory system that is expectorated through the mouth.

6. Acetone is called _____ or ketone body.

7. A substance that appears in urine from the rapid breakdown of fat for energy is _____.

8. Sugar in the urine is called glycosuria or _____.

9. _____ is blood in the urine.

Circle the BEST Answer

10. Specimens are collected and tested for all of these reasons *except*
    A. To measure the specimen
    B. To prevent diseases
    C. To detect diseases
    D. To treat diseases

11. When you are collecting a specimen, which of these is *incorrect*?
    A. Use a clean container for each specimen
    B. Gloves are not needed
    C. Do not touch the inside of the container or lid
    D. Place the specimen container in a plastic bag

12. A urine specimen may be placed in a paper bag to
    A. Prevent embarrassing the person
    B. Protect the specimen from light
    C. Follow Standard Precautions
    D. Keep the specimen sterile

13. A random urine specimen is collected
    A. First thing in the morning
    B. After meals
    C. At any time
    D. At bedtime

14. When a person is collecting a random urine specimen, ask the person to put the toilet tissue in
    A. The wastebasket or toilet
    B. The specimen container
    C. The specimen pan
    D. Any of the above

15. When obtaining a midstream specimen, the perineal area is cleaned to
    A. Remove all microbes from the area
    B. Reduce the number of microbes in the urethral area
    C. Follow Standard Precautions and the Bloodborne Pathogen Standard
    D. Reduce infection during the specimen collection

16. When collecting a midstream specimen, which of these is correct?
    A. Collect the entire amount of urine voided
    B. Collect about 4 oz (120 ml) of urine
    C. Have the person void and then pass the receptacle into the stream of urine
    D. Collect several specimens and mix them together

17. When collecting a 24-hour urine specimen, the urine is kept
    A. Chilled on ice or refrigerated during the time
    B. At room temperature
    C. In a sterile container at the nurses' station
    D. In a drainage collection bag at the bedside

18. A 24-hour urine specimen collection is started
    A. At the beginning of a shift
    B. After a meal
    C. At night
    D. After the person voids and that urine is discarded

19. At the end of a 24-hour specimen collection
    A. The person voids and that urine is saved
    B. Write down any missed or spilled urine
    C. Record the amount of urine collected
    D. The person voids and that urine is discarded

20. When collecting a double-voided specimen, the first specimen is
    A. Discarded without testing
    B. Mixed with the second specimen collected
    C. Tested in case you cannot obtain a second specimen
    D. Sent to the laboratory

21. Which of these tests is best if done with a double-voided specimen?
    A. Test for pH
    B. Test for blood
    C. Test for melena
    D. Test for glucose and ketones

22. When you test urine with a reagent strip, it is important that you
    A. Follow the manufacturer's instructions
    B. Use a sterile urine specimen
    C. Wear sterile gloves
    D. Make sure the urine is cold

23. When you are assigned to strain a person's urine, you
    A. Have the person void directly into the strainer
    B. Send all urine to the lab
    C. Have the person void into the receptacle and then pour the urine through the strainer
    D. Discard the strainer if it contains any stones

24. If a warm stool specimen is required, it is
    A. Placed it in an insulated container
    B. Taken to the laboratory at once
    C. Tested at once on the nursing unit
    D. Taken at once to the storage area for transport to the laboratory

25. When collecting a stool specimen, ask the person to
    A. Void and have a bowel movement in a bedpan
    B. Use only a bedpan or commode to collect the specimen
    C. Urinate into the toilet and collect the stool in the specimen pan
    D. Place the toilet tissue in the bedpan, commode, or specimen pan with the stool

26. When collecting the stool specimen
    A. Pour it into the specimen container
    B. Use your gloved hand to obtain a specimen to place in the container
    C. Use a tongue blade to take about 2 tablespoons of stool from the middle of the formed stool
    D. Use a tongue blade to place the entire stool specimen in the container

27. When you test a stool specimen for blood
    A. It must be sent to the laboratory
    B. The specimen must be sterile
    C. You will need to test the entire stool specimen
    D. Use a tongue blade to obtain a small of amount of stool

28. A sputum specimen is more easily collected
    A. Upon awakening   C. At bedtime
    B. After eating   D. After activity

29. Before obtaining a sputum specimen, ask the person to
    A. Rinse the mouth with clear water
    B. Brush the teeth and use mouthwash
    C. Cough and discard the first sputum expectorated
    D. Sit in an upright position to loosen secretions

30. Postural drainage is used when collecting a sputum specimen to
    A. Collect sterile specimens
    B. Make the sputum specimen more liquid
    C. Stimulate coughing
    D. Help secretions drain by gravity

Fill in the Blanks

31. When collecting urine specimens, what observations are reported and recorded?
    A. _____
    B. _____
    C. _____
    D. _____
    E. _____

32. How much urine is collected for a random urine specimen? _____

33. When collecting a midstream urine specimen, the person starts to void and then stops _____. After the specimen container is positioned, the person _____.

34. When you are obtaining a midstream specimen from a female, spread the labia with your thumb and index finger with your _____ hand.

35. When cleaning the female perineum for a midstream specimen, clean from _____.

36. When cleaning the male perineum for a midstream specimen, clean the penis starting _____ _____.

37. When you make labels for a 24-hour urine collection to place in the room and bathroom, what information is marked? _____ _____

38. Another name for a double-voided specimen is a _____ _____

39. When collecting a double-voided specimen, the second voiding is collected _____ minutes after the first voiding.

40. Urine pH measures if the urine is _____ or _____.

41. When you use reagent strips, you read the strip by comparing it with the _____ .

42. When you strain urine, you are looking for stones that can develop in the _____ _____.

43. The strainer or gauze is placed in the specimen container if any_____ _____ appear.

44. Stool specimens are studied and checked for:
    A. _____
    B. _____
    C. _____
    D. _____
    E. _____

45. After collecting a stool specimen, place the container in a _____.

46. When you are delegated to collect a stool specimen, what observations are reported and recorded?
    A. _____
    B. _____
    C. _____
    D. _____

47. When stools are black and tarry, there is bleeding in the _____
    _____.

48. Blood in the stool that is hidden is called _____.

49. Mouthwash is not used before a sputum specimen is collected because it _____.

50. When you are delegated to collect a sputum specimen, report and record:
    A. _____
    B. _____
    C. _____
    D. _____
    E. _____
    F. _____
    G. _____
    H. _____
    I. _____

51. When you are assisting a person to collect a sputum specimen, ask the person to take 2 or 3 _____ and _____ the sputum.

Crossword

Fill in the crossword by answering the clues below with the words from this list:

Calculi

Dysuria

Expectorated

Labia

Midstream

Occult

Postural

Random

Specimens

Suctioning

ACROSS

1. Samples
3. Urine specimen that can be collected at any time
6. Hidden, as in blood in stool
8. Position with head lower than body used to cause fluid to flow down
9. Folds of tissue on each side of the vagina
10. Pain when urinating

DOWN

2. Expelled, as in sputum through the mouth
4. Urine specimen that is collected after the person starts to void
5. Stones that develop in kidneys, ureters, or bladder
7. Removal of sputum from the trachea with a machine

Optional Learning Exercises

52. If you are collecting a midstream specimen, what should you do if it is hard for the person to stop the stream of urine? _____

53. You are caring for a person who is having a 24-hour urine specimen test. He tells you he forgot to save a specimen an hour ago. What should you do and why? _____

54. When collecting a double-voided specimen, why do you test the first specimen? _____

55. When collecting a double-voided specimen, what can you do to help the person void 30 minutes after the first voiding? _____

56. What is normal pH for urine? _____
What can cause changes in the normal pH? _____

57. When the body cannot use sugar for energy, it uses fat. When this happens, _____ appear in the urine.

58. Why is privacy important when collecting a sputum specimen? _____
_____

Independent Learning Activities

Answer these questions about collecting specimens.

- What specimens may be collected by nursing assistants in your state?
- What special training is given to make sure nursing assistants understand how to collect specimens?
- Ask permission to look at specimen containers used in your clinical site.
- Are any directions included with the containers?
- Where is information about collecting specimens kept at the clinical site?

31 Admitting, Transferring, and Discharging Persons

Key Terms
Admission   Discharge   Transfer

Fill in the Blanks: Key Terms

1. _____ is moving a person from one room or nursing unit to another.

2. The official entry of a person into a nursing center is _____.

3. _____ occurs with the official departure of a person from a nursing center.

Circle the BEST Answer

4. Usually, _____ is a happy time.
   A. Admission   C. Transfer
   B. Discharge   D. Home care

5. What staff member starts the admissions process?
   A. The doctor
   B. The nurse
   C. The admissions coordinator
   D. The activities director

6. When a person with dementia is admitted to a nursing center, the person
   A. Is usually depressed
   B. May have an increase in confusion
   C. May have a decrease in confusion
   D. Usually feels safer in the new setting

7. Persons admitted to rehabilitation and subacute care units are
   A. Usually admitted by the RN
   B. Usually admitted by the nursing assistant
   C. Admitted by the nursing assistant if the person's condition is stable and the person has no discomfort or distress
   D. Never admitted by the nursing assistant

8. If a person being admitted is arriving by stretcher, you should
   A. Raise the bed to its highest level
   B. Leave the bed closed
   C. Raise the head of the bed to Fowler's position
   D. Lower the bed to its lowest level

9. During admission, you can help the person feel more comfortable by
   A. Offering the person and the family beverages to drink
   B. Introducing nearby residents
   C. Assisting the person to hang pictures or display photos
   D. All of the above

10. When weighing a resident, have the person
    A. Wear socks and shoes and bathrobe
    B. Remove regular clothes and wear a gown or pajamas
    C. Wear regular street clothes
    D. Remove clothing after weighing and then weigh the clothes

11. A chair scale is used when
    A. A person can transfer from a wheelchair to the chair scale
    B. A person cannot stand
    C. A person can stand and walk independently
    D. A person is in the supine position

12. When a person cannot stand on the scale to have the height measured
    A. Ask the person or the family the height of the person
    B. Have the person sit in a chair and use a tape measure from head to toe to measure the person
    C. Position the person in supine position and measure with a tape measure
    D. Estimate the height of the person by observing him or her

13. When a person is being transferred, who is informed?
    A. The doctor
    B. The social worker
    C. The family and business office
    D. The person's roommate

14. When you are transferring a person, you should do all of these except
    A. Identify the person by checking the ID bracelet with the transfer slip
    B. Explain the reasons for the transfer
    C. Collect the person's personal belongings and bedside equipment
    D. Introduce the person to the receiving nurse

15. If a person wishes to leave the center without the doctor's permission, you should
    A. Tell the person this is not allowed
    B. Prevent the person from leaving
    C. Tell the nurse immediately
    D. Try to convince the person to stay

16. When you are assisting a person who is being discharged, you should
    A. Check all drawers and closet
    B. Check off the clothing list and personal belongings list
    C. Help the person dress as needed
    D. All of the above

Fill in the Blanks

17. OBRA has standards for transfers and discharges. List the ways these standards affect the person's rights.
    A. Reasons for _____ and _____ are part of the person's _____.
    B. The _____ and _____ are told of transfer or discharge plans.
    C. A procedure is followed if the person _____ _____.
    D. An _____ often works with the person and family to ensure that the _____.

18. When you are delegated to assist with admissions, transfers, or discharges, what information do you need from the nurse?
    A. _____
    B. _____
    C. _____
    D. _____
    E. _____
    F. _____
    G. _____
    H. _____
    I. _____

19. When a person is being admitted, what identifying information is obtained?
    A. _____
    B. _____
    C. _____
    D. _____
    E. _____
    F. _____

20. During admission, why does the person have a photo taken and receive an ID bracelet?
    _____

21. When you are asked to admit a person, what can you do to make a good first impression?
    A. _____
    B. _____
    C. _____
    D. _____
    E. _____

22. Why is it important to have a person urinate before being weighed? _____

23. What is done to the balance scale before having the person step on?
    A. _____
    B. _____
    C. _____

24. When measuring a person in the supine position, the ruler is placed _____ _____.

25. If you transfer a person to a new unit, you can help the person by introducing the person to _____ _____.

26. When a person is discharged, the nurse will tell you when _____ and how to _____ .

27. When you assist with a discharge, you should report and record:
    A. _____
    B. _____
    C. _____
    D. _____
    E. _____
    F. _____

28. To help the person and family cope with admission, transfer, and discharge, you should:
    A. Be _____
    B. Be _____
    C. Handle _____
    D. Treat _____

Nursing Assistant Skills Video Exercise
View the portions of the Measurements video that apply to this chapter and answer these questions.

29. How did the nursing assistant aid Mr. Bernardo's stability while measuring his weight? _____ _____

Optional Learning Exercises
Rosa Romirez, age 65, had a stroke (CVA) last week and is being admitted to a rehabilitation unit in the nursing care center where you work. Answer questions 30–34.

30. Because you know Mrs. R. is arriving by wheelchair, you leave the bed _____ and _____ the bed to its _____.

31. The nurse instructs you to collect the needed equipment to admit a new person. You collect:
    A. _____
    B. _____
    C. _____
    D. _____
    E. _____
    F. _____
    G. _____
    H. _____
    I. _____
    J. _____

32. When Mrs. R. arrives with her husband, it may help them feel more comfortable if you offer them _____

33. You greet Mrs. Romirez by name and ask her if a certain _____ _____ .

34. Mrs. R. has some weakness on her left side and cannot stand alone but can safely transfer from the wheelchair to chairs or the bed. The nurse tells you to weigh Mrs. R. with the _____ scale.

When you arrive at work one day, you are told Mrs. Romirez is being transferred to another unit and you are asked to assist. Answer these questions 35–37 about transferring her:

35. When you transport Mrs. R. in a wheelchair, she is covered with a _____ _____ .

36. What items are taken with Mrs. R. to the new unit?
_____
_____
_____

37. What information is recorded and reported about the transfer?
A. _____
B. _____
C. _____
D. _____
E. _____
F. _____
G. _____

Several weeks later, you are sent to the unit where Mrs. R. is living and find she is going home. Answer questions 38–39 about her discharge:

38. Mrs. R. tells you she and her family have been taught about her _____, _____, and _____ _____ .

39. Good communication skills should be used when assisting with the discharge. When Mrs. R. and her family leave, you should _____ _____ .

Independent Learning Activities

Have a discussion with 3 or 4 classmates to share experiences you have had with admissions to care facilities. You may have had personal experience, or you may have observed a friend or family member being admitted. If you have not had this experience, perhaps you can relate the feelings you have had when visiting a doctor's office. Use these questions during the discussion:

- Who was the first person you met when you arrived to be admitted? How were you greeted? Did you feel welcome?
- How did you arrive at your room? Were you escorted, or did you have to find your way?
- How long did you wait in the room before a staff member came to admit you? How did this affect your feelings about the place?
- How were you addressed? First name? Last name? Did anyone ask you what you preferred?
- What information were you given to make you feel more comfortable? What printed information was provided?
- Overall, how did the admission procedure affect your feelings about the facility? Negative? Positive?
- How will your personal experience and the experiences of others in this group affect your approach to new persons in a care facility?

32 Wound Care

Key Terms

Abrasion
Arterial ulcer
Chronic wound
Circulatory ulcer
Clean-contaminated wound
Clean wound
Closed wound
Contaminated wound
Contusion
Dehiscence

Diabetic foot ulcer
Dirty wound
Edema
Embolus
Evisceration
Full-thickness wound
Gangrene
Incision
Infected wound
Intentional wound

Laceration
Open wound
Partial-thickness wound
Penetrating wound
Phlebitis
Pressure ulcer
Puncture wound
Purulent drainage
Sanguineous drainage
Serosanguineous drainage

Serous drainage
Skin tear
Stasis ulcer
Thrombus
Trauma
Ulcer
Unintentional wound
Vascular ulcer
Venous ulcer
Wound

Fill in the Blanks: Key Terms

1. A _____ is a break or rip in the skin that separates the epidermis from underlying skin.

2. An open wound with clean, straight edges, usually produced with a sharp instrument, is an _____ _____.

3. A shallow or deep, crater-like sore of the skin or mucous membrane is an _____.

4. When tissues are injured but the skin is not broken, it is a _____.

5. _____ is thick green, yellow, or brown drainage.

6. When the dermis and epidermis of the skin are broken, it is called a _____.

7. A _____ is a break in the skin or mucous membrane.

8. A wound that is not infected and microbes have not entered the wound is a _____.

9. An _____ is a partial-thickness wound caused by the scraping away or rubbing of the skin.

10. A _____ is an open wound on the foot caused by complications from diabetes.

11. Thin, watery drainage that is blood-tinged is called _____.

12. An _____ is a wound that contains large amounts of bacteria and that shows signs of infection; dirty wound.

13. An open sore on the lower legs or feet caused by decreased blood flow is a _____ _____.

14. Another name for a blood clot is a _____ _____.

15. _____ is an inflammation of a vein.

16. A wound with a high risk of infection is a _____ _____.

17. A condition in which there is death of tissue is _____ _____.

18. An injury usually from unrelieved pressure that damages the skin and underlying tissues is a _____; decubitus ulcer, bedsore, or pressure sore.

19. A _____ is an open wound with torn tissues and jagged edges.

20. A wound resulting from trauma is an _____ _____.

21. An _____ is an open wound on the lower legs and feet caused by poor arterial blood flow.

22. Clear, watery fluid is _____.

23. A blood clot that travels through the vascular system until it lodges in a distant vessel is called an _____ _____.

24. An infected wound is a _____.

25. A wound that occurs from surgical entry of the urinary, reproductive, respiratory, or gastrointestinal system is a _____.

26. A _____ is a wound that does not heal easily.

27. An open sore on the lower legs or feet caused by poor blood flow through the veins is a _____ _____; stasis ulcer.

28. An open wound made by a sharp object is a _____. The entry of the skin and underlying tissues may be intentional or unintentional.

29. A wound created for therapy is an _____ _____.

30. A _____ is an open wound in which the skin and underlying tissues are pierced.

31. _____ is the separation of wound layers.

32. A circulatory ulcer is also called a _____ _____.

33. Swelling that is caused by fluid collecting in tissues is _____.

34. A _____ occurs when the dermis, epidermis, and subcutaneous tissue are penetrated. Muscle and bone may be involved.

35. An accident or violent act that injures the skin, mucous membranes, bones, and internal organs is called _____.

36. The separation of the wound along with the protrusion of abdominal organs is _____ _____.

37. A _____ is another name for a venous ulcer.

38. Bloody drainage is called _____ _____.

39. A closed wound caused by a blow to the body is a _____.

40. An _____ occurs when the skin or mucous membrane is broken.

Circle the BEST Answer

41. The skin
    A. Is the body's first line of defense
    B. Protects the body from microbes
    C. Is easily injured in older and disabled persons
    D. All of the above

42. When you inspect a resident's elbow, you find some of the skin is rubbed away. You would report this to the nurse as an
    A. Laceration   C. Contusion
    B. Abrasion   D. Incision

43. When you look at a resident's arm that caught on the wheelchair, the tissue is torn with jagged edges. You know this is a
    A. Puncture wound   C. Penetrating wound
    B. Abrasion   D. Laceration

44. Which of these *would not* place a person at risk for skin tears?
    A. The person is obese
    B. The person requires complete help in moving
    C. The person has poor nutrition
    D. The person has altered mental awareness

45. Applying lotion will help prevent skin breakdown or skin tears because it may prevent
    A. Loss of fatty layer under the skin
    B. General thinning of the skin
    C. Dryness of the skin
    D. Moisture in areas of the body where perspiration occurs

46. A pressure ulcer occurs because
    A. The person repositions himself or herself in the bed or chair
    B. The person drinks too many fluids
    C. Skin and underlying tissue is damaged by unrelieved pressure
    D. The person is repositioned too frequently

47. The first sign of a pressure ulcer in an area would be
    A. Skin has a color change to red, blue, or purple
    B. Swelling in the area
    C. A break in the skin
    D. Exposed tissue and some drainage from the area

48. Mrs. Greene keeps sliding down in bed. The nurse tells you to raise the head of the bed no more than 30 degrees. This position will help prevent tissue damage caused by
    A. Pressure over hard surfaces
    B. Shearing
    C. Poor body mechanics
    D. Poor fluid balance

49. Pressure ulcers can occur
    A. Over bony areas such as the hips
    B. Underneath the breasts
    C. Between abdominal folds
    D. All of the above

50. When following a repositioning schedule, the person should be repositioned
    A. According to the schedule in the person's care plan
    B. Every 2 hours
    C. Every 15 minutes
    D. As often as you have time

51. One way to prevent friction in the bed is to
    A. Use soap when cleansing the skin
    B. Rub or massage reddened areas
    C. Use pillows and blankets to prevent skin from being in contact with skin
    D. Powder sheets lightly

52. Bed cradles are used to
    A. Position the person in good body alignment
    B. Prevent pressure on the legs and feet
    C. Keep the heels off the bed
    D. Distribute body weight evenly

53. When the person is using an eggcrate-type mattress, it is covered with a special cover and
    A. Only a bottom sheet
    B. A bottom sheet and a waterproof pad
    C. A bottom sheet and a draw sheet
    D. Waterproof materials, a lift sheet, and a bottom sheet

54. Ulcers of the feet and legs are caused by
    A. Poorly fitted shoes
    B. Decreased blood flow through arteries or veins
    C. Increased activity
    D. Increased fluid intake

55. A measure to prevent venous (stasis) ulcers is
    A. Use elastic or rubber band–type garters to hold the person's socks in place
    B. Keep the person's feet flat on the floor while sitting in a chair
    C. Apply elastic stockings or elastic wraps to legs
    D. Massage the legs and feet
56. Elastic stockings
    A. Are removed every 8 hours for 30 minutes
    B. Are applied after the person has been out of bed for 30 minutes or more
    C. Normally cause the person to complain of tingling or numbness in the feet
    D. Are removed only at bedtime or for a bath or shower
57. When applying elastic stockings, all of these are correct except
    A. Position the person in the chair
    B. Turn the stocking inside out down to the heel
    C. Grasp the stocking top and slip it over the foot and heel
    D. Remove twists, creases, or wrinkles
58. Elastic bandages are
    A. Applied loosely to prevent discomfort
    B. Applied starting at the hip
    C. Used with persons with venous ulcers
    D. Used with persons with arterial ulcers
59. When applying elastic bandages, you should
    A. Apply the bandage so that it completely covers the fingers or toes
    B. First apply the bandage to the smallest part of the wrist, foot, ankle, or knee
    C. Secure the bandage at the back of the leg with a safety pin
    D. Remove the bandage only when it becomes loose or falls off the extremity
60. Common causes of arterial ulcers are
    A. Poor blood flow through the veins
    B. Leg or foot surgery
    C. Smoking, high blood pressure, and diabetes
    D. Surgery on bones and joints
61. When caring for a person at risk for arterial ulcers, you should do all of these except
    A. Remind the person to sit with the legs uncrossed
    B. Assist the person to apply garters to hold up socks or hose
    C. Make sure the shoes fit well
    D. Encourage the person to stop smoking
62. It is important to check the feet of a diabetic every day because
    A. The person may not feel pain if he or she has an injury to a foot
    B. Tissue and cells do not get needed oxygen and nutrients to heal
    C. Injuries do not heal well
    D. All of the above
63. During wound healing, what phase is happening when the wound is about 1 year old?
    A. Initial phase
    B. Inflammatory phase
    C. Maturation phase
    D. Proliferative phase

64. The nurse tells you to make sure Mrs. Reynolds supports her abdominal wound when she coughs. The nurse wants this done to protect against
    A. Secondary intention healing
    B. Infection
    C. Scarring
    D. Dehiscence
65. When you are caring for Mrs. Reynolds, you notice thin, watery drainage that is blood-tinged. When you report your observations, you would tell the nurse that the wound has _____ drainage.
    A. Purulent
    B. Serosanguineous
    C. Serous
    D. Sanguineous
66. Which of these methods used in wound care will prevent microbes from entering a draining wound?
    A. Wet-to-dry dressings
    B. A Hemovac suction device
    C. A Penrose drain
    D. Nonadherent gauze
67. When wet-to-dry dressings are used, they
    A. Absorb dead tissue, which is removed when dressings are dry
    B. Are kept moist
    C. Allow air to reach the wound, but fluids and bacteria cannot
    D. Do not stick to the wound
68. Plastic and paper tape may be used to secure a dressing
    A. Because they allow movement of the body part
    B. When the dressing must be changed frequently
    C. If the person is allergic to adhesive tape
    D. Because they stick well to the skin
69. If you care for a person who has Montgomery ties to secure a dressing, you should
    A. Replace the cloth ties when you give care
    B. Tell the nurse if the adhesive strips are soiled
    C. Replace the adhesive strips each time you give care
    D. Retie the cloth ties when you reposition the person
70. If you are assigned to change a dressing, which of these is important information to have?
    A. What kind of medication the person receives
    B. The person's diagnosis
    C. When pain medication was given and how long until it takes effect
    D. All of the above
71. You can make the person more comfortable when changing a dressing by doing all of the following except
    A. Control your nonverbal communication when looking at the wound
    B. Avoid body language that indicates the wound is unpleasant
    C. Encourage the person to look at the wound
    D. Make sure the person does not see the old dressing when it is removed

72. When you are assigned to change dressings, you should
    A. Follow Standard Precautions and Bloodborne Pathogen Standard
    B. Use sterile technique
    C. Wear gloves only to remove old dressings
    D. Use one pair of gloves throughout the dressing change
73. A binder promotes healing because it will
    A. Prevent infection
    B. Prevent drainage
    C. Reduce or prevent swelling
    D. Prevent bleeding
74. A binder should be applied
    A. With firm, even pressure over the area
    B. And secured with safety pins positioned where they are easy to reach
    C. Very loosely to prevent interfering with movement
    D. Only once a day and removed only during AM care
75. Which of these measures *will not* be helpful when a person has a wound?
    A. Tell the person the wound looks fine and he or she shouldn't be upset
    B. Encourage the person to eat well so that the body can heal better
    C. Remove any soiled dressings from the room as soon as possible
    D. Allow pain medications to take effect before giving wound care

Fill in the Blanks

76. What are common causes of wounds?
    A. _____
    B. _____
    C. _____
    D. _____
    E. _____

77. You can cause a skin tear when moving, repositioning, and transferring by holding on to a person's arm or leg _____.

78. List ways to prevent skin tears in the following:
    A. Keep the person hydrated by _____
    B. What kind of clothing would be helpful? _____
    C. Nail care of the person _____
    D. Lift and turn the person with a _____
    E. Support the arms and legs with _____
    F. Pad _____
    G. Your fingernails _____ and _____.

79. Skin tears are portals _____.

80. Name the stage of pressure ulcer described in each of these:
    A. The skin is gone, and underlying tissues are exposed. _____
    B. The skin is red with light skin, or red, blue, or purple with dark skin. The color does not return to normal when the skin is relieved of pressure. _____
    C. Muscle and bone are exposed and damaged. Drainage is likely. _____
    D. The wound may involve an abrasion, blister, or shallow crater. _____

81. You can help prevent shearing by raising the head of the bed only _____. The care plan tells you:
    A. _____
    B. _____
    C. _____

82. If a person sitting in a chair is able to move, remind the person to shift position every _____ to decrease pressure on _____.

83. Explain how these protective devices help prevent pressure ulcers:
    A. Bed cradle prevents pressure on _____.
    B. Heel and elbow protectors prevent _____ and _____.
    C. Heel and foot elevators raise _____.
    D. Eggcrate-type pads distribute _____.
    E. Special beds distribute _____. There is little pressure on _____.

84. When the person has circulatory ulcers, report any _____.

85. You are caring for a person with a disease that affects venous circulation. You notice her toenails are long and sharp. You should _____.

86. Elastic stockings help prevent the development of thrombi because the elastic _____.

87. When you are delegated to apply elastic stockings, what observations should you report and record?
    A. _____
    B. _____
    C. _____
    D. _____
    E. _____
    F. _____
    G. _____
    H. _____
    I. _____

88. When you apply elastic bandages, the fingers or toes are exposed to allow _____.

89. After applying elastic bandages, you should check the fingers or toes for _____ _____. Also ask about _____ _____. If any of these are noted, you should _____ _____.

90. What two diseases are common causes of arterial ulcers?
_____
_____

91. When a person has diabetes, what complications can occur with the following?
A. Nerves: The person does not feel _____ _____. The person can develop _____ _____.
B. Blood vessels: Blood flow _____. What can occur?
_____

92. Explain what can happen if a person with diabetes has these foot problems:
A. Corns and calluses _____ _____
B. Ingrown toenails _____ _____
C. Hammer toes _____ _____
D. Dry and cracked skin _____ _____

93. With primary intention healing, the wound edges are held together with _____ _____.

94. Secondary intention healing is used for _____ _____wounds. Because healing takes longer, the threat of _____ _____ is great.

95. What should you do if you find a person's wound has dehiscence or evisceration? _____ _____

96. What observations would you make about wound appearance?
A. _____
B. _____
C. _____
D. _____
E. _____

97. When you are delegated to change a dressing, what should you do if the old dressings stick to the wound?
_____

98. If the person has drainage from a wound, how is it measured?
A. _____
B. _____
C. _____

99. What are purposes of a transparent adhesive film dressing?
A. _____
B. _____
C. _____
D. _____

100. What is the difference between wet-to-dry dressings and wet-to-wet dressings?
_____
_____

101. When taping a dressing in place, the tape should not encircle the entire body part because _____ _____.

102. When delegated to apply dressings, list what observations should be reported and recorded.
A. _____
B. _____
C. _____
D. _____
E. _____
F. _____
G. _____
H. _____
I. _____
J. _____
K. _____
L. _____
M. _____

Labeling
Answer questions 103 and 104 using the following illustration.

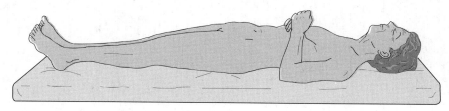

103. Name this position. _____

104. Place an "X" on each of the 5 pressure points. Name the bony point for each one.
    A. _____
    B. _____
    C. _____
    D. _____
    E. _____

Answer questions 105 and 106 using the following illustration.

105. Name this position. _____

106. Place an "X" on each of the 7 pressure points. Name the bony point(s) for each one.
    A. _____
    B. _____
    C. _____
    D. _____
    E. _____
    F. _____
    G. _____

Answer questions 107 and 108 using the following illustration.

107. Name this position. _____

108. Place an "X" on each of the 6 pressure points. Name the bony point for each one.
    A. _____
    B. _____
    C. _____
    D. _____
    E. _____
    F. _____

Answer questions 109 and 110 using the following illustration.

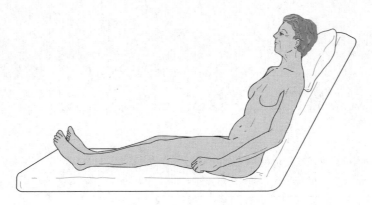

109. Name this position. _____

110. Place an "X" on each of the 3 pressure points. Name the bony point for each one.
   A. _____
   B. _____
   C. _____

Answer questions 111 and 112 using the following illustration.

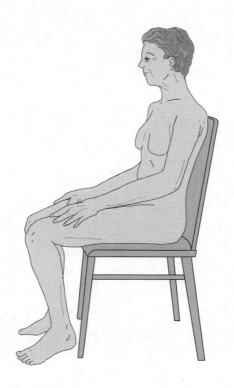

111. Name this position. _____

112. Place an "X" on each of the 5 pressure points. Name the bony point for each one.
   A. _____
   B. _____
   C. _____
   D. _____
   E. _____

Crossword

Fill in the crossword by answering the clues below with the words from this list:

Adhesive
Anti-embolism
Bed cradle
Bony prominence
Eggcrate-type
Footboard
Gauze
Hemoglobin

Hemovac
Infection
Montgomery ties
Penrose
Sutures
T-binder
Trochanter roll

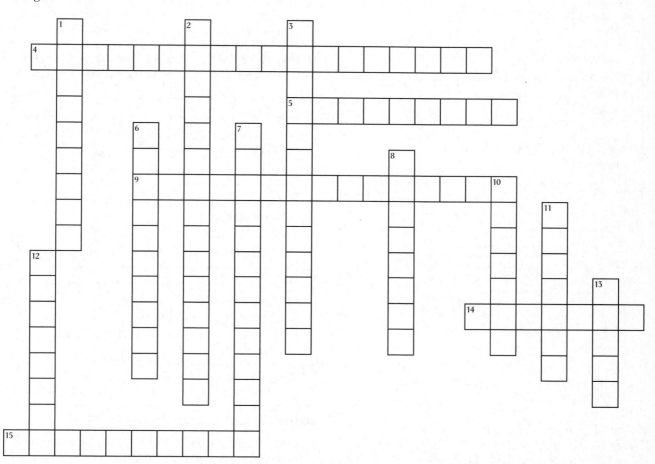

The words used in this crossword are found in the chapter but are not in the key terms. Some of the words were defined in other chapters.

ACROSS

4. Area where the bone sticks out or projects from the flat surface of the body.
5. Disease state resulting from the invasion and growth of microorganisms in the body.
9. Consists of adhesive strips and cloth ties. Designed to hold dressings in place.
14. Closed drainage system that removes drainage from a wound with suction.
15. Metal frame placed on a bed and over the person.

DOWN

1. Device placed at the foot of the mattress to prevent plantar flexion.
2. Device that prevents the hips and legs from turning outward.
3. Stockings that prevents the development of thrombi.
6. Substance in red blood cells that carries oxygen and gives blood its color.
7. Matters made of foam with peaks in the matters to distribute the person's weight.
8. Binder that holds dressings in place after rectal or perineal surgeries.
10. Stitches used to close a wound.
11. Rubber tube that drains onto a dressing from a wound.
12. Tape that sticks well to skin but can irriate skin.
13. Type of dressing that absorbs moisture. Comes in rolls, squares, rectangles, and pads.

Nursing Assistant Skills Video Exercise
View the **Preventing and Treating Pressure Ulcers** *video to answer these questions.*

113. A pressure ulcer can be life-threatening.
    A. True
    B. False

114. Nursing assistants play an important role in helping prevent pressure ulcers.
    A. True
    B. False

115. A bony prominence is _____
    _____.

116. Pressure ulcers develop when preventative care measures are practiced.
    A. True
    B. False

117. List the factors that place Mr. Raider at risk for pressure ulcers:
    A. _____
    B. _____
    C. _____
    D. _____
    E. _____

118. Which factors place Mrs. Jensen at risk for pressure ulcers?
    A. _____
    B. _____
    C. _____
    D. _____

119. When you are delegated measures to prevent pressure ulcers, you need to obtain specific instructions from the _____ and the _____.

Optional Learning Exercises
You are assigned to care for Mrs. Stevens. She is 87 years old and has diabetes and high blood pressure. She walks with difficulty and spends most of her day sitting in her chair. She is somewhat overweight and tells you she had a knee replacement 5 years ago and had phlebitis after surgery. The nurse tells you to watch carefully for signs of circulatory ulcers. Answer questions 120–122.

120. What risk factors does Mrs. Stevens have that place her at risk for circulatory ulcers?
    A. _____
    B. _____
    C. _____
    D. _____
    E. _____
    F. _____
    G. _____

121. What signs and symptoms may be present if Mrs. Stevens has venous ulcers?
    _____
    _____

122. If arterial ulcers develop, they are usually found _____
    _____.

Mr. Hawkins, age 74, was in an automobile accident and has a wound on his leg that is large and open. It has become infected, and he is being treated with antibiotics. When you are talking with him, he tells you he has smoked for 55 years and has poor circulation in his legs. He lives alone and generally eats takeout foods or eats cereal when he is at home. Answer questions 123–126.

123. Why is he receiving antibiotics?
    _____

124. What side effect of the antibiotics can cause a problem that could interfere with healing?
    _____

125. What factors would increase Mr. Hawkins' risk for complications?
    A. _____
    B. _____
    C. _____
    D. _____

126. What is missing in Mr. Hawkins' diet that is needed to help in healing the wound?
    _____

You are assisting the nurse with wound care. She is changing dressings for two different persons. Mrs. Henderson has a wound that has a large of amount of drainage. Mr. Wendel has a drain in his wound that is attached to suction. Answer questions 127–131.

127. Why does the nurse weigh Mrs. Henderson's new dressings before applying them to the wound and weigh the old dressings when they are removed?
    _____

128. How does she find out the amount of drainage from Mr. Wendel's wound?
    _____

129. What other ways can be used to measure drainage in old dressings?
    A. _____
    B. _____
    C. _____
    D. _____
    E. _____
    F. _____

130. When you are changing a nonsterile dressing, why do you need two pairs of gloves?

_____

_____

_____

131. When a wound is infected and has poor circulation, the wound may be left open at first and then closed later. This type of wound healing is called healing through _____. This type of healing combines _____ and _____ _____ intention healing.

Independent Learning Activities

Take turns with a classmate and carry out these exercises. They will help you understand how a person who cannot move without help feels when pressure is unrelieved. NOTE: These exercises work best if the person wears thin clothes so the discomfort is more noticeable.

- Place a pencil or similar hard object on the seat of a chair and have a classmate sit on the object for 10 minutes. Keep time, and remind the person not to move, to make it more uncomfortable. Remember, persons at risk for pressure ulcers often are unable to change position without assistance.
- Position a classmate in bed, making sure the bedclothes are wrinkled to form lumps under bony pressure points. (For example, place a wrinkle under the sacrum in the supine position, or under the hip or shoulders in the lateral position.)

Answer these questions about the exercises done.

- How long did it *seem* when you were waiting for 10 minutes to pass?
- How many times did you begin to reposition yourself without thinking about it?
- How did the pressure areas feel when you completed the 10 minutes? What color was the area?
- How will this exercise affect your care of persons who cannot move?

Key Terms

Compress	Cyanosis	Hyperthermia	Pack
Constrict	Dilate	Hypothermia	

Fill in the Blanks: Key Terms

1. A body temperature that is much higher than the person's normal range is _____ _____.

2. _____ means to narrow.

3. A treatment that involves wrapping a body part with a wet or dry application is a _____.

4. A _____ is a soft pad applied over a body area.

5. _____ means to expand or open wider.

6. _____ occurs when the body temperature is very low.

7. A bluish color is _____.

Circle the BEST Answer

8. Before you apply heat applications, it is important to know if
   A. A nurse is available to answer questions and supervise you
   B. Your state allows you to perform the procedure
   C. The procedure is in your job description
   D. All of the above

9. Heat applications can be applied
   A. Only to extremities
   B. To areas with metal implants
   C. To almost any body part
   D. To persons who have difficulty sensing heat or pain

10. When heat is applied to the skin
    A. Blood vessels in the area dilate
    B. Tissues have less oxygen
    C. Blood flow decreases
    D. Blood vessels constrict

11. When heat is applied too long, a complication that occurs is
    A. Blood vessels dilate
    B. Blood flow increases
    C. Blood vessels constrict
    D. More nutrients reach the area

12. Moist heat applications have cooler temperatures than dry heat applications because
    A. Dry heat penetrates more deeply
    B. Dry heat cannot cause burns
    C. Heat penetrates deeper with a moist application
    D. Moist heat has a slower effect than dry heat

13. When heat is applied in an area, which of these is an expected response?
    A. The skin is red and warm
    B. The skin is pale, white, or gray
    C. The person begins to shiver
    D. The area is excessively red

14. The care plan states that the resident receives a heat application of 110° F. As a nursing assistant, you know that you should
    A. Measure the temperature carefully before applying to the person
    B. Not apply an application that is above 106° F
    C. Ask the person if the application is too warm
    D. Apply the application and remind the person not to remove the application

15. Heat and cold applications are applied for no longer than
    A. 1 hour   C. 15 to 20 minutes
    B. 30 minutes   D. 4 hours

16. When a hot or cold application is in place, you should check the area
    A. Every 15 to 20 minutes
    B. Every 5 minutes
    C. About every 30 minutes
    D. Once an hour

17. When hot compresses are in place, you may apply an aquathermia pad over the compress
    A. To keep the compress wet
    B. To protect the area from injury
    C. To measure the temperature of the compress
    D. To maintain the correct temperature of the compress

18. A hot soak is applied
    A. By putting the body part into water
    B. By applying a soft pad to a body part
    C. And is covered with plastic wrap
    D. Only until the water temperature cools down

19. When giving a sitz bath
    A. Stay with the person if he or she is weak or unsteady
    B. Observe for signs of weakness, faintness, or fatigue
    C. Prevent the person from chills and burns
    D. All of the above

20. Hot packs may be heated by all of these methods except
    A. Boiling in water for a few minutes
    B. Squeezing, kneading, or striking the pack
    C. Sterilizing in an autoclave
    D. Warming in a microwave oven

21. When you use an aquathermia pad
    A. The pad temperature will cool off after about 20 to 30 minutes
    B. The temperature is maintained by the flow of water through the pad
    C. It is a form of moist heat
    D. You do not need to check the person as often as with other heat applications
22. When a cold application is applied, the numbing effect helps to
    A. Reduce or relieve pain in the part
    B. Constrict blood vessels
    C. Decrease blood flow
    D. Cool the body part
23. Which of these cold applications is moist?
    A. Ice bag
    B. Ice collar
    C. Ice glove
    D. Cold compress
24. You should remove the heat or cold application if
    A. The skin is red and warm with a heat application
    B. The person tells you the cold application has numbed the area and relieved some pain
    C. The skin appears pale, white, gray, or bluish in color
    D. The person is slightly chilled and asks for another blanket
25. When a person has hyperthermia, ice packs are applied to all of these areas *except*
    A. The abdomen
    B. The head
    C. The underarms
    D. The groin

Fill in the Blanks

26. What are the effects of heat applications?
    A. _____
    B. _____
    C. _____
    D. _____
    E. _____

27. When you are caring for a confused person and heat or cold is applied, how can you know if the person is in pain? _____

28. What are the advantages of dry heat applications?
    A. _____
    B. _____

29. Give an example of a dry heat application. _____
    _____

30. When the nurse delegates you to prepare a warm soak, what is the temperature range that is correct?
    _____

31. When you are giving a sitz bath, what observations should be reported to the nurse?
    _____

32. When using an aquathermia pad, you should make sure the hoses do not have kinks or air bubbles to allow the water to _____.
33. Name uses for cold applications:
    A. _____
    B. _____
    C. _____
    D. _____
    E. _____
34. When you prepare an ice bag, collar, or glove, remove the excess air by _____
    _____.
35. When a heat or cold compress is in place, it usually needs to be changed every 5 minutes because it
    _____.
36. When a cooling blanket is being used, _____
    _____ are checked often.
37. To promote comfort and safety, what can be done for the person before and during the application of heat or cold?
    A. _____
    B. _____
    C. _____
    D. _____
38. How can you manage your time to stay in or near the person's room during a heat or cold application?
    A. _____
    B. _____
    C. _____
    D. _____
    E. _____
    F. _____

Optional Learning Exercises
SITUATION: The nurse instructs you to apply a cold pack to a resident who has twisted her ankle. Use the information you learned in this chapter to answer questions 39–47 about carrying out this treatment.

39. What is the purpose of the cold application for this injury?
    _____
    _____

40. What can you use to make a cool dry application to the ankle if no commercial packs are available?
    _____

41. Why do you squeeze the application tightly after filling it with ice?
    _____
    _____

42. How will you protect the person's skin?
    _____

43. How often do you check the application?
_____

44. What signs and symptoms would be important when you check the area?
_____

45. What should you do if they are present?
_____

46. How long should you leave the application in place?
_____

47. What happens if you leave it too long?
_____

Independent Learning Exercises

Role-play this situation with a classmate. One of you should act as the person, and one should act as the nursing assistant. Work together to answer the questions for each role.

Situation: Mr. Chavez is 45 years old and has a reddened area on his left calf. The doctor has ordered moist warm compresses to the area, and the nurse has delegated this task to you.

As the Nursing Assistant:
- What questions would you ask the nurse before you applied the compresses?
- What temperature range is used for this compress?
- How did you check the temperature of the compresses?
- How did you keep the compress at the correct temperature?
- How often did you check the compress? What did you observe when you checked the area?

As Mr. Chavez:
- How was the treatment explained to you?
- How were you positioned? How did the nursing assistant check to see if you were comfortable?
- How did the compress feel? Was the temperature maintained? How?
- How often was the compress checked?

34 Hearing, Speech, and Vision Problems

Key Terms

Aphasia
Blind
Braille
Broca's aphasia
Cerumen

Deafness
Expressive aphasia
Expressive-receptive aphasia
Global aphasia

Hearing loss
Low vision
Mixed aphasia
Motor aphasia
Receptive aphasia

Tinnitus
Vertigo
Wernicke's aphasia

Fill in the Blanks: Key Terms

1. _____ is a touch reading and writing system that uses raised dots for each letter of the alphabet.

2. Another name for receptive aphasia is _____ _____.

3. Another name for earwax is _____ _____.

4. _____ is dizziness.

5. A ringing, roaring, or hissing sound in the ears is _____.

6. The inability to have normal speech; a language disorder resulting from damage to parts of the brain responsible for language is _____.

7. _____ is not being able to hear the normal range of sounds associated with normal hearing.

8. _____ is difficulty expressing or sending out thoughts; motor aphasia, Broca's aphasia.

9. Eyesight that cannot be corrected with eyeglasses, contact lenses, medicine, or surgery is _____ _____.

10. _____ is also called expressive aphasia or Broca's aphasia.

11. A hearing loss in which it is impossible for the person to understand speech through hearing alone is _____.

12. Another name for expressive aphasia or motor aphasia is _____.

13. _____ is also called expressive-receptive aphasia or mixed aphasia.

14. The absence of sight is _____.

15. Difficulty expressing or sending out thought and difficulty understanding language is _____ _____.

16. Another name for expressive aphasia or Broca's aphasia is _____.

17. Difficulty understanding language is _____ _____; also called Wernicke's aphasia.

Circle the BEST Answer

18. If a person has chronic otitis media, the person may develop
    A. Vertigo
    B. Permanent hearing loss
    C. Diarrhea
    D. Nausea and vomiting

19. How would you know whether a person with dementia has otitis media?
    A. The person would tell you he or she has pain
    B. The person would not be able to hear you
    C. You might notice the person tugging or pulling at one or both ears
    D. The person would have tinnitus

20. If you are caring for a person who has Meniere's disease, it is important to
    A. Prevent falls
    B. Assist the person to move quickly
    C. Keep the lights in the room very bright
    D. Encourage the person to be active

21. Which of these is a preventable cause of hearing loss?
    A. Aging
    B. Heredity
    C. Exposure to very loud music
    D. Birth defects

22. When you are caring for a person with a hearing loss, which of these would *not* help communication?
    A. Gain the person's attention by lightly touching the person's arm
    B. Speak as loudly as possible
    C. Do not cover your mouth or eat while talking
    D. Use gestures and facial expressions to give useful clues

23. A person with a hearing loss may
    A. Answer questions or respond inappropriately
    B. Think others are mumbling or slurring words
    C. Shun social events to avoid embarrassment
    D. All of the above

24. When you are caring for a person with a hearing aid, follow the nurse's instructions before
    A. Turning the hearing aid off at night
    B. Inserting a new battery if needed
    C. Cleaning the hearing aid
    D. Removing the battery at night

25. If a person has expressive aphasia, he or she
    A. Would not understand simple language
    B. Would speak in complete sentences
    C. Would have difficulty hearing what was said
    D. Might speak in single words or put words in the wrong order
26. When a person cannot communicate, he or she may be
    A. Frustrated   C. Depressed
    B. Angry   D. All of the above
27. An effective measure to use when caring for a speech-impaired person is to
    A. Speak in a child-like way
    B. Ask the person questions to which you know the answer
    C. Use long, involved sentences
    D. Make sure the TV or radio is loud
28. When a person has glaucoma, he or she may have difficulty seeing objects
    A. That are far away
    B. To the right or left of the person
    C. Directly in front of the person
    D. That are bright colors
29. Which of these is *not* a risk factor for glaucoma?
    A. Everyone over 60 years of age
    B. Caucasians and Asians over 40 years of age
    C. Those with a family history of glaucoma
    D. Those who have eye diseases or eye injuries
30. Cataracts most commonly are caused by
    A. Aging
    B. Injury
    C. Increased pressure in the eye
    D. Surgery
31. When a person has had eye surgery for cataracts, the care includes
    A. Remove the eye shield or patch for naps and at night
    B. Have the person cover the eye during a shower or shampoo
    C. Do not let the person bend at the waist or pick up objects from the floor
    D. Place the overbed table on the operative side
32. After cataract surgery, report to the nurse if
    A. The person complains of eye pain or blurred vision
    B. Glasses need to be cleaned
    C. The person asks for equipment to clean contact lenses
    D. The person asks for help with basic needs
33. If a person has dry, age-related macular degeneration (AMD)
    A. It can be treated with surgery
    B. The person will need to use eye drops for the rest of his or her life
    C. The person will eventually be blind
    D. The person will need to wear corrective glasses to see clearly
34. Which of these measures can reduce the risk of AMD?
    A. Exposing the eyes to sunlight
    B. Eating a healthy diet high in green leafy vegetables and fish
    C. Eating a diet high in red meats
    D. Decreasing the amount of exercise

35. Diabetic retinopathy is the result of
    A. High blood pressure
    B. Tiny blood vessels in the retina are damaged as a complication of diabetes
    C. Pressure increases in the eye
    D. The lens become cloudy
36. A person who is legally blind
    A. Is totally unable to see anything
    B. May sense some light but has no usable vision
    C. May have some usable vision but cannot read newsprint
    D. All of the above may be true
37. When you enter the room of a blind person, you should first
    A. Touch the person to let him or her know you are there
    B. Speak loudly to make sure the person knows you are there
    C. Make sure the lights are bright
    D. Identify yourself; give your name, title, and reason for being there
38. When a person is blind, you should avoid
    A. Rearranging furniture and equipment
    B. Using words such as "see," "look," or "read"
    C. Letting the person moving about
    D. Letting the person perform self-care
39. When you assist a blind person to walk, it is best if you
    A. Walk slightly behind the person
    B. Walk slightly ahead of the person
    C. Grasp the person's arm firmly to guide him or her
    D. Walk very slowly to allow the person to take small steps
40. If a blind person uses a cane, you can assist by
    A. Grasping the person by the arm holding the cane
    B. Coming up behind the person and grasping his or her elbow
    C. Giving the person verbal cues to avoid objects in the way
    D. Asking if you can assist before trying to help
41. If a blind person uses a guide dog, it is correct to
    A. Take the person by the arm on the side opposite from the dog
    B. Not pet or feed the dog
    C. Give the dog commands to avoid danger
    D. All of the above
42. Eyeglasses should be cleaned with
    A. Cleaning solution or clear water
    B. Boiling water
    C. Detergent
    D. Dry cleansing tissues
43. When cleaning an artificial eye, you should
    A. Wash the prosthesis with mild soap and warm water
    B. Wash the eyelid and eyelashes with warm water
    C. Rinse the eye with sterile water before the person inserts the eye
    D. All of the above

Fill in the Blanks

44. Otitis media often begins with _____ _____.

45. If a person has chronic otitis media, it can cause permanent _____.

46. When a person has Meniere's disease, attacks can occur _____ or just _____ _____.

47. With Meniere's disease, the person should not walk alone in case _____ _____.

48. What are examples of noises that can cause hearing loss?
    A. _____
    B. _____
    C. _____
    D. _____

49. When persons are 85 years of age or older, about _____ have a hearing loss.

50. Symptoms of hearing loss include:
    A. _____
    B. _____
    C. _____
    D. _____
    E. _____
    F. _____
    G. _____
    H. _____
    I. _____
    J. _____
    K. _____

51. If a woman is speaking to a person who is hard of hearing, why should she adjust the pitch of her voice?
    _____
    _____

52. Why is it important for a person with a hearing loss to see your face when you are speaking to the person?
    _____

53. What are common causes of speech disorders?
    A. _____
    B. _____
    C. _____

54. If a person has apraxia, the brain _____ _____ _____.

55. Measures you can use to communicate with a speech-impaired person are
    A. Listen, and give _____ _____
    B. Repeat _____
    C. Write down _____
    D. Allow the person _____
    E. Watch _____

56. When a person has expressive aphasia, the person knows what _____ _____. Thinking is _____.

57. When a person has receptive aphasia, the person may speak in _____ that have no _____.

58. Symptoms of glaucoma include
    A. Peripheral _____
    B. Blurred _____
    C. Halos _____

59. Drugs and surgery are used with glaucoma to _____.

60. Most cataracts are caused by _____. Other risk factors are
    A. _____
    B. _____
    C. _____
    D. _____
    E. _____

61. When you are caring for a person after cataract surgery, an eye shield is worn as directed and is worn for _____.

62. When assisting a blind or visually impaired person, what can be done to provide a consistent mealtime setting?
    A. _____
    B. _____
    C. _____
    D. _____
    E. _____
    F. _____

63. A person with age-related macular degeneration (AMD) would develop a blind spot _____.

64. Which type of AMD is the more severe form?
    _____

65. Everyone with diabetes is at risk for _____ _____.

66. How can a person with low vision use a computer as an adaptive device?

    A. _____

    B. _____

67. The legally blind person sees at 20 feet what a person with normal vision sees at _____

    _____.

68. When you orient a person to the room, why do you let the person move about the room? _____

    _____

Optional Learning Exercises

Mr. Herman is an 85-year-old man with a hearing loss that has developed as he has gotten older. Answer these questions about his care:

69. Two nursing assistants are caring for Mr. Herman, a male and a female. They notice that he answers questions asked by the male nursing assistant more quickly. What is the likely reason for this?

    _____

    _____

70. The nursing assistants have found that Mr. H. is alert and oriented. They are surprised when Joan, another nursing assistant, tells them he is "senile." Why would Joan make this statement?

    _____

    _____

71. Mr. H. says he is too tired to go to the game room for a party. He says no one likes him. What are some reasons for his actions and statements?

    A. Tired because _____

    B. No one likes him _____

72. When giving care, the nursing assistant turns off the TV and radio in Mr. H.'s room. Why is this done?

    _____

You are caring for Mrs. Sanchez, who is legally blind because of glaucoma. Answer these questions about her care:

73. When you enter the room, you notice that Mrs. Sanchez is looking at her mail with a magnifying glass. How is this possible since you thought she was blind?

    _____

    _____

74. When you enter the room, Mrs. S. asks you to adjust the blinds. Why?

    _____

    _____

75. When you are helping Mrs. S. move about the room, you are careful not to leave her in the middle of the room. Why?

    _____

    _____

Independent Learning Activities

Cover your ears so that you cannot hear clearly. Use one of these methods or one that you devise:

- Commercial earplugs
- Cotton plugs in ears
- Cover ears with earmuffs or similar devices

Keep you ears covered and hearing muffled for at least 1 hour as you go about your daily activities. A wise student will not wear earplugs during class time! Answer these questions about the experience:

- How did you find yourself compensating for the hearing loss? Turning up the TV or radio? Asking others to write out information? Staying away from others? Getting angry or frustrated?
- When you could not understand someone, what did you do? Ask him or her to repeat? Ask him or her to speak louder? Answer even if you were unsure of what was said? Not respond at all?
- If you answered when unsure, what was your response? Did you tend to agree or disagree with the speaker? Why?
- What methods listed in the chapter were helpful? What other methods did you use to understand what was being said? Watching the speaker? Cupping your hand around ears?
- How will this experience assist you when you care for a person with a hearing loss?

Cover your eyes with a blindfold so you cannot see. Keep the blindfold on for at least 1 hour as you go about your normal activities. Have someone act as a guide during this time. In addition to your normal activities, include the activities listed. Answer these questions about the experience:

- Go outside with your guide and cross a street.
- Visit a store or restaurant with your guide.
- Eat a simple snack or meal.
- Go to the toilet, wash your hands, and comb your hair.
- Have your guide take you to a public area, place you in a chair or on a benchs and leave you alone for 5-10 minutes.

NOTE: *You may wish to carry out this exercise using the blindfold and using this alternate method. If you wear glasses, cover the lenses with a heavy coating of petroleum jelly. This will simulate the vision experienced by a person with cataracts. Answer these questions for both experiences:*

- How did you feel when you were unable to see what was going on around you? What noises or other sensory stimulants did you notice?
- When you were crossing the street, how did you feel? Safe? Frightened?
- When you were in a public area, what did you notice? How did you feel? How did others respond to you?
- How comfortable did you feel about eating when you could not see the food? How were you able to locate the food? What problems did you have?
- How did you manage in the bathroom? Were you able to find the equipment you needed? How competent did you feel about carrying out hand washing and grooming without seeing?
- What were your feelings when left alone in a public area for 5-10 minutes? How long did it *seem* to be before your guide returned? What concerns did you have? Safety? Fear of injury? Desertion?
- How will this experience assist you when caring for a person with a vision loss?

Have a group discussion with your classmates who have all carried out the exercises to simulate vision and hearing problems. Answer these questions:

- Which disability did you find the most difficult to tolerate? Why?
- If you had to live with one of these disabilities, which one would you choose? Why?
- What happened during these exercises that surprised you about being unable to see or hear? How does this discovery change your attitude about the disabilities?

35 Common Health Problems

Key Terms

Amputation
Arthritis
Arthroplasty
Benign tumor
Cancer

Closed fracture
Compound fracture
Fracture
Hemiplegia
Hyperglycemia

Hypoglycemia
Malignant tumor
Metastasis
Open fracture
Paraplegia

Quadriplegia
Simple fracture
Stomatitis
Tumor
Tetraplegia

Fill in the Blanks: Key Terms

1. _____ is another name for quadriplegia.

2. The spread of cancer to other body parts is _____ _____.

3. A new growth of abnormal cells, which may be benign or malignant, is a _____.

4. When the bone is broken but the skin is intact, it is called a simple fracture or a _____ _____.

5. _____ is joint inflammation.

6. Low sugar in the blood is _____ _____.

7. An inflammation of the mouth is _____.

8. A _____ is a tumor that does not spread to other body parts.

9. Paralysis and loss of sensation of the arms, legs, and trunk is _____.

10. An _____ is the surgical replacement of a joint.

11. Another name for an open fracture is a _____ _____.

12. _____ means high sugar in the blood.

13. A malignant tumor is _____.

14. An _____ is the removal of all or part of an extremity.

15. A _____ is another name for a closed fracture.

16. A broken bone is a _____.

17. A tumor that invades and destroys nearby tissue and can spread to other body parts is _____ _____.

18. _____ is paralysis on one side of the body.

19. Paralysis of the legs is _____.

20. When a broken bone has come through the skin, it is called a compound fracture or _____.

Circle the BEST Answer

21. Benign tumors
   A. Do not spread to other body parts
   B. Invade healthy tissue
   C. Spread to other parts of the body
   D. Divide in an orderly and controlled way

22. Risk factors that cause cancer include all of these *except*
   A. Exposure to sun and tanning booths
   B. Smoking
   C. A diet high in fresh fruits and vegetables
   D. Close relatives with certain types of cancer

23. If you care for a person who is receiving radiation therapy to treat cancer, you might expect the person to
   A. Have pain related to the therapy
   B. Need extra rest because of fatigue
   C. Be at risk for bleeding and infections
   D. Complain of flu-like symptoms—for example, chills, fever, muscle aches

24. Chemotherapy involves
   A. X-ray beams aimed at the tumor
   B. Giving drugs that prevent the production of certain hormones
   C. Therapy to help the immune system
   D. Giving drugs that kill cells

25. You are giving care to Mrs. Ferris, a resident who is receiving chemotherapy. She tells you she is upset because her hair is falling out. You know that
   A. The hair often falls out when a person receives chemotherapy
   B. This is a result of her illness
   C. You should report this to the nurse immediately because it means her chemotherapy is not working
   D. It is best to change the subject to keep Mrs. Ferris from getting upset

26. When hormone therapy is used to treat cancer, a woman may experience
   A. Fatigue and fluid retention
   B. Changes in fertility
   C. Weight gain, hot flashes, nausea and vomiting
   D. All of the above

27. A person with cancer may complain of constipation because of
   A. The side effects of pain-relief drugs
   B. Pain
   C. Rest and exercise
   D. Fluids and nutrition

28. When a person having treatment for cancer expresses anger, fear, and depression, you can help the most by
    A. Telling the person not to worry or get upset
    B. Give the person privacy and time alone
    C. Being there when needed and listening to the person
    D. Changing the subject to distract the person

29. Osteoarthritis differs from rheumatoid arthritis because osteoarthritis
    A. Is an inflammatory disease
    B. Occurs with aging
    C. Causes the person to not feel well
    D. Occurs on both sides of the body

30. When you are caring for a person with osteoarthritis, which of these would be most helpful to the person?
    A. Allow the person to stay in bed all day
    B. Keep the room cool, because osteoarthritis improves with cold temperatures
    C. Help the person use good body mechanics and posture and get regular rest
    D. Tell the person not to exercise, because that will prevent healing

31. You are caring for a person who has rheumatoid arthritis, and the person has a flare-up of the disease. You should do all of these *except*
    A. Make sure the person exercises more frequently
    B. Position the person in good body alignment
    C. Encourage the person to rest more than usual
    D. Apply splints to support affected joints

32. When caring for a person who has had a hip replacement (arthroplasty), which of these measures would be *incorrect*?
    A. Have a high, firm chair for the person to use when out of bed
    B. Remove the abductor splint when turning the person in bed
    C. Remind the person not to cross his or her legs
    D. Make sure the person has a raised toilet seat

33. Which of these will help strengthen bones in a person at risk for osteoporosis?
    A. Bedrest
    B. Decreased calcium intake
    C. Exercise weight-bearing joints
    D. Smoking and alcohol

34. Which of these *is not* a sign or symptom of a fracture?
    A. Full range of motion in the affected limb
    B. Bruising and color change in the skin in the area
    C. Pain and tenderness
    D. Swelling

35. When a person has a newly applied plaster cast, it will dry in
    A. 2 to 4 hours   C. 24 to 48 hours
    B. 3 to 4 days   D. 12 to 24 hours

36. You can prevent flat spots on the cast by
    A. Positioning the cast on a hard, flat surface
    B. Supporting the entire cast with pillows
    C. Using your fingertips to lift the cast
    D. Cover the cast with a blanket

37. If a person complains of numbness in a part that is in a cast, you should
    A. Tell the person to move the limb a little to relieve the numbness
    B. Reposition the person to help the numbness
    C. Gently rub the exposed toes or fingers to relieve the numbness
    D. Report immediately, because it may mean there is pressure on a nerve or reduced blood flow to the part

38. If a person is in traction and you are giving care, it would be correct to
    A. Put bottom linens on the bed from the top down
    B. Remove the weights while you are giving care
    C. Turn the person from side to side to change the bed and give care
    D. Assist the person to use the commode chair to avoid walking very far

39. When caring for a person who has had surgery to repair a hip fracture, the operated leg should be
    A. Abducted at all times
    B. Adducted at all times
    C. Exercised with range-of-motion exercises every 4 hours
    D. Positioned to keep the hip in external rotation

40. If you assist a person to get up to a chair after hip surgery, you should
    A. Place the chair on the affected side
    B. Have the person stand on the operative side
    C. Place the person in a low, soft chair
    D. Remind the person not to cross the legs

41. If a person complains of pain in the amputated part, you should
    A. Report this immediately to the nurse
    B. Tell the person that he is confused
    C. Reassure the person that this is a normal reaction
    D. Tell the person this feeling will go away shortly

42. Which of these people are at higher risk for stroke?
    A. A 79-year-old man with hypertension and diabetes
    B. A 50-year-old woman who smokes and is slightly overweight
    C. A 70-year-old African-American man who has high blood pressure and diabetes
    D. A 75-year-old Asian man who is inactive, has normal blood pressure, and has diabetes

43. If a person who has had a stroke ignores the weaker side of the body, it is probably because the person has
    A. Lost movement on that side
    B. Lost feeling on that side
    C. A loss of vision on that side
    D. All of the above

44. When a person who has a stroke has urinary incontinence, you can expect that
    A. Bladder training will restore normal function
    B. The person will always be incontinent
    C. Bladder training will help the person regain the highest possible level of function
    D. Bladder training will not help

45. A safety concern for a person with Parkinson's disease would be
   A. Changes in speech
   B. Swallowing and chewing problems
   C. A mask-like expression
   D. Emotional changes
46. A person with relapsing-remitting multiple sclerosis is likely to
   A. Recover quickly from the disease
   B. Have symptoms that gradually disappear with partial or complete recovery
   C. Have a series of attacks that cause more symptoms to occur
   D. Be given medication to cure the disease
47. A person with amyotrophic lateral sclerosis (ALS) would be
   A. Confused and disoriented
   B. Able to walk with assistance even as the disease progresses
   C. Incontinent of bladder and bowel functions
   D. Unable to move the arms, legs, and body
48. A person who has a spinal cord injury in the lumbar region will likely have
   A. Quadriplegia   C. Hemiplegia
   B. Paraplegia   D. Tetraplegia
49. When caring for a person with paralysis, it is important to include
   A. Turning and repositioning at least every 2 hours
   B. Maintaining muscle function and preventing contractures
   C. Giving emotional and psychological support
   D. All of the above
50. Autonomic dysreflexia occurs in a person who has paralysis
   A. Of any kind
   B. Above the mid-thoracic level
   C. In the lumbar region
   D. That is incomplete
51. If you are caring for a person with autonomic dysreflexia, report to the nurse at once if
   A. The person has sweating above the level of injury
   B. The blood pressure is low
   C. The person complains of pain below the level of the injury
   D. The person has sweating below the level of the injury
52. If a person is at risk for autonomic dysreflexia, only the nurse should
   A. Give basic care
   B. Make sure the catheter is draining and the tubing is not kinked
   C. Reposition the person at least every 2 hours
   D. Check for fecal impactions or give an enema
53. The most common cause of chronic obstructive pulmonary disease (COPD) is
   A. Family history
   B. Respiratory infections
   C. Cigarette smoking
   D. Exercise

54. When a person has COPD, it interferes with
   A. Oxygen and carbon dioxide exchange in the lungs
   B. Airflow in the lungs
   C. Elasticity in the airways and alveoli
   D. All of the above
55. If a person has chronic bronchitis, a common symptom is
   A. Wheezing and tightening in the chest
   B. Shortness of breath on exertion
   C. A smoker's cough in the morning
   D. A high temperature for several days
56. Asthma is caused by
   A. Smoking and second-hand smoke
   B. Air pollutants and irritants
   C. Cold air
   D. All of the above
57. If an older person has influenza, he or she may
   A. Have a body temperature below normal
   B. Have an increased appetite
   C. Feel more energy than usual
   D. Have no symptoms of illness
58. Which of these symptoms is more likely to be from a cold rather than the flu?
   A. Sinus congestion
   B. High fever (100° to 102° F)
   C. Fatigued for 2 to 3 weeks
   D. Bronchitis or pneumonia
59. The flu vaccine would be recommended for all of these persons *except*
   A. A man with diabetes and chronic heart disease
   B. A woman with an immune system disease
   C. A healthy 30-year-old
   D. A 75-year-old man in good health
60. When a person has pneumonia, fluid intake is increased to
   A. Decrease the amount of bacteria in the lungs
   B. Dilute medication given to treat the disease
   C. Thin secretions
   D. Decrease inflammation of the breathing passages
61. Breathing is easier for a person with pneumonia when the person is positioned in
   A. Semi-Fowler's position
   B. Side-lying position
   C. Supine position
   D. A soft chair
62. When you care for a person with tuberculosis, you should
   A. Wash your hands if you have contact with sputum
   B. Flush tissues down the toilet
   C. Remind the person to cover the mouth and nose with tissues when coughing and sneezing
   D. All of the above
63. The leading cause of death in the United States is
   A. Cardiovascular disorders
   B. Hypertension
   C. Cancer
   D. Chronic obstructive pulmonary disease (COPD)

64. Hypertension (high blood pressure) is a condition in which
    A. The systolic pressure is 120 mm Hg or higher and diastolic is 70 or higher
    B. The systolic pressure is 100 mm Hg or higher and diastolic is 60 or higher
    C. The systolic pressure is 140 mm Hg or higher and diastolic is 90 or higher
    D. The systolic pressure is 140 mm Hg or higher and diastolic is 60 or higher

65. A risk factor for hypertension that cannot change is
    A. Stress
    B. Being overweight
    C. Age
    D. Lack of exercise

66. The most common cause of coronary artery disease is
    A. Lack of exercise
    B. Atherosclerosis
    C. Family history
    D. Stress

67. When a person has angina pectoris, the chest pain occurs when
    A. Oxygen does not reach the lungs
    B. There is reduced blood flow to the heart
    C. Blood pressure is too high
    D. Heart muscle dies

68. If a person has angina pain, it will usually be relieved by
    A. Resting for about 3 to15 minutes
    B. Taking narcotic drugs
    C. Using oxygen therapy
    D. Getting up and walking for exercise

69. If a person takes a nitroglycerin tablet when an angina attack occurs, you should
    A. Give the person a large glass of water to swallow the pill
    B. Take the pills back to the nurses' station
    C. Make sure the person tells the nurse a pill was taken
    D. Encourage the person to walk around

70. When a myocardial infarction occurs, it means that
    A. A part of the heart muscle dies
    B. The heart muscle is not receiving enough oxygen
    C. The pain is relieved by rest
    D. Blood backs up into the lungs

71. If a person complains of pain in the back, neck, jaw, or stomach, you should get help because the person
    A. Is having an angina attack
    B. Has indigestion
    C. May be having a heart attack
    D. May be having a stroke

72. When heart failure occurs, the person may have
    A. Fluid in the lungs
    B. Swelling in the feet and ankles
    C. Confusion, dizziness, and fainting
    D. All of the above

73. An older person with heart failure is at risk for
    A. Contractures
    B. Skin breakdown
    C. Fractures
    D. Urinary tract infections

74. Women have a higher risk of urinary tract infections because of
    A. Hormone levels in the body
    B. The short female urethra
    C. Bacteria
    D. Prostrate gland secretions

75. If a person has cystitis, you should
    A. Restrict fluid intake
    B. Assist the person to ambulate frequently
    C. Keep the person on bedrest
    D. Encourage the person to drink 2000 ml per day

76. If a man has benign prostatic hypertrophy (BPH), he will probably
    A. Be incontinent of urine
    B. Have frequent urination at night
    C. Have increased urinary output
    D. Have renal failure

77. After surgery to correct BPH, the care plan may include
    A. A balanced diet to prevent constipation
    B. Increased activity with an exercise plan
    C. Restricted fluid intake
    D. Care of the surgical incision

78. If you are caring for a person with renal calculi, you will be expected to
    A. Restrict the person's fluid intake
    B. Keep the person on bedrest
    C. Strain all urine
    D. All of the above

79. When you care for a person with acute renal failure, the care plan will include
    A. Increasing fluid intake to 2000 to 3000 ml per day
    B. Measuring and recording urine output every hour
    C. Making sure the person does not drink any fluids
    D. Measuring weight weekly

80. Chronic renal failure
    A. Occurs suddenly
    B. Generally improves and kidney function returns to normal within 1 year
    C. Occurs when nephrons of the kidney are destroyed over many years
    D. Has very little effect on the person's overall health

81. If a person has chronic renal failure, which of these would be included in the care plan?
    A. A diet high in protein, potassium, and sodium
    B. Plenty of exercise
    C. Measures to prevent itching
    D. Frequent bathing with soap

82. An obese 50-year-old woman with hypertension is diagnosed with diabetes. She most likely has
    A. Type 1
    B. Type 2
    C. Gestational
    D. None of the above

83. A person with diabetes complains of thirst and frequent urination. You notice the person has a flushed face and slow, deep, and labored respirations. It is likely the person has
    A. Hyperglycemia
    B. Hypoglycemia
    C. Diabetic coma
    D. An infection

84. A risk factor for gastroesophageal reflux disease (GERD) is
    A. Eating small, frequent meals
    B. Lying down after eating a large meal
    C. Maintaining normal weight
    D. Respiratory illnesses
85. Diverticular disease may occur because of
    A. A high-fiber diet
    B. Regular bowel movements
    C. Aging
    D. Infections
86. Vomiting can be life-threatening when it
    A. Is caused by an infection
    B. Is aspirated and obstructs the airway
    C. Contains undigested food
    D. Has a bitter taste
87. If vomitus looks like coffee grounds, you should report to the nurse because
    A. It signals bleeding
    B. The person may need a change in diet
    C. This indicates an infection
    D. The person may need pain medication
88. When hepatitis is contracted by eating or drinking food or water contaminated by feces, it is
    A. Hepatitis A   C. Hepatitis C
    B. Hepatitis B   D. Hepatitis D

89. A person with hepatitis will need good skin care because
    A. Of muscles aches
    B. The person will have itching and skin rash
    C. Of nausea and vomiting
    D. Of diarrhea or constipation
90. The HIV virus *is not* spread by
    A. Blood   C. Sneezing or coughing
    B. Semen   D. Breast milk
91. To protect yourself from HIV and AIDS, you should
    A. Avoid all body fluids when giving care
    B. Refuse to care for persons diagnosed with these diseases
    C. Follow Standard Precautions and the Bloodborne Pathogen Standard when giving care
    D. Always use sterile technique when giving care
92. A woman who complains about a frothy, thick, foul-smelling, yellow vaginal discharge most likely has
    A. Gonorrhea
    B. Genital warts
    C. Syphilis
    D. Trichomoniasis

Matching
Match the related symptom with the form of chronic obstructive pulmonary disorder (COPD).
93. _____Person develops a barrel chest
94. _____Mucus and inflamed breathing passages obstruct airflow
95. _____Alveoli become less elastic
96. _____Air passages narrow
97. _____First symptom is often a smoker's cough in morning
98. _____Normal O$_2$ and CO$_2$ exchange cannot occur in affected alveoli
99. _____Allergies and air pollutants are common causes

A. Chronic bronchitis
B. Emphysema
C. Asthma

Match the symptom listed with disorder of coronary artery disease.
100. _____Chest pain occurs with exertion
101. _____Blood flow to the heart is suddenly blocked
102. _____Blood backs up into the venous system
103. _____Fluid occurs in the lungs
104. _____Rest and nitroglycerin often relieve the symptoms
105. _____Pain is described as crushing, stabbing, or squeezing

A. Angina
B. Myocardial infarction
C. Heart failure

Match the symptom listed with either hypoglycemia or hyperglycemia.
106. _____Trembling; shakiness
107. _____Sweet breath odor
108. _____Tingling around mouth
109. _____Cold, clammy skin
110. _____Slow, deep, and labored respirations
111. _____Headache
112. _____Flushed face
113. _____Frequent urination

A. Hypoglycemia
B. Hyperglycemia

Match each statement with the correct type of hepatitis.

114. _____This hepatitis occurs in a person infected with hepatitis B
115. _____Caused by poor sanitation, crowded living conditions
116. _____Caused by HBV
117. _____Person may have virus but no symptoms
118. _____Ingested by eating from contaminated food or water
119. _____Serious liver damage may show up years later

A. Hepatitis A
B. Hepatitis B
C. Hepatitis C
D. Hepatitis D

Match each statement with the correct sexually transmitted disease.

120. _____Surgical removal if ointment is not effective
121. _____Sores may have a watery discharge
122. _____May have vaginal bleeding
123. _____Urinary urgency and frequency
124. _____Treated with anti-viral drugs
125. _____May not show symptoms

A. Herpes
B. Genital warts
C. Gonorrhea
D. Chlamydia

Fill in the Blanks

126. Signs and symptoms of cancer include:
    A. _____
    B. _____
    C. _____
    D. _____
    E. _____
    F. _____
    G. _____
    H. _____
    I. _____
    J. _____

127. With radiation therapy, skin care measures are needed at the treatment site because of:
    A. _____
    B. _____

128. Chemotherapy has the following uses when treating cancer:
    A. _____
    B. _____
    C. _____

129. When chemotherapy is used, what side effects can occur?
    A. _____
    B. _____
    C. _____

130. If you are caring for a person with osteoarthritis, exercise is important because it:
    A. _____
    B. _____
    C. _____

131. Rest and joint care are also used to treat osteoarthritis. Explain how these treatments help.
    A. Regular rest _____
    B. Cane and walkers _____
    C. Splints _____

132. Which type of arthritis generally develops between the ages of 20 and 50?
    _____

133. If a person has hip replacement surgery, what measures are needed to protect the hip?
    A. _____
    B. _____
    C. _____
    D. _____
    E. _____
    F. _____
    G. _____

134. List how these risks factors affect developing osteoporosis.
    A. Women risk increases_____
    B. Family _____
    C. Weight _____

135. How is calcium lost from bone? _____
    _____ What happens to the bone when calcium is lost? _____

136. If a person has a cast on a fracture, what do these symptoms mean?
    A. Pain _____
    B. Swelling and a tight cast _____
    C. Pale skin _____
    D. Odor _____
    E. Numbness _____
    F. Cool skin _____

137. What disorders increase the risk for stroke?
    A. _____
    B. _____
    C. _____
    D. _____

138. What are the warning signs of stroke?
    A. _____
    B. _____
    C. _____
    D. _____
    E. _____

139. What signs and symptoms of Parkinson's disease may cause falls and injury?
    A. _____
    B. _____
    C. _____
    D. _____

140. Which type of multiple sclerosis causes the person's condition to gradually decline with more and more symptoms and no remissions?

    _____
    _____

141. What affect does amyotrophic lateral sclerosis (ALS) have on
    A. Mind, intelligence, memory_____
    B. Senses _____
    C. Bowel and bladder functions _____
    _____
    D. Motor nerve cells _____
    _____

142. If a person has paralysis, you may need to check the person often if he or she is unable to _____
    _____.

143. Range-of-motion exercises are important when caring for a person with paralysis because they will
    _____ and _____
    _____.

144. If the nurse delegates you to raise the head of the bed 45 degrees or more for a person with a spinal cord injury, he or she may have signs or symptoms of _____
    _____.

145. What changes occur in the lungs when a person has chronic obstructive pulmonary disease (COPD)?
    A. _____
    B. _____
    C. _____
    D. _____

146. What is the best way to prevent COPD?
    _____

147. If an older person has pneumonia, what may mask typical symptoms?
    A. _____
    B. _____

148. Why does tuberculosis (TB) sometimes become active as a person ages?

    _____
    _____

149. What signs and symptoms occur with TB?
    A. _____
    B. _____
    C. _____
    D. _____
    E. _____

150. How do these risk factors increase blood pressure?
    A. Stress _____
    B. Tobacco _____
    C. High-salt diet _____
    D. Excessive alcohol _____
    E. Lack of exercise _____

151. Pain from angina is usually relieved by _____ and taking _____.

152. The goals of cardiac rehabilitation are:
    A. _____
    B. _____
    C. _____

153. When left-sided heart failure occurs, blood _____
    _____. What effect does this have on the rest of the body?
    A. Brain _____
    B. Kidneys _____
    C. Skin _____
    D. Blood pressure _____

154. When right-sided heart failure occurs, the signs and symptoms in the previous question occur. In addition, what happens to these areas?
    A. Feet and ankles _____
    B. Liver _____
    C. Abdomen _____

155. Older persons with heart failure are at increased risk for pressure ulcers because of:
    A. _____
    B. _____
    C. _____

156. Why are older persons at high risk for urinary tract infections (UTIs)?
    A. _____
    B. _____
    C. _____
    D. _____

157. After a transurethral resection of the prostate (TURP), the person's care plan may include:
    A. _____
    B. _____
    C. _____
    D. _____
    E. _____

158. What are the risk factors of developing renal calculi?
    A. Age, race, sex_____
    B. _____
    C. _____
    D. _____

159. A person with renal calculi is encouraged to drink 2000 to 3000 ml of fluid a day to help _____ _____.

160. When acute renal failure occurs, two phases occur. Name and explain these phases:
    A. _____. Urine output is _____ _____. Phase lasts _____ _____.
    B. _____. Urine output is _____ _____. Phase lasts _____.

161. Signs and symptoms of chronic renal failure appear when _____ _____.

162. You may need to assist a person in chronic renal failure with nutritional needs. List what is needed in these areas:
    A. Diet _____
    B. Fluid intake _____ _____

163. A person with _____ diabetes will be treated with healthy eating, exercise, and, sometimes, oral drugs.

164. A person with _____ diabetes will be treated with daily insulin therapy, healthy eating, and exercise.

165. What life-style changes may be needed to treat gastroesophageal reflux disease (GERD)?
    A. _____
    B. _____
    C. _____
    D. _____
    E. _____

166. Risk factors for diverticular disease are:
    A. _____
    B. _____
    C. _____

167. What can you do to make a person more comfortable after the person has vomited?
    A. _____
    B. _____
    C. _____
    D. _____

168. What ways are communicable diseases transmitted from one person to another?
    A. _____
    B. _____
    C. _____
    D. _____
    E. _____

169. To protect yourself when caring for a person with hepatitis, you should follow _____ _____.

170. List the characteristics of the types of hepatitis:
    A. Hepatitis A is spread by the _____ _____ route.
    B. Hepatitis B is present in the _____ _____.
    C. Hepatitis C can be transmitted even when the infected person has no _____ _____.
    D. Hepatitis D occurs only in people with _____ _____.
    E. Hepatitis E is not common in _____ _____.

171. Acquired immunodeficiency syndrome (AIDS) is caused by a _____ that attacks the _____.

172. A threat to the health team when caring for a person with AIDS is from _____ _____.

173. Sexually transmitted diseases (STDs) are spread by _____ _____.

174. The use of _____ helps prevent the spread of STDs.

Optional Learning Exercises
Mrs. Myers is a 62-year-old who is having chemotherapy to treat cancer. She has not been eating well and complains of feeling very tired. When you are assisting her with personal care, you notice a large amount of hair on her pillow. Answer questions 175 through 177 about Mrs. Myers and her care.

175. Mrs. Myers probably is not eating well because the chemotherapy _____ the gastrointestinal tract and causes _____ _____ and _____.

176. She may also have _____, which is called stomatitis. You can help her relieve the discomfort and eat better when you provide good _____.

177. What is causing Mrs. Myers to lose her hair? _____ _____ What is this condition called? _____

You are caring for two persons who have arthritis. Read the information about each of them and answer questions 178 through 180 about these two persons.
Mr. Miller is 78 years old. He worked in construction for many years, where he did heavy physical work. He complains about pain in his hips and his right knee. His fingers are deformed by the arthritis and interfere with good range of motion. Ms. Haxton is 40 years old. She has swelling, warmth, and tenderness in her wrists, several finger joints on both hands, and both knees. She tells you that she has had arthritis for 10 years and it "comes and goes." At present, Ms. Haxton is complaining about pain in the affected joints, has a temperature of 100.2° F, and states she is very tired.

178. Mr. Miller has _____.
    What time of day is he likely to have more joint stiffness? _____

179. It is cold and raining. Which of these persons is likely to be more affected?
    _____

180. Ms. Haxton has _____. She is likely to complain of not feeling well because the arthritis affects _____ as well as joints.

You are caring for several persons with diabetes as follows:
75-year-old African-American man
45-year-old white, obese woman
32-year-old pregnant woman
60-year-old Hispanic woman with hypertension
14-year-old girl who has lost 15 pounds
Answer questions 181 through 185 about these persons.

181. Which of these persons is most likely to have diabetes type 2? (3)
    _____

182. The 32-year-old probably has _____
    _____. She is at risk to develop _____
    _____ later in life.

183. The 14-year-old probably has _____
    _____.

184. Which type of diabetes develops rapidly?
    _____.

185. _____ is treated with daily insulin therapy. _____ is treated with oral drugs. Both types include healthy _____ and _____ in treatment.

Independent Learning Exercises
Many people have had a fracture at some time. If you have had a broken bone, answer these questions about the experience:
- Did you know the bone was broken right away? Several hours later? Days later? How did you find out?
- What symptoms did you have? Describe the pain.
- What treatment was done? A cast? Surgery? Pins, plates, screws, traction?
- How did the fracture affect your day-to-day life? Work? School? Leisure activities?
- What changes were needed for you to carry out ADL? How much help did you need from others? How did the need for help make you feel?
- How was your mobility affected? Walking? Getting out of bed or out of chair? Driving?
- What discomfort did you have during the healing process? With the cast or surgical site?
- What permanent or long-range problems happened? Periodic pain? Limited mobility?

If you have never had a fracture, try this experiment to get a small sample of how a fracture may interfere with your life. Make an immobilizer for your leg. Use one of the methods suggested, or devise one of your own.
- Find four pieces of sturdy cardboard that are long enough to reach from the ankle to mid-thigh. Place them on the front, back, and sides of the leg and secure with elastic bandages or cloth strips. You should not be able to bend your knee.
- Use several layers of newspaper or magazines and wrap around leg from ankle to knee. Secure with elastic bandages or cloth strips. You should not be able to bend the knee.

After the "cast" is in place, leave it on for 1 to 2 hours and go about your normal routine. Answer these questions about what you experienced:
- How much did the "cast" interfere with your routine?
- How did the cast interfere with your ADL? Driving? Walking? Working?
- What other problems did you have with the cast?
- How did you feel when you were in the cast? Awkward? Embarrassed?
- How do you think this short experience will help you care for someone with a cast?

Try these experiments to understand how these diseases affect the body or the person:

- **Osteoporosis**: Fold a piece of standard 8×10-inch paper in half the long way three times. (It will now be about 1×10 inches) Now try to tear it in half along the fold and along the 1-inch edge. What happens? Unfold the paper once (it will be 2×10 inches), and cut pieces out along all of the edges. This step will make the paper porous much like the bone becomes with osteoporosis. Refold the paper to the 1×10-inch size, and try to tear it again. What happens now?
- **Coronary artery disease**: Use a straw to drink water. Now, put small pieces of paper towel into the end of the straw, and try to drink again. What happens? Add more paper, and try to drink again. How does this experiment relate to coronary artery disease?

36 Mental Health Problems

Key Terms

Anxiety
Compulsion
Defense mechanism
Delusion
Delusion of grandeur
Delusion of persecution

Emotional illness
Hallucination
Mental
Mental disorder
Mental health
Mental illness

Obsession
Panic
Paranoia
Phobia
Psychiatric disorder
Psychosis

Stress
Stressor
Withdrawal syndrome

Fill in the Blanks: Key Terms

1. When a person has an exaggerated belief about one's own importance, wealth, power, or talents, it is called _____.

2. Mental illness, emotional disorder, or psychiatric disorder is also a _____ _____.

3. A _____ is the event or factor that causes stress.

4. The person's physical and mental response after stopping or severely reducing the intake of a substance that was used regularly is _____ _____.

5. _____ is relating to the mind. It is something that exists in the mind or is performed by the mind.

6. A recurrent, unwanted thought, idea, or dread is an _____.

7. The response or change in the body caused by any emotional, physical, social, or economic factor is _____.

8. _____ is a vague, uneasy feeling that occurs in response to stress.

9. _____ is another name for mental illness, mental disorder, or psychiatric disorder.

10. A _____ is an intense fear, panic, or dread.

11. A false belief is a _____.

12. _____ is a disturbance in the ability to cope or adjust to stress; behavior and functioning are impaired. This condition is also called a mental disorder, an emotional illness, or a psychiatric disorder.

13. A state of severe mental impairment is _____ _____.

14. A _____ is seeing, hearing, or feeling something that is not real.

15. _____ is a disorder of the mind. The person has false beliefs and suspicion about a person or situation.

16. The uncontrolled performance of an act is _____.

17. _____ is when the person copes with and adjusts to the stresses of everyday living in ways accepted by society.

18. _____ is a false belief that one is being mistreated, abused, or harassed.

19. An intense and sudden feeling of fear, anxiety, terror, or dread is _____.

20. _____ is another name for mental illness, mental disorder, or emotional disorder.

21. A _____ is an unconscious reaction that blocks unpleasant or threatening feelings.

Circle the BEST Answer

22. Which of these statements about anxiety is *not* true?
    A. Anxiety often occurs when needs are not met
    B. Anxiety is always abnormal
    C. Increases in pulse, respirations, and blood pressure may be caused by anxiety
    D. Anxiety is a response to stress

23. An unhealthy coping mechanism would be
    A. Talking about the problem
    B. Playing music
    C. Smoking
    D. Exercising

24. Panic is
    A. The highest level of anxiety
    B. A disorder that occurs gradually
    C. A psychosis
    D. Vague, normal response to stress

25. A person you are caring for tells you he is the president of the United States. He has a delusion of grandeur, which is a part of
    A. Obsessive-compulsive disorder
    B. Phobias
    C. Bipolar disorders
    D. Schizophrenia

26. A person with bipolar disorder may
    A. Be more depressed than manic
    B. Be more manic than depressed
    C. Alternate between depression and mania
    D. Have any of the above
27. A major risk of a depressive episode is that the person
    A. Is very sad
    B. May be a suicide risk
    C. Has depressed body functions
    D. Cannot concentrate
28. If an older person is depressed, it may be wrongly diagnosed as a
    A. Cognitive disorder
    B. Physical problem
    C. Hormonal change
    D. Side effect of drugs
29. A person with an antisocial personality disorder may
    A. Be suspicious and distrust others
    B. Have violent behavior
    C. See, hear, or feel something that is not real
    D. Blame others for actions and behaviors
30. An adult is considered an alcoholic if
    A. The person enjoys a glass of wine with dinner
    B. The person becomes "high" or drunk after one or two drinks
    C. The person cannot stop drinking once drinking has begun
    D. He or she drinks only liquor with a high alcohol content
31. Alcohol can be more dangerous for an older person because
    A. The person has been drinking for a long period
    B. The person eats a poor diet
    C. Older people tend to take more drugs that may be harmful when taken with alcohol
    D. He or she is more likely to lie about alcohol intake than a young person
32. When a person is addicted to drugs, he or she
    A. Takes the drug only as prescribed
    B. Takes smaller and smaller amounts to get the same affect
    C. Is taking only illegal drugs
    D. Continues to use the substance even when he or she knows the drug makes a situation worse
33. Safety measures are included in the care plan of a person with mental health problems if
    A. Communication is a problem
    B. The person is anxious
    C. Suicide is a risk
    D. The person does not learn from experiences or punishment

Fill in the Blanks

34. What are causes of mental health disorders?
    A. _____
    B. _____
    C. _____
    D. _____
    E. _____

35. Name the defense mechanism being used in these situations.
    A. A girl fails a test. She blames the other girl for not helping her study. _____
    B. A man does not like his boss. He buys the boss an expensive Christmas present. _____
    C. A girl complains of a stomachache so she will not have to read aloud. _____
    D. A child is angry with his teacher. He hits his brother. _____
    E. A woman misses work frequently and is often late. She gets a bad evaluation. She says that the boss does not like her. _____
36. Below are examples of problems that occur with schizophrenia. Name each one.
    A. A man believes his neighbor is poisoning his water. _____
    B. A woman says that voices told her to set fire to her apartment. _____
    C. A man believes that he is a doctor. _____
    D. A woman tells you she owns three BMW cars and is the president of MacDonald's. _____
37. If a person talks about or tries to commit suicide, you should _____. Do not leave _____.
38. A person who greatly admires and loves family and friends and suddenly shifts to intense anger and dislike may have a _____.
39. Alcoholism includes these symptoms:
    A. _____
    B. _____
    C. _____
    D. _____
40. When tissues do not get the substance being abused, how does the body respond? (What signs and symptoms occur?)
    A. _____
    B. _____
    C. _____
    D. _____
    E. _____
    F. _____
41. When a person has mental health problems, quality of life must be met. Which right is being protected in each of these examples?
    A. All harmful items are removed from the person's setting. _____
    B. When the person says or does something, you share it only with the nurse. _____
    C. The person is given very simple choices so that he or she still feels in control. _____
    D. You report bruises or other signs that the person is not well cared for. _____

Crossword

Fill in the crossword by answering the clues below with the words from this list:

Agoraphobia   Mysophobia
Algophobia   Nyctophobia
Aquaphobia   Pyrophobia
Claustrophobia   Xenophobia

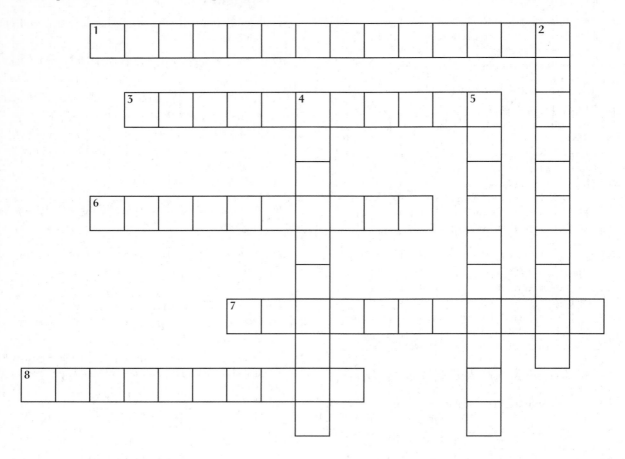

ACROSS
1. Fear of being trapped in an enclosed or narrow space
3. Fear of night or darkness
6. Fear of the slightest uncleanliness
7. Fear of being in an open, crowded, or public place
8. Fear of strangers

DOWN
2. Fear of pain or seeing others in pain
4. Fear of fire
5. Fear of water

Optional Learning Exercises

42. Mr. Johnson is very worried about his surgery tomorrow. You notice that he is talking very fast and is sweating. You give him directions to collect a urine specimen. Five minutes later, he turns on his call light to ask you to repeat the directions. He tells you he is using the toilet "all the time" because he has diarrhea and frequent urination. The nurse tells you that all of these things are signs and symptoms of _____
_____.

43. You are assigned to care for Mrs. Grand, a new resident. She is getting ready to go to the dining room. You assist her to get dressed, and she tells you she wants to wash her hands before going to the dining room. She goes to the bathroom and washes her hands for several minutes. As she leaves the room, she stops to turn off the light. Then she tells you she must wash her hands again. She repeats washing her hands and turning the lights on and off 4 or 5 times. You report this to the nurse who tells you that Mrs. Grand has

_____.

Independent Learning Activities

Try this experiment with a group of classmates. Make up labels with various roles for "staff members" and "mentally ill" persons. A list is provided, but you may add or subtract according to the size of your group. Make sure that the group includes a mixture of people with mental health problems and staff or visitors.

Doctor	A person with bipolar disorder
Nurse	A person with delusions of grandeur
Visitor	A person with obsessive compulsive disorder
Nursing assistant	A person with schizophrenia with paranoia
Recreational therapist	A person with hallucinations
Dietitian	A person with anorexia nervosa

Attach a label to each person so that he or she cannot read it. (It may be placed on the back or the forehead.) Have everyone move about the group, and talk to each other based on how the person thinks he or she should approach the person with a certain "label." Continue the experiment for about 15 minutes, and then use these questions to guide a group discussion:

- How did you feel talking to a person with a mental health disorder?
- How were the people with a mental health disorder approached? How quickly were the "mentally ill" able to sense that this was their label? What cues did they receive from others?
- How quickly did "staff members" recognize the label they had? What cues did they receive from others?
- In what ways did the approach of others cause people to respond in a way expected?
- Did the people with mental health problems show signs of the illness based on the reaction of others?
- What did the group learn about approaching a person with a mental health problem?

Consider this situation and answer these questions concerning how you would feel about caring for a person with a mental health problem.
Situation: Marion Cross, age 65, is a patient in an acute care hospital with a diagnosis of pneumonia. The nurse tells you that Mrs. Cross has a history of schizophrenia. You are assigned to provide AM care for Mrs. Cross.

- How would you approach Mrs. Cross when you enter her room? How would your knowledge about her mental health problem affect your initial contact with her?
- What would you do if Mrs. Cross told you she sees an elephant in the room? What would you say to her?
- How would you react if Mrs. Cross told you that she owns Disney World and goes there free anytime she wants? How would you respond?
- How would you provide good oral hygiene if Mrs. Cross refuses to cooperate because she is sure the staff is trying to poison her? What could you try that might be helpful?
- What would you do if Mrs. Cross curls up in a tight ball and refuses to talk or cooperate during AM care? What could you do to maintain her hygiene?
- How would you feel about caring for a person with abnormal behavior? Why?

37 Confusion and Dementia

Key Terms

Cognitive function   Delusion   Hallucination   Sundowning
Delirium   Dementia   Pseudodementia

Fill in the Blanks: Key Terms

1. A false belief is a _____.

2. Seeing, hearing, or feeling something that is not real is _____.

3. Increased signs, symptoms, and behavior of AD during hours of darkness is _____ _____.

4. _____ is a state of temporary but acute mental confusion that comes on suddenly.

5. The loss of cognitive function and social function caused by changes in the brain is _____ _____.

6. _____ is a false disorder of the mind.

7. _____ involves memory, thinking, reasoning, ability to understand, judgment, and behavior.

Circle the BEST Answer

8. Confusion caused by aging
   A. Occurs suddenly
   B. Is caused by reduced blood flow to the brain
   C. Can be cured
   D. Is usually temporary

9. When a person is confused, it is helpful if you
   A. Repeat the date and time as often as necessary
   B. Change the routine each day to stimulate the person
   C. Keep the drapes pulled during the day
   D. Give complex answers to questions

10. Hearing and vision decrease with confusion, so you should
    A. Speak in a loud voice
    B. Write out directions to the person
    C. Face the person and speak clearly
    D. Keep the lighting dim in the room

11. Dementia can be caused by
    A. Infections
    B. Depression
    C. Heart, lung, and blood vessel problems
    D. All of the above

12. Dementia
    A. Is a normal part of aging
    B. Causes the person to have difficulty with common tasks
    C. Is always temporary and can be cured
    D. Affects most older people

13. The most common type of permanent dementia is
    A. Alzheimer's disease   C. Depression
    B. Dementia   D. Delirium

14. The classic sign of Alzheimer's disease (AD) is
    A. Forgetting simple tasks
    B. Gradual loss of short-term memory
    C. Acute confusion and delirium
    D. Wandering and sundowning

15. In stage 1 of AD (mild), the person may
    A. Walk slowly with a shuffling gait
    B. Be totally incontinent
    C. Blame others for mistakes
    D. Become agitated and may be violent

16. In stage 2 of AD (moderate), the person may
    A. Have difficulty performing everyday tasks
    B. Need assistance with activities of daily living
    C. Be disoriented to time and place
    D. Have seizures

17. In stage 3 of AD (severe), the person may
    A. Forget recent events
    B. Lose impulse control and use foul language or have poor table manners
    C. Be less interested in things or be less outgoing
    D. Be disoriented to person, time, and place

18. When a person wanders, the major concern is
    A. The person's comfort
    B. The person is at risk for life-threatening accidents
    C. Inconvenience of the family or facility
    D. Making sure the person gets enough rest and sleep

19. When sundowning occurs, it may be related to
    A. Being tired or hungry
    B. Having poor judgment
    C. Impaired vision or hearing
    D. The person looking for something or someone

20. Too much stimuli from being asked too many questions all at once can overwhelm a person and cause
    A. Delusions
    B. Catastrophic reactions
    C. Hallucinations
    D. Sundowning

21. A caregiver may cause agitation and restlessness by
    A. Calling the person by name
    B. Selecting tasks and activities specific to the person's cognitive abilities and interests
    C. Encouraging activity early in the day
    D. Insisting the person hurry to complete care quickly

22. When you are caring for a person with AD, it is helpful if you
    A. Give the person simple choices during basic care
    B. Play loud, familiar TV programs during meals and care activities
    C. Encourage late afternoon or early evening exercise and activity
    D. Restrain a person who insists on going outside

23. When a person with AD screams, it may be because the person
    A. Has hearing and vision problems
    B. Is trying to communicate
    C. Has too much stimulation in the environment
    D. All of the above

24. If a person with AD displays sexual behaviors, the nurse may tell you to
    A. Tell the person this behavior is not acceptable
    B. Make sure the person has good hygiene to prevent itching
    C. Avoid caring for the person
    D. Ignore the behavior because the disease causes it

25. What should you do when a person repeats the same motions or repeats the same words over and over?
    A. Remind the person to stop the repeating
    B. Report this to the nurse immediately
    C. Take the person for a walk or distract the person with music or picture books
    D. Isolate the person in his or her room until the repeating behavior stops

26. A person with AD is encouraged to take part in therapies and activities that
    A. Increase the level of confusion
    B. Help the person feel useful, worthwhile, and active
    C. Will prevent aggressive behaviors
    D. Improve physical problems such as incontinence and contractures

27. How do AD special care units differ from other areas of a care facility?
    A. Complete care is provided
    B. Entrances and exits are locked
    C. Meals are served in the person's room
    D. No activities are provided

28. A person with AD no longer stays in a secured unit when
    A. The condition improves
    B. The family requests a move to another unit
    C. The person cannot sit or walk and is in bed
    D. Aggressive behaviors disrupt the unit

29. A family who cares for a person with dementia at home
    A. May feel anger and resentment toward the person
    B. May feel guilty
    C. Needs assistance from others to cope with the person
    D. All of the above

Fill in the Blanks

30. Cognitive function involves:
    A. _____
    B. _____
    C. _____
    D. _____
    E. _____
    F. _____

31. When caring for a confused person, how can you help the person know the date and time?
    A. _____
    B. _____

32. How can you help the confused person maintain the day-night cycle?
    A. _____
    B. _____
    C. _____

33. What senses decrease with changes in the nervous system from aging?
    _____

34. Give examples of how early warnings signs of dementia may be seen in these areas:
    A. Memory: _____
    B. Doing tasks: _____
    C. Language: _____
    D. Judgment: _____

35. What substances can cause dementia?
    _____

36. Pseudodementia can occur with _____ and _____.

37. The most common mental health problem in older persons is _____.

38. A person with mild cognitive impairment has ongoing _____. The person does not have other losses like _____.

39. Alzheimer's disease (AD) damages brain cells that control these functions:
    A. _____
    B. _____
    C. _____
    D. _____
    E. _____
    F. _____
    G. _____
    H. _____

40. Which of the seven stages of AD are described in the following examples?
    A. Person cannot walk without help. _____
    _____
    B. Person may need help choosing correct clothes to wear. _____
    C. Person shows no signs of memory problems. _____
    D. Family, friends, and others notice problems. _____
    E. Person has problems with shopping, paying bills, and managing money. _____ _____
    F. Person may forget names but recognizes faces. _____
    G. Person does not know where to find keys, eyeglasses, or other objects. _____ _____

41. The Safe Return program will help an AD person who has the behavior of _____ _____.

42. Which behavior of AD is described in the following examples?
    A. Confusion and restlessness increase after dark. _____
    B. Too much stimuli may trigger this behavior. _____
    C. The person may use this behavior to communicate as the disease progresses. _____ _____
    D. The person may walk into traffic or go out not properly dressed for the weather. _____ _____
    E. The person repeats the same words or motions over and over. _____ _____
    F. The person may have false beliefs about who he or she is or who the caregiver may be. _____ _____
    G. The person may pace, hit, or yell. _____ _____
    H. The person touches self or others in a sexual way that is inappropriate. _____ _____
    I. The person complains of feeling bugs crawling or seeing animals that are not there. _____
    J. The person hits, pinches, grabs, bites, or swears at others. _____

43. When a person has dementia or AD, what is the reason these may be part of the care plan?
    A. Approach the person from the front. _____
    B. Provide plastic eating and drinking utensils. _____
    C. Respond to door alarms at once. _____
    D. Do not argue with a person who wants to leave. _____
    E. Do not ask a person to tell you what is bothering him or her. _____ _____
    F. Turn off TV or movies when violent or disturbing programs are on. _____
    G. Use night-lights so the person can see. _____
    H. Promote exercise and activity during the day. _____
    I. Have equipment ready for any procedure. _____

44. Validation therapy is based on these principles:
    A. _____
    B. _____
    C. _____
    D. _____
    E. _____
    F. _____

Optional Learning Exercises
You are caring for Mr. Harris, a 78-year-old who is confused. You know there are ways to help a person be more oriented. Answer questions 45 through 47 about ways to help a confused person.

45. How can you help orient Mr. Harris to who he is every time you are in contact with him? _____

46. What are two ways you can help orient Mr. Harris to time?
    A. _____
    B. _____

47. What are ways you can maintain the day-night cycle when dressing Mr. Harris? _____

You are caring for Mrs. Matthews, an 82-year-old resident. The nurse tells you she lived with her daughter for the past 2 years, but the family is now concerned for her safety. She left the home when the temperature was 35° F and was found 2 miles away, wearing a light sweater. On another occasion, she turned on the gas stove and could not remember how to turn it off. Sometimes, she did not recognize her daughter and resisted getting a bath or changing clothes. Since admission to the care facility, she tells everyone she must leave to go to her birthday party. She brushes her arms and legs and tells you that "bugs" are crawling on her. Answer questions 48 through 52 about Mrs. Matthews and her care.

48. Why would Mrs. Matthews be most likely in a special care unit in the nursing facility?

49. It is likely that Mrs. Matthews has what disease?

50. Mrs. Matthews is probably in stage _____ of the disease. What activities would indicate she is in this stage?
   A. _____
   B. _____
   C. _____
   D. _____
   E. _____

51. How often will the health team review Mrs. Matthews' need to stay on this unit? _____ Why is this done? _____

52. The nurse may encourage Mrs. Matthews' daughter to join a _____ group. How can this be helpful to the daughter?

Independent Learning Activities
Consider the situation and answer the questions about how you would feel.
Situation: Imagine you are in a strange country where people talk to you but you do not understand what they are saying. They use strange tools to eat, and you cannot figure out how to use them. They try to feed you food you do not recognize. Sometimes these people seem friendly and caring, but at other times, they become angry because you are not doing what they ask you to do. You become frightened when they try to remove your clothes and take you in a room to shower you. You become frightened and upset because you do not know what will happen next. At times, other strangers come to your room and bring gifts. They talk kindly to you, but you do not know them. They seem upset when you do not respond to their gifts and gestures. The doors and windows in this country are all locked, and you cannot find a way out so that you can go home.
- How does this situation relate to the information in this chapter?
- How would you react if you were the person in this situation? Why?
- What methods might you use to try to communicate with the person in this situation?
- Why would the person want to go home? What does "home" mean to him or her?
- How will this exercise help you when you care for a person who is confused?

Consider the situation and answer the questions about how you would care for a person who has dementia.
Situation: You are assigned to care for Ronald Myers, 85, who has Alzheimer's disease. He often wanders from room to room and tries to open the outside doors. He frequently becomes agitated and restless, especially in the evening. Most of the time, Mr. Myers is unable to feed himself and is often incontinent. He keeps repeating, "Help me, help me" all day.
- How do you feel about caring for a person like this? Frightened? Angry? Impatient? How do you deal with your feelings so that you can give care to the person?
- At what stage of Alzheimer's disease is Mr. Myers? What signs and symptoms support your answer?
- Why would it be ineffective to remind Mr. Myers of the date and time during your shift? Why is this a good technique with some confused persons and not with others?
- Why does Mr. Myers become more agitated toward evening? What is this called?
- What methods could you use to make sure Mr. Myers receives the care needed to maintain good personal hygiene? How could you get him to cooperate or participate in his care?
- What parts of Mr. Myers' behavior would be most difficult for you to tolerate? What would you do if you found yourself becoming irritated and angry with Mr. Myers?
- What information in this chapter has helped you understand persons like Mr. Myers better? How will this information help you give better care to these persons and to maintain their quality of life?

Developmental Disabilities

Key Terms

Developmental disability   Diplegia   Spastic

Fill in the Blanks: Key Terms

1. When similar body parts are affected on both sides of the body, it is called _____.

2. The uncontrolled contractions of skeletal muscles is _____.

3. A disability that occurs before 22 years of age is _____.

Circle the Best Answer

4. A developmental disability (DD)
   A. Always occurs at birth
   B. Is usually temporary
   C. Limits function in three or more life skills
   D. Is present before the age of 12

5. Developmentally disabled adults
   A. Need life-long assistance, support, and special services
   B. Usually can live independently after they become adults
   C. Always need to be in long-term care in special centers
   D. Generally outgrow the problems as they mature

6. A person is considered to have intellectual disabilities if
   A. The IQ score is below 70
   B. The person has difficulty understanding the behavior of others
   C. The person is limited in the skills needed to live, work, and play
   D. All of the above

7. The Arc of the United States is a national organization
   A. Related to Alzheimer's disease
   B. Dealing with intellectual disabilities
   C. That provides care for people with physical disability
   D. For persons with cerebral palsy

8. Down syndrome (DS) is caused by
   A. An extra 21st chromosome
   B. Head injury during birth
   C. Diseases of the mother during pregnancy
   D. Lack of oxygen to the brain

9. A person with Down syndrome is at risk for
   A. Cerebral palsy   C. Leukemia
   B. Diplegia   D. Poor nutrition

10. Cerebral palsy is a group of disorders involving
    A. Intellectual disabilities
    B. Muscle weakness or poor muscle control
    C. Abnormal genes from one or both parents
    D. An increased risk of developing leukemia

11. When a person has spastic cerebral palsy, the symptoms include
    A. Constant, slow, weaving or writhing motions
    B. Uncontrolled contractions of skeletal muscles
    C. Using little or no eye contact
    D. A strong attachment to a single item, idea, activity, or person

12. A person with autism may
    A. Dislike being held or cuddled
    B. Have bladder and bowel control problems
    C. Have generalized seizures
    D. Have diplegia or hemiplegia

13. An adult with autism
    A. Needs to develop social and work skills
    B. Will outgrow the condition
    C. Will always live in group homes or residential care centers
    D. Will have severe physical problems

14. Spina bifida occurs
    A. At birth, as a result of injury during delivery
    B. Because of traumatic injury in childhood
    C. During the first month of pregnancy
    D. As a result of child abuse

15. Which of these types of spina bifida causes the person to have leg paralysis and lack of bowel and bladder control?
    A. Spina bifida cystica
    B. Myelomeningocele
    C. Spina bifida occulta
    D. Meningocele

16. A shunt placed in the brain of a child with hydrocephalus will
    A. Relieve pressure on the brain
    B. Drain fluid from the brain to the abdomen
    C. Reduce the intellectual disabilities or neurological damage that may occur with hydrocephalus
    D. All of the above

17. Which of these statements about persons with a developmental disability *is not* true?
    A. All persons with a disability will always need to live with family or in a nursing-care center
    B. The Americans with Disabilities Act of 1990 protects the rights of persons with developmental disabilities
    C. When a person with a developmental disability needs care in a nursing center, OBRA protects his or her rights
    D. The developmental disability will affect the person and the family throughout life

Fill in the Blanks

18. A developmental disability is present when function is limited in three or more of these life skills:
    A. _____
    B. _____
    C. _____
    D. _____
    E. _____
    F. _____
    G. _____

19. What genetic conditions can cause intellectual disabilities?
    A. _____
    B. _____
    C. _____
    D. _____
    E. _____

20. Intellectual disabilities may be caused after birth by childhood diseases such as
    A. _____
    B. _____
    C. _____
    D. _____
    E. _____
    F. _____

21. According to the Arc of the United States, intellectual disabilities involve the condition being present before _____.

22. The Arc believes that persons with intellectual disabilities have the right to:
    A. _____
    B. _____
    C. _____
    D. _____
    E. _____
    F. _____
    G. _____
    H. _____

23. If a child has Down syndrome (DS), what features are present in these areas?
    A. Head: _____
    B. Eyes: _____
    C. Tongue: _____
    D. Nose: _____
    E. Hands and fingers: _____

24. Persons with Down syndrome need therapy in these areas:
    A. _____
    B. _____
    C. _____
    D. _____

25. The usual cause of cerebral palsy is a lack of _____.

26. Which type of cerebral palsy is described in each example?
    A. Arm and leg on one side are paralyzed.
       _____
    B. Muscles contract or shorten. They are stiff and cannot relax. _____
    C. Both arms and both legs are paralyzed.
       _____
    D. Person has constant, slow, weaving or writhing motions. _____
    E. Both arms or both legs are paralyzed.
       _____

27. The goal for a person with cerebral palsy is to be _____

28. A person with autism has:
    A. _____
    B. _____
    C. _____

29. Spina bifida is a defect of the _____.

30. Children with spina bifida may having difficulty learning because of problems with:
    A. _____
    B. _____
    C. _____
    D. _____

31. Which type of spina bifida would cause the problems in each of the examples given?
    A. The person has leg paralysis and a lack of bowel and bladder control. _____
    B. The person may have no symptoms. _____
    C. Nerve damage usually does not occur, and surgery corrects the defect. _____

32. If a hydrocephalus is not treated, pressure increases in the head and causes _____ and _____.

Optional Learning Exercises

Mr. Murphy is one of the residents you care for. He has Down syndrome. Answer questions 33 through 35 that relate to this person.

33. Mr. Murphy is 40 years old. What disease is a risk for an adult with Down syndrome?
    _____

34. Mr. Murphy is encouraged to eat a well-balanced diet and to attend regular exercise classes. Including these in the care plan will help prevent the problems of _____ and _____.

35. What two therapies may help Mr. Murphy communicate more clearly? _____ and _____

You care for Mary Reynolds, who has cerebral palsy.
Answer questions 36 and 37 about Ms. Reynolds.

36. It is difficult to feed Ms. Reynolds because she drools, grimaces, and moves her head constantly. You know that she does this because she has a type of cerebral palsy called _____.

37. Because Ms. Reynolds remains in bed or a special chair all the time, she is at special risk for _____ _____ because of immobility. She needs to be repositioned at least every _____.

Independent Learning Activities

Many communities have services available to families with children and adults who are developmentally disabled. Some communities have sheltered workshops, day care, sheltered living centers, or physical and occupational therapy programs available. If your community has these services, ask permission to visit them and observe the persons being served there. Answer these questions when you observe in the agency:

- What age-groups are served in this program?
- What activities are available to the group?
- What training is required for the people who work there?
- How do the persons in the program act? Happy? Bored? Withdrawn? Other reactions?
- What other services are available to these individuals in the agency? In the community?
- Where do the persons in this program live? With family? Group homes? Other?

Do you know a family who has a developmentally disabled family member? Ask the family if they will answer these questions about living with this person:

- How old is the developmentally disabled person? Where does the person live?
- What abilities does the person have? What disabilities interfere with the activities of daily living for the person?
- What therapies are being done to help the person reach his or her highest level of function?
- What community programs have been helpful for the person?
- How does this person's disability affect the family? Physically? Emotionally? Financially? Day-to-day activities?

39 Rehabilitation and Restorative Care

Key Terms

Activities of daily living Disability
Prosthesis

Rehabilitation Restorative nursing care
Restorative aide

Fill in the Blanks: Key Terms

1. A nursing assistant with special training in restorative nursing and rehabilitation skills is a _____ _____.

2. _____ are activities usually done during a normal day in a person's life.

3. An artificial replacement for a missing body part is a _____.

4. Care that helps persons regain their health, strength, and independence is _____ _____.

5. A _____ is any lost, absent, or impaired physical or mental function.

6. The process of restoring the disabled person to the highest possible level of physical, psychological, social, and economic functioning is _____ _____.

Circle the BEST Answer

7. The focus of rehabilitation is to
   A. Improve abilities
   B. Restore function to normal
   C. Help the person regain health and strength
   D. Prevent injury

8. Restorative nursing promotes
   A. Self-care, elimination, and positioning
   B. Mobility, communication, and cognitive function
   C. Helping regain health, strength, and independence
   D. All of the above

9. If you are a restorative aide, it means you have
   A. Special training in restorative nursing and rehabilitation skills
   B. Taken required classes for restorative aides
   C. Passed a special test to show you can perform these duties
   D. The most seniority at the facility

10. When assisting with rehabilitation and restorative care, it is important to
    A. Give complete care to prevent exertion by the person
    B. Make sure you do everything for the person
    C. Encourage the person to perform ADL to the extent possible
    D. Complete care quickly

11. Which of these would be most helpful for a person receiving rehabilitative care?
    A. Give the person pity or sympathy when tasks are difficult
    B. Remind the person not to try new skills or those that are difficult
    C. Give praise when even a little progress is made
    D. Encourage the person to perform ADL quickly

12. Complications can be prevented by
    A. Doing all ADL for the person
    B. Allowing the person to decide if he or she wants to move or exercise
    C. Making sure the person is in good alignment, is turned and repositioned, and has range-of-motions exercises
    D. Making sure rehabilitation is fast-paced

13. Rehabilitation begins
    A. After the person has recovered
    B. When the person first seeks health care
    C. When the person asks for help
    D. When a discharge date has been set

14. Self-help devices help meet the goal of
    A. Recovery of all normal abilities
    B. Self-care
    C. Living alone
    D. Dependence on others

15. When dysphagia occurs after a stroke, a person may need
    A. Exercises to improve swallowing
    B. A dysphagia diet
    C. Enteral nutrition
    D. All of the above

16. A rehabilitation plan includes information to meet
    A. Only physical care needs
    B. Only ambulation needs
    C. Physical, psychological, social, and economic needs
    D. Only psychological and social needs

17. The rehabilitation team meets to evaluate the person's progress
    A. Every 90 days
    B. Often, to change the plan as needed
    C. Every week
    D. Only when requested by the family or person

18. OBRA requires that nursing centers
    A. Have a full-time physical therapist
    B. Provide rehabilitation services
    C. Provide physical care only
    D. Employ full-time occupational and speech therapists

Fill in the Blanks

19. Restorative nursing programs do the following:
   A. _____
   B. _____

20. A person in rehabilitation needs to adjust in these areas:
   A. _____
   B. _____
   C. _____
   D. _____

21. Rehabilitation takes longer in which age-group? _____ What are reasons for this?
   A. Changes affect _____
   B. Chronic _____
   C. Risk for _____

22. What are some self-help devices that will assist in self-feeding?
   A. _____
   B. _____
   C. _____

23. The goal for a prosthesis is to _____
   _____
   _____.

24. When you are assisting with rehabilitation and restorative care, why should you practice the task that the person must perform? _____
   _____

25. When assisting with rehabilitation and restorative care, what complications can be prevented if you report early signs and symptoms? _____
   _____

26. What can you do to promote the person's quality of life?
   A. _____
   B. _____
   C. _____
   D. _____
   E. _____
   F. _____
   G. _____

Optional Learning Exercises

Mrs. Mercer is 82 years old. She is a resident in a rehabilitation unit because she had a stroke that has caused weakness on her left side. Although she is right-handed, she needs to learn to use several self-help devices as she relearns ways to carry out ADL. She often becomes angry or depressed. Answer questions 27 through 32 about Mrs. Mercer and her care.

27. Mrs. Mercer is having difficulty with controlling urinary and bowel elimination. What would be the goal of her care for these problems?
   _____
   Her plan of care would include programs for
   _____.

28. What should you do to prepare Mrs. Mercer's food at mealtime so she can feed herself?
   _____
   _____

29. Mrs. Mercer can brush her teeth but needs help getting prepared. What should you do to get her ready to brush her teeth?
   _____
   _____

30. Why does she need help at mealtime and to brush her teeth?
   _____
   _____

31. Mrs. Mercer needs help to get in and out of bed. When helping her transfer, you remember to position the chair on her _____ side.

32. When Mrs. Mercer becomes discouraged because progress is slow, how can you help her? You can stress _____ and focus on _____
   _____.

Independent Learning Activities

Role-play the situation with a classmate. Answer the questions about how you felt when you played Mrs. Leeds to understand how a person with a disability feels. Use your non-dominant hand to attempt the activities she must do. Situation: Mary Leeds is 62 and had a stroke last month. She has weakness on her dominant side and has been admitted to a rehabilitation unit to relearn activities of daily living (ADL). She is practicing eating by using a spoon to place fluids and food in her mouth. She is also learning to button clothing.

- How well could you hold the spoon with your non-dominant hand?
- What problems did you having controlling the spoon?
- How rapidly could you eat? What type of food was easier to eat?
- How well were you able to button your clothing? What techniques did you find that made you more successful?
- How did this experience make you feel? How will it affect the way you interact with persons who have similar disabilities?

With your instructor's permission, borrow a wheelchair from your school to use for 1-2 hours. Have a classmate push you around in the chair in a grocery store or mall or in your school. You must stay in the chair for the entire time to experience the feelings of a person who must use a wheelchair. Use a handicap-equipped bathroom during this experience.

- How comfortable was the wheelchair? Did you use any special padding or cushion in the seat?
- What difficulties were encountered moving about? Doorways? Steps? Aisles? Crowds? How did you deal with any difficulties?
- How accessible was the handicap-equipped bathroom? How much room was available for you to transfer from the wheelchair to the toilet?
- How did other people treat you? How many spoke to you? How many talked to your classmate and avoided you?
- How did this experience make you feel? How will it affect the way you interact with a person in a wheelchair?

Key Terms

Anaphylaxis	First aid	Respiratory arrest	Shock
Convulsion	Hemorrhage	Seizure	Sudden cardiac arrest
Fainting			

Fill in the Blanks: Key Terms

1. In _____, breathing stops but the heart still pumps for several minutes.

2. The sudden loss of consciousness from an inadequate blood supply to the brain is _____.

3. When the heart and breathing stop suddenly and without warning, it is _____.

4. _____ is a condition that results when there is not enough blood supply to organs and tissues.

5. Emergency care given to an ill or injured person before medical help arrives is _____ _____.

6. A convulsion may also be called a _____ _____.

7. _____ is the excessive loss of blood in a short period.

8. Violent and sudden contractions or tremors of muscles is a seizure or a _____.

9. A life-threatening sensitivity to an antigen is _____ _____.

Circle the BEST Answer

10. When an emergency occurs, the nurse determines when to
    A. Call the doctor for orders
    B. Activate the EMS system
    C. Call the supervisor
    D. Assist the person to bed

11. If you find a person lying on the floor, you should
    A. Keep the person lying down
    B. Help the person back to bed
    C. Elevate the head
    D. Help the person to a chair

12. If the nurse instructs you to activate the EMS system, you should do all of these *except*
    A. Tell the operator your location
    B. Explain to the operator what has happened
    C. Describe aid that is being given
    D. Hang up as soon as you have finished giving the information

13. It is important to restore breathing and circulation quickly because
    A. The lungs will be damaged
    B. The person will lose consciousness
    C. Brain and other organ damage occur within minutes
    D. Hemorrhage will occur

14. Which of these *is not* a major sign of sudden cardiac arrest (SCA)?
    A. Complaints of chest pain
    B. No pulse
    C. No breathing
    D. No response

15. The purpose of the head tilt-chin lift method is to
    A. Make the person more comfortable
    B. Open the airway
    C. Practice Standard Precautions
    D. Stimulate the heart to beat

16. To determine whether the person is breathing
    A. Ask the person if he or she can take a deep breath
    B. Pinch the person's nostrils shut with your thumb and index finger
    C. Look to see if the person's chest rises and falls
    D. Remove the dentures

17. When you use mouth-to-mouth breathing, you should
    A. Allow the person's chin to relax against the neck
    B. Place your mouth loosely over the person's mouth
    C. Blow into the person's mouth slowly; you should see the chest rise
    D. Apply pressure on the chin to close the mouth

18. Mouth-to-nose breathing is used when
    A. You cannot ventilate through the person's mouth
    B. You want to avoid contact with body fluids
    C. Giving rescue breaths to a child
    D. Chest compressions are not needed

19. Before starting chest compressions
    A. Make sure the person is breathing
    B. Check for a pulse
    C. Wait 30 seconds to see if the person regains consciousness
    D. Turn the person to the side

20. When CPR is started, you first give
    A. 5 chest compressions
    B. 2 breaths
    C. 5 breaths
    D. 15 chest compressions

21. The purpose of chest compressions is to
    A. Deflate the lungs
    B. Increase oxygen in the blood
    C. Force blood through the circulatory system
    D. Help the heart work more effectively

22. For chest compressions to be effective, the person must be
    A. In prone position
    B. On a soft surface
    C. Supine on a hard, flat surface
    D. In a semi-Fowler's position
23. When preparing to give chest compressions, locate the hands
    A. On the sternum between the nipples
    B. On the lower half of the sternum
    C. Side by side over the sternum
    D. Slightly below the end of the sternum
24. When giving chest compressions to an adult, depress the sternum
    A. About 1 to 1½ inches
    B. About ½ to 1 inch
    C. About 1½ to 2 inches
    D. About 2 to 2½ inches
25. CPR is done when the person
    A. Does not respond when you shout, "Are you OK?"
    B. Is not breathing
    C. Is unconscious
    D. Does not respond, is not breathing, and has no pulse
26. If the person is not breathing or not breathing adequately, give 2 breaths that
    A. Last about 1 second each
    B. Last about 5 seconds each
    C. Last 5 to 10 seconds each
    D. Last 15 seconds each
27. When performing one-rescuer CPR, chest compressions are at a rate of
    A. 15 compressions per minute
    B. 100 compressions per minute
    C. 60 compressions per minute
    D. 12 compressions per minute
28. When performing one-rescuer CPR, check for a carotid pulse, breathing, coughing, and moving every
    A. 5 minutes
    B. 100 compressions
    C. Few minutes
    D. 4 cycles of 15 compressions and 2 breaths
29. Side-lying position is the recovery position when the person is breathing and has a pulse but is not responding, because
    A. The position helps keep the airway open
    B. It prevents aspiration
    C. The person can breathe more easily
    D. All of the above
30. When an automated external defibrillator (AED) is used, it
    A. Stops the heart
    B. Slows the heartbeat down
    C. Stops ventricular fibrillation and restores a regular heartbeat
    D. Starts the heartbeat
31. Which of these is a sign of internal hemorrhage?
    A. Steady flow of blood from a wound
    B. Pain, shock, vomiting blood, or coughing up blood
    C. Bleeding that occurs in spurts
    D. Dried blood at the site of an injury

32. To control external bleeding, you should do all of these *except*
    A. Remove any objects that have pierced or stabbed the person
    B. Place a sterile dressing directly over the wound
    C. Apply pressure with your hand directly over the bleeding site
    D. Bind the wound when bleeding stops
33. If a person is in shock, it is helpful if you
    A. Have the person sit in a chair
    B. Keep the person cool by removing some of the clothing
    C. Stay calm; this helps the person feels more secure
    D. Give the person something to drink or eat
34. Anaphylactic shock occurs because of
    A. Hemorrhage
    B. An allergy to foods, insects, chemicals, or drugs
    C. Sudden cardiac arrest
    D. Seizures
35. If a person has a seizure, you should
    A. Place an object between the teeth
    B. Distract the person to stop the seizure
    C. Position the person in bed
    D. Move furniture, equipment, and sharp objects away from the person
36. If you are assisting a person with burns
    A. Remove burned clothing
    B. Cover the burn wounds with a sterile or clean, cool, moist covering
    C. Give the person plenty of fluids
    D. Apply oils or ointments to the burns
37. If a person tells you she feels faint
    A. Have the person lie down in a supine position
    B. Let the person walk around to increase circulation
    C. Have the person sit or lie down before fainting occurs
    D. If the person is lying down, raise the head with pillows
38. When a stroke occurs, position the person in the recovery position
    A. On the affected side
    B. On the unaffected side
    C. In the supine position
    D. In a semi-Fowler's position

Fill in the Blanks

39. If you activate the EMS system, what information should you give to the operator?
    A. _____
    B. _____
    C. _____
    D. _____
    E. _____
    F. _____
40. Chain of Survival actions are:
    A. _____
    B. _____
    C. _____
    D. _____

41. CPR means _____ .

42. Basic life support (BLS) has four parts. They are:
    A. _____
    B. _____
    C. _____
    D. _____

43. When performing the head tilt-chin lift method, explain how you tilt the head and lift the chin:
    A. Tilt: _____
    B. Place: _____
    C. Lift: _____

44. When you are trying to determine if a person is breathing, explain what you do when you:
    A. Look: _____
    B. Listen: _____
    C. Feel: _____

45. When you perform mouth-to-mouth breathing, it is likely you will have contact with _____ .

46. If a person has a mouth that is severely injured and you need to perform rescue breathing, you will use _____ .

47. To find the carotid pulse, place _____ . Slide your fingers down _____ .

48. When giving CPR, give compressions at the rate of _____ .

49. Give _____ compressions followed by _____ rescue breaths.

50. When giving two-person CPR, change positions every ___ minutes or after ___ cycles of ____ compressions and ___ breaths.

51. If direct pressure does not stop hemorrhage, apply pressure over the artery _____ .

52. List the signs and symptoms of shock:
    A. _____
    B. _____
    C. _____
    D. _____
    E. _____
    F. _____
    G. _____

53. Anaphylaxis is an emergency because it occurs within _____ .

54. Penicillin causes _____ shock in many people.

55. Describe the two phases of a generalized tonic-clonic seizure:
    A. Tonic phase: _____
    B. Clonic phase: _____

56. The following relate to the emergency care of a person having a seizure:
    A. How do you protect the person's head? _____
    B. How is the person positioned? _____
    C. Why is furniture moved? _____
    D. What times are noted? _____

57. Partial-thickness burns involve the _____ .

58. Full-thickness burns involve _____ .

59. A _____ burn is very painful because _____ .

60. Common causes of fainting are:
    A. _____
    B. _____
    C. _____
    D. _____

61. What signs or symptoms will be present on the affected side with a stroke?
    A. _____
    B. _____

Optional Learning Exercises
You are visiting a neighbor, and she is washing dishes. As she washes a glass, it shatters and she sustains a deep cut on her wrist. Answer questions 62 through 67 about how you would respond.

62. How would you determine whether the bleeding was from an artery or vein? _____

63. Your neighbor is crying and walking around the room. What is the best thing you can do to help her? _____

64. Clean rubber gloves are lying on the counter. How can they be useful to you? _____

65. What materials in the home could be used to place over the wound? _____

66. Your neighbor is restless and has a rapid and weak pulse. You notice her skin is cold, moist, and pale. These signs indicate she may be in _____.

67. Her wound is still bleeding, and she loses consciousness. What should you do before you continue to give first aid? _____

Independent Learning Activities

You have learned some basic emergency care in this chapter. Find out where in your community a more advanced first aid course is available. Answer these questions about the course:
- What agency or agencies offer a course in first aid?
- How long does the course last? How much does it cost?
- Who may take the course? The public? Medical personnel? Others, such as police, firefighters, etc?
- What subjects are covered in the course?
- Would taking this course help you on your job? In your family? In your community?

Most health care facilities require employees to take a course in basic CPR. You may be required to take CPR as part of this course. Answer these questions about CPR training in your community:
- What agency or agencies offer CPR courses?
- How long does the course take? How much does it cost?
- Who can take the courses? The public? Medical personnel? Are different classes offered to the medical personnel? If so, what is the difference?
- How often does the person need to be re-certified? How does the re-certification course differ from the beginning class?

41 The Dying Person

Key Terms

Advance directive   Reincarnation   Rigor mortis   Terminal illness
Postmortem

Fill in the Blanks: Key Terms

1. The stiffness or rigidity of skeletal muscles that occurs after death is _____.

2. An _____ is a document stating a person's wishes about health care when that person cannot make his or her own decisions.

3. After death is _____.

4. An illness or injury for which there is no reasonable expectation of recovery is a _____.

5. _____ is the belief that the spirit or soul is reborn in another human body or in another form of life.

Circle the BEST Answer

6. When a person has a terminal illness
   A. The doctor is able to accurately predict when the person will die
   B. Modern medicine can cure the disease
   C. The person may live longer than expected or die sooner that expected
   D. He or she will die when expected

7. Practices and attitudes among people from India include
   A. Placing small pillows under the body's neck, feet, and wrists
   B. Wearing white clothing for mourning
   C. Providing a time and place for prayer is essential for the family and the person
   D. Having an aversion to death

8. A group that believes in reincarnation would be
   A. Hindus   C. Christians
   B. Chinese   D. Jews

9. Children between ages 3 and 5 years see death as
   A. Final
   B. Punishment for being bad
   C. Suffering and pain
   D. A reunion with those who have died

10. Older persons see death as
    A. A temporary state
    B. Freedom from pain, suffering, and disability
    C. Something that happens to other people
    D. Something that affects plans, hopes, dreams, and ambitions

11. In which stage of dying does the person make promises and make "just one more" request?
    A. Acceptance   C. Depression
    B. Anger   D. Bargaining

12. If a dying person begins to talk about worries and concerns, you should
    A. Call a spiritual leader
    B. Tell the nurse
    C. Be there and listen quietly
    D. Change the subject to more pleasant topics

13. When a person is dying, care should be given
    A. Only if the person requests it
    B. To meet basic needs
    C. Often, to keep the person active
    D. Only while the person is conscious

14. Because vision fails as death approaches, you should
    A. Explain what you are doing to the person when you are in the room
    B. Have the room very brightly lit
    C. Turn out all the lights
    D. Keep the eyes covered at all times

15. Hearing is one of the last functions lost, so it is important to
    A. Speak in a normal voice
    B. Offer words of comfort
    C. Provide reassurance and explanations about care
    D. All of the above

16. As death nears, oral hygiene is
    A. Given routinely
    B. Given more frequently when taking oral fluids is difficult
    C. Given very infrequently to avoid disturbing the person
    D. Never given because the person cannot swallow

17. Which of these *does not* occur as death nears?
    A. Body temperature rises
    B. The skin is cool, pale, and mottled
    C. Perspiration decreases
    D. Circulation fails

18. Because of breathing difficulties, the dying person is generally more comfortable in
    A. The supine position
    B. A side-lying position
    C. A prone position
    D. A semi-Fowler's position

19. When a person is dying, you can help the family by
    A. Allowing the family to stay as long as they wish
    B. Staying away from the room and delay giving care
    C. Telling the family that they need to leave so you can give care
    D. Telling the family that the person dying is not in pain

20. The goal of hospice is to
    A. Cure the person
    B. Improve the dying person's quality of life
    C. Provide life-saving measures
    D. Help the family seek hospitals or clinics that specialize in the disease of the dying person
21. If a person has a living will, it instructs doctors
    A. To start measures that will save the person's life
    B. To start CPR whenever necessary
    C. Not to start measures that prolong dying
    D. To activate the EMS system for a person
22. If the doctor writes a "do not resuscitate" (DNR) order, it means that
    A. The person will not be resuscitated
    B. The person will be resuscitated if it is an emergency
    C. The doctor will decide whether or not to resuscitate
    D. The RN may decide that in a particular situation resuscitation is needed
23. A sign that death is near would be
    A. Deep, rapid respirations
    B. The blood pressure begins to fall
    C. Muscles tense and contract in spasms
    D. Peristalsis increases
24. When the family wishes to see the body after death
    A. It should be positioned in normal alignment
    B. It should be positioned to appear comfortable and natural
    C. Soiled areas are bathed and cleaned
    D. All of the above
25. When you are assisting with postmortem care, you should
    A. Place the body in good alignment in supine position without pillows
    B. Tape all jewelry in place
    C. Gently pull eyelids over the eyes
    D. Dress the person in the person's regular clothing
26. An ID tag is attached to the big toe or
    A. Wrist   C. Upper arm
    B. Ankle   D. Upper leg
27. The Dying Person's Bill of Rights includes all of these except
    A. The right to freedom from restraint
    B. The right to laugh
    C. The right to hear the truth
    D. The right to be in denial

Fill in the Blanks

28. It is important to examine your own feelings about death because they will affect _____.

29. When you understand the dying process, you can approach the dying person with _____.

30. Religious beliefs strengthen when dying, and it often provides _____.

31. Adults fear death because they fear:
    A. _____
    B. _____
    C. _____
    D. _____
    E. _____
    F. _____
    G. _____
32. Name the five stages of dying.
    A. _____
    B. _____
    C. _____
    D. _____
    E. _____
33. When caring for a dying person do not ask questions that need long answers because _____.
34. Because crusting and irritation of the nostrils can occur, you should _____.
35. What kinds of elimination problems are common in the dying person? _____
36. You can promote comfort by providing:
    A. _____
    B. _____
    C. _____
    D. _____
    E. _____
37. List the service that hospice provides to these persons or groups:
    A. Dying person: _____
    B. Survivors: _____
    C. Health team: _____
38. The Patient Self-Determination Act and OBRA give two rights that affect the rights of a dying person. They are:
    A. _____
    B. _____
39. A living will instructs doctors:
    A. _____
    B. _____
40. When a person cannot make health care decisions, the authority to do so is given to the person with _____.

41. What are the signs that death is near?
    A. _____
    B. _____
    C. _____
    D. _____
    E. _____
    F. _____

42. The signs of death include no _____,
    no _____, and no _____.
    The pupils are _____ and _____.

43. When assisting with postmortem care, you need this
    information from the nurse:
    A. _____
    B. _____
    C. _____
    D. _____
    E. _____

44. The right to confidentiality before and after death
    provides that _____
    _____
    _____.

Optional Learning Exercises
You are assigned to care for Mrs. Adams, who is dying.
Answer questions 45 through 52 regarding this situation.

45. You find Mrs. Adams crying in her room. When you
    ask her what is wrong, she tells you no one gave her
    fresh water this morning and she has not had her bath
    yet. She tells you just to go away. What stage of dying
    is she displaying? _____

46. Later in the day, Mrs. Adams tells you she can't wait
    until she is better to go home and plant her garden.
    She states that she knows the tests done last week
    were wrong and she will recover quickly from her
    illness. Now what stage is she displaying?
    _____ Why is she displaying two
    different stages so rapidly? _____
    _____

47. A minister comes to visit Mrs. Adams while you are
    giving care. What should you do?
    _____
    _____

48. You are working one night and find Mrs. Adams
    awake during the night. She asks you to sit with her.
    She begins to talk about her fears, worries, and
    anxieties. What are two things you can do to convey
    caring to her?
    _____
    _____

49. As Mrs. Adams becomes weaker, a family member is
    always at her bedside. When they ask to assist with
    her care, you know that this is acceptable because
    _____
    _____.

50. Mrs. Adams has very irregular breathing that becomes
    deeper and then stops for a period of time. This
    pattern of breathing, called _____
    _____, occurs because the
    _____ fails as
    death nears.

51. Mrs. Adams dies while you are working, and the
    nurse asks you to assist with postmortem care. As you
    clean soiled areas, you assist the nurse to turn the
    body and air is expelled. This occurs because
    _____
    _____.

52. You wear gloves during postmortem care because they
    will _____
    _____.

Independent Learning Activities
It is important to explore your own beliefs about death and dying before you care for persons who are dying. Answer
these questions to understand your own feelings.
- Have you attended a funeral or visited a funeral home? How did you feel?
- Has anyone close to you died? How did you assist with any of the funeral arrangements? What kinds of preparation
  did the family do?
- What cultural or religious practices in your family affect death and funeral arrangements? How do you think these
  practices will affect you when you care for those who are dying?
- Have you ever been present when someone died? In your personal life? As a student? At your job? How did you
  respond? What were you asked to do in this situation?
- What is your personal belief about a living will? How will you respond if a person or family refuses a feeding tube or a
  ventilator? How will you respond if they ask to have these measures discontinued and the person dies?
- What is your personal belief about a "Do Not Resuscitate" order? How would you feel if a person you are caring for
  has this order? How will you respond when the person dies and no effort is made to help the person?

Relieving Choking—The Responsive Adult or Child (Over 1 Year of Age)

Name: _____   Date: _____

Procedure	S	U	Comments
1. Asked the person is he or she was choking.	___	___	_____
2. If yes, gave abdominal thrusts:			
a. Stood behind the person.	___	___	_____
b. Wrapped your arms around the person's waist.	___	___	_____
c. Made a fist with one hand.	___	___	_____
d. Placed thumb side of fist against the abdomen. The fist was in the middle above the navel and below the end of the sternum (breastbone).	___	___	_____
e. Grasped the fist with other hand.	___	___	_____
f. Pressed fist and hand into the person's abdomen with a quick, upward thrust.	___	___	_____
g. Repeated thrusts until the object was expelled or the person lost consciousness.	___	___	_____
3. Lowered the unresponsive person to the floor or ground. Positioned the person supine.	___	___	_____
4. Activated the EMS system or the center's emergency response system.	___	___	_____
5. Removed a foreign object if seen:			
a. Opened the airway with the head tilt-chin lift method.	___	___	_____
b. Looked in the mouth for a foreign object.	___	___	_____
c. Grasped and removed the object if it was within reach.	___	___	_____
6. Opened the airway with the head tilt-chin lift method.	___	___	_____
7. Gave 1 or 2 rescue breaths.	___	___	_____
8. Repositioned the person's head if the chest did not rise. Gave 1 or 2 rescue breaths.	___	___	_____
9. Gave up to 5 abdominal thrusts.	___	___	_____
10. Repeated steps 5 through 9 until rescue breathing was effective:			
a. Removed a foreign object if seen:			
(1) Opened the airway with the head tilt-chin lift method.	___	___	_____
(2) Looked in the mouth for a object.	___	___	_____
(3) Grasped and removed the object if it was within reach.	___	___	_____
b. Opened the airway with the head tilt-chin lift method.	___	___	_____
c. Gave 1 or 2 rescue breaths.	___	___	_____
d. Repositioned the person's head if the chest did not rise. Gave 1 or 2 rescue breaths.	___	___	_____
e. Gave up to 5 abdominal thrusts.	___	___	_____
11. Did the following if the person became unresponsive:			
a. Made sure the EMS system was activated.	___	___	_____
b. Started CPR.	___	___	_____

Date of Satisfactory Completion _____   Instructor's Initials _____

Using a Fire Extinguisher

Name: _____   Date: _____

Procedure	**S**	**U**	**Comments**
1. Pulled the fire alarm.	_____	_____	_____
2. Got the nearest fire extinguisher.	_____	_____	_____
3. Carried it upright.	_____	_____	_____
4. Took it to the fire.	_____	_____	_____
5. Removed the safety pin.	_____	_____	_____
6. Directed the hose at the base of the fire.	_____	_____	_____
7. Pushed the handle or lever down.	_____	_____	_____
8. Swept the hose slowly back and forth at the base of the fire.	_____	_____	_____

Date of Satisfactory Completion_____   Instructor's Initials _____

Applying a Transfer/Gait Belt

Name: _____   Date: _____

	S	U	Comments

Quality of Life
- Knocked before entering the person's room
- Addressed the person by name
- Introduced yourself by name and title
- Explained the procedure to the person before beginning and during the procedure
- Protected the person's rights during the procedure
- Handled the person gently during the procedure

Procedure
1. Saw *Promoting Safety and Comfort: Transfer/Gait Belts*
2. Practiced hand hygiene.
3. Identified the person. Checked the ID bracelet against the assignment sheet. Called the person by name.
4. Provided for privacy.
5. Assisted the person to a sitting position.
6. Applied the belt around the person's waist over clothing. Did not apply it over bare skin.
7. Tightened the belt so it was snug. It should not have caused discomfort or impaired breathing. You were able to slide 4 fingers (your open, flat hand) under the belt.
8. Made sure that a woman's breasts were not caught under the belt.
9. Placed the buckle off center in the front or in the back for the person's comfort. The buckle was not over the spine.

Date of Satisfactory Completion_____   Instructor's Initials _____

Helping the Falling Person

Name: _____   Date: _____

Procedure	S	U	Comments
1. Stood with your feet apart. Kept your back straight.	___	___	_____
2. Brought the person close to your body as fast as possible. Used the transfer/gait belt. Or wrapped your arms around the person's waist. If necessary, you could have also held the person under the arms.	___	___	_____
3. Moved your leg so the person's buttocks rested on it. Moved the leg near the person.	___	___	_____
4. Lowered the person to the floor. The person slid down your leg to the floor. You were bent at your hips and knees as you lowered the person.	___	___	_____
5. Called a nurse a to check the person. Stayed with the person.	___	___	_____
6. Helped the nurse return the person to bed.	___	___	_____

Post-Procedure

	S	U	Comments
7. Provided for comfort.	___	___	_____
8. Placed the signal light within reach.	___	___	_____
9. Raised or lowered the bed rails. Followed the care plan.	___	___	_____
10. Completed a safety check of the room.	___	___	_____
11. Reported and recorded the following:			
a. How the fall occurred.	___	___	_____
b. How far the person walked.	___	___	_____
c. How activity was tolerated before the fall.	___	___	_____
d. Complained before the fall.	___	___	_____
e. How much help the person needed while walking.	___	___	_____
12. Completed an incident report.	___	___	_____

Date of Satisfactory Completion_____   Instructor's Initials _____

Applying Restraints

Name: _____   Date: _____

	S	U	Comments

Quality of Life
- Knocked before entering the person's room
- Addressed the person by name
- Introduced yourself by name and title
- Explained the procedure to the person before beginning and during the procedure
- Protected the person's rights during the procedure
- Handled the person gently during the procedure

Pre-Procedure
1. Followed *Delegation Guidelines*:
   Applying Restraints
   Saw *Promoting Safety and Comfort*:
   Applying Restraints
2. Collected the following as instructed by the nurse:
   - Correct type and size of restraints
   - Padding for bony areas
   - Bed rail pads or gap protectors (if needed)
3. Practiced hand hygiene.
4. Identified the person. Checked the ID bracelet against the assignment sheet.
   Called the person by name.
5. Provided for privacy.

Procedure
6. Made sure the person was comfortable and in good alignment.
7. Put the bed rail pads or gap protectors (if needed) on the bed if the person was in bed. Followed the manufacturer's instructions.
8. Padded bony areas. Followed the nurse's instructions and the care plan.
9. Read the manufacturer's instructions.
   Noted the front and back of the restraint.
10. *For wrist restraints:*
    a. Applied the restraint following the manufacturer's instructions. Placed the soft part toward the skin.
    b. Secured the restraint so it was snug but not tight. Made sure you could slide 1 or 2 fingers under the restraint. Followed the manufacturer's instructions. Adjusted the straps if the restraint was too loose or too tight. Checked for snugness again.
    c. Tied the straps to the movable part of the bed frame out of the person's reach. Used a center-approved tie. Left 1 or 2 inches of slack in the straps.
    d. Repeated steps for the other wrist:
       (1) Applied the restraint following the manufacturer's instructions. Placed the soft part toward the skin.
       (2) Secured the restraint so it is snug but not tight. Made sure you could slide 1 or 2 fingers under the restraint. Followed the manufacturer's instructions. Adjusted the straps if the restraint was too loose or too tight. Checked for snugness again.
       (3) Tied the straps to the movable part of the bed frame out of the person's reach. Used a center-approved tie. Left 1 or 2 inches of slack in the straps.

Date of Satisfactory Completion_____ Instructor's Initials _____

Procedure—cont'd	S	U	Comments

11. For mitt restraints:

a. Made sure the person's hands were clean and dry.

b. Applied the mitt restraint. Followed the manufacturer's instructions.

c. Tied the straps to the movable part of the bed frame. Used a center-approved tie. Left 1 to 2 inches of slack in the straps.

d. Made sure the restraint was snug. Slid 1 or 2 fingers between the restraint and the wrist. Followed the manufacturer's instructions. Adjusted the straps if the restraint was too loose or too tight. Checked for snugness again.

e. Repeated steps for the other hand:

  (1) Applied the mitt restraint. Followed the manufacturer's instructions.

  (2) Tied the straps to the movable part of the bed frame. Used a center-approved tie. Left 1 to 2 inches of slack in the straps.

  (3) Made sure the restraint was snug. Slid 1 to 2 fingers between the restraint and the wrist. Followed the manufacturer's instructions. Adjusted the straps if the restraint was too loose or too tight. Checked for snugness again.

12. For a belt restraint:

a. Assisted the person to a sitting position.

b. Applied the restraint with your free hand. Followed the manufacturer's instructions.

c. Removed wrinkles or creases from the front and back of the restraint.

d. Brought the ties through the slots in the belt.

e. Helped the person lie down if he or she was in bed.

f. Secured the straps to the movable part of the bed frame out of the person's reach or to the chair or wheelchair. Used a center-approved tie. Left 1 to 2 inches of slack in the straps.

g. Made sure the belt was snug. Slid an open hand between the restraint and the person. Adjusted the restraint if it was too loose or too tight. Checked for snugness again.

13. For a vest restraint:

a. Assisted the person to a sitting position.

b. Applied the restraint with your free hand. Followed the manufacturer's instructions. The "V" part of the vest crossed in front.

c. Made sure the vest was free of wrinkles in the front and back.

d. Helped the person lie down if he or she was in bed.

e. Brought the straps through the slots.

f. Made sure the person was comfortable and in good alignment.

g. Secured the straps to the chair or to the movable part of the bed frame. If secured to the bed frame, the straps were secured at waist level out of the person's reach. Used a center-approved tie. Left 1 to 2 inches of slack in the straps.

h. Made sure the vest was snug. Slid an open hand between the restraint and the person. Adjusted the restraint if it was too loose or too tight. Checked for snugness again.

Date of Satisfactory Completion _____   Instructor's Initials _____

Procedure—cont'd   S   U   **Comments**

14. *Foe a jacket restraint:*
    a. Assisted the person to a sitting position.
    b. Applied the restraint with your free hand.
       Followed the manufacturer's instructions. Remembered,
       the jacket opening goes in the back.
    c. Closed the back with the zipper, ties, or hook and
       loop closures.
    d. Made sure the side seams were under the arms.
       Removed any wrinkles in the front and back.
    e. Helped the person lie down if he or she was in bed.
    f. Made sure the person was comfortable and in
       good alignment.
    g. Secured the straps to the chair or to the movable
       part of the bed frame. If secured to the bed frame,
       the straps were secured at waist level out of the
       person's reach. Used a center-approved knot.
       Left 1 to 2 inches of slack in the straps.
    h. Made sure the jacket was snug. Slid an open hand
       between the restraint and the person.
       Adjusted the restraint if it was too tight.
       Checked for snugness again.

Post-Procedure
15. Positioned the person as the nurse directed.
16. Provided for comfort.
17. Placed the signal light within the person's reach.
18. Raised or lowered bed rails. Followed the care plan
    and the manufacturer's instructions for the restraint.
19. Unscreened the person.
20. Completed a safety check of the room.
21. Decontaminated your hands.
22. Checked the person and the restraint at least every
    15 minutes. Reported and recorded your observations:
    a. For wrist and mitt restraints: checked the pulse,
       color, and temperature of the restrained parts.
    b. For vest, jacket, and belt restraints: checked the
       person's breathing. *Called for the nurse at once if the
       person was not breathing or was having problems breathing.*
       Made sure the restraint was properly positioned
       in the front and back.
23. Did the following at least every 2 hours:
    a. Removed the restraint.
    b. Repositioned the person.
    c. Met food, fluid, hygiene, and elimination needs.
    d. Gave skin care.
    e. Performed range-of-motion exercises or helped the
       person walk. Followed the care plan.
    f. Provided for comfort.
    g. Reapplied the restraints.
24. Completed a safety check of the room.
25. Reported and recorded your observations and the care given.

Date of Satisfactory Completion_____ Instructor's Initials _____

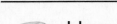

Hand Washing (NNAAP™)

Name: _____   Date: _____

Procedure	S	U	Comments
1. Saw *Promoting Safety and Comfort: Hand Hygiene*	___	___	_____
2. Made sure you had soap, paper towels, an orange stick or nail file, and a wastebasket. Collected missing items.	___	___	_____
3. Pushed your watch up your arm 4-5 inches. If your uniform sleeves were long, pushed them up too.	___	___	_____
4. Stood away from the sink so your clothes did not touch the sink. Stood so the soap and faucet were easy to reach.	___	___	_____
5. Turned on and adjusted the water until it felt warm.	___	___	_____
6. Wet your wrists and hands. Kept your hands lower than your elbows. Was sure to wet the area 3 to 4 inches above your wrists.	___	___	_____
7. Applied about 1 teaspoon of soap to your hands.	___	___	_____
8. Rubbed your palms together and interlaced your fingers to work up a good lather. This step lasted at least 15 seconds or the amount of time required by your state competency test.	___	___	_____
9. Washed each hand and wrist thoroughly. Cleaned between the fingers.	___	___	_____
10. Cleaned under the fingernails. Rubbed your fingertips against your palms.	___	___	_____
11. Cleaned under fingernails with a nail file or orange stick. This step was done for the first hand washing of the day and when hands were highly soiled.	___	___	_____
12. Rinsed your wrists and hands well. Water flowed from the arms to the hands.	___	___	_____
13. Repeated, if needed:			
a. Applied about 1 teaspoon of soap to your hands.	___	___	_____
b. Rubbed your palms together and interlaced your fingers to work up a good lather. This step lasted at least 15 seconds or the amount of time required by your state competency test.	___	___	_____
c. Washed each hand and wrist thoroughly. Cleaned well between the fingers.	___	___	
d. Cleaned under the fingernails. Rubbed your fingertips against your palms.	___	___	_____
e. Cleaned under the fingernails with a nail file or orange stick. This step was done for the first hand washing of the day and when your hands were highly soiled.	___	___	_____
f. Rinsed your wrists and hands well. Water flowed from the arms to the hands.	___	___	_____
14. Dried your wrists and hands well with paper towels. Patted dry. Started at fingertips.	___	___	_____
15. Discarded the paper towels.	___	___	_____
16. Turned off faucets with clean paper towels. This prevented you from contaminating your hands. Used a clean paper towel for each faucet.	___	___	_____
17. Discarded the paper towels into the wastebasket.	___	___	_____

Date of Satisfactory Completion_____   Instructor's Initials _____

Removing Gloves

Name: _____   Date: _____

Procedure

	S	U	Comments
1. Saw *Promoting Safety and Comfort: Gloves*	____	____	_____
2. Made sure that glove touched only glove.	____	____	_____
3. Grasped a glove just below the cuff. Grasped it on the outside.	____	____	_____
4. Pulled the glove down over your hand so it was inside out.	____	____	_____
5. Held the removed glove with your other gloved hand.	____	____	_____
6. Reached inside the other glove. Used the first two fingers of the ungloved hand.	____	____	_____
7. Pulled the glove down (inside out) over your hand and the other glove.	____	____	_____
8. Discarded the gloves. Followed center policy.	____	____	_____
9. Decontaminated your hands.	____	____	_____

Date of Satisfactory Completion _____   Instructor's Initials _____

Donning and Removing a Gown

Name: _____   Date: _____

Procedure	S	U	Comments
1. Removed your watch and all jewelry.	____	____	_____
2. Rolled up uniform sleeves.	____	____	_____
3. Practiced hand hygiene.	____	____	_____
4. Held a clean gown out in front of you. Allowed it to unfold. Did not shake the gown.	____	____	_____
5. Put your hands and arms through the sleeves.	____	____	_____
6. Made sure the gown covered you from your neck to your knees. It covered your arms to the end of your wrists	____	____	_____
7. Tied the strings at the back of the neck.	____	____	_____
8. Overlapped the back of the gown. Made sure it covered your uniform. The gown was snug, not loose.	____	____	_____
9. Tied the waist strings. Tied them at the back or the side. Did not tie them in front.	____	____	_____
10. Put on the gloves. Provided care.	____	____	_____
11. Removed and discarded the gloves. Decontaminated your hands.	____	____	_____
12. Removed and discarded the goggles or face shield if worn.	____	____	_____
13. Removed the gown:			
a. Untied the neck and waist strings. Did not touch the front of the gown.			
b. Pulled the gown down from each shoulder toward the same hand.	____	____	_____
c. Turned the gown inside out as it was removed. Held it at the inside shoulder seams and brought your hands together.	____	____	_____
14. Held and rolled up the gown away from you. Kept it inside out.	____	____	_____
15. Discarded the gown. Followed center policy.	____	____	_____
16. Removed and discarded the mask if worn. (NOTE: A respirator was removed outside the room.)	____	____	_____
17. Decontaminated your hands.	____	____	_____

Date of Satisfactory Completion _____   Instructor's Initials _____

Donning and Removing a Mask

Name: _____   Date: _____

Procedure

	S	U	Comments
1. Practiced hand hygiene.	___	___	_____
2. Put on a gown if required.	___	___	_____
3. Picked up a mask by its upper ties. Did not touch the part that covered your face.	___	___	_____
4. Placed the mask over your nose and mouth.	___	___	_____
5. Placed the upper strings above your ears. Tied them at the back in the middle of your head.	___	___	_____
6. Tied the lower strings at the back of your neck. The lower part of the mask was under your chin.	___	___	_____
7. Pinched the metal band around you nose. The top of the mask was snug over your nose. If you were wearing eyeglasses, the mask was snug under the bottom of the eyeglasses.	___	___	_____
8. Made sure the mask was snug over your face and under your chin.	___	___	_____
9. Put on goggles or a face shield if needed and not part of the mask.	___	___	_____
10. Decontaminated your hands. Put on gloves.	___	___	_____
11. Provided care. Avoided coughing, sneezing, and unnecessary talking.	___	___	_____
12. Changed the mask if it became wet or contaminated.	___	___	_____
13. Removed the mask. (NOTE: A respirator was removed outside of the room.)			
a. Removed the gloves. Also removed the goggles or face shield and gown if worn.	___	___	_____
b. Untied the lower strings of the mask.	___	___	
c. Untied the top strings.	___	___	_____
d. Held the top strings. Removed the mask.	___	___	_____
14. Discarded the mask. Followed center policy.	___	___	_____
15. Decontaminated your hands.	___	___	_____

Date of Satisfactory Completion_____ Instructor's Initials _____

Sterile Gloving

Name: _____   Date: _____

Procedure	S	U	Comments

1. Followed *Delegation Guidelines:*
   Assisting With Sterile Procedures
   Saw *Promoting Safety and Comfort*:
   • *Assisting With Sterile Procedures*
   • *Sterile Gloving*
	_____	_____	_____

2. Practiced hand hygiene.	_____	_____	_____
3. Inspected the package of sterile gloves for sterility:			
a. Checked the expiration date.	_____	_____	_____
b. Saw if the package was dry.	_____	_____	_____
c. Checked for tears, holes, punctures, and watermarks.	_____	_____	_____
4. Arranged a work surface:			
a. Made sure you had enough room.	_____	_____	_____
b. Arranged the work surface at waist level and within your vision.	_____	_____	_____
c. Cleaned and dried the work surface.	_____	_____	_____
d. Did not reach over or turn your back on the work surface.	_____	_____	_____
5. Opened the package. Grasped the flaps. Gently peeled them back.	_____	_____	_____
6. Removed the inner package. Placed it on the work surface.	_____	_____	_____
7. Read the manufacturer's instructions on the inner package. It may be labeled with *left, right, up,* and *down*.	_____	_____	_____
8. Arranged the inner package for left, right, up, and down. The left glove was on your left. The right glove was on your right. The cuffs were near you with the fingers pointing away from you.	_____	_____	_____
9. Grasped the folded edges of the inner package. Used the thumb and index finger of each hand.	_____	_____	_____
10. Folded back the inner package to expose the gloves. Did not touch or otherwise contaminate the inside of the package or the gloves. The inside of the inner package is a sterile field.	_____	_____	_____
11. Noted that each glove had a cuff about 2-3 inches wide. The cuffs and insides of the gloves are *not considered sterile*.	_____	_____	_____
12. Put on the right glove if you were right-handed. Put on the left glove if you were left-handed:			
a. Picked up the glove with your other hand. Used your thumb, index, and middle fingers.	_____	_____	_____
b. Touched only the cuff and inside of the glove.	_____	_____	_____
c. Turned the hand to be gloved palm side up.	_____	_____	_____
d. Lifted the cuff up. Slid your fingers and hand into the glove.	_____	_____	_____
e. Pulled the glove up over your hand. If some fingers got stuck, left them that way until the other glove was on. *Did not use your ungloved hand to straighten the glove. Did not let the outside of the glove touch any non-sterile surface.*	_____	_____	_____
f. Left the cuff turned down.	_____	_____	_____

Date of Satisfactory Completion_____   Instructor's Initials _____

Procedure—cont'd

	S	U	Comments
13. Put on the other glove. Used your gloved hand:			
a. Reached under the cuff of the second glove. Used the four fingers of your gloved hand. Kept your gloved thumb close to your gloved palm.	_____	_____	_____
b. Pulled on the second glove. Your gloved hand did not touch the cuff or any surface. Held the thumb of your first gloved hand away from the gloved palm.	_____	_____	_____
14. Adjusted each glove with the other hand. The gloves were smooth and comfortable.	_____	_____	_____
15. Slid your fingers under the cuffs to pull them up.	_____	_____	_____
16. Touched only sterile items.	_____	_____	_____
17. Removed the gloves.	_____	_____	_____
18. Decontaminated your hands.	_____	_____	_____

Date of Satisfactory Completion_____ Instructor's Initials _____

Raising the Person's Head and Shoulders

Name: _____   Date: _____

	S	U	Comments

Quality of Life
- Knocked before entering the person's room   ___ ___ _____
- Addressed the person by name   ___ ___ _____
- Introduced yourself by name and title   ___ ___ _____
- Explained the procedure to the person before beginning and during the procedure   ___ ___ _____
- Protected the person's rights during the procedure   ___ ___ _____
- Handled the person gently during the procedure   ___ ___ _____

Pre-Procedure
1. Followed *Delegation Guidelines*:
   - *Preventing Work-Related Injuries*
   - *Moving Persons in Bed*
   Saw *Promoting Safety and Comfort*:
   - *Safe Resident Handling, Moving, and Transfers*
   - *Preventing Work-Related Injuries*   ___ ___ _____
2. Asked a co-worker to assist if needed help.   ___ ___ _____
3. Practiced hand hygiene.   ___ ___ _____
4. Identified the person. Checked the ID bracelet against the assignment sheet. Called the person by name.   ___ ___ _____
5. Provided for privacy.   ___ ___ _____
6. Locked the bed wheels.   ___ ___ _____
7. Raised the bed for body mechanics. Bed rails were up if used.   ___ ___ _____

Procedure
8. Asked your co-worker to stand on the other side of the bed. Lowered the bed rail if up.   ___ ___ _____
9. Asked the person to put the near arm under your near arm and behind your shoulder. His or her hand rested on top of your shoulder. If you stood on the right side, the person's right hand rested on your shoulder. The person did the same with your co-worker. The person's left hand rested on your co-worker's left shoulder.   ___ ___ _____
10. Put your arm nearest the person under his or her arm. Your hand was on the person's shoulder. Your co-worker did the same.   ___ ___ _____
11. Put your free arm under the person's neck and shoulders. Your co-worker did the same.   ___ ___ _____
12. Helped the person pull up to a sitting or semi-sitting position on the "count of 3."   ___ ___ _____
13. Used the arm and hand that supported the person's neck and shoulders to give care. Your co-worker supported the person.   ___ ___ _____
14. Helped the person lie down. Provided support with your locked arm. Supported the person's neck and shoulders with your other arm. Your co-worker did the same.   ___ ___ _____

Post-Procedure
15. Provided for comfort.   ___ ___ _____
16. Placed the signal light within reach.   ___ ___ _____
17. Lowered the bed to its lowest position.   ___ ___ _____
18. Raised or lowered bed rails. Followed the care plan.   ___ ___ _____
19. Unscreened the person.   ___ ___ _____
20. Completed a safety check of the room.   ___ ___ _____
21. Decontaminated your hands.   ___ ___ _____
22. Reported and recorded your observations.   ___ ___ _____

Date of Satisfactory Completion_____   Instructor's Initials _____

Moving the Person Up in Bed

Name: _____   Date: _____

	S	U	Comments

Quality of Life
- Knocked before entering the person's room
- Addressed the person by name
- Introduced yourself by name and title
- Explained the procedure to the person before beginning and during the procedure
- Protected the person's rights during the procedure
- Handled the person gently during the procedure

Pre-Procedure
1. Followed *Delegation Guidelines*:
   - *Preventing Work-Related Injuries*
   - *Moving Persons in Bed*
   Saw *Promoting Safety and Comfort*:
   - *Safe Resident Handling, Moving, and Transfers*
   - *Preventing Work-Related Injuries*
   - *Moving the Person Up in Bed*
2. Asked a co-worker to assist if needed help.
3. Practiced hand hygiene.
4. Identified the person. Checked the ID bracelet against the assignment sheet. Called the person by name.
5. Provided for privacy.
6. Locked the bed wheels.
7. Raised the bed for body mechanics. Bed rails were up if used.

Procedure
8. Lowered the head of the bed to a level appropriate for the person. It was as flat as possible.
9. Stood on one side of the bed. Your co-worker stood on the other side.
10. Lowered the bed rails if up.
11. Removed pillows as directed by the nurse. Placed a pillow upright against the headboard if the person could be without it.
12. Stood with a wide base of support. Pointed the foot near the head of the bed toward the head of the bed. Faced the head of the bed.
13. Bent your hips and knees. Kept your back straight.
14. Placed one arm under the person's shoulders and one arm under the thighs. Your co-worker did the same. Grasped each other's forearms.
15. Asked the person to grasp the trapeze.
16. Had the person flex both knees.
17. Explained the following:
    a. You will count "1, 2, 3."
    b. The move will be on "3."
    c. On "3," the person pushes against the bed with the feet if able. And the person pulls up with the trapeze.
18. Moved the person to the head of the bed on the count of "3." Shifted your weight from your rear leg to your front leg. Your co-worker did the same.
19. Repeated steps 12 through 18 if necessary:
    a. Stood with a wide base of support. Pointed the foot near the head of the bed toward the head of the bed. Faced the head of the bed.
    b. Bent your hips and knees. Kept your back straight.

Date of Satisfactory Completion _____   Instructor's Initials _____

Procedure—cont'd   S   U   **Comments**

  c. Placed one arm under the person's shoulder and
    one arm under the thighs. Your co-worker did
    the same. Grasped each other's forearms.   ____ ____ _____
  d. Asked the person to grasp the trapeze.   ____ ____ _____
  e. Had the person flex both knees.   ____ ____ _____
  f. Explained the following:
    (1) You will count "1, 2, 3."   ____ ____ _____
    (2) The move will be on "3."   ____ ____ _____
    (3) On "3," the person pushes against the bed with
      the feet if able. And the person pulls up
      with the trapeze.   ____ ____ _____
  g. Moved the person to the head of the bed on the
    count of "3." Shifted your weight from your rear
    leg to your front leg. Your co-worker did the same. ____ ____ _____

Post-Procedure
20. Put the pillow under the person's head and shoulders.
    Straightened linens.   ____ ____ _____
21. Positioned the person in good alignment.   ____ ____ _____
22. Provided for comfort.   ____ ____ _____
23. Placed the signal light within reach.   ____ ____ _____
24. Raised the head of the bed to a level appropriate for the person. ____ ____ _____
25. Lowered the bed to its lowest position.   ____ ____ _____
26. Raised or lowered bed rails. Followed the care plan. ____ ____ _____
27. Unscreened the person.   ____ ____ _____
28. Completed a safety check of the room.   ____ ____ _____
29. Decontaminated your hands.   ____ ____ _____
30. Reported and recorded your observations.   ____ ____ _____

Date of Satisfactory Completion_____   Instructor's Initials _____

Moving the Person Up in Bed With an Assist Device

Name: _____ Date: _____

	S	U	Comments

Quality of Life
- Knocked before entering the person's room
- Addressed the person by name
- Introduced yourself by name and title
- Explained the procedure to the person before beginning and during the procedure
- Protected the person's rights during the procedure
- Handled the person gently during the procedure

Pre-Procedure
1. Followed *Delegation Guidelines*:
   - *Preventing Work-Related Injuries*
   - *Moving Persons in Bed*
   Saw *Promoting Safety and Comfort*:
   - *Safe Resident Handling, Moving, and Transfers*
   - *Preventing Work-Related Injuries*
   - *Moving the Person Up in Bed*
   - *Moving the Person Up in Bed With an Assist Device*
2. Asked a co-worker to assist if needed help.
3. Practiced hand hygiene.
4. Identified the person. Checked the ID bracelet against the assignment sheet. Called the person by name.
5. Provided for privacy.
6. Locked the bed wheels.
7. Raised the bed for body mechanics. Bed rails were up if used.

Procedure
8. Lowered the head of the bed to a level appropriate for the person. It was as flat as possible.
9. Stood on one side of the bed. Your co-worker stood on the other side.
10. Lowered the bed rails if up.
11. Removed pillows as directed by the nurse. Placed a pillow upright against the headboard if the person could be without it.
12. Stood with a wide base of support. Pointed the foot near the head of the bed toward the head of the bed. Faced that direction.
13. Rolled the sides of the assist device up close to the person. (NOTE: Omitted this step if the device had handles.)
14. Grasped the rolled-up assist device firmly near the person's shoulders and hips. Or grasped it by the handles. Supported the head.
15. Bent your hips and knees.
16. Moved the person up in bed on the count of "3." Shifted your weight from your rear leg to your front leg.
17. Repeated steps 12 through 16 if necessary:
    a. Stood with a wide base of support. Pointed the foot near the head of the bed toward the head of the bed. Faced that direction.
    b. Rolled the sides of the assist device up close to the person. (NOTE: Omitted this step if the device had handles.)

Date of Satisfactory Completion_____ Instructor's Initials _____

Procedure—cont'd	S	U	Comments

Procedure—cont'd

   c. Grasped the rolled-up assist device firmly near the
person's shoulders and hips. Or grasped it by the handles.   ____ ____ _____

   d. Bent your hips and knees.   ____ ____ _____

   e. Moved the person up in bed on the count of "3."
Shifted your weight from your rear leg to your front leg.   ____ ____ _____

18. Unrolled the assist device. (*Note:* Omitted this step if the
device had handles.)   ____ ____ _____

Post-Procedure

19. Put the pillow under the person's head and shoulders.
20. Positioned the person in good alignment.
21. Provided for comfort.
22. Placed the signal light within reach.
23. Raised the head of the bed to a level appropriate for the person.
24. Lowered the bed to its lowest position.
25. Raised or lowered bed rails. Followed the care plan.
26. Unscreened the person.
27. Completed a safety check of the room.
28. Decontaminated your hands.
29. Reported and recorded your observations.

Date of Satisfactory Completion_____ Instructor's Initials _____

Moving the Person to the Side of the Bed

Name: _____   Date: _____

	S	U	Comments

Quality of Life
- Knocked before entering the person's room
- Addressed the person by name
- Introduced yourself by name and title
- Explained the procedure to the person before beginning and during the procedure
- Protected the person's rights during the procedure
- Handled the person gently during the procedure

Pre-Procedure
1. Followed *Delegation Guidelines*:
   - *Preventing Work-Related Injuries*
   - *Moving Persons in Bed*

   Saw *Promoting Safety and Comfort*:
   - *Safe Resident Handling, Moving, and Transfers*
   - *Preventing Work-Related Injuries*
   - *Moving the Person to the Side of the Bed*
2. Asked a co-worker to assist if using an assist device.
3. Practiced hand hygiene.
4. Identified the person. Checked the ID bracelet against the assignment sheet. Called the person by name.
5. Provided for privacy.
6. Locked the bed wheels.
7. Raised the bed for body mechanics. Bed rails were up if used.

Procedure
8. Lowered the head of the bed to a level appropriate for the person. It was as flat as possible.
9. Stood on the side of the bed to which you moved the person.
10. Lowered the bed rails if bed rails were used. (Both bed rails were lowered for step 15.)
11. Removed pillows as directed by the nurse.
12. Stood with your feet about 12 inches apart. One foot was in front of the other. Flexed your knees.
13. Crossed the person's arms over the person's chest.
14. *Method 1: Moving the person in segments:*
    a. Placed your arm under the person's neck and shoulders. Grasped the far shoulder.
    b. Placed your other arm under the mid-back.
    c. Moved the upper part of the person's body toward you. Rocked backward and shifted your weight to your rear leg.
    d. Placed one arm under the person's waist and one under the thighs.
    e. Rocked backward to move the lower part of the person toward you.
    f. Repeated the procedure for the legs and feet. Your arms should have been under the person's thighs and calves.
15. *Method 2: Moving the person with a drawsheet:*
    a. Rolled up the drawsheet close to the person.
    b. Grasped the rolled-up drawsheet near the person's shoulders and hips. Your co-worker did the same. Supported the person's head.

Date of Satisfactory Completion_____   Instructor's Initials _____

Procedure—cont'd   S   U   **Comments**

    c. Rocked backward on the count of "3," moving
       moved the person toward you. Your co-worker
       rocked backward slightly and then forward toward
       you with arms kept straight.   ____ ____ _____
    d. Unrolled the drawsheet. Removed any wrinkles.   ____ ____ _____

Post-Procedure

16. Positioned the person in good alignment.   ____ ____ _____
17. Provided for comfort.   ____ ____ _____
18. Placed the signal light within reach.   ____ ____ _____
19. Lowered the bed to its lowest position.   ____ ____ _____
20. Raised or lowered bed rails. Followed the care plan. ____ ____ _____
21. Unscreened the person.   ____ ____ _____
22. Completed a safety check of the room.   ____ ____ _____
23. Decontaminated your hands.   ____ ____ _____
24. Reported and recorded your observations.   ____ ____ _____

Date of Satisfactory Completion _____ Instructor's Initials _____

Turning and Repositioning the Person (NNAAP™)

Name: _____ Date: _____

	S	U	Comments

Quality of Life
- Knocked before entering the person's room
- Addressed the person by name
- Introduced yourself by name and title
- Explained the procedure to the person before beginning and during the procedure
- Protected the person's rights during the procedure
- Handled the person gently during the procedure

Pre-Procedure
1. Followed *Delegation Guidelines*:
   - *Preventing Work-Related Injuries*
   - *Moving Persons in Bed*
   - *Turning Persons*
   Saw *Promoting Safety and Comfort*:
   - *Safe Resident Handling, Moving, and Transfers*
   - *Preventing Work-Related Injuries*
   - *Moving the Person to the Side of the Bed*
   - *Turning Persons*
2. Practiced hand hygiene.
3. Identified the person. Checked the ID bracelet against the assignment sheet. Called the person by name.
4. Provided for privacy.
5. Locked the bed wheels.
6. Raised the bed for body mechanics. Bed rails were up if used.

Procedure
7. Lowered the head of the bed to a level appropriate for the person. It was as flat as possible.
8. Stood on the side of the bed opposite to where you turned the person. The far bed rail was up if used.
9. Lowered the bed rails near you if used.
10. Moved the person to the side near you.
11. Crossed the person's arms over the person's chest. Crossed the leg near you over the far leg.
12. *Turned the person away from you:*
    a. Stood with a wide base of support. Flexed the knees.
    b. Placed one hand on the person's shoulder. Placed the other on the hip near you.
    c. Pushed the person gently toward the other side of the bed. Shifted your weight from your rear leg to your front leg.
13. *Turned the person toward you:*
    a. Raised the bed rail if used.
    b. Went to the other side of the bed. Lowered the bed rail if used.
    c. Stood with a wide base of support. Flexed your knees.
    d. Placed one hand on the person's far shoulder. Placed the other on the far hip.
    e. Rolled the person toward you gently.
14. Positioned the person. Followed the nurse's directions, the care plan, and these common measures:
    a. Placed a pillow under the head and neck.
    b. Adjusted the shoulder. The person did not lie on an arm.

Date of Satisfactory Completion_____ Instructor's Initials _____

Procedure—cont'd   S   U   **Comments**

   c. Placed a pillow under the upper hand and arm.   _____ _____ _____

   d. Positioned a pillow against the back.   _____ _____ _____

   e. Flexed the upper knee. Positioned the upper
      leg in front of the lower leg.   _____ _____ _____

   f. Supported the upper leg and thigh on pillows.
      Made sure the ankle was supported.   _____ _____ _____

Post-Procedure

15. Provided for comfort.   _____ _____ _____

16. Placed the signal light within reach.   _____ _____ _____

17. Lowered the bed to its lowest position.   _____ _____ _____

18. Raised or lowered bed rails. Followed the care plan.   _____ _____ _____

19. Unscreened the person.   _____ _____ _____

20. Completed a safety check of the room.   _____ _____ _____

21. Decontaminated your hands.   _____ _____ _____

22. Reported and recorded your observations.   _____ _____ _____

Date of Satisfactory Completion _____   Instructor's Initials _____

Logrolling the Person

Name: _____   Date: _____

Quality of Life	S	U	Comments
• Knocked before entering the person's room	___	___	_____
• Addressed the person by name	___	___	_____
• Introduced yourself by name and title	___	___	_____
• Explained the procedure to the person before beginning and during the procedure	___	___	_____
• Protected the person's rights during the procedure	___	___	_____
• Handled the person gently during the procedure	___	___	_____

Pre-Procedure

1. Followed *Delegation Guidelines*:
   - *Preventing Work-Related Injuries*
   - *Moving Persons in Bed*
   - *Turning Persons*

   Saw *Promoting Safety and Comfort*:
   - *Safe Resident Handling, Moving, and Transfers*
   - *Preventing Work-Related Injuries*
   - *Turning Persons*
   - *Logrolling*
2. Asked a co-worker to help you.
3. Practiced hand hygiene.
4. Identified the person. Checked the ID bracelet against the assignment sheet. Called the person by name.
5. Provided for privacy.
6. Locked the bed wheels.
7. Raised the bed for body mechanics. Bed rails were up if used.

Procedure

8. Made sure the bed was flat.
9. Stood on the side opposite to which you turned the person. Your co-worker stood on the other side.
10. Lowered the bed rails if used.
11. Moved the person as a unit to the side of the bed near you. Used the assist device.
12. Placed the person's arms across the chest. Placed a pillow between the knees.
13. Raised the bed rail if used.
14. Went to the other side.
15. Stood near the shoulders and chest. Your co-worker stood near the hips and thighs.
16. Stood with a broad base of support. One foot was in front of the other.
17. Asked the person to hold his or her body rigid.
18. Rolled the person toward you. Or used the assist device. Turned the person as a unit.
19. Positioned the person in good alignment. Used pillows as directed by the nurse and the care plan. Followed these common measures (unless the spinal cord was involved):
    a. One pillow against the back for support.
    b. One pillow under the head and neck if allowed.
    c. One pillow or a folded bath blanket between the legs.
    d. A small pillow under the upper arm and hand.

Date of Satisfactory Completion _____ Instructor's Initials _____

	S	U	Comments
Post-Procedure			
20. Provided for comfort.	_____	_____	_____
21. Placed the signal light within reach.	_____	_____	_____
22. Lowered the bed to its lowest position.	_____	_____	_____
23. Raised or lowered bed rails. Followed the care plan.	_____	_____	_____
24. Unscreened the person.	_____	_____	_____
25. Completed a safety check of the room.	_____	_____	_____
26. Decontaminated your hands.	_____	_____	_____
27. Reported and recorded your observations.	_____	_____	_____

Date of Satisfactory Completion _____ Instructor's Initials _____

Sitting on the Side of the Bed (Dangling)

Name: _____   Date: _____

	S	U	Comments

Quality of Life
- Knocked before entering the person's room
- Addressed the person by name
- Introduced yourself by name and title
- Explained the procedure to the person before beginning and during the procedure
- Protected the person's rights during the procedure
- Handled the person gently during the procedure

Pre-Procedure
1. Followed *Delegation Guidelines*:
   - *Preventing Work-Related Injuries*
   - *Dangling*

   Saw *Promoting Safety and Comfort*:
   - *Safe Resident Handling, Moving, and Transfers*
   - *Preventing Work-Related Injuries*
   - *Dangling*
2. Practiced hand hygiene.
3. Identified the person. Checked the ID bracelet against the assignment sheet. Called the person by name.
4. Provided for privacy.
5. Decided what side of the bed to use.
6. Moved furniture to provide moving space.
7. Locked the bed wheels.
8. Raised the bed for body mechanics. Bed rails were up if used.

Procedure
9. Lowered the bed rail if up.
10. Positioned the person in a side-lying position facing you. The person lay on the strong side.
11. Raised the head of the bed to a sitting position.
12. Stood by the person's hips. Faced the foot of the bed.
13. Stood with your feet apart. The foot near the head of the bed was in front of the other foot.
14. Slid one arm under the person's neck and shoulders. Grasped the far shoulder. Placed your other hand over the thighs near the knees.
15. Pivoted toward the foot of the bed while moving the person's legs and feet over the side of the bed. As the legs went over the edge of the mattress, the trunk was upright.
16. Asked the person to hold onto the edge of the mattress. This supported the person in the sitting position.
17. Did not leave the person alone. Provided support if necessary.
18. Checked the person's condition:
    a. Asked how the person felt. Asked if the person felt dizzy or light-headed.
    b. Checked pulse and respiration.
    c. Checked for difficulty breathing.
    d. Noted if the skin was pale or bluish in color *(cyanosis)*.
19. Helped the person lie down if necessary.
20. Reversed the procedure to return the person to bed.
21. Lowered the head of the bed after the person returned to bed. Helped him or her move to the center of the bed.
22. Positioned the person in good alignment.

Date of Satisfactory Completion_____   Instructor's Initials _____

	S	U	Comments

Post-Procedure

23. Provided for comfort.
24. Placed the signal light within reach.
25. Lowered the bed to its lowest position.
26. Raised or lowered bed rails. Followed the care plan.
27. Returned furniture to its proper place.
28. Unscreened the person.
29. Completed a safety check of the room.
30. Decontaminated your hands.
31. Reported and recorded your observations.

Date of Satisfactory Completion _____ Instructor's Initials _____

Transferring a Person to a Chair or Wheelchair (NNAAP™)

Name: _____   Date: _____

Quality of Life	S	U	Comments

Quality of Life
- Knocked before entering the person's room
- Addressed the person by name
- Introduced yourself by name and title
- Explained the procedure to the person before beginning and during the procedure
- Protected the person's rights during the procedure
- Handled the person gently during the procedure

Pre-Procedure
1. Followed *Delegation Guidelines*:
   - *Preventing Work-Related Injuries*
   - *Transferring Persons*
   Saw *Promoting Safety and Comfort*:
   - *Transfer/Gait Belts*
   - *Safe Resident Handling, Moving, and Transfers*
   - *Preventing Work-Related Injuries*
   - *Transferring Persons*
   - *Chair or Wheelchair Transfers*
2. Collected:
   - Wheelchair or arm chair
   - Bath blanket
   - Lap blanket
   - Robe and non-skid footwear
   - Paper or sheet
   - Transfer belt (if needed)
   - Seat cushion (if needed)
3. Practiced hand hygiene.
4. Identified the person. Checked the ID bracelet against the assignment sheet. Called the person by name.
5. Provided for privacy.
6. Decided what side of the bed to use. Moved furniture for a safe transfer.

Procedure
7. Placed the chair near the bed on the person's strong side. The arm of the chair almost touched the bed.
8. Placed a folded bath blanket or cushion on the seat (if needed).
9. Locked the wheelchair wheels. Raised the footplates. Removed or swung the front rigging out of the way.
10. Lowered the bed to its lowest position. Locked the bed wheels.
11. Fan-folded top linens to the foot of the bed.
12. Placed the paper or sheet under the person's feet. Put footwear on the person.
13. Helped the person sit on the side of bed. His or her feet touched the floor.
14. Helped the person put on a robe.
15. Applied the transfer belt if needed.
16. *Method 1: Using a transfer belt:*
    a. Stood in front of the person.
    b. Had the person hold onto the mattress.
    c. Made sure the person's feet were flat on the floor.
    d. Had the person lean forward.
    e. Grasped the transfer belt at each side. Grasped the handles or grasped the belt from underneath.

Date of Satisfactory Completion_____   Instructor's Initials _____

Procedure—cont'd   S   U   **Comments**

f. Prevented the person from sliding or falling by
doing one of the following:
(1) Braced your knees against the person's knees.
Blocked his or her feet with your feet.   _____ _____ _____
(2) Used the knee and foot of one leg to block the
person's weak leg or foot. Placed your other foot
slightly behind your own for balance.   _____ _____ _____
(3) Straddled your legs around the person's weak leg.   _____ _____ _____
g. Explained the following:
(1) You will count "1, 2, 3."   _____ _____ _____
(2) The move will be on "3."   _____ _____ _____
(3) On "3," the person pushes down on the mattress
and stands.   _____ _____ _____
h. Asked the person to push down on the mattress and
to stand on the count of "3."   _____ _____ _____
i. Pulled the person to a standing position as you
straightened your knees.   _____ _____ _____

17. *Method 2: No transfer belt:* (NOTE: Used this method only
if directed be the nurse and the care plan.)
a. Followed steps 16, a-c:
(1) Stood in front of the person.   _____ _____ _____
(2) Had the person hold onto the mattress.   _____ _____ _____
(3) Made sure the person's feet were flat on the floor.   _____ _____ _____
b. Placed your hands under the person's arms. Your hands
were around the person's shoulder blades.   _____ _____ _____
c. Had the person lean forward.   _____ _____ _____
d. Prevented the person from sliding or falling by
doing one of the following:
(1) Braced your knees against the person's knees.
Blocked his or her feet with your feet.   _____ _____ _____
(2) Used the knee and foot of one leg to block the
person's weak leg or foot. Placed your other
foot slightly behind you for balance.   _____ _____ _____
(3) Straddled your legs around the person's weak leg.   _____ _____ _____
e. Explained the "count of 3."
1. You will count "1, 2, 3."   _____ _____ _____
2. The move will be on "3."   _____ _____ _____
3. On "3," the person pushes down on the mattress
and stands.   _____ _____ _____
f. Asked the person to push down on the mattress and
to stand on the count of "3." Pulled the person up
into a standing position as you straightened your knees.   _____ _____ _____

18. Supported the person in the standing position. Held the
transfer belt, or kept hands around the person's
shoulder blades. Continued to prevent the person
from sliding or falling.   _____ _____ _____
19. Turned the person so he or she could grasp the
far arm of the chair. The legs touched the edge of the chair.   _____ _____ _____
20. Continued to turn the person until the other armrest
was grasped.   _____ _____ _____
21. Lowered him or her into the chair as you bent your
hips and knees. The person assisted by leaning forward
and bending the elbows and knees.   _____ _____ _____
22. Made sure the buttocks were to the back of the seat.
Positioned person in good alignment.   _____ _____ _____

Date of Satisfactory Completion_____   Instructor's Initials _____

Procedure—cont'd

	S	U	Comments
23. Attached the wheelchair front rigging. Positioned the person's feet on the wheelchair footplates.			
24. Covered the person's lap and legs with a lap blanket. Kept the blanket off the floor and the wheels.	___	___	_____
25. Removed the transfer belt if used.	___	___	_____
26. Positioned the chair as the person preferred. Locked the wheelchair wheels according to the care plan.	___	___	_____

Post-Procedure

	S	U	Comments
27. Provided for comfort.	___	___	_____
28. Placed the signal light within reach.	___	___	_____
29. Unscreened the person.	___	___	_____
30. Completed a safety check of the room.	___	___	_____
31. Decontaminated your hands.	___	___	_____
32. Reported and recorded your observations.	___	___	_____

Date of Satisfactory Completion_____   Instructor's Initials _____

Transferring a Person From a Chair or Wheelchair to Bed

Name: _____   Date: _____

	S	U	Comments

Quality of Life
- Knocked before entering the person's room
- Addressed the person by name
- Introduced yourself by name and title
- Explained the procedure to the person before beginning and during the procedure
- Protected the person's rights during the procedure
- Handled the person gently during the procedure

Pre-Procedure
1. Followed *Delegation Guidelines:*
   - *Preventing Work-Related Injuries*
   - *Transferring Persons*
   Saw *Promoting Safety and Comfort*:
   - *Transfer/Gait Belts*
   - *Safe Resident Handling, Moving, and Transfers*
   - *Preventing Work-Related Injuries*
   - *Transferring Persons*
   - *Chair or Wheelchair Transfers*
2. Collected a transfer belt if needed.
3. Practiced hand hygiene.
4. Identified the person. Checked the ID bracelet against the assignment sheet. Called the person by name.
5. Provided for privacy.

Procedure
6. Moved furniture for moving space.
7. Raised the head of the bed to a sitting position. The bed was in the lowest position.
8. Moved the signal light so it was on the strong side when the person was in bed.
9. Positioned the chair or wheelchair so the person's strong side was next to the bed. Had a co-worker help you if necessary.
10. Locked the wheelchair and the bed wheels.
11. Removed and folded the lap blanket.
12. Removed the person's feet from the footplates. Raised the footplates. Removed or swung the front rigging out of the way.
13. Applied the transfer belt (if needed).
14. Made sure the person's feet were flat on the floor.
15. Stood in front of the person.
16. Asked the person to hold onto the armrest. Or placed your arms under the person's arms. Your hands were around the shoulder blades.
17. Had the person lean forward.
18. Grasped the transfer belt on each side if used. Grasped underneath the belt.
19. Prevented the person from sliding or falling by doing one of the following:
    a. Braced your knees against the person's knees. Blocked his or her feet with your feet.
    b. Used the knee and foot of one leg to block the person's weak leg or foot. Placed your other foot slightly behind your own for balance.
    c. Straddled your legs around the person's weak leg.

Date of Satisfactory Completion _____ Instructor's Initials _____

Procedure—cont'd   S   U   **Comments**

20. Explained the following:
    a. You will count "1, 2, 3."
    b. The move will be on "3."
    c. On "3," the person pushes down on the mattress and stands.
21. Asked the person to push down on the armrests on the count of "3." Pulled the person to a standing position as you straightened your knees.
22. Supported the person in the standing position. Held the transfer belt, or kept hands around the person's shoulder blades. Continued to prevent the person from sliding or falling.
23. Turned the person so he or she could reach the edge of the mattress. The legs touched the mattress.
24. Continued to turn the person until he or she reached the mattress with both hands.
25. Lowered him or her into the bed as you bent your hips and knees. The person assisted by leaning forward and bending the elbows and knees.
26. Removed the transfer belt.
27. Removed the robe and footwear.
28. Helped the person lie down.

Post-Procedure
29. Provided for comfort.
30. Placed the signal light within reach and other needed items within reach.
31. Raised or lowered bed rails. Followed the care plan.
32. Arranged furniture to meet the person's needs.
33. Unscreened the person.
34. Completed a safety check of the room.
35. Decontaminated your hands.
36. Reported and recorded your observations.

Date of Satisfactory Completion_____ Instructor's Initials _____

Transferring the Person Using a Mechanical Lift

Name: _____   Date: _____

Quality of Life	S	U	Comments

Quality of Life
- Knocked before entering the person's room
- Addressed the person by name
- Introduced yourself by name and title
- Explained the procedure to the person before beginning and during the procedure
- Protected the person's rights during the procedure
- Handled the person gently during the procedure

Pre-Procedure
1. Followed *Delegation Guidelines:*
   - *Preventing Work-Related Injuries*
   - *Transferring Persons*
   - *Using Mechanical Lifts*
   Saw *Promoting Safety and Comfort*:
   - *Safe Resident Handling, Moving, and Transfers*
   - *Preventing Work-Related Injuries*
   - *Transferring Persons*
   - *Using Mechanical Lifts*
2. Asked a co-worker to help you.
3. Collected:
   - Mechanical lift
   - Arm chair or wheelchair
   - Footwear
   - Bath blanket or cushion
   - Lap blanket
4. Practiced hand hygiene.
5. Identified the person. Checked the ID bracelet against the assignment sheet. Called the person by name.
6. Provided for privacy.

Procedure
7. Raised the bed for body mechanics. Bed rails were up if used.
8. Lowered the head of the bed to a level appropriate for the person. It was as flat as possible.
9. Stood on one side of the bed. Your co-worker stood on the other side.
10. Lowered the bed rails if up.
11. Centered the sling under the person. To position the sling, turned the person from side to side as if making an occupied bed. Positioned the sling according to the manufacturer's instructions.
12. Positioned the person in semi-Fowler's position.
13. Placed the chair at the head of the bed. It was even with the headboard and about 1 foot away from the bed. Placed a folded bath blanket or cushion in the chair.
14. Locked the bed wheels. Lowered the bed to its lowest position.
15. Raised the lift so you could position it over the person.
16. Positioned the lift over the person.
17. Locked the lift wheels in position.
18. Attached the sling to the swivel bar.
19. Raised the head of the bed to a sitting position.
20. Crossed the person's arms over the chest. He or she held onto the straps or chains but not the swivel bar.
21. Raised the lift high enough until the person and the sling were free of the bed.

Date of Satisfactory Completion_____   Instructor's Initials _____

Procedure—cont'd

	S	U	Comments
22. Had your co-worker support the person's legs as you moved the lift and the person away from the bed.			
23. Positioned the lift so the person's back was toward the chair.	___	___	___
24. Positioned the chair so you could lower the person into it.	___	___	___
25. Lowered the person into the chair. Guided the person into the chair.	___	___	___
26. Lowered the swivel bar to unhook the sling. Removed the sling from under the person unless otherwise indicated.	___	___	___
27. Put footwear on the person. Positioned the person's feet on the wheelchair footplates.	___	___	___
28. Covered the person's lap and legs with a lap blanket. Kept it off the floor and wheels.	___	___	___
29. Positioned the chair as the person preferred. Locked the wheelchair wheels according to the care plan.	___	___	___

Post-Procedure

	S	U	Comments
30. Provided for comfort.	___	___	___
31. Placed the signal light within reach and other needed items within reach.	___	___	___
32. Unscreened the person.	___	___	___
33. Completed a safety check of the room.	___	___	___
34. Decontaminated your hands.	___	___	___
35. Reported and recorded your observations.	___	___	___
36. Reversed the procedure to return the person to bed.	___	___	___

Date of Satisfactory Completion _____   Instructor's Initials _____

Transferring the Person to and From the Toilet

Name: _____   Date: _____

Quality of Life	S	U	Comments
• Knocked before entering the person's room	___	___	_____
• Addressed the person by name	___	___	_____
• Introduced yourself by name and title	___	___	_____
• Explained the procedure to the person before beginning and during the procedure	___	___	_____
• Protected the person's rights during the procedure	___	___	_____
• Handled the person gently during the procedure	___	___	_____

Pre-Procedure
1. Followed *Delegation Guidelines:*
   • *Preventing Work-Related Injuries*
   • *Transferring Persons*
   Saw *Promoting Safety and Comfort:*
   • *Transfer/Gait Belts*
   • *Safe Resident Handling, Moving, and Transfers*
   • *Preventing Work-Related Injuries*
   • *Transferring Persons*
   • *Chair or Wheelchair Transfers*
   • *Transferring the Person To and From a Toilet*   ___ ___ _____
2. Practiced hand hygiene.   ___ ___ _____

Procedure
3. Had the person wear non-skid footwear.   ___ ___ _____
4. Positioned the wheelchair next to the toilet if there was enough room. If not, positioned the chair at a right angle (90 degrees) to the toilet. Best if the person's strong side was near the toilet.   ___ ___ _____
5. Locked the wheelchair wheels.   ___ ___ _____
6. Raised the footplates. Removed or swung the front rigging out of the way.   ___ ___ _____
7. Applied the transfer belt.   ___ ___ _____
8. Helped the person unfasten clothing.   ___ ___ _____
9. Used the transfer belt to help the person stand and to turn to the toilet. The person used the grab bars to turn to the toilet.   ___ ___ _____
10. Supported the person with the transfer belt while he or she lowered clothing. Or had the person hold onto the grab bars for support. Lowered the person's pants and undergarments.   ___ ___ _____
11. Used the transfer belt to lower the person onto the toilet seat. Made sure he or she was properly positioned on the toilet.   ___ ___ _____
12. Removed the transfer belt.   ___ ___ _____
13. Told the person you will stay nearby. Reminded the person to use the signal light or call for you when help is needed. Stayed with the person if required by the care plan.   ___ ___ _____
14. Closed the bathroom door to provide privacy.   ___ ___ _____
15. Stayed near the bathroom. Completed other tasks in the person's room. Checked on the person every 5 minutes.   ___ ___ _____
16. Knocked on the bathroom door when the person called for you.   ___ ___ _____
17. Helped with wiping, perineal care, flushing, and hand washing as needed. Wore gloves and practiced hand hygiene after removing the gloves.   ___ ___ _____
18. Applied the transfer belt.   ___ ___ _____
19. Used the transfer belt to help the person stand.   ___ ___ _____
20. Helped the person raise and secure clothing.   ___ ___ _____

Date of Satisfactory Completion_____   Instructor's Initials _____

Procedure—cont'd	S	U	Comments
21. Used the transfer belt to transfer the person to the wheelchair.	___	___	_____
22. Made sure the person's buttocks were to the back of the seat. Positioned the person in good alignment.	___	___	_____
23. Positioned the person's feet on the footplates.	___	___	_____
24. Covered the person's lap and legs with a lap blanket. Kept the blanket off the floor and wheels.	___	___	_____
25. Positioned the chair as the person preferred. Locked the wheelchair wheels according to the care plan.	___	___	_____

Post-Procedure

	S	U	Comments
26. Provided for comfort.	___	___	_____
27. Placed the signal light and other needed items within the person's reach.	___	___	_____
28. Unscreened the person.	___	___	_____
29. Completed a safety check of the room.	___	___	_____
30. Practiced hand hygiene.	___	___	_____
31. Reported and recorded your observations.	___	___	_____

Date of Satisfactory Completion _____   Instructor's Initials _____

Moving the Person to a Stretcher

Name: _____   Date: _____

	S	U	Comments

Quality of Life
- Knocked before entering the person's room
- Addressed the person by name
- Introduced yourself by name and title
- Explained the procedure to the person before beginning and during the procedure
- Protected the person's rights during the procedure
- Handled the person gently during the procedure

Pre-Procedure
1. Followed *Delegation Guidelines:*
   - *Preventing Work-Related Injuries*
   - *Transferring Persons*
   Saw *Promoting Safety and Comfort*:
   - *Safe Resident Handling, Moving, and Transfers*
   - *Preventing Work-Related Injuries*
   - *Transferring Persons*
   - *Moving the Person to a Stretcher*
2. Asked 1 or 2 staff members to help.
3. Collected:
   - Stretcher covered with a sheet or bath blanket
   - Bath blanket
   - Pillow(s) if needed
   - Slide sheet, slide board, drawsheet, or other assist device
4. Practiced hand hygiene.
5. Identified the person. Checked the ID bracelet against the assignment sheet. Called the person by name.
6. Provided for privacy.
7. Raised the bed and stretcher for body mechanics.

Procedure
8. Positioned yourself and co-worker:
   a. One or two workers on the side of the bed where the stretcher was.
   b. One worker stood on the other side of the bed.
9. Lowered the head of the bed. It was as flat as possible.
10. Lowered the bed rails if used.
11. Covered the person with a bath blanket. Fan-folded top linens to the foot of the bed.
12. Positioned the assist device. Or loosened the drawsheet on each side.
13. Used the assist device to move the person to the side of the bed where the stretcher would be.
14. Protected the person from falling. Held the far arm and leg.
15. Had your co-workers position the stretcher next to the bed. They stood behind the stretcher.
16. Locked the bed and stretcher wheels.
17. Grasped the assist device.
18. Transferred the person to the stretcher on the count of "3." Centered the person on the stretcher.
19. Placed a pillow or pillows under the person's head and shoulders if allowed. Raised the head of the stretcher if allowed.
20. Covered the person. Provided privacy.
21. Fastened the safety straps. Raised the side rails.
22. Unlocked the stretcher wheels. Transported the person.

Date of Satisfactory Completion_____   Instructor's Initials _____

	S	U	Comments

Post-Procedure
23. Decontaminated your hands.
24. Reported and recorded:
- The time of the transport
- Where the person was transported to
- Who went with him of her
- How the transfer was tolerated
25. Reversed the procedure to return the person to bed.

Date of Satisfactory Completion _____ Instructor's Initials _____

Making a Closed Bed

Name: _____　　Date: _____

	S	U	Comments
Quality of Life			
• Knocked before entering the person's room	___	___	_____
• Addressed the person by name	___	___	_____
• Introduced yourself by name and title	___	___	_____
• Explained the procedure to the person before beginning and during the procedure	___	___	_____
• Protected the person's rights during the procedure	___	___	_____
• Handled the person gently during the procedure	___	___	_____

Pre-Procedure

	S	U	Comments
1. Followed *Delegation Guidelines: Making Beds* Saw *Promoting Safety and Comfort: Making Beds*	___	___	_____
2. Practiced hand hygiene.	___	___	_____
3. Collected clean linen:			
• Mattress pad (if needed)	___	___	_____
• Bottom sheet (flat or fitted)	___	___	_____
• Plastic draw sheet or waterproof pad (if needed)	___	___	_____
• Cotton drawsheet (if needed)	___	___	_____
• Top sheet	___	___	_____
• Blanket	___	___	_____
• Bedspread	___	___	_____
• Two pillowcases	___	___	_____
• Bath towel(s)	___	___	_____
• Hand towel	___	___	_____
• Washcloth	___	___	_____
• Gown	___	___	_____
• Bath blanket	___	___	_____
• Gloves	___	___	_____
• Laundry bag	___	___	_____
4. Placed linen on a clean surface.	___	___	_____
5. Raised the bed for body mechanics.	___	___	_____

Procedure

	S	U	Comments
6. Put on gloves.	___	___	_____
7. Removed linen. Rolled each piece away from you. Placed each piece in a laundry bag. (*NOTE:* Discarded incontinence products or disposable bed protectors in the trash. Did not put them in the laundry bag.)	___	___	_____
8. Cleaned the bed frame and mattress if this was part of your job.	___	___	_____
9. Removed and discarded gloves. Decontaminated your hands.	___	___	_____
10. Moved the mattress to the head of the bed.	___	___	_____
11. Put the mattress pad on the mattress. It was even with the top of the mattress.	___	___	_____
12. Placed the bottom sheet on the mattress pad:			
a. Unfolded it lengthwise.	___	___	_____
b. Placed the center crease in the middle of the bed.	___	___	_____
c. Positioned the lower edge even with the bottom of the mattress.	___	___	_____
d. Placed the large hem at the top and the small hem at the bottom.	___	___	_____
e. Faced hem-stitching downward, away from the person.	___	___	_____
13. Opened the sheet. Fan-folded it to the other side of the bed.	___	___	_____
14. Tucked the top of the sheet under the mattress. The sheet was tight and smooth.	___	___	_____

Date of Satisfactory Completion_____　Instructor's Initials _____

Procedure—cont'd

	S	U	Comments
15. Made a mitered corner if using a flat sheet.			
16. Placed the plastic drawsheet on the bed. It was in the middle of the mattress. Or put the waterproof pad on the bed.			
17. Opened the plastic drawsheet. Fan-folded it to the other side of the bed.			
18. Placed a cotton drawsheet over the plastic drawsheet. It covered the entire plastic drawsheet.			
19. Opened the cotton drawsheet. Fan-folded it to the other side of the bed.			
20. Tucked both drawsheets under the mattress. Or tucked each in separately.			
21. Went to the other side of the bed.			
22. Mitered the top corner of the flat bottom sheet.			
23. Pulled the bottom sheet tight so there were no wrinkles. Tucked in the sheet.			
24. Pulled the drawsheets tight so there were no wrinkles. Tucked both in together or separately.			
25. Went to the other side of the bed.			
26. Put the top sheet on the bed:			
a. Unfolded it lengthwise.			
b. Placed the center crease in the middle.			
c. Placed the large hem even with the top of the mattress.			
d. Opened the sheet. Fan-folded it to the other side.			
e. Faced hem-stitching outward, away from the person.			
f. Did not tuck the bottom in yet.			
g. Never tucked top linens in on the sides.			
27. Placed the blanket on the bed:			
a. Unfolded it so the center crease was in the middle.			
b. Put the upper hem about 6 to 8 inches from the top of the mattress.			
c. Opened the blanket. Fan-folded it to the other side.			
d. Turned the top sheet down over the blanket. Hem-stitching was down, away from the person. (*NOTE:* Followed center procedure.)			
28. Placed the bedspread on the bed:			
a. Unfolded it so the center crease was in the middle.			
b. Placed the upper hem even with the top of the mattress.			
c. Opened and fan-folded the spread to the other side.			
d. Made sure the spread facing the door was even. It covered all top linens.			
29. Tucked in top linens together at the foot of the bed. They were smooth and tight. Made a mitered corner.			
30. Went to the other side.			
31. Straightened all top linen. Worked from the head of the bed to the foot.			
32. Tucked in top linens together at the foot of the bed. Made a mitered corner.			
33. Turned the top hem of the spread under the blanket to make a cuff. (*NOTE:* Followed center procedure.)			
34. Turned the top sheet down over the spread. Hem-stitching was down. (*NOTE:* Not done in some centers.) The spread covered the pillow, and it was tucked under the pillow.			
35. Put the pillowcases on the pillow following center policy. Folded extra material under the pillow at the seam end of the pillowcase.			

Date of Satisfactory Completion_____ Instructor's Initials _____

Procedure—cont'd	S	U	Comments
36. Placed the pillow on the bed. The open end of the pillowcase was away from the door. The seam was toward the head of the bed.	_____	_____	_____

Post-Procedure

	S	U	Comments
37. Provided for comfort. (*NOTE:* Omitted this step if the bed was prepared for a new person.)	_____	_____	_____
38. Attached the signal light to the bed. Or placed it within the person's reach.	_____	_____	_____
39. Lowered bed to its lowest position. Locked the bed wheels.	_____	_____	_____
40. Put the towels, washcloth, gown or pajamas, and bath blanket in the bedside stand.	_____	_____	_____
41. Completed a safety check of the room.	_____	_____	_____
42. Followed center policy for dirty linen.	_____	_____	_____
43. Decontaminated your hands.	_____	_____	_____

Date of Satisfactory Completion_____   Instructor's Initials _____

Making an Open Bed

Name: _____   Date: _____

	S	U	Comments
Quality of Life			
• Knocked before entering the person's room	___	___	_____
• Addressed the person by name	___	___	_____
• Introduced yourself by name and title	___	___	_____
• Explained the procedure to the person before beginning and during the procedure	___	___	_____
• Protected the person's rights during the procedure	___	___	_____
• Handled the person gently during the procedure	___	___	_____

Procedure

1. Followed *Delegation Guidelines:*
   Making Beds
   Saw *Promoting Safety and Comfort:*
   Making Beds
2. Practiced hand hygiene.
3. Collected linen for a closed bed.
4. Made a closed bed:
   a. Placed linen on a clean surface.
   b. Raised the bed for body mechanics.
   c. Put on gloves.
   d. Removed linen. Rolled each piece away from you. Placed each piece in a laundry bag. (*NOTE:* Discarded incontinence products or disposable bed protectors in the trash. Did not put them in the laundry bag.)
      (1) Cleaned the bed frame and mattress if this was part of your job.
      (2) Removed and discarded gloves.
      (3) Decontaminated your hands.
   e. Moved the mattress to the head of the bed.
   f. Put the mattress pad on the mattress. It was even with the top of the mattress.
   g. Placed the bottom sheet on the mattress pad:
      (1) Unfolded it lengthwise.
      (2) Placed the center crease in the middle of the bed.
      (3) Positioned the lower edge even with the bottom of the mattress.
      (4) Placed the large hem at the top and the small hem at the bottom.
      (5) Faced hem-stitching downward, away from the person.
   h. Opened the sheet. Fan-folded it to the other side of the bed.
   i. Tucked the top of the sheet under the mattress. The sheet was tight and smooth.
   j. Made a mitered corner if using a flat sheet.
   k. Placed the plastic drawsheet on the bed. It was in the middle of the mattress. Or put the waterproof pad on the bed.
   l. Opened the plastic drawsheet. Fan-folded it to the other side of the bed.
   m. Placed a cotton drawsheet over the plastic drawsheet. It covered the entire plastic drawsheet.
   n. Opened the cotton drawsheet. Fan-folded it to the other side of the bed.
   o. Tucked both drawsheets under the mattress. Or tucked each in separately.
   p. Went to the other side of the bed.
   q. Mitered the top corner of the flat bottom sheet.

Date of Satisfactory Completion_____   Instructor's Initials _____

Procedure—cont'd   S   U   **Comments**

r. Pulled the bottom sheet tight so there were no wrinkles. Tucked in the sheet.

s. Pulled the drawsheets tight so there were no wrinkles. Tucked both in together or separately.

t. Went to the other side of the bed.

u. Put the top sheet on the bed:
(1) Unfolded it lengthwise.
(2) Placed the center crease in the middle.
(3) Placed the large hem even with the top of the mattress.
(4) Opened the sheet. Fan-folded it to the other side.
(5) Faced hem-stitching outward, away from the person.
(6) Did not tuck the bottom in yet.
(7) Never tucked top linens in on the sides.

v. Placed the blanket on the bed:
(1) Unfolded it so the center crease was in the middle.
(2) Put the upper hem about 6 to 8 inches from the top of the mattress.
(3) Opened the blanket. Fan-folded it to the other side.
(4) Turned the top sheet down over the blanket. Hem-stitching was down, away from the person. (*NOTE:* Followed center procedure.)

w. Placed the bedspread on the bed:
(1) Unfolded it so the center crease was in the middle.
(2) Placed the upper hem even with the top of the mattress.
(3) Opened and fan-folded the spread to the other side.
(4) Made sure the spread facing the door was even. It covered all top linens.

x. Tucked in top linens together at the foot of the bed. They were smooth and tight.

y. Made a mitered corner.

z. Went to the other side.

aa. Straightened all top linen. Worked from the head of the bed to the foot.

bb. Tucked in top linens together at the foot of the bed. Made a mitered corner.

cc. Turned the top hem of the spread under the blanket to make a cuff. (*NOTE:* Followed center procedure.)

dd. Turned the top sheet down over the spread.

ee. Hem-stitching was down. (*NOTE:* Not done in some centers.) The spread covered the pillow, and it was tucked under the pillow.

ff. Put the pillowcases on the pillows, followed center policy. Folded extra material under the pillow at the seam end of the pillowcase.

gg. Placed the pillow on the bed. The open end of the pillowcase was away from the door. The seam was toward the head of the bed.

5. Fan-folded top linens to the foot of the bed.
6. Attached the signal light to the bed.
7. Lowered the bed to its lowest position.
8. Put the towels, washcloth, gown or pajamas, and bath blanket in the bedside stand.

Post-Procedure
9. Provided for comfort.
10. Completed a safety check of the room.
11. Followed center policy for dirty linen.
12. Decontaminated your hands.

Date of Satisfactory Completion _____ Instructor's Initials _____

Making an Occupied Bed (NNAAP™)

Name: _____   Date: _____

	S	**U**	**Comments**

Quality of Life
- Knocked before entering the person's room
- Addressed the person by name
- Introduced yourself by name and title
- Explained the procedure to the person before beginning and during the procedure
- Protected the person's rights during the procedure
- Handled the person gently during the procedure

Pre-Procedure
1. Followed *Delegation Guidelines:*
   Making Beds
   Saw *Promoting Safety and Comfort:*
   - *Making Beds*
   - *The Occupied Bed*
2. Practiced hand hygiene.
3. Collected the following:
   - Gloves
   - Laundry bag
   - Clean linen
4. Placed linen on a clean surface.
5. Identified the person. Checked the ID bracelet against the assignment sheet. Called the person by name.
6. Provided for privacy.
7. Removed the signal light.
8. Raised the bed for body mechanics. Bed rails were up if used.
9. Lowered the head of the bed. It was as flat as possible.

Procedure
10. Decontaminated your hands. Put on gloves.
11. Loosened top linens at the foot of the bed.
12. Removed the bedspread. Then removed the blanket. Placed each over the chair.
13. Covered the person with a bath blanket. Used the blanket in the bedside stand:
    a. Unfolded a bath blanket over the top sheet.
    b. Asked the person to hold onto the bath blanket. If he or she could not, tucked the top part under the person's shoulders.
    c. Grasped the top sheet under the bath blanket at the shoulders. Brought the sheet down to the foot of the bed. Removed the sheet from under the blanket.
14. Lowered the bed rail near you, if up.
15. Positioned the person on the side of the bed away from you. Adjusted the pillow for comfort.
16. Loosened bottom linens from the head to the foot of the bed.
17. Fan-folded bottom linens one at a time toward the person. Started with the cotton drawsheet. If reused the mattress pad, did not fan-fold it.
18. Placed a clean mattress pad on the bed Unfolded it lengthwise. The center crease was in the middle. Fan-folded the top part toward the person. If reused the mattress pad, straightened and smoothed any wrinkles.
19. Placed the bottom sheet on the mattress pad. Hem-stitching was away from the person. Unfolded the sheet so the crease was in the middle. The small hem was even with the bottom of the mattress. Fan-folded the top part toward the person.

Date of Satisfactory Completion_____   Instructor's Initials _____

Procedure—cont'd   S   U   **Comments**

20. Made a mitered corner at the head of the bed. Tucked the
    sheet under the mattress from the head to the foot.   _____   _____   _____

21. Pulled the plastic drawsheet toward you over the bottom
    sheet. Tucked excess material under the mattress.
    Did the following for a clean plastic drawsheet:
    a. Placed the plastic drawsheet on the bed. It was in
       the middle of the mattress.   _____   _____   _____
    b. Fan-folded the part toward the person.   _____   _____   _____
    c. Tucked in excess fabric.   _____   _____   _____

22. Placed the cotton drawsheet over the plastic drawsheet.
    It covered the entire plastic drawsheet. Fan-folded the
    top part toward the person. Tucked in excess fabric.   _____   _____   _____

23. Raised the bed rail if used. Went to the other side,
    and lowered the bed rail.   _____   _____   _____

24. Explained to the person that he or she will roll over
    a "bump." Assured the person that he or she would not fall. _____   _____   _____

25. Helped the person turn to the other side. Adjusted the
    pillow for comfort.   _____   _____   _____

26. Loosened bottom linens. Removed one piece at a time.
    Placed each piece in the laundry bag. (NOTE: Discarded
    disposable bed protectors and incontinence products in
    the trash. Did not put them in the laundry bag.)   _____   _____   _____

27. Removed and discarded the gloves. Decontaminated
    your hands.   _____   _____   _____

28. Straightened and smoothed the mattress pad.   _____   _____   _____

29. Pulled the clean bottom sheet toward you. Made a mitered
    corner at the top. Tucked the sheet under the mattress
    from the head to the foot of the bed.   _____   _____   _____

30. Pulled the drawsheets tightly toward you. Tucked both
    under together or separately.   _____   _____   _____

31. Positioned the person supine in the center of the bed.
    Adjusted the pillow for comfort.   _____   _____   _____

32. Put the top sheet on the bed. Unfolded it lengthwise.
    The crease was in the middle. The large hem was even with
    the top of the mattress. Hem-stitching was on the outside. _____   _____   _____

33. Asked the person to hold onto the top sheet so you could
    remove the bath blanket. Or tucked the top sheet under
    the person's shoulders. Removed the bath blanket.   _____   _____   _____

34. Placed the blanket on the bed. Unfolded it so the center
    crease was in the middle and it covered the person.
    The upper hem was 6 to 8 inches from the top of the mattress. _____   _____   _____

35. Placed the bedspread on the bed. Unfolded it so the
    center crease was in the middle and it covered the person.
    The top hem was even with the mattress top.   _____   _____   _____

36. Turned the top hem of the spread under the blanket
    to make a cuff.   _____   _____   _____

37. Brought the top sheet down over the spread to form a cuff. _____   _____   _____

38. Went to the foot of the bed.   _____   _____   _____

39. Made a toe pleat. Made a 2-inch pleat across the foot
    of the bed. The pleat was about 6-8 inches from the
    foot of the bed.   _____   _____   _____

40. Lifted the mattress corner with one arm. Tucked all top
    linen under the mattress together. Made a mitered corner. _____   _____   _____

41. Raised the bed rail if used. Went to the other side, and
    lowered the bed rail if used.   _____   _____   _____

42. Straightened and smoothed top linens.   _____   _____   _____

Date of Satisfactory Completion_____   Instructor's Initials _____

Procedure—cont'd

	S	U	Comments
43. Tucked the top linens under the bottom of the mattress. Made a mitered corner.	___	___	_____
44. Changed the pillowcase(s).	___	___	_____

Post-Procedure

	S	U	Comments
45. Provided for comfort.	___	___	_____
46. Placed the signal light within reach.	___	___	_____
47. Lowered bed to its lowest position. Locked the bed wheels.	___	___	_____
48. Raised or lowered bed rails. Followed the care plan.	___	___	_____
49. Put the towels, washcloth, gown or pajamas, and bath blanket in the bedside stand.	___	___	_____
50. Unscreened the person.	___	___	_____
51. Completed a safety check of the room.	___	___	_____
52. Followed center policy for dirty linen.	___	___	_____
53. Decontaminated your hands.	___	___	_____

Date of Satisfactory Completion_____ Instructor's Initials _____

Making a Surgical Bed

Name: _____   Date: _____

Procedure	S	U	Comments

1. Followed *Delegation Guidelines:*
   Making Beds
   Saw *Promoting Safety and Comfort:*
   • *Making Beds*
   • *Surgical Bed*   _____ _____ _____
2. Practiced hand hygiene.   _____ _____ _____
3. Collected the following:
   • Gloves   _____ _____ _____
   • Laundry bag   _____ _____ _____
   • Equipment requested by the nurse   _____ _____ _____
4. Placed linen on a clean surface.   _____ _____ _____
5. Removed the signal light.   _____ _____ _____
6. Raised the bed for body mechanics.   _____ _____ _____
7. Removed all linens from the bed. Wore gloves.   _____ _____ _____
8. Made a closed bed. Did not tuck top linens under the
   mattress:
   a. Moved the mattress to the head of the bed.   _____ _____ _____
   b. Put the mattress pad on the mattress. It was even
      with the top of the mattress.   _____ _____ _____
   c. Placed the bottom sheet on the mattress pad:
      (1) Unfolded it lengthwise.   _____ _____ _____
      (2) Placed the center crease in the middle of the bed. _____ _____ _____
      (3) Positioned the lower edge even with the bottom
          of the mattress.   _____ _____ _____
      (4) Placed the large hem at the top and the small
          hem at the bottom.   _____ _____ _____
      (5) Faced hem-stitching downward.   _____ _____ _____
   d. Opened the sheet. Fan-folded it to the other side of the bed. _____ _____ _____
   e. Tucked the top of the sheet under the mattress.
      The sheet was tight and smooth.   _____ _____ _____
   f. Made a mitered corner if using a flat sheet.   _____ _____ _____
   g. Placed the plastic drawsheet on the bed. It was in the
      middle of the mattress. Or put the waterproof pad
      on the bed.   _____ _____ _____
   h. Opened the plastic drawsheet. Fan-folded it to the
      other side of the bed.   _____ _____ _____
   i. Placed a cotton drawsheet over the plastic drawsheet.
      It covered the entire plastic drawsheet.   _____ _____ _____
   j. Opened the cotton drawsheet. Fan-folded it to the
      other side of the bed.   _____ _____ _____
   k. Tucked both drawsheets under the mattress.
      Or tucked each in separately.   _____ _____ _____
   l. Went to the other side of the bed.   _____ _____ _____
   m. Mitered the top corner of the flat bottom sheet.   _____ _____ _____
   n. Pulled the bottom sheet tight so there were no wrinkles.
      Tucked in the sheet.   _____ _____ _____
   o. Pulled the drawsheets tight so there were no wrinkles.
      Tucked both in together or separately.   _____ _____ _____
   p. Went to the other side of the bed.   _____ _____ _____
   q. Put the top sheet on the bed:
      (1) Unfolded it lengthwise.   _____ _____ _____
      (2) Placed the center crease in the middle.   _____ _____ _____
      (3) Placed the large hem even with the top of the mattress. _____ _____ _____
      (4) Opened the sheet. Fan-folded it to the other side. _____ _____ _____
      (5) Faced hem-stitching outward, away from the person. _____ _____ _____

Date of Satisfactory Completion_____   Instructor's Initials _____

Procedure—cont'd

	S	U	Comments
9. Folded all top linens at the foot of the bed back onto the bed. The fold was even with the edge of the mattress.	___	___	_____
10. Fan-folded linen lengthwise to the side of the bed farthest from the door.	___	___	_____
11. Put the pillowcase(s) on the pillow.	___	___	_____
12. Placed the pillow(s) on a clean surface.	___	___	_____
13. Left the bed in its highest position.	___	___	_____
14. Left both bed rails down.	___	___	_____
15. Put the towels, washcloth, gown or pajamas, and bath blanket in the bedside stand.	___	___	_____
16. Moved furniture away from the bed. Allowed room for the stretcher and the staff.	___	___	_____
17. Did not attach the signal light to the bed.	___	___	_____
18. Completed a safety check of the room.	___	___	_____
19. Followed center policy for dirty linen.	___	___	_____
20. Decontaminated your hands.	___	___	_____

Date of Satisfactory Completion_____   Instructor's Initials _____

Assisting the Person to Brush and Floss the Teeth

Name: _____   Date: _____

	S	U	Comments

Quality of Life
- Knocked before entering the person's room
- Addressed the person by name
- Introduced yourself by name and title
- Explained the procedure to the person before beginning and during the procedure
- Protected the person's rights during the procedure
- Handled the person gently during the procedure

Pre-Procedure
1. Followed *Delegation Guidelines:*
   Oral Hygiene
   Saw *Promoting Safety and Comfort:*
   Oral Hygiene
2. Practiced hand hygiene.
3. Collected the following:
   - Toothbrush
   - Toothpaste
   - Mouthwash (or solution noted in care plan)
   - Dental floss (if used)
   - Water glass with cool water
   - Straw
   - Kidney basin
   - Hand towel
   - Paper towels
   - Gloves
4. Placed the paper towels on the overbed table. Arranged items on the top of them.
5. Identified the person. Checked the ID bracelet against the assignment sheet. Called the person by name.
6. Provided for privacy.
7. Positioned the person so he or she could brush with ease.

Procedure
8. Lowered the bed rail near you if up.
9. Placed the towel over the person's chest. This protected garments and linens from spills.
10. Adjusted the overbed table in front of the person.
11. Allowed the person to perform oral hygiene. This included brushing the teeth, rinsing the mouth, flossing, and using mouthwash or other solution.
12. Removed the towel when the person was done.
13. Moved the overbed table to the side of the bed.

Post-Procedure
14. Provided for comfort.
15. Placed the signal light within reach.
16. Raised or lowered bed rails. Followed the care plan.
17. Cleaned and returned items to their proper place. Wore gloves.
18. Wiped off the overbed table with the paper towels. Discarded the paper towels.
19. Removed the gloves. Decontaminated your hands.
20. Unscreened the person.
21. Completed a safety check of the room.
22. Followed center policy for dirty linen.
23. Decontaminated your hands.
24. Reported and recorded your observations.

Date of Satisfactory Completion _____ Instructor's Initials _____

Brushing and Flossing the Person's Teeth (NNAAP™)

Name: _____   Date: _____

Quality of Life   S   U   **Comments**
- Knocked before entering the person's room
- Addressed the person by name
- Introduced yourself by name and title
- Explained the procedure to the person before beginning and during the procedure
- Protected the person's rights during the procedure
- Handled the person gently during the procedure

Pre-Procedure
1. Followed *Delegation Guidelines:*
   Oral Hygiene
   Saw *Promoting Safety and Comfort:*
   Oral Hygiene
2. Practiced hand hygiene.
3. Collected the following:
   - Toothbrush
   - Toothpaste
   - Mouthwash (or solution noted in care plan)
   - Dental floss (if used)
   - Water glass with cool water
   - Straw
   - Kidney basin
   - Hand towel
   - Paper towels
   - Gloves
4. Placed the paper towels on the overbed table. Arranged items on the top of them.
5. Identified the person. Checked the ID bracelet against the assignment sheet. Called the person by name.
6. Provided for privacy.
7. Raised the bed for body mechanics. Bed rails were up if used.

Procedure
8. Lowered the bed rail near you if up.
9. Assisted the person to a sitting position or to a side-lying position near you.
10. Placed the towel across the person's chest.
11. Adjusted the overbed table so you could reach it with ease.
12. Decontaminated your hands. Put on gloves.
13. Held the toothbrush over the kidney basin. Poured some water over the brush.
14. Applied toothpaste to the brush.
15. Brushed the teeth gently.
16. Brushed the tongue gently.
17. Let the person rinse the mouth with water. Held the kidney basin under the person's chin. Repeated as needed.
18. Flossed the person's teeth (optional):
    a. Broke off an 18-inch piece of floss from the dispenser.
    b. Held the floss between the middle fingers of each hand.
    c. Stretched the floss with your thumb.
    d. Started at the upper back tooth on the right side. Worked around to the left side.
    e. Moved the floss gently up and down between the teeth. Moved the floss up and down against the side of the tooth. Worked from the top of the crown to the gum line.

Date of Satisfactory Completion_____   Instructor's Initials _____

Procedure—cont'd   S   U   **Comments**

    f. Moved to a new section of floss after every second tooth.   _____ _____ _____

    g. Flossed the lower teeth. Used up and down motions as for
       the upper teeth. Started on the right side. Worked around
       to the left side.   _____ _____ _____

19. Allowed the person to use mouthwash or other solution.
     Held the kidney basin under the chin.   _____ _____ _____

20. Wiped the person's mouth. Removed the towel.   _____ _____ _____

21. Removed and discarded the gloves. Decontaminated
     your hands.   _____ _____ _____

Post-Procedure

22. Provided for comfort.   _____ _____ _____

23. Placed the signal light within reach.   _____ _____ _____

24. Lowered the bed to its lowest position.   _____ _____ _____

25. Raised or lowered bed rails. Followed the care plan.   _____ _____ _____

26. Cleaned and returned equipment to its proper place.
     Wore gloves.   _____ _____ _____

27. Wiped off the overbed table with the paper towels.
     Discarded the paper towels.   _____ _____ _____

28. Removed the gloves. Decontaminated your hands.   _____ _____ _____

29. Unscreened the person.   _____ _____ _____

30. Completed a safety check of the room.   _____ _____ _____

31. Followed center policy for dirty linen.   _____ _____ _____

32. Decontaminated your hands.   _____ _____ _____

33. Reported and recorded your observations.   _____ _____ _____

Date of Satisfactory Completion _____   Instructor's Initials _____

Providing Mouth Care for the Unconscious Person

Name: _____   Date: _____

	S	U	Comments

Quality of Life
- Knocked before entering the person's room
- Addressed the person by name
- Introduced yourself by name and title
- Explained the procedure to the person before beginning and during the procedure
- Protected the person's rights during the procedure
- Handled the person gently during the procedure

Pre-Procedure
1. Followed *Delegation Guidelines:*
   Oral Hygiene
   Saw *Promoting Safety and Comfort:*
   - *Oral Hygiene*
   - *Mouth Care for the Unconscious Person*
2. Practiced hand hygiene.
3. Collected the following:
   - Cleaning agent (checked the care plan)
   - Sponge swabs
   - Padded tongue blade
   - Water glass or cup with cool water
   - Hand towel
   - Kidney basin
   - Lip lubricant
   - Paper towels
   - Gloves
4. Placed the paper towels on the overbed table. Arranged items on the top of them.
5. Identified the person. Checked the ID bracelet against the assignment sheet. Called the person by name.
6. Provided for privacy.
7. Raised the bed for body mechanics. Bed rails were up if used.

Procedure
8. Lowered the bed rail near you if up.
9. Decontaminated your hands. Put on gloves.
10. Positioned the person in a side-lying position near you. Turned his or her head well to the side.
11. Placed the towel under the person's face.
12. Placed the kidney basin under the chin.
13. Separated the upper and lower teeth. Used the padded tongue blade. Was gentle. Never used force. If you had problems, asked the nurse for help.
14. Cleaned the mouth using sponge swaps moistened with the cleaning agent:
    a. Cleaned the chewing and inner surfaces of the teeth.
    b. Cleaned the gums and outer surfaces of the teeth.
    c. Swabbed the roof of the mouth, inside of the cheeks, and the lips.
    d. Swabbed the tongue.
    e. Moistened a clean swab with water. Swabbed the mouth to rinse.
    f. Placed used swabs in the kidney basin.
15. Applied lubricant to the lips.
16. Removed the kidney basin and supplies.

Date of Satisfactory Completion _____   Instructor's Initials _____

Procedure—cont'd	S	U	Comments
17. Wiped the person's mouth. Removed the towel.	___	___	_____
18. Removed and discarded the gloves. Decontaminated your hands.	___	___	_____

Post-Procedure

	S	U	Comments
19. Provided for comfort.	___	___	_____
20. Placed the signal light within reach.	___	___	_____
21. Lowered the bed to its lowest position.	___	___	_____
22. Raised or lowered bed rails. Followed the care plan.	___	___	_____
23. Cleaned and returned equipment to its proper place. Discarded disposable items. (Wore gloves.)	___	___	_____
24. Wiped off the overbed table with the paper towels. Discarded the paper towels.	___	___	_____
25. Removed the gloves. Decontaminated your hands.	___	___	_____
26. Unscreened the person.	___	___	_____
27. Completed a safety check of the room.	___	___	_____
28. Told the person that you were leaving the room. Told him or her when you would return.	___	___	_____
29. Followed center policy for dirty linen.	___	___	_____
30. Decontaminated your hands.	___	___	_____
31. Reported and recorded your observations.	___	___	_____

Date of Satisfactory Completion_____ Instructor's Initials _____

Providing Denture Care (NNAAP™)

Name: _____   Date: _____

	S	U	Comments

Quality of Life
- Knocked before entering the person's room
- Addressed the person by name
- Introduced yourself by name and title
- Explained the procedure to the person before beginning and during the procedure
- Protected the person's rights during the procedure
- Handled the person gently during the procedure

Pre-Procedure
1. Followed *Delegation Guidelines:*
   Oral Hygiene
   Saw *Promoting Safety and Comfort:*
   - *Oral Hygiene*
   - *Denture Care*
2. Practiced hand hygiene.
3. Collected the following:
   - Denture brush or toothbrush (for cleaning dentures)
   - Denture cup labeled with the person's name and room and bed number
   - Denture cleaning agent
   - Soft-bristled toothbrush or sponge swabs (for oral hygiene)
   - Toothpaste
   - Water glass with cool water
   - Straw
   - Mouthwash (or other noted solution)
   - Kidney basin
   - Two hand towels
   - Gauze squares
   - Paper towels
   - Gloves
4. Placed the paper towels on the overbed table. Arranged items on the top of them.
5. Identified the person. Checked the ID bracelet against the assignment sheet. Called the person by name.
6. Provided for privacy.
7. Raised the bed for body mechanics.

Procedure
8. Lowered the bed rail near you if up.
9. Decontaminated your hands. Put on gloves.
10. Placed the towel over the person's chest.
11. Asked the person to remove the dentures. Carefully placed them in the kidney basin.
12. Removed the dentures if the person could not do so.
    Used gauze square to get a good grip on the slippery dentures:
    a. Grasped the denture with your thumb and index finger. Moved it up and down slightly to break the seal. Gently removed the denture. Placed it in the kidney basin.
    b. Grasped and removed the lower denture with your thumb and index finger. Turned it slightly, and lifted it out of the person's mouth. Placed it in the kidney basin.
13. Followed the care plan for raising side rails.
14. Took the kidney basin, denture cup, denture brush, and denture cleaning agent to the sink.
15. Lined the sink with a towel. Filled the sink halfway with water.

Date of Satisfactory Completion_____   Instructor's Initials _____

Procedure—cont'd   S   U   **Comments**

16. Rinsed each denture under warm running water.
    (Some state competency tests require cool water.)   ____   ____   _____
17. Returned dentures to the kidney basin or denture cup.   ____   ____   _____
18. Applied the denture cleaning agent to the brush.   ____   ____   _____
19. Brushed the dentures.   ____   ____   _____
20. Rinsed the dentures under running water. Used warm or
    cool water as directed by the cleaning agent manufacturer.
    (Some state competency tests require cool water.)   ____   ____   _____
21. Rinsed the denture cup. Placed dentures in the denture cup.
    Covered the dentures with cool water.   ____   ____   _____
22. Cleaned the kidney basin.   ____   ____   _____
23. Took the denture cup and kidney basin to the overbed table.____   ____   _____
24. Lowered the bed rail if up.   ____   ____   _____
25. Positioned the person for oral hygiene.   ____   ____   _____
26. Cleaned the person's gums and tongue, used toothpaste and
    the toothbrush (or sponge swab).   ____   ____   _____
27. Had the person use mouthwash (or noted solution). Held the
    kidney basin under the chin.   ____   ____   _____
28. Asked the person to insert the dentures. Inserted them if
    the person could not:
    a. Held the upper denture firmly with your thumb and index
       finger. Raised the upper lip with the other hand.
       Inserted the denture. Gently pressed on the denture with
       your index fingers to make sure it was in place.   ____   ____   _____
    b. Held the lower denture with your thumb and index finger.
       Pulled the lower lip down slightly. Inserted the denture.
       Gently pressed down on it to make sure it was in place. ____   ____   _____
29. Placed the denture cup in the top drawer of the bedside stand
    if the dentures were not worn. If not worn, the dentures
    were in water or in a denture soaking solution.   ____   ____   _____
30. Wiped the person's mouth. Removed the towel.   ____   ____   _____
31. Removed the gloves. Decontaminated your hands.   ____   ____   _____

Post-Procedure
32. Assisted with hand washing.   ____   ____   _____
33. Provided for comfort.   ____   ____   _____
34. Placed the signal light within reach.   ____   ____   _____
35. Lowered the bed to its lowest position.   ____   ____   _____
36. Raised or lowered bed rails. Followed the care plan.   ____   ____   _____
37. Cleaned and returned equipment to its proper place.
    Discarded disposable items. (Wore gloves.)   ____   ____   _____
38. Wiped off the overbed table with the paper towels.
    Discarded the paper towels.   ____   ____   _____
39. Removed the gloves. Decontaminated your hands.   ____   ____   _____
40. Unscreened the person.   ____   ____   _____
41. Completed a safety check of the room.   ____   ____   _____
42. Followed center policy for dirty linen.   ____   ____   _____
43. Decontaminated your hands.   ____   ____   _____
44. Reported and recorded your observations.   ____   ____   _____

Date of Satisfactory Completion_____   Instructor's Initials _____

Giving a Complete Bed Bath (NNAAP™)

Name: _____　　Date: _____

	S	U	Comments

Quality of Life
- Knocked before entering the person's room
- Addressed the person by name
- Introduced yourself by name and title
- Explained the procedure to the person before beginning and during the procedure
- Protected the person's rights during the procedure
- Handled the person gently during the procedure

Pre-Procedure
1. Followed *Delegation Guidelines:*
   Bathing
   Saw *Promoting Safety and Comfort:*
   Bathing
2. Practiced hand hygiene.
3. Identified the person. Checked the ID bracelet against the assignment sheet. Called the person by name.
4. Collected clean linen for a closed bed and placed linen on a clean surface:
   - Mattress pad (if needed)
   - Bottom sheet
   - Plastic drawsheet or waterproof pad (if used)
   - Cotton drawsheet (if needed)
   - Top sheet
   - Blanket
   - Bedspread
   - Two pillowcases
   - Gloves
   - Laundry bag
5. Collected the following:
   - Wash basin
   - Soap
   - Bath thermometer
   - Orange stick or nail file
   - Washcloth
   - Two bath towels and two hand towels
   - Bath blanket
   - Clothing or sleepwear
   - Lotion
   - Powder
   - Deodorant or antiperspirant
   - Brush and comb
   - Other grooming items as requested
   - Paper towels
   - Gloves
6. Covered the overbed table with paper towels. Arranged items on the overbed table. Adjusted the height as needed.
7. Provided for privacy.
8. Raised the bed for body mechanics. Bed rails were up if used.

Procedure
9. Removed the signal light.
10. Decontaminated your hands. Put on gloves.
11. Covered the person with a bath blanket. Removed top linens.
12. Lowered the head of the bed. It was as flat as possible. The person had at least one pillow.

Date of Satisfactory Completion_____　Instructor's Initials _____

Procedure—cont'd	S	U	Comments

13. Filled the wash basin ⅔ (two-thirds) full with water.
    Water temperature was 110°-115° F (43.3°-46.1° C) for adults.
    Measured water temperature. Used the bath thermometer.
    Or tested the water by dipping your elbow or inner
    wrist into the basin.
14. Placed the basin on the overbed table.
15. Lowered the bed rail near you if up.
16. Placed a hand towel over the person's chest.
17. Made a mitt with the washcloth. Used a mitt for the entire bath.
18. Washed around the person's eyes with water. Did not use soap:
    a. Cleaned the far eye. Gently wiped from the inner to the outer
       aspect of the eye with a corner of the mitt.
    b. Cleaned around the eye near you. Used a clean part of the
       washcloth for each stroke.
19. Asked the person if you should use soap to wash the face.
20. Washed the face, ears, and neck. Rinsed and patted dry with
    the towel on the chest.
21. Helped the person move to the side of the bed near you.
22. Removed the sleepwear. Did not expose the person.
23. Placed a bath towel lengthwise under the far arm.
24. Supported the arm with your palm under the person's elbow.
    His or her forearm rested on your forearm.
25. Washed the arm, shoulder, and underarm. Used long, firm
    strokes. Rinsed and patted dry.
26. Placed the basin on the towel. Put the person's hand into
    the water. Washed it well. Cleaned under the fingernails
    with an orange stick or nail file.
27. Had the person exercise the hand and fingers.
28. Removed the basin. Dried the hand well. Covered the arm
    with the bath blanket.
29. Repeated for the near arm:
    a. Placed a bath towel lengthwise under the near arm.
    b. Supported the arm with your palm under the person's
       elbow. His or her forearm rested on your forearm.
    c. Washed the arm, shoulder, and under arm. Used long,
       firm strokes. Rinsed and patted dry.
    d. Placed the basin on the towel. Put the person's hand
       into the water. Washed it well. Cleaned under the
       fingernails with an orange stick or nail file.
    e. Had the person exercise the hand and fingers.
    f. Removed the basin. Dried the hand well. Covered the
       arm with the bath blanket.
30. Placed a bath towel over the chest crosswise. Held the towel
    in place. Pulled the bath blanket from under the towel to
    the waist.
31. Lifted the towel slightly, and washed the chest. Did not
    expose the person. Rinsed and patted dry, especially
    under the breasts.
32. Moved the towel lengthwise over the chest and abdomen.
    Did not expose the person. Pulled the bath blanket down
    to the pubic area.
33. Lifted the towel slightly, and washed the abdomen.
    Rinsed and patted dry.
34. Pulled the bath blanket up to the shoulders; covered
    both arms. Removed the towel.

Date of Satisfactory Completion_____ Instructor's Initials _____

Procedure—cont'd

	S	U	Comments

35. Changed soapy or cool water. Measured water temperature (110°-115° F or 43.3°-46.1° C) for adults. Used the bath thermometer. Or tested the water by dipping your elbow or inner wrist into the basin. If bed rails were used, raised the bed rail near you before you left the bedside. Lowered it when you returned.

36. Uncovered the far leg. Did not expose the genital area. Placed a towel lengthwise under the foot and leg.

37. Bent the knee, and supported the leg with your arm. Washed it with long, firm strokes. Rinsed and patted dry.

38. Placed the basin on the towel near the foot.

39. Lifted the leg slightly. Slid the basin under the foot.

40. Placed the foot in the basin. Used an orange stick or nail file to clean under toenails if necessary. If the person could not bend the knees:

   a. Washed the foot. Carefully separated the toes. Rinsed and patted dry.

   c. Cleaned under the toenails with the orange stick or nail file if necessary.

41. Removed the basin. Dried the leg and foot. Applied lotion to the foot if directed by the nurse and care plan. Covered the leg with the bath blanket. Removed the towel.

42. Repeated for the near leg:

   a. Uncovered the near leg. Did not expose the genital area. Placed a towel lengthwise under the foot and leg.

   b. Bent the knee and supported the leg with your arm. Washed it with long, firm strokes. Rinsed and patted dry.

   c. Placed the basin on the towel near the foot.

   d. Lifted the leg slightly. Slid the basin under the foot.

   e. Placed the foot in the basin. Used an orange stick or nail file to clean under toenails if necessary. If the person could not bend the knee:

     (1) Washed the foot. Carefully separated the toes. Rinsed and patted dry.

     (2) Cleaned under the toenails with an orange stick or nail file if necessary.

   f. Removed the basin. Dried the leg and foot. Applied lotion to the foot if directed by the nurse and care plan. Covered the leg with the bath blanket. Removed the towel.

43. Changed the water. Measured water temperature (110°-115° F or 43.3°-46.1° C) for adults. Used the bath thermometer. Or tested the water by dipping your elbow or inner wrist into the basin. If bed rails were used, raised the bed rail near you before you left the bedside. Lowered it when you returned.

44. Turned the person onto the side away from you. The person was covered with the bath blanket.

45. Uncovered the back and buttocks. Did not expose the person. Placed a towel lengthwise on the bed along the back.

46. Washed the back. Worked from the back of the neck to the lower end of the buttocks. Used long, firm, continuous strokes. Rinsed and dried well.

47. Gave a back massage. The person may have wanted the back massage after the bath.

Date of Satisfactory Completion _____ Instructor's Initials _____

Procedure—cont'd	S	U	Comments
48. Turned the person onto his or her back.	___	___	_____
49. Changed the water for perineal care. Measured water temperature (110°-115° F or 43.3°-46.1° C) for adults. Used the bath thermometer. Or tested the water by dipping your elbow or inner wrist into the basin. (Some state competency tests also required changing gloves and hand hygiene at this time.) If bed rails were used, raised the bed rail near you before you left the bedside. Lowered it when you returned.	___	___	_____
50. Allowed the person to wash the genital area. Adjusted the overbed table so he or she could reach the wash basin, soap, and towels with ease. Placed the signal light within reach. Asked the person to signal when finished. Made sure the person understood what to do.	___	___	_____
51. Removed the gloves. Decontaminated your hands.	___	___	_____
52. Answered the signal light promptly. Knocked before entering the room. Provided perineal care if the person could not do so. (Decontaminated your hands and wore gloves for perineal care.)	___	___	_____
53. Gave a back massage if you had not already done so.	___	___	_____
54. Applied deodorant or antiperspirant. Applied lotion and powder as requested. Saw *Promoting Safety and Comfort: Bathing.*	___	___	_____
55. Put clean garments on the person.	___	___	_____
56. Combed and brushed the hair.	___	___	_____
57. Made the bed.	___	___	_____

Post-Procedure

	S	U	Comments
58. Provided for comfort.	___	___	_____
59. Placed the signal light within reach.	___	___	_____
60. Lowered the bed to its lowest position.	___	___	_____
61. Raised or lowered bed rails. Followed the care plan.	___	___	_____
62. Emptied and cleaned the wash basin. Returned it and other supplies to their proper place.	___	___	_____
63. Wiped off the overbed table with the paper towels. Discarded the paper towels.	___	___	_____
64. Unscreened the person.	___	___	_____
65. Completed a safety check of the room.	___	___	_____
66. Followed center policy for dirty linen.	___	___	_____
67. Decontaminated your hands.	___	___	_____
68. Reported and recorded your observations.	___	___	_____

Date of Satisfactory Completion_____   Instructor's Initials _____

Assisting With a Partial Bath

Name: _____   Date: _____

	S	U	Comments

Quality of Life
- Knocked before entering the person's room
- Addressed the person by name
- Introduced yourself by name and title
- Explained the procedure to the person before beginning and during the procedure
- Protected the person's rights during the procedure
- Handled the person gently during the procedure

Pre-Procedure
1. Followed *Delegation Guidelines:*
   Bathing
   Saw *Promoting Safety and Comfort:*
   Bathing
2. Did the following:
   a. Practiced hand hygiene.
   b. Identified the person. Checked the ID bracelet against the assignment sheet. Called the person by name.
   c. Collected clean linen for a closed bed, and placed linen on a clean surface:
      - Mattress pad (if needed)
      - Bottom sheet
      - Plastic drawsheet or waterproof pad (if used)
      - Cotton drawsheet (if needed)
      - Top sheet
      - Blanket
      - Bedspread
      - Two pillowcases
      - Gloves
      - Laundry bag
   d. Collected the following:
      - Wash basin
      - Soap
      - Bath thermometer
      - Orange stick or nail file
      - Washcloth
      - Two bath towels and two hand towels
      - Bath blanket
      - Clothing or sleepwear
      - Lotion
      - Powder
      - Deodorant or antiperspirant
      - Brush and comb
      - Other grooming items as requested
      - Paper towels
      - Gloves
   e. Covered the overbed table with paper towels. Arranged items on the overbed table. Adjusted the height as needed.
   f. Provided for privacy.

Procedure
3. Made sure the bed was in the lowest position.
4. Decontaminated your hands. Put on gloves.
5. Covered the person with a bath blanket. Removed top linens.

Date of Satisfactory Completion_____   Instructor's Initials _____

Procedure—cont'd	S	U	Comments
6. Filled the wash basin $2/3$ (two-thirds) full with water. Water temperature was 110°-115° F (43.3°-46.1° C) for adults. Measured water temperature with the bath thermometer. Or tested the water by dipping your elbow or inner wrist into the basin.			
7. Placed the basin on the overbed table.	___	___	___
8. Positioned the person in Fowler's position. Or assisted him or her to sit at the bedside.	___	___	___
9. Adjusted the overbed table so the person could reach the basin and supplies.	___	___	___
10. Helped the person undress. Provided for privacy and warmth with a bath blanket.	___	___	___
11. Asked the person to wash easy-to-reach body parts. Explained that you would wash the back and areas the person could not reach.	___	___	___
12. Placed the signal light within reach. Asked him or her to signal when help was needed or bathing was complete.	___	___	___
13. Left the room after decontaminating your hands.	___	___	___
14. Returned when the signal light was on. Knocked before entering. Decontaminated your hands.	___	___	___
15. Changed the bath water. Measured bath water temperature (110°-115° F or 43.3°-46.1° C) for adults. Used the bath thermometer. Or tested the water by dipping your elbow or inner wrist into the basin.	___	___	___
16. Raised the bed for body mechanics. The far bed rail was up if used.	___	___	___
17. Asked what was washed. Put on gloves. Washed and dried areas the person could not reach. The face, hands, underarms, back, buttocks, and perineal area were washed for the partial bath.	___	___	___
18. Removed the gloves. Decontaminated your hands.	___	___	___
19. Gave a back massage.	___	___	___
20. Applied lotion, powder, and deodorant or antiperspirant as requested.	___	___	___
21. Helped the person put on clean garments.	___	___	___
22. Assisted with hair care and other grooming needs.	___	___	___
23. Assisted the person to a chair. (Lowered the bed if the person transferred to a chair.) Or turned the person onto the side away from you.	___	___	___
24. Made the bed. (Raised the bed for body mechanics.)	___	___	___

Post-Procedure

	S	U	Comments
25. Provided for comfort.	___	___	___
26. Placed the signal light within reach.	___	___	___
27. Lowered the bed to its lowest position.	___	___	___
28. Raised or lowered bed rails. Followed the care plan.	___	___	___
29. Emptied and cleaned the wash basin. Returned it and other supplies to their proper place.	___	___	___
30. Wiped off the overbed table with the paper towels. Discarded the paper towels.	___	___	___
31. Unscreened the person.	___	___	___
32. Completed a safety check of the room.	___	___	___
33. Followed center policy for dirty linen.	___	___	___
34. Decontaminated your hands.	___	___	___
35. Reported and recorded your observations.	___	___	___

Date of Satisfactory Completion_____ Instructor's Initials _____

Assisting With a Tub Bath or Shower

Name: _____   Date: _____

	S	U	Comments

Quality of Life
- Knocked before entering the person's room
- Addressed the person by name
- Introduced yourself by name and title
- Explained the procedure to the person before beginning and during the procedure
- Protected the person's rights during the procedure
- Handled the person gently during the procedure

Pre-Procedure
1. Followed *Delegation Guidelines:*
   - *Bathing*
   - *Tub Baths and Showers*

   Saw *Promoting Safety and Comfort*:
   - *Bathing*
   - *Tub Baths and Showers*
2. Reserved the bathtub or shower.
3. Practiced hand hygiene.
4. Identified the person. Checked the ID bracelet against the assignment sheet. Called the person by name.
5. Collected the following:
   - Washcloth and two bath towels
   - Soap
   - Bath thermometer
   - Clothing or sleepwear
   - Grooming items as requested
   - Robe and non-skid footwear
   - Rubber bath mat if needed
   - Disposable bath mat
   - Gloves
   - Wheelchair, shower chair, transfer bench, and so on as needed

Procedure
6. Placed items in the tub or shower room. Used the space provided or a chair.
7. Cleaned and disinfected the tub or shower.
8. Placed a rubber bathmat in the tub or on the shower floor. Did not block the drain.
9. Placed the disposable bathmat on the floor in front of the tub or shower.
10. Placed the OCCUPIED sign on the door.
11. Returned to the person's room. Provided for privacy. Decontaminated your hands.
12. Helped the person sit on the side of the bed.
13. Helped the person put on a robe and non-skid footwear. Or the person left on clothing.
14. Assisted or transported the person to the tub room or shower.
15. Had the person sit on a chair if he or she walked to the tub or shower room.
16. Provided for privacy.
17. *For a tub bath:*
    a. Filled the tub halfway with warm water (105° F; 40.5° C).
    b. Measured water temperature with bath thermometer. Or checked the digital display.

Date of Satisfactory Completion_____   Instructor's Initials _____

Procedure—cont'd	S	U	Comments

18. *For a shower:*
   a. Turned on the shower.
   b. Adjusted water temperature and pressure. Checked the digital display.
19. Helped the person undress and removed footwear.
20. Helped the person into the tub or shower. Positioned the shower chair, and locked the wheels.
21. Assisted with washing as necessary. Wore gloves.
22. Asked the person to use the signal light when done or when help was needed. Reminded the person that a tub bath lasts no longer than 20 minutes.
23. Placed a towel across the chair.
24. Left the room if the person could bathe alone. If not, stayed in the room or nearby. Removed the gloves and decontaminated your hands if you left the room.
25. Checked the person at least every 5 minutes.
26. Returned when he or she signaled for you. Knocked before entering.
27. Turned off the shower, or drained the tub. Covered the person while the tub drained.
28. Helped the person out of the shower or tub and onto a chair.
29. Helped the person dry off. Patted gently. Dried under the breasts, between skin folds, in the perineal area, and between the toes.
30. Assisted with lotion an other grooming items as needed.
31. Helped the person dress and put on footwear.
32. Helped the person return to the room. Provided for privacy.
33. Assisted the person to a chair or into bed.
34. Provided a back massage if the person returned to bed.
35. Assisted with hair care and other grooming needs.

Post-Procedure
36. Provided for comfort.
37. Placed the signal light within reach.
38. Raised or lowered bed rails. Followed the care plan.
39. Unscreened the person.
40. Completed a safety check of the room.
41. Cleaned and disinfected the tub or shower. Removed soiled linen. Wore gloves for this step.
42. Discarded disposable items. Put the UNOCCUPIED sign on the door. Returned supplies to their proper place.
43. Followed center policy for dirty linen.
44. Decontaminated your hands.
45. Reported and recorded your observations.

Date of Satisfactory Completion_____ Instructor's Initials _____

Giving a Back Massage

Name: _____   Date: _____

	S	U	Comments

Quality of Life
- Knocked before entering the person's room
- Addressed the person by name
- Introduced yourself by name and title
- Explained the procedure to the person before beginning and during the procedure
- Protected the person's rights during the procedure
- Handled the person gently during the procedure

Pre-Procedure
1. Followed *Delegation Guidelines:*
   The Back Massage
   Saw *Promoting Safety and Comfort:*
   The Back Massage
2. Practiced hand hygiene.
3. Identified the person. Checked the ID bracelet against the assignment sheet. Called the person by name.
4. Collected the following:
   - Bath blanket
   - Bath towel
   - Lotion
5. Provided for privacy.
6. Raised the bed for body mechanics. Bed rails were up if used.

Procedure
7. Lowered the bed rail near you if up.
8. Positioned the person in the prone or side-lying position. The back was toward you.
9. Exposed the back, shoulders, upper arms, and buttocks. Covered the rest of the body with the bath blanket.
10. Laid the towel on the bed along the back (if the person was in the side-lying position).
11. Warmed the lotion.
12. Explained that the lotion may feel cool and wet.
13. Applied lotion to the lower back area.
14. Stroked up from the buttocks to the shoulders. Then stroked down over the upper arms. Stroked up the upper arms, across the shoulders, and down the back to the buttocks. Used firm strokes. Kept your hands in contact with the person's skin.
15. Repeated stroking up from the buttocks to the shoulders. Then stroked down over the upper arms. Stroked up the upper arms, across the shoulders, and down the back to the buttocks. Used firm strokes. Kept your hands in contact with the person's skin. Continued this for at least 3 minutes.
16. Kneaded the back:
    a. Grasped the skin between your thumb and fingers.
    b. Kneaded half of the back. Started at the buttocks and moved up to the shoulder. Then kneaded down from the shoulder to the buttocks.
    c. Repeated on the other half of the back.
17. Applied lotion to bony areas. Used circular motions with the tips of your fingers. (Did not massage reddened bony areas.)
18. Used fast movements to stimulate. Used slow movements to relax the person.

Date of Satisfactory Completion_____   Instructor's Initials _____

Procedure—cont'd   S   U   **Comments**

19. Stroked with long, firm movements to end the massage.
    Told the person you were finishing.   ___ ___ _____

20. Straightened and secured clothing or sleepwear.   ___ ___ _____

21. Covered the person. Removed the towel and bath blanket. ___ ___ _____

Post-Procedure

22. Provided for comfort.   ___ ___ _____

23. Placed the signal light within reach.   ___ ___ _____

24. Lowered the bed to its lowest position.   ___ ___ _____

25. Raised or lowered bed rails. Followed the care plan.   ___ ___ _____

26. Returned lotion to its proper place.   ___ ___ _____

27. Unscreened the person.   ___ ___ _____

28. Completed a safety check of the room.   ___ ___ _____

29. Followed center policy for dirty linen.   ___ ___ _____

30. Decontaminated your hands.   ___ ___ _____

31. Reported and recorded your observations.   ___ ___ _____

Date of Satisfactory Completion_____   Instructor's Initials _____

Giving Female Perineal Care (NNAAP™)

Name: _____   Date: _____

	S	U	Comments

Quality of Life
- Knocked before entering the person's room
- Addressed the person by name
- Introduced yourself by name and title
- Explained the procedure to the person before beginning and during the procedure
- Protect the person's rights during the procedure
- Handled the person gently during the procedure

Pre-Procedure
1. Followed *Delegation Guidelines:*
   Perineal Care
   Saw *Promoting Safety and Comfort:*
   Perineal Care
2. Practiced hand hygiene.
3. Collected the following:
   - Soap or other cleaning agent as directed
   - At least 4 washcloths
   - Bath towel
   - Bath blanket
   - Bath thermometer
   - Wash basin
   - Waterproof pad
   - Gloves
   - Paper towels
4. Covered the overbed table with paper towels. Arranged items on top of them.
5. Identified the person. Checked the ID bracelet against the assignment sheet. Called her by name.
6. Provided for privacy.
7. Raised the bed for body mechanics. Bed rails were up if used.

Procedure
8. Lowered the bed rail near you if up.
9. Decontaminated your hands. Put on gloves.
10. Covered the person with a bath blanket. Moved top linens to the foot of the bed.
11. Positioned the person on her back.
12. Draped the person.
13. Raised the bed rail if used.
14. Filled the wash basin. Water temperature was 105°-109° F (40.5°-42.7° C). Measured water temperature according to center policy.
15. Placed the basin on the overbed table.
16. Lowered the bed rail if up.
17. Helped the person flex her knees and spread her legs. Or helped her spread her legs as much as possible with the knees straight.
18. Placed a waterproof pad under her buttocks.
19. Folded the corner of the bath blanket between her legs onto her abdomen.
20. Wet the washcloths.
21. Squeezed out water from a washcloth. Made a mitted washcloth. Applied soap.
22. Spread the labia. Cleaned downward from front to back with one stroke.

Date of Satisfactory Completion _____   Instructor's Initials _____

Procedure—cont'd

	S	U	Comments
23. Repeated until area clean. Used a clean part of the washcloth for each stroke. Used more than one washcloth if needed:	___	___	_____
a. Squeezed out water from washcloth. Made a mitted washcloth. Applied soap.	___	___	_____
b. Separated the labia. Cleaned downward from front to back with one stroke.	___	___	_____
24. Rinsed the perineum with a clean washcloth. Separated the labia. Stroked downward from front to back. Repeated as necessary. Used a clean part of the washcloth for each stroke. Used more than one washcloth if needed.	___	___	_____
25. Patted the area dry with the towel. Dried from front to back.	___	___	_____
26. Folded the blanket back between her legs.	___	___	_____
27. Helped the person lower her legs and turn onto her side away from you.	___	___	_____
28. Applied soap to a mitted washcloth.	___	___	_____
29. Cleaned the rectal area. Cleaned from the vagina to the anus with one stroke.	___	___	_____
30. Repeated until the area was clean. Used a clean part of the washcloth for each stroke. Used more than one washcloth if needed:			
a. Applied soap to a mitted washcloth.	___	___	_____
b. Cleaned the rectal area. Cleaned from the vagina to the anus with one stroke.	___	___	_____
31. Rinsed the rectal area with a washcloth. Stroked from the vagina to the anus. Repeated as necessary. Used a clean part of the washcloth for each stroke. Used more than one washcloth if needed.	___	___	_____
32. Patted the area dry with the towel. Dried from front to back.	___	___	_____
33. Removed the waterproof pad.	___	___	_____
34. Provided clean and dry linens and incontinence products as needed.	___	___	_____
35. Removed and discarded the gloves. Decontaminated your hands.	___	___	_____

Post-Procedure

	S	U	Comments
36. Covered the person. Removed the bath blanket.	___	___	_____
37. Provided for comfort.	___	___	_____
38. Placed the signal light within reach.	___	___	_____
39. Lowered the bed to its lowest position.	___	___	_____
40. Raised or lowered bed rails. Followed the care plan.	___	___	_____
41. Emptied and cleaned the wash basin. Wore gloves.	___	___	_____
42. Returned the basin and supplies to their proper place.	___	___	_____
43. Wiped off the overbed table with the paper towels. Discarded the paper towels.	___	___	_____
44. Removed the gloves. Decontaminated your hands.	___	___	_____
45. Unscreened the person.	___	___	_____
46. Completed a safety check of the room.	___	___	_____
47. Followed center policy for dirty linen.	___	___	_____
48. Decontaminated your hands.	___	___	_____
49. Reported and recorded your observations.	___	___	_____

Date of Satisfactory Completion_____   Instructor's Initials _____

Giving Male Perineal Care (NNAAP™)

Name: _____   Date: _____

	S	U	Comments

Quality of Life
- Knocked before entering the person's room
- Addressed the person by name
- Introduced yourself by name and title
- Explained the procedure to the person before beginning and during the procedure
- Protected the person's rights during the procedure
- Handled the person gently during the procedure

Pre-Procedure
1. Followed *Delegation Guidelines:*
   Perineal Care
   Saw *Promoting Safety and Comfort:*
   Perineal Care
2. Practiced hand hygiene.
3. Collected the following:
   - Soap or other cleaning agent as directed
   - At least 4 washcloths
   - Bath towel
   - Bath blanket
   - Bath thermometer
   - Wash basin
   - Waterproof pad
   - Gloves
   - Paper towels
4. Covered the overbed table with paper towels. Arranged items on top of them.
5. Identified the person. Checked the ID bracelet against the assignment sheet. Called him by name.
6. Provided for privacy.
7. Raised the bed for body mechanics. Bed rails were up if used.

Procedure
8. Lowered the bed rail near you if up.
9. Decontaminated your hands. Put on gloves.
10. Covered the person with a bath blanket. Moved top linens to the foot of the bed.
11. Positioned the person on his back.
12. Draped the person.
13. Raised the bed rail if used.
14. Filled the wash basin. Water temperature was 105°-109° F (40.5°-42.7° C). Measured water temperature according to center policy.
15. Placed the basin on the overbed table.
16. Lowered the bed rail if up.
17. Retracted the foreskin if the person was not circumcised.
18. Grasped the penis.
19. Cleaned the tip. Used a circular motion. Started at the meatus of the urethra, and worked outward. Repeated as needed. Used a clean part of the washcloth each time.
20. Rinsed the area with another washcloth.
21. Returned the foreskin to its natural position.
22. Cleaned the shaft of the penis. Used firm downward strokes. Rinsed the area.

Date of Satisfactory Completion_____   Instructor's Initials _____

Procedure—cont'd	**S**	**U**	**Comments**
23. Helped the person flex his knees and spread his legs. Or helped him spread his legs as much as possible with his knees straight.	____	____	_____
24. Cleaned the scrotum. Rinsed well. Observed for redness and irritation of the skin folds.	____	____	_____
25. Patted dry the penis and the scrotum. Used the towel.	____	____	_____
26. Folded the blanket back between his legs.	____	____	_____
27. Helped the person lower his legs and turn onto his side away from you.	____	____	_____
28. Cleaned the rectal area:			
a. Applied soap to a mitted washcloth.	____	____	_____
b. Cleaned from behind scrotum to the anus with one stroke.	____	____	_____
c. Repeated until the area was clean. Used a clean part of the washcloth for each stroke. Used more than one washcloth if needed.	____	____	_____
d. Rinsed the rectal area with a washcloth. Stroked from the scrotum to the anus. Repeated as necessary. Used a clean part of the washcloth for each stroke. Used more than one washcloth if needed.	____	____	_____
e. Patted the area dry with the towel.	____	____	_____
29. Removed the waterproof pad.	____	____	_____
30. Provided clean and dry linens and incontinence products as needed.	____	____	_____
31. Removed and discarded the gloves. Decontaminated your hands.	____	____	_____

Post-Procedure

	S	**U**	**Comments**
32. Covered the person. Removed the bath blanket.	____	____	_____
33. Provided for comfort.	____	____	_____
34. Placed the signal light within reach.	____	____	_____
35. Lowered the bed to its lowest position.	____	____	_____
36. Raised or lowered bed rails. Followed the care plan.	____	____	_____
37. Emptied and cleaned the wash basin. Wore gloves.	____	____	_____
38. Returned the basin and supplies to their proper place.	____	____	_____
39. Wiped off the overbed table with the paper towels. Discarded the paper towels.	____	____	_____
40. Removed the gloves. Decontaminated your hands.	____	____	_____
41. Unscreened the person.	____	____	_____
42. Completed a safety check of the room.	____	____	_____
43. Followed center policy for dirty linen.	____	____	_____
44. Decontaminated your hands.	____	____	_____
45. Reported and recorded your observations.	____	____	_____

Date of Satisfactory Completion_____   Instructor's Initials _____

Brushing and Combing the Person's Hair

Name: _____   Date: _____

Quality of Life	**S**	**U**	**Comments**
• Knocked before entering the person's room	___	___	_____
• Addressed the person by name	___	___	_____
• Introduced yourself by name and title	___	___	_____
• Explained the procedure to the person before beginning and during the procedure	___	___	_____
• Protected the person's rights during the procedure	___	___	_____
• Handled the person gently during the procedure	___	___	_____

Pre-Procedure

1. Followed *Delegation Guidelines:*
   Brushing and Combing Hair
   Saw *Promoting Safety and Comfort:*
   Brushing and Combing Hair ___ ___ _____
2. Practiced hand hygiene. ___ ___ _____
3. Identified the person. Checked the ID bracelet against the assignment sheet. Called the person by name. ___ ___ _____
4. Asked the person how to style hair. ___ ___ _____
5. Collected the following:
   • Comb and brush ___ ___ _____
   • Bath towel ___ ___ _____
   • Other hair items as requested ___ ___ _____
6. Arranged items on the bedside stand. ___ ___ _____
7. Provided for privacy. ___ ___ _____

Procedure

8. Lowered the bed rail if up. ___ ___ _____
9. Helped the person to the chair. The person put on a robe and non-skid footwear while up. (If the person was in bed, raised the bed for body mechanics. Bed rails were up if used. Lowered the bed rail near you. Assisted the person to a semi-Fowler's position if allowed.) ___ ___ _____
10. Placed a towel across the person's back and shoulders or across the pillow. ___ ___ _____
11. Asked the person to remove eyeglasses. Put them in the eyeglass case. Put the case inside the bedside stand. ___ ___ _____
12. *Brushed and combed hair that was not matted or tangled*:
    a. Used the comb to part the hair:
       (1) Parted hair down the middle into two sides. ___ ___ _____
       (2) Divided one side into two smaller sections. Used comb for this step. ___ ___ _____
    b. Brushed one of the small sections of hair. Started at the scalp, and brushed toward the hair ends. Did the same for the other small section of hair. ___ ___ _____
    c. Repeated for the other side:
       (1) Divided other side into two smaller sections. Used comb for this step. ___ ___ _____
       (2) Brushed one of the small sections of hair. Started at the scalp, and brushed toward the hair ends. Did the same for the other small section of hair. ___ ___ _____
13. *Brushed and combed matted and tangled hair*:
    a. Took a small section of hair near the ends. ___ ___ _____
    b. Combed or brushed through to the hair ends. ___ ___ _____
    c. Added small sections of hair as you worked up to the scalp. ___ ___ _____
    d. Combed or brushed through each longer section to the hair ends. ___ ___ _____
    e. Brushed or combed from the scalp to the hair ends. ___ ___ _____

Date of Satisfactory Completion_____   Instructor's Initials _____

Procedure—cont'd	**S**	**U**	**Comments**
14. Styled the hair as the person preferred.	_____	_____	_____
15. Removed the towel.	_____	_____	_____
16. Allowed the person to put on the eyeglasses.	_____	_____	_____

Post-Procedure

	S	**U**	**Comments**
17. Provided for comfort.	_____	_____	_____
18. Placed the signal light within reach.	_____	_____	_____
19. Lowered the bed to its lowest position.	_____	_____	_____
20. Raised or lowered bed rails. Followed the care plan.	_____	_____	_____
21. Cleaned and returned hair care items to their proper place.	_____	_____	_____
22. Unscreened the person.	_____	_____	_____
23. Completed a safety check of the room.	_____	_____	_____
24. Followed center policy for dirty linen.	_____	_____	_____
25. Decontaminated your hands.	_____	_____	_____

Date of Satisfactory Completion_____ Instructor's Initials _____

Shampooing the Person's Hair (NNAAP™)

Name: _____   Date: _____

	S	U	Comments
Quality of Life			
• Knocked before entering the person's room			
• Addressed the person by name			
• Introduced yourself by name and title			
• Explained the procedure to the person before beginning and during the procedure			
• Protected the person's rights during the procedure			
• Handled the person gently during the procedure			

Pre-Procedure

1. Followed *Delegation Guidelines: Shampooing* Saw *Promoting Safety and Comfort: Shampooing*
2. Practiced hand hygiene.
3. Collected the following:
   - Two bath towels
   - Washcloth
   - Shampoo
   - Hair conditioner (if requested)
   - Bath thermometer
   - Pitcher or hand-held nozzle (if needed)
   - Shampoo tray (if needed)
   - Basin or pan (if needed)
   - Waterproof pad (if needed)
   - Gloves (if needed)
   - Comb and brush
   - Hair dryer
4. Arranged items nearby.
5. Identified the person. Checked the ID bracelet against the assignment sheet. Called the person by name.
6. Provided for privacy.
7. Raised the bed for body mechanics for a shampoo in bed. Bed rails were up if used.
8. Decontaminated your hands.

Procedure

9. Lowered the bed rail near you if up.
10. Covered the person's chest with a bath towel.
11. Brushed and combed hair to remove snarls and tangles.
12. Positioned the person for the method you used. To shampoo the person in bed:
    a. Lowered the head of the bed and removed the pillow.
    b. Placed the waterproof pad and shampoo tray under the head and shoulders.
    c. Supported the head and neck with a folded towel if necessary.
13. Raised the bed rail if used.
14. Obtained water. Water temperature was 105° F (40.5° C). Tested water temperature according to center policy.
15. Lowered the bed rail near you if up.
16. Put on gloves (if needed).
17. Asked the person to hold a washcloth over the eyes. It did not cover the nose and mouth. (*NOTE:* A damp washcloth is easier to hold. It will not slip. However, some state competency tests require a dry washcloth.)
18. Used the pitcher or nozzle to wet the hair.

Date of Satisfactory Completion_____   Instructor's Initials _____

Procedure—cont'd	S	U	Comments
19. Applied a small amount of shampoo.	___	___	_____
20. Worked up a lather with both hands. Started at the hairline. Worked toward the back of the head.	___	___	_____
21. Massaged the scalp with your fingertips. Did not scratch the scalp.	___	___	_____
22. Rinsed the hair until the water ran clear.	___	___	_____
23. Repeated:			
a. Applied a small amount of shampoo.	___	___	_____
b. Worked up a lather with both hands. Started at the hairline. Worked toward the back of the head.	___	___	_____
c. Massaged the scale with your fingertips. Did not scratch the scalp.	___	___	_____
d. Rinsed the hair until the water ran clear.	___	___	_____
24. Applied conditioner. Followed directions on the container.	___	___	_____
25. Squeezed water from the person's hair.	___	___	_____
26. Covered the hair with a bath towel.	___	___	_____
27. Removed the shampoo tray and waterproof pad.	___	___	_____
28. Dried the person's face with the towel. Used the towel on the person's chest.	___	___	_____
29. Helped the person raise the head if appropriate. For the person in bed, raised the head of the bed.	___	___	_____
30. Rubbed the hair and scalp with the towel. Used the second towel if the first one was wet.	___	___	_____
31. Combed the hair to remove snarls and tangles.	___	___	_____
32. Dried and styled hair as quickly as possible.	___	___	_____
33. Removed and discarded the gloves if used. Decontaminated your hands.	___	___	_____

Post-Procedure

	S	U	Comments
34. Provided for comfort.	___	___	_____
35. Placed the signal light within reach.	___	___	_____
36. Lowered the bed to its lowest position.	___	___	_____
37. Raised or lowered bed rails. Followed the care plan.	___	___	_____
38. Unscreened the person.	___	___	_____
39. Completed a safety check of the room.	___	___	_____
40. Cleaned and returned equipment to its proper place. Remembered to clean the brush and comb.	___	___	_____
41. Followed center policy for dirty linen.	___	___	_____
42. Decontaminated your hands.	___	___	_____

Date of Satisfactory Completion_____   Instructor's Initials _____

Shaving the Person's Face With a Safety Razor

Name: _____   Date: _____

	S	U	Comments

Quality of Life
- Knocked before entering the person's room
- Addressed the person by name
- Introduced yourself by name and title
- Explained the procedure to the person before beginning and during the procedure
- Protected the person's rights during the procedure
- Handled the person gently during the procedure

Pre-Procedure
1. Followed *Delegation Guidelines:*
   Shaving
   Saw *Promoting Safety and Comfort:*
   Shaving
2. Practiced hand hygiene.
3. Collected the following:
   - Wash basin
   - Bath towel
   - Hand towel
   - Washcloth
   - Safety razor
   - Mirror
   - Shaving cream, soap, or lotion
   - Shaving brush
   - After-shave or lotion
   - Tissues or paper towels
   - Paper towels
   - Gloves
4. Arranged paper towels and supplies on the overbed table.
5. Identified the person. Checked the ID bracelet against the assignment sheet. Called the person by name.
6. Provided for privacy.
7. Raised the bed for body mechanics. Bed rails were up if used.

Procedure
8. Filled the wash basin with warm water.
9. Placed the basin on the overbed table.
10. Lowered the bed rail near you if up.
11. Decontaminated your hands. Put on gloves.
12. Assisted the person to semi-Fowler's position if allowed or to the supine position.
13. Adjusted lighting to clearly see the person's face.
14. Placed the bath towel over the person's chest and shoulders.
15. Adjusted the overbed table for easy reach.
16. Tightened the razor blade to the shaver.
17. Washed the person's face. Did not dry.
18. Wet the washcloth or towel. Wrung it out.
19. Applied the washcloth or towel to the face for a few minutes.
20. Applied shaving cream with your hands. Or used a shaving brush to apply lather.
21. Held the skin taut with one hand.
22. Shaved in the direction of hair growth. Used shorter strokes around the chin and lips.
23. Rinsed the razor often. Wiped it with tissues or paper towels.
24. Applied direct pressure to any bleeding areas.
25. Washed off any remaining shaving cream or soap. Patted dry with a towel.

Date of Satisfactory Completion_____   Instructor's Initials _____

Procedure—cont'd   S   U   **Comments**

26. Applied after-shave or lotion if requested.   _____   _____   _____
27. Removed the towel and gloves. Decontaminated your hands.   _____   _____   _____

Post-Procedure

28. Provided for comfort.   _____   _____   _____
29. Placed the signal light within reach.   _____   _____   _____
30. Lowered the bed to its lowest position.   _____   _____   _____
31. Raised or lowered bed rails. Followed the care plan. _____   _____   _____
32. Cleaned and returned equipment and supplies to their proper
    place. Discarded disposable items. Wore gloves.   _____   _____   _____
33. Wiped off the overbed table with paper towels. Discarded the
    paper towels.
34. Removed the gloves. Decontaminated your hands.   _____   _____   _____
35. Unscreened the person.   _____   _____   _____
36. Completed a safety check of the room.   _____   _____   _____
37. Followed center policy for dirty linen.   _____   _____   _____
38. Decontaminated your hands.   _____   _____   _____
39. Reported nicks, cuts, irritation, or bleeding to the nurse
    at once. Also reported and recorded other observations.   _____   _____   _____

Date of Satisfactory Completion_____   Instructor's Initials _____

Giving Nail and Foot Care (NNAAP™)

Name: _____   Date: _____

	S	U	Comments

Quality of Life
- Knocked before entering the person's room
- Addressed the person by name
- Introduced yourself by name and title
- Explained the procedure to the person before beginning and during the procedure
- Protected the person's rights during the procedure
- Handled the person gently during the procedure

Pre-Procedure
1. Followed *Delegation Guidelines:*
   Nail and Foot Care
   Saw *Promoting Safety and Comfort:*
   Nail and Foot Care
2. Practiced hand hygiene.
3. Collected the following:
   - Wash basin or whirlpool foot bath
   - Soap
   - Bath thermometer
   - Bath towel
   - Hand towel
   - Washcloth
   - Kidney basin
   - Nail clippers
   - Orange stick
   - Emery board or nail file
   - Lotion for the hands
   - Lotion or petroleum jelly for the feet
   - Paper towels
   - Bathmat
   - Gloves
4. Arranged paper towels and supplies on the overbed table.
5. Identified the person. Checked the ID bracelet against the assignment sheet. Called the person by name.
6. Provided for privacy.
7. Assisted the person to the bedside chair. Placed the signal light within reach.

Procedure
8. Placed the bathmat under the feet.
9. Filled the wash basin or whirlpool foot bath ²⁄₃ (two-thirds) full with water. The nurse told you what water temperature to use. (Measured water temperature with a bath thermometer. Or tested it by dipping your elbow or inner wrist into the basin. Followed center policy.)
10. Placed the basin or foot both on the bathmat.
11. Helped the person put the feet into the basin or foot bath. Made sure both feet were completely covered by water.
12. Adjusted the overbed table in front of the person.
13. Filled the kidney basin ²⁄₃ (two-thirds) full with water. The nurse told you what water temperature to use. (Measured water temperature with a bath thermometer. Or tested it by dipping your elbow or inner wrist into the basin. Followed center policy.)
14. Placed the kidney basin on the overbed table.
15. Placed the person's fingers into the basin. Positioned the arms for comfort.

Date of Satisfactory Completion_____   Instructor's Initials _____

Procedure—cont'd	**S**	**U**	**Comments**
16. Allowed the fingers to soak for 5-10 minutes. Allowed the feet to soak for 15-20 minutes. Rewarmed water as needed.	_____	_____	_____
17. Decontaminated your hands. Put on gloves.	_____	_____	_____
18. Removed the kidney basin.	_____	_____	_____
19. Cleaned under the fingernails with the orange stick. Used a towel to wipe the orange stick after each nail.	_____	_____	_____
20. Dried the hands and between the fingers thoroughly.	_____	_____	_____
21. Clipped fingernails straight across with the nail clippers.	_____	_____	_____
22. Shaped nails with an emery board or nail file. Nails were smooth with no rough edges.	_____	_____	_____
23. Pushed cuticles back with the orange stick or a wash cloth.	_____	_____	_____
24. Applied lotion to the hands. Warmed the lotion before applying it.	_____	_____	_____
25. Moved the overbed table to the side.	_____	_____	_____
26. Washed the feet and between the toes with soap and a washcloth. Rinsed the feet and between the toes.	_____	_____	_____
27. Removed the feet from the basin or foot bath. Dried thoroughly, especially between the toes.	_____	_____	_____
28. Applied lotion or petroleum jelly to the tops and soles of the feet. Did not apply between the toes. Warmed lotion before applying it. Removed excess lotion or petroleum jelly with a towel.	_____	_____	_____
29. Removed and discarded the gloves. Decontaminated your hands.	_____	_____	_____
30. Helped the person put on non-skid footwear.	_____	_____	_____
Post-Procedure			
31. Provided for comfort.	_____	_____	_____
32. Placed the signal light within reach.	_____	_____	_____
33. Raised or lowered bed rails. Followed the care plan.	_____	_____	_____
34. Cleaned and returned equipment and supplies to their proper place. Discarded disposable items. Wore gloves.	_____	_____	_____
35. Removed the gloves. Decontaminated your hands.	_____	_____	_____
36. Unscreened the person.	_____	_____	_____
37. Completed a safety check of the room.	_____	_____	_____
38. Followed center policy for dirty linen.	_____	_____	_____
39. Decontaminated your hands.	_____	_____	_____
40. Reported and recorded your observations.	_____	_____	_____

Date of Satisfactory Completion _____ Instructor's Initials _____

Undressing the Person

Name: _____   Date: _____

Quality of Life	S	U	Comments
• Knocked before entering the person's room			
• Addressed the person by name			
• Introduced yourself by name and title			
• Explained the procedure to the person before beginning and during the procedure			
• Protected the person's rights during the procedure			
• Handled the person gently during the procedure			

Pre-Procedure

1. Followed *Delegation Guidelines: Dressing and Undressing*
2. Practiced hand hygiene.
3. Collected a bath blanket and clothing requested by the person.
4. Identified the person. Checked the ID bracelet against the assignment sheet. Called the person by name.
5. Provided for privacy.
6. Raised the bed for body mechanics for a shampoo in bed. Bed rails were up if used.
7. Lowered the bed rail on the person's weak side.
8. Positioned him or her supine.
9. Covered the person with a bath blanket. Fan-folded linens to the foot of the bed.

Procedure

10. Removed garments that opened in the back:
    a. Raised the head and shoulders. Or turned him or her onto the side away from you.
    b. Undid buttons, zippers, ties, or snaps.
    c. Brought the sides of the garment to the sides of the person. If he or she was in a side-lying position, tucked the far side under the person. Folded the near side onto the chest.
    d. Positioned the person supine.
    e. Slid the garment off the shoulder on the strong side. Removed it from the arm.
    f. Slid the garment off the shoulder on the weak side. Removed it from the arm.
11. Removed garments that opened in the front:
    a. Undid buttons, zippers, ties, or snaps.
    b. Slid the garment off the shoulder and arm on the strong side.
    c. Assisted the person to sit up, or raised the head and shoulders. Brought the garment over to the weak side.
    d. Lowered the head and shoulders. Removed the garment from the weak side.
    e. If you could not raise the head and shoulders:
       (1) Turned the person toward you. Tucked the removed part under the person.
       (2) Turned him or her onto the side away from you.
       (3) Pulled the side of the garment out from under the person. Made sure he or she was not lying on it when supine.
       (4) Returned the person to the supine position.
       (5) Removed the garment from the weak side.
12. Removed pullover garments:
    a. Undid any buttons, zippers, ties, or snaps.
    b. Removed the garment from the strong side.

Date of Satisfactory Completion_____   Instructor's Initials _____

Procedure—cont'd   S   U   **Comments**

   c. Raised the head and shoulders. Or turned the person onto
     the side away from you.   ____ ____ _____
   d. Removed the garment from the weak side.   ____ ____ _____
   e. Brought the garment over the person's head.   ____ ____ _____
   f. Positioned him or her in the supine position.   ____ ____ _____
13. Removed pants or slacks:
   a. Removed footwear.   ____ ____ _____
   b. Positioned the person supine.   ____ ____ _____
   c. Undid buttons, zippers, ties, snaps, or buckles.   ____ ____ _____
   d. Removed the belt.   ____ ____ _____
   e. Asked the person to lift the buttocks off the bed. Slid the
     pants down over the hips and buttocks. Had the person
     lower the hips and buttocks.   ____ ____ _____
   f. If the person could not raise the hips off the bed:
     (1) Turned the person toward you.   ____ ____ _____
     (2) Slid the pants off the hip and buttocks on the
       strong side.   ____ ____ _____
     (3) Turned the person away from you.   ____ ____ _____
     (4) Slid the pants off the hip and buttocks on the
       weak side.   ____ ____ _____
   g. Slid the pants down the legs and over the feet.   ____ ____ _____
14. Dressed the person. Followed the procedure: *Dressing the Person*. ____ ____ _____

Post-Procedure
15. Provided for comfort.   ____ ____ _____
16. Placed the signal light within reach.   ____ ____ _____
17. Lowered the bed to its lowest position.   ____ ____ _____
18. Raised or lowered bed rails. Followed the care plan.   ____ ____ _____
19. Unscreened the person.   ____ ____ _____
20. Completed a safety check of the room.   ____ ____ _____
21. Followed center policy for soiled clothing.   ____ ____ _____
22. Decontaminated your hands.   ____ ____ _____
23. Reported and recorded your observations.   ____ ____ _____

Date of Satisfactory Completion_____ Instructor's Initials _____

Dressing the Person (NNAAP™)

Name: _____ Date: _____

Quality of Life	S	U	Comments
• Knocked before entering the person's room			
• Addressed the person by name			
• Introduced yourself by name and title			
• Explained the procedure to the person before beginning and during the procedure			
• Protected the person's rights during the procedure			
• Handled the person gently during the procedure			

Pre-Procedure

1. Followed *Delegation Guidelines:* *Dressing and Undressing*
2. Practiced hand hygiene.
3. Asked the person what he or she would like to wear.
4. Collected a bath blanket and clothing requested by the person.
5. Identified the person. Checked the ID bracelet against the assignment sheet. Called the person by name.
6. Provided for privacy.
7. Raised the bed for body mechanics for a shampoo in bed. Bed rails were up if used.
8. Lowered the bed rail (if up) on the person's strong side.
9. Positioned the person supine.
10. Covered the person with a bath blanket. Fan-folded linens to the foot of the bed.
11. Undressed the person. Followed the procedure: *Undressing the Person.*

Procedure

12. Put on garments that opened in the back:
    a. Slid the garment onto the arm and shoulder of the weak side.
    b. Slid the garment onto the arm and shoulder of the strong arm.
    c. Raised the person's head and shoulders.
    d. Brought the sides to the back.
    e. If you could not raise the person's head and shoulders:
       (1) Turned the person toward you.
       (2) Brought one side of the garment to the person's back.
       (3) Turned the person away from you.
       (4) Brought the other side to the person's back.
    f. Fastened buttons, ties, snaps, zippers, or other closures.
    g. Positioned the person supine.
13. Put on garments that opened in the front:
    a. Slid the garment onto the arm and shoulder on the weak side.
    b. Raised the head and shoulders. Brought the side of the garment around to the back. Lowered the person down. Slid the garment arm onto the arm and shoulder of the strong arm.
    c. If the person could not raise the head and shoulders:
       (1) Turned the person away from you.
       (2) Tucked the garment under the person.
       (3) Turned the person toward you.
       (4) Pulled the garment out from under the person.
       (5) Turned the person back to the supine position.
       (6) Slid the garment over the arm and shoulder of the strong arm.
    d. Fastened buttons, ties, snaps, zippers, or other closures.

Date of Satisfactory Completion _____ Instructor's Initials _____

Procedure—cont'd	**S**	**U**	**Comments**
14. Put on pullover garments:			
a. Positioned the person supine.	_____	_____	_____
b. Brought the neck of the garment over the head.	_____	_____	_____
c. Slid the head and shoulder of the garment onto the weak side.	_____	_____	_____
d. Raised the person's head and shoulders.	_____	_____	_____
e. Brought the garment down.	_____	_____	_____
f. Slid the arm and shoulder of the garment onto the strong side.	_____	_____	_____
g. If the person could not assume a semi-sitting position:			
(1) Turned the person away from you.	_____	_____	_____
(2) Tucked the garment under the person.	_____	_____	_____
(3) Turned the person toward you.	_____	_____	_____
(4) Pulled the garment out from under the person.	_____	_____	_____
(5) Positioned the person supine.	_____	_____	_____
(6) Slid the arm and shoulder of the garment onto the strong side.	_____	_____	_____
h. Fastened buttons, ties, snaps, zippers, or other closures.	_____	_____	_____
15. Put on pants or slacks:			
a. Slid the pants over the feet and up the legs.	_____	_____	_____
b. Asked the person to raise the hips and buttocks off the bed.	_____	_____	_____
c. Brought the pants up over the buttocks and hips.	_____	_____	_____
d. Asked the person to lower the hips and buttocks.	_____	_____	_____
e. If the person could not raise the hips and buttocks:			
(1) Turned the person onto the strong side (away from you).	_____	_____	_____
(2) Pulled the pants over the buttock and hip on the weak side.	_____	_____	_____
(3) Turned the person onto the weak side (toward you).	_____	_____	_____
(4) Pulled the pants over the buttock and hip on the strong side.	_____	_____	_____
(5) Positioned the person supine.	_____	_____	_____
f. Fastened buttons, ties, snaps, zipper, belt buckle, or other closure.	_____	_____	_____
16. Put socks and non-skid footwear on the person.	_____	_____	_____
17. Helped the person get out of bed. If the person stayed in bed, covered the person. Removed the bath blanket.	_____	_____	_____
Post-Procedure			
18. Provided for comfort.	_____	_____	_____
19. Placed the signal light within reach.	_____	_____	_____
20. Lowered the bed to its lowest position.	_____	_____	_____
21. Raised or lowered bed rails. Followed the care plan.	_____	_____	_____
22. Unscreened the person.	_____	_____	_____
23. Completed a safety check of the room.	_____	_____	_____
24. Followed center policy for soiled clothing.	_____	_____	_____
25. Decontaminated your hands.	_____	_____	_____
26. Reported and recorded your observations.	_____	_____	_____

Date of Satisfactory Completion_____   Instructor's Initials _____

Changing the Gown of the Person With an IV

Name: _____   Date: _____

Quality of Life	S	U	Comments

Quality of Life
- Knocked before entering the person's room
- Addressed the person by name
- Introduced yourself by name and title
- Explained the procedure to the person before beginning and during the procedure
- Protected the person's rights during the procedure
- Handled the person gently during the procedure

Pre-Procedure
1. Followed *Delegation Guidelines:*
   Changing Hospital Gowns
   Saw *Promoting Safety and Comfort:*
   Changing Hospital Gowns
2. Practiced hand hygiene.
3. Collected a clean gown and a bath blanket.
4. Identified the person. Checked the ID bracelet against the assignment sheet. Called the person by name.
5. Provided for privacy.
6. Raised the bed for body mechanics.
   Bed rails were up if used.

Procedure
7. Lowered the bed rail near you (if up).
8. Covered the person with a bath blanket. Fan-folded linens to the foot of the bed.
9. Untied the gown. Freed parts the person was lying on.
10. Removed the gown from the arm *with no IV.*
11. Gathered up the sleeve of the arm *with the IV.* Slid it over the IV site and tubing. Removed the arm and hand from the sleeve.
12. Kept the sleeve gathered. Slid your arm along the tubing to the bag.
13. Removed the bag from the pole. Slid the bag and tubing through the sleeve. Did not pull on the tubing. Kept the bag above the person.
14. Hung the IV bag on the pole.
15. Gathered the sleeve of the clean gown that went on the arm with the IV infusion.
16. Removed the bag from the pole. Slipped the sleeve over the bag at the shoulder part of the gown. Hung the bag.
17. Slid the gathered sleeve over the tubing, hand, arm, and IV site. Then slid it onto the shoulder.
18. Put the other side of the gown on the person. Fastened the gown.
19. Covered the person. Removed the bath blanket.

Post-Procedure
20. Provided for comfort.
21. Placed the signal light within reach.
22. Lowered the bed to its lowest position.
23. Raised or lowered bed rails. Followed the care plan.
24. Unscreened the person.
25. Completed a safety check of the room.
26. Followed center policy for dirty linens.
27. Decontaminated your hands.
28. Asked the nurse to check the flow rate.
29. Reported and recorded your observations.

Date of Satisfactory Completion_____   Instructor's Initials _____

Giving the Bedpan (NNAAP™)

Name: _____   Date: _____

Quality of Life	S	U	Comments

Quality of Life
- Knocked before entering the person's room
- Addressed the person by name
- Introduced yourself by name and title
- Explained the procedure to the person before beginning and during the procedure
- Protected the person's rights during the procedure
- Handled the person gently during the procedure

Pre-Procedure
1. Followed *Delegation Guidelines:*
   Bedpans
   Saw *Promoting Safety and Comfort:*
   Bedpans
2. Provided for privacy.
3. Practiced hand hygiene.
4. Put on gloves.
5. Collected the following:
   - Bedpan
   - Bedpan cover
   - Toilet tissue
   - Waterproof pad (if required by center)
6. Arranged equipment on the chair or bed.

Procedure
7. Warmed and dried the bedpan if necessary.
8. Lowered the bed rail near you (if up).
9. Positioned the person supine. Raised the head of the bed slightly.
10. Folded the top linens and gown out of the way. Kept the lower body covered.
11. Asked the person to flex the knees and raise the buttocks by pushing against the mattress with his or her feet.
12. Slid your hand under the lower back. Helped raise the buttocks. If used waterproof pad, placed it under the person's buttocks.
13. Slid the bedpan under the person.
14. If the person did not assist in getting on the bedpan:
    a. Placed the waterproof pad under the person's buttocks if using one.
    b. Turned the person onto the side away from you.
    c. Placed the bedpan firmly against the buttocks.
    d. Pushed the bedpan down and toward the person.
    e. Held the bedpan securely. Turned the person onto his or her back.
    f. Made sure the bedpan was centered under the person.
15. Covered the person.
16. Raised the head of the bed so the person was in a sitting position.
17. Made sure the person was correctly positioned on the bedpan.
18. Raised the bed rail if used.
19. Paced the toilet tissue and signal light within reach.
20. Asked the person to signal when done or when help was needed.
21. Removed the gloves. Decontaminated your hands.
22. Left the room, and closed the door.
23. Returned when the person signaled. Or checked on the person every 5 minutes. Knocked before entering.

Date of Satisfactory Completion_____   Instructor's Initials _____

Procedure—cont'd   S   U   Comments

24. Decontaminated your hands. Put on gloves.
25. Raised the bed for body mechanics. Lowered the bed rail (if used) and the head of the bed.
26. Asked the person to raise the buttocks. Removed the bedpan. Or held the bedpan and turned him or her onto the side away from you.
27. Cleaned the genital area if the person did not do so. Cleaned from front (urethra) to back (anus) with toilet tissue. Used fresh tissue for each wipe. Provided perineal care if needed. Removed and discarded the waterproof pad if used.
28. Covered the bedpan. Took it to the bathroom. Raised the bed rail (if used) before leaving the bedside.
29. Noted the color, amount, and character of the urine or feces.
30. Emptied the bedpan contents into the toilet and flushed.
31. Rinsed the bedpan. Poured the rinse into the toilet and flushed.
32. Cleaned the bedpan with a disinfectant.
33. Removed soiled gloves. Practiced hand hygiene, and put on clean gloves.
34. Returned the bedpan and clean cover to the bedside stand.
35. Assisted with hand washing.
36. Removed the gloves. Decontaminated your hands.

Post-Procedure
37. Provided for comfort.
38. Placed the signal light within reach.
39. Lowered the bed to its lowest position.
40. Raised or lowered bed rails. Followed the care plan.
41. Unscreened the person.
42. Completed a safety check of the room.
43. Followed center policy for soiled linens.
44. Decontaminated your hands.
45. Reported and recorded your observations.

Date of Satisfactory Completion_____ Instructor's Initials _____

Giving the Urinal

Name: _____   Date: _____

	S	U	Comments

Quality of Life

- Knocked before entering the person's room
- Addressed the person by name
- Introduced yourself by name and title
- Explained the procedure to the person before beginning and during the procedure
- Protected the person's rights during the procedure
- Handled the person gently during the procedure

Pre-Procedure

1. Followed *Delegation Guidelines:*
   Urinals
   Saw *Promoting Safety and Comfort:*
   Urinals
2. Provided for privacy.
3. Determined if the man will stand, sit, or lie in bed.
4. Practiced hand hygiene.
5. Put on gloves.
6. Collected the following:
   - Urinal
   - Non-skid footwear if the person stood to void.

Procedure

7. Gave him the urinal if he was in bed. Reminded him to tilt the bottom down to prevent spills.
8. If he stood:
   a. Helped him sit on the side of the bed.
   b. Put non-skid footwear on him.
   c. Helped him stand. Provided support if he was unsteady.
   d. Gave him the urinal.
9. Positioned the urinal if necessary. Positioned the penis in the urinal if he could not do so.
10. Placed the signal light within reach. Asked him to signal when done or when he needed help.
11. Provided for privacy.
12. Removed the gloves. Decontaminated your hands.
13. Left the room, and closed the door.
14. Returned when he signaled. Or checked on the person every 5 minutes. Knocked before entering.
15. Decontaminated your hands. Put on gloves.
16. Closed the cap on the urinal. Took it to the bathroom.
17. Noted the color, amount, and character of the urine.
18. Emptied the urinal into the toilet and flushed.
19. Rinsed the urinal with cold water. Poured rinse into the toilet and flushed.
20. Cleaned the urinal with a disinfectant.
21. Returned the urinal to its proper place.
22. Removed soiled gloves. Practiced hand hygiene and put on clean gloves.
23. Assisted with hand washing.
24. Removed the gloves. Decontaminated your hands.

Date of Satisfactory Completion_____   Instructor's Initials _____

	S	U	Comments

Post-Procedure
25. Provided for comfort.
26. Placed the signal light within reach.
27. Raised or lowered bed rails. Followed the care plan.
28. Unscreened the person.
29. Completed a safety check of the room.
30. Followed center policy for soiled linens.
31. Decontaminated your hands.
32. Reported and recorded your observations.

Date of Satisfactory Completion_____ Instructor's Initials _____

Helping the Person to the Commode

Name: _____   Date: _____

Quality of Life	S	U	Comments

Quality of Life
- Knocked before entering the person's room
- Addressed the person by name
- Introduced yourself by name and title
- Explained the procedure to the person before beginning and during the procedure
- Protected the person's rights during the procedure
- Handled the person gently during the procedure

Pre-Procedure
1. Followed *Delegation Guidelines:*
   Commodes
   Saw *Promoting Safety and Comfort:*
   Commodes
2. Provided for privacy.
3. Practiced hand hygiene.
4. Put on gloves.
5. Collected the following:
   - Commode
   - Toilet tissue
   - Bath blanket
   - Transfer belt
   - Robe and non-skid footwear

Procedure
6. Brought the commode next to the bed. Removed the chair seat and container lid.
7. Helped the person sit on the side of the bed. Lowered the bed rail if used.
8. Helped the person put on a robe and non-skid footwear.
9. Assisted the person to the commode. Used the transfer belt.
10. Covered the person with a bath blanket for warmth.
11. Placed the toilet tissue and signal light within reach.
12. Asked the person to signal when done or when help was needed. (Stayed with the person if necessary. Was respectful. Provided as much privacy as possible.)
13. Removed the gloves. Decontaminated your hands.
14. Left the room. Closed the door.
15. Returned when he signaled. Or checked on the person every 5 minutes. Knocked before entering.
16. Decontaminated your hands. Put on gloves.
17. Helped the person clean the genital area as needed. Removed the gloves, and practiced hand hygiene.
18. Helped the person back to bed using the transfer belt. Removed the transfer belt, robe, and footwear. Raised the bed rail if used.
19. Put on clean gloves. Removed and covered the commode container. Cleaned the commode.
20. Took the container to the bathroom.
21. Observed urine and feces for color, amount, and character.
22. Emptied the container contents into the toilet and flushed.
23. Rinsed the container. Poured rinse into the toilet and flushed.
24. Cleaned and disinfected the container.
25. Returned the container to the commode. Returned other supplies to their proper place.

Date of Satisfactory Completion_____   Instructor's Initials _____

Procedure—cont'd

	S	U	Comments
26. Removed soiled gloves. Practiced hand hygiene and put on clean gloves.			
27. Assisted with hand washing.	___	___	_____
28. Removed the gloves. Decontaminated your hands.	___	___	_____

Post-Procedure

	S	U	Comments
29. Provided for comfort.			
30. Placed the signal light within reach.	___	___	_____
31. Raised or lowered bed rails. Followed the care plan.	___	___	_____
32. Unscreened the person.	___	___	_____
33. Completed a safety check of the room.	___	___	_____
34. Followed center policy for soiled linens.	___	___	_____
35. Decontaminated your hands.	___	___	_____
36. Reported and recorded your observations.	___	___	_____

Date of Satisfactory Completion_____ Instructor's Initials _____

Giving Catheter Care (NNAAP™)

Name: _____   Date: _____

Quality of Life	S	U	Comments

Quality of Life
- Knocked before entering the person's room
- Addressed the person by name
- Introduced yourself by name and title
- Explained the procedure to the person before beginning and during the procedure
- Protected the person's rights during the procedure
- Handled the person gently during the procedure

Pre-Procedure
1. Followed *Delegation Guidelines:*
   Catheter
   Saw *Promoting Safety and Comfort:*
   Catheters
2. Practiced hand hygiene.
3. Collected the following:
   - Items for perineal care:
     —Soap or other cleaning agent as directed
     —At least 4 washcloths
     —Bath towel
     —Bath thermometer
     —Wash basin
     —Waterproof pad
     —Paper towels
   - Gloves
   - Bath blanket
4. Identified the person. Checked the ID bracelet against the assignment sheet. Called the person by name.
5. Provided for privacy.
6. Raised the bed for body mechanics. Bed rails were up if used.

Procedure
7. Lowered the bed rail near you if used.
8. Decontaminated your hands. Put on gloves.
9. Covered the person with a bath blanket. Fan-folded top linens to the foot of the bed.
10. Draped the person for perineal care.
11. Folded back the bath blanket to expose the genital area.
12. Placed the waterproof pad under the buttocks. Asked the person to flex the knees and raise the buttocks off the bed.
13. Separated the labia (female). With an uncircumcised male, retracted the foreskin. Checked for crusts, abnormal drainage, or secretions.
14. Gave perineal care.
15. Applied soap to clean, wet washcloth.
16. Held the catheter near the meatus.
17. Cleaned the catheter from the meatus down the catheter about 4 inches. Cleaned downward, away from the meatus with 1 stroke. Did not tug or pull on the catheter. Repeated as needed with a clean area of the washcloth. Used a clean washcloth if needed.
18. Rinsed the catheter with a clean washcloth. Rinsed from the meatus down the catheter about 4 inches. Rinsed downward, away from the meatus with 1 stroke. Did not tug or pull on the catheter. Repeated as needed with a clean area of the washcloth. Used a clean washcloth if needed.
19. Patted the perineal area dry. Dried from front to back.

Date of Satisfactory Completion_____   Instructor's Initials _____

Procedure—cont'd

20. Returned the foreskin to its natural position.
21. Secured the catheter. Coiled and secured tubing.
22. Removed the waterproof pad.
23. Covered the person. Removed the bath blanket.
24. Removed the gloves. Decontaminated your hands.

Post-Procedure

25. Provided for comfort.
26. Placed the signal light within reach.
27. Lowered the bed to its lowest position.
28. Raised or lowered bed rails. Followed the care plan.
29. Cleaned and returned equipment to its proper place. Discarded disposable items. (Wore gloves for this step.)
30. Removed the gloves. Decontaminated your hands.
31. Unscreened the person.
32. Completed a safety check of the room.
33. Followed center policy for soiled linens.
34. Decontaminated your hands.
35. Reported and recorded your observations.

S   U   Comments

Date of Satisfactory Completion_____ Instructor's Initials _____

Changing a Leg Bag to a Drainage Bag

Name: _____   Date: _____

	S	U	Comments

Quality of Life
- Knocked before entering the person's room
- Addressed the person by name
- Introduced yourself by name and title
- Explained the procedure to the person before beginning and during the procedure
- Protected the person's rights during the procedure
- Handled the person gently during the procedure

Pre-Procedure
1. Followed *Delegation Guidelines:*
   Drainage Systems
   Saw *Promoting Safety and Comfort:*
   Drainage Systems
2. Practiced hand hygiene.
3. Collected the following:
   - Gloves
   - Drainage bag and tubing
   - Antiseptic wipes
   - Waterproof pad
   - Sterile cap and plug
   - Catheter clamp
   - Paper towels
   - Bedpan
   - Bath blanket
4. Arranged paper towels and equipment on the overbed table.
5. Identified the person. Checked the ID bracelet against the assignment sheet. Called the person by name.
6. Provided for privacy.

Procedure
7. Had the person sit on the side of the bed.
8. Decontaminated your hands. Put on gloves.
9. Exposed the catheter and leg bag.
10. Clamped the catheter. This prevented urine from draining from the catheter into the drainage tubing.
11. Allowed urine to drain from below the clamp into the drainage tubing. This emptied the lower end of the catheter.
12. Helped the person lie down.
13. Raised the bed rails if used. Raised the bed for body mechanics.
14. Lowered the bed rail near you if up.
15. Covered the person with a bath blanket. Exposed the catheter and leg bag.
16. Placed the waterproof pad under the person's leg.
17. Opened the antiseptic wipes. Put them on paper towels.
18. Opened the package with the sterile cap and plug. Placed the package on the paper towels. Did not let anything touch the sterile cap or plug.
19. Opened the package with the drainage bag and tubing.
20. Attached the drainage bag to the bed frame.
21. Disconnected the catheter from the drainage tubing. Did not allow anything to touch the ends.
22. Inserted the sterile plug into the catheter end. Touched only the end of the plug. Did not touch the part that went inside the catheter. (If you contaminated the end of the catheter, wiped the end with an antiseptic wipe. Did so before you inserted the sterile plug.)

Date of Satisfactory Completion_____   Instructor's Initials _____

Procedure—cont'd

	S	U	Comments
23. Placed the sterile cap on the end of the leg bag drainage tube. (If you contaminated the tubing end, wiped the end with an antiseptic wipe. Did so before you applied the sterile cap.)	___	___	_____
24. Removed the cap from the new drainage tubing.	___	___	_____
25. Removed the sterile plug from the catheter.	___	___	_____
26. Inserted the end of the drainage tubing into the catheter.	___	___	_____
27. Removed the clamp from the catheter.	___	___	_____
28. Looped the drainage tubing on the bed. Secured the tubing to the mattress.	___	___	_____
29. Removed the leg bag. Placed it in the bedpan.	___	___	_____
30. Removed and discarded the waterproof pad.	___	___	_____
31. Covered the person. Removed the bath blanket.	___	___	_____
32. Took the bedpan to the bathroom.	___	___	_____
33. Removed the gloves. Practiced hand hygiene.	___	___	_____

Post-Procedure

	S	U	Comments
34. Provided for comfort.	___	___	_____
35. Placed the signal light within reach.	___	___	_____
36. Lowered the bed to its lowest position.	___	___	_____
37. Raised or lowered bed rails. Followed the care plan.	___	___	_____
38. Unscreened the person.	___	___	_____
39. Put on clean gloves. Discarded disposable items.	___	___	_____
40. Emptied the drainage bag.	___	___	_____
41. Discarded the drainage tubing and bag following center policy. Or cleaned the bag following center policy.	___	___	_____
42. Cleaned and disinfected the bedpan. Placed it in a clean cover.	___	___	_____
43. Returned the bedpan and other supplies to their proper place.	___	___	_____
44. Removed the gloves. Decontaminated your hands.	___	___	_____
45. Completed a safety check of the room.	___	___	_____
46. Followed center policy for soiled linens.	___	___	_____
47. Decontaminated your hands.	___	___	_____
48. Reported and recorded your observations.	___	___	_____

Date of Satisfactory Completion _____ Instructor's Initials _____

Emptying a Urinary Drainage Bag

Name: _____   Date: _____

	S	U	Comments

Quality of Life
- Knocked before entering the person's room
- Addressed the person by name
- Introduced yourself by name and title
- Explained the procedure to the person before beginning and during the procedure
- Protected the person's rights during the procedure
- Handled the person gently during the procedure

Pre-Procedure
1. Followed *Delegation Guidelines:*
   Drainage Systems
   Saw *Promoting Safety and Comfort:*
   Drainage Systems
2. Collected the following:
   - Graduate (measuring container)
   - Gloves
   - Paper towels
3. Practiced hand hygiene.
4. Identified the person. Checked the ID bracelet against the assignment sheet. Called the person by name.
5. Provided for privacy.

Procedure
6. Put on the gloves.
7. Placed paper towel on the floor. Placed graduate on top of it.
8. Positioned the graduate under the collection bag.
9. Opened the clamp on the drain.
10. Allowed all urine to drain into the graduate. Did not let the drain touch the graduate.
11. Closed and positioned the clamp.
12. Measured the urine.
13. Removed and discarded the paper towel.
14. Emptied the contents of the graduate into the toilet and flushed.
15. Rinsed the graduate. Emptied the rinse into the toilet and flushed.
16. Cleaned and disinfected the graduate.
17. Returned the graduate to its proper place.
18. Removed the gloves. Practiced hand hygiene.
19. Recorded the time and amount on the intake and output (I&O) record.

Post-Procedure
20. Provided for comfort.
21. Placed the signal light within reach.
22. Unscreened the person.
23. Completed a safety check of the room.
24. Reported and recorded the amount and other observations.

Date of Satisfactory Completion _____   Instructor's Initials _____

Applying a Condom Catheter

Name: _____ Date: _____

	S	U	Comments

Quality of Life
- Knocked before entering the person's room
- Addressed the person by name
- Introduced yourself by name and title
- Explained the procedure to the person before beginning and during the procedure
- Protected the person's rights during the procedure
- Handled the person gently during the procedure

Pre-Procedure
1. Followed *Delegation Guidelines:*
   Condom Catheters
   Saw *Promoting Safety and Comfort:*
   Condom Catheters
2. Practiced hand hygiene.
3. Collected the following:
   - Condom catheter
   - Elastic tape
   - Drainage bag or leg bag
   - Cap for the drainage bag
   - Basin of warm water
   - Soap
   - Towel and washcloth
   - Bath blanket
   - Gloves
   - Waterproof pad
   - Paper towels
4. Arranged paper towels and equipment on the overbed table.
5. Identified the person. Checked the ID bracelet against the assignment sheet. Called the person by name.
6. Provided for privacy.
7. Raised the bed for body mechanics. Bed rails were up if used.

Procedure
8. Lowered the bed rail near you if up.
9. Decontaminated your hands. Put on the gloves.
10. Covered the person with a bath blanket. Lowered top linens to the knees.
11. Asked the person to raise his buttocks off the bed. Or turned him onto his side away from you.
12. Slid the waterproof pad under his buttocks.
13. Had the person lower his buttocks. Or turned him onto his back.
14. Secured the drainage bag to the bed frame. Or had a leg bag ready. Closed the drain.
15. Exposed the genital area.
16. Removed the condom catheter:
    a. Removed the tape. Rolled the sheath off the penis.
    b. Disconnected the drainage tubing from the condom. Capped the drainage tube.
    c. Discarded the tape and condom.
17. Provided perineal care. Observed the penis for reddened areas, skin breakdown, and irritations.
18. Removed the protective backing from the condom. This exposed the adhesive strip.
19. Held the penis firmly. Rolled the condom onto the penis. Left a 1-inch space between the penis and the end of the catheter.

Date of Satisfactory Completion _____ Instructor's Initials _____

Procedure—cont'd	S	U	Comments

20. Secured the condom:
  a. For a self-adhering condom:
    • Pressed the condom to the penis.
  b. For a condom secured with elastic tape:
    • Applied elastic tape in a spiral.
    • Did not apply tape completely around the penis.
21. Made sure the penis tip did not touch the condom. Made sure the condom was not twisted.
22. Connected the condom to the drainage tubing. Coiled and secured excess tubing on the bed. Or attached a leg bag.
23. Removed the waterproof pad and gloves. Discarded them. Practiced hand hygiene.
24. Covered the person. Removed the bath blanket.

Post-Procedure

25. Provided for comfort.
26. Placed the signal light within reach.
27. Lowered the bed to its lowest position.
28. Raised or lowered bed rails. Followed the care plan.
29. Unscreened the person.
30. Decontaminated your hands. Put on clean gloves.
31. Measured and recorded the amount of urine in the bag. Cleaned or discarded the collection bag.
32. Cleaned and returned the wash basin and other equipment. Returned items to their proper place.
33. Removed the gloves. Decontaminated your hands.
34. Completed a safety check of the room.
35. Reported and recorded your observations.

Date of Satisfactory Completion_____ Instructor's Initials _____

Giving a Cleansing Enema

Name: _____   Date: _____

	S	U	Comments

Quality of Life
- Knocked before entering the person's room
- Addressed the person by name
- Introduced yourself by name and title
- Explained the procedure to the person before beginning and during the procedure
- Protected the person's rights during the procedure
- Handled the person gently during the procedure

Pre-Procedure
1. Followed *Delegation Guidelines:*
   Enemas
   Saw *Promoting Safety and Comfort:*
   Enemas
2. Practiced hand hygiene.
3. Collected the following before going to the person's room:
   - Disposable enema kit as directed by the nurse (enema bag, tube, clamp, and waterproof pad)
   - Bath thermometer
   - Waterproof pad (if not part of the enema kit)
   - Water-soluble lubricant
   - 3 to 5 ml (1 teaspoon) castile soap or 1 to 2 teaspoons of salt
   - IV pole
4. Arranged collected items in the person's room or bathroom.
5. Decontaminated your hands.
6. Identified the person. Checked the ID bracelet against the assignment sheet. Called the person by name.
7. Put on gloves.
8. Collected the following:
   - Bedpan and cover or commode
   - Gloves
   - Toilet tissue
   - Bath blanket
   - Robe and non-skid footwear
   - Paper towels
9. Provided for privacy.
10. Raised the bed for body mechanics. Bed rails were up if used.

Procedure
11. Lowered the bed rail near you if up.
12. Removed the gloves and decontaminated your hands. Put on clean gloves.
13. Covered the person with a bath blanket. Fan-folded top linens to the foot of the bed.
14. Positioned the IV pole so the enema bag was 12 inches above the anus. Or it was at the height directed by the nurse.
15. Raised the bed rail if used.
16. Prepared the enema:
    a. Closed the clamp on the tube.
    b. Adjusted water flow until it was lukewarm.
    c. Filled the enema bag for the amount ordered.
    d. Measured water temperature with the bath thermometer. It was 105° F (40.5° C) for adults or center policy.
    e. Prepared the solution as directed by the nurse:
       (1) Tap water: added nothing.
       (2) Saline enema: added salt as directed.
       (3) Soapsuds enema: added castile soap as directed.

Date of Satisfactory Completion_____   Instructor's Initials _____

Procedure—cont'd   S   U   **Comments**

   f. Stirred the solution with the bath thermometer. If suds,
      scooped them off.
   g. Sealed the bag.
   h. Hung the bag on the IV pole.
17. Lowered the bed rail near you if up.
18. Positioned the person in Sims' position or in left
     side-lying position.
19. Placed a waterproof pad under the buttocks.
20. Exposed the anal area.
21. Placed the bedpan behind the person.
22. Positioned the enema tube in the bedpan. Removed the
     cap from the tubing.
23. Opened the clamp. Allowed solution to flow through the tube
     to remove air. Clamped the tube.
24. Lubricated the tube 3 to 4 inches from the tip.
25. Separated the buttocks to see the anus.
26. Asked the person to take a deep breath through the mouth.
27. Inserted the tube gently 3 to 4 inches into the adult's rectum.
     Did this when the person was exhaling. Stopped if the person
     complained of pain, you felt resistance, or bleeding occurred.
28. Checked the amount of solution in the bag.
29. Unclamped the tube. Gave the solution slowly.
30. Asked the person to take slow, deep breaths. This helped
     the person relax.
31. Clamped the tube if the person needed to defecate, had
     cramping, or started to expel solution. Unclamped when
     symptoms subsided.
32. Gave the amount of solution ordered. Stopped if the person
     did not tolerate the procedure.
33. Clamped the tube before it emptied. This prevented air from
     entering the bowel.
34. Held toilet tissue around the tube and against the anus.
     Removed the tube.
35. Discarded toilet tissue into the bedpan.
36. Wrapped the tubing tip with paper towels. Placed it inside
     the enema bag.
37. Helped the person onto the bedpan. Raised the head of
     the bed, and raised the bed rail if used. Or assisted the person
     to the bathroom or commode. The person wore a robe and
     non-skid footwear while up. The bed was in the
     lowest position.
38. Placed the signal light and toilet tissue within reach.
     Reminded the person not to flush the toilet.
39. Discarded disposable items.
40. Removed the gloves. Decontaminated your hands.
41. Left the room if the person could be left alone.
42. Returned when the person signaled Or checked on the person
     every 5 minutes. Knocked before entering.
43. Decontaminated your hands. Put on gloves. Lowered the
     bed rail if up.
44. Observed enema results for amount, color, consistency, shape,
     and odor. Called the nurse to observe results.
45. Provided perineal care as needed.
46. Removed the waterproof pad.

Date of Satisfactory Completion _____ Instructor's Initials _____

Procedure—cont'd

	S	U	Comments
47. Emptied, cleaned, and disinfected equipment. Flushed the toilet after the nurse observed the results.	___	___	_____
48. Returned equipment to its proper place.	___	___	_____
49. Removed the gloves, and practiced hand hygiene.	___	___	_____
50. Assisted with hand washing. Wore gloves for this step.	___	___	_____
51. Covered the person. Removed the bath blanket.	___	___	_____

Post-Procedure

	S	U	Comments
52. Provided for comfort.	___	___	_____
53. Placed the signal light within reach.	___	___	_____
54. Lowered the bed to its lowest position.	___	___	_____
55. Raised or lowered bed rails. Followed the care plan.	___	___	_____
56. Unscreened the person.	___	___	_____
57. Completed a safety check of the room.	___	___	_____
58. Followed center policy for dirty linen and used supplies.	___	___	_____
59. Decontaminated your hands.	___	___	_____
60. Reported and recorded your observations.	___	___	_____

Date of Satisfactory Completion_____ Instructor's Initials _____

Giving a Small-Volume Enema

Name: _____   Date: _____

Quality of Life	S	U	Comments
• Knocked before entering the person's room	_____	_____	_____
• Addressed the person by name	_____	_____	_____
• Introduce yourself by name and title	_____	_____	_____
• Explained the procedure to the person before beginning and during the procedure	_____	_____	_____
• Protected the person's rights during the procedure	_____	_____	_____
• Handled the person gently during the procedure	_____	_____	_____

Pre-Procedure

1. Followed *Delegation Guidelines:*
   Enemas
   Saw *Promoting Safety and Comfort:*
   Enemas   _____ _____ _____
2. Practiced hand hygiene.   _____ _____ _____
3. Collected the following before going to the person's room:
   • Small-volume enema   _____ _____ _____
   • Waterproof pad   _____ _____ _____
4. Arranged items in the person's room.   _____ _____ _____
5. Decontaminated your hands.   _____ _____ _____
6. Identified the person. Checked the ID bracelet against the
   assignment sheet. Called the person by name.   _____ _____ _____
7. Put on gloves.   _____ _____ _____
8. Collected the following:
   • Bedpan and cover or commode   _____ _____ _____
   • Waterproof pad   _____ _____ _____
   • Toilet tissue   _____ _____ _____
   • Gloves   _____ _____ _____
   • Robe and non-skid footwear   _____ _____ _____
   • Bath blanket   _____ _____ _____
9. Provided for privacy.   _____ _____ _____
10. Raised the bed for body mechanics.
    Bed rails were up if used.   _____ _____ _____

Procedure

11. Lowered the bed rail near you if up.   _____ _____ _____
12. Removed the gloves and decontaminated your hands.
    Put on clean gloves.   _____ _____ _____
13. Covered the person with a bath blanket. Fan-folded top
    linens to the foot of the bed.   _____ _____ _____
14. Positioned the person in Sims' position or in left
    side-lying position.   _____ _____ _____
15. Placed a waterproof pad under the buttocks.   _____ _____ _____
16. Exposed the anal area.   _____ _____ _____
17. Placed the bedpan near the person.   _____ _____ _____
18. Removed the cap from the enema tip.   _____ _____ _____
19. Separated the buttocks to see the anus.   _____ _____ _____
20. Asked the person to take a deep breath through the mouth.   _____ _____ _____
21. Inserted the enema tip 2 inches into the rectum. Did this when
    the person was exhaling. Stopped if the person complained
    of pain, you felt resistance, or bleeding occurred.   _____ _____ _____
22. Squeezed and rolled the bottle gently. Released pressure
    on the bottle after you removed the tip from the rectum.   _____ _____ _____
23. Placed the bottle into the box, tip first.   _____ _____ _____

Date of Satisfactory Completion _____   Instructor's Initials _____

Procedure—cont'd S U Comments

24. Helped the person onto the bedpan; raised the head of the bed.
    Raised or lowered bed rails according to the care plan.
    Or assisted the person to the bathroom or commode.
    The person wore a robe and non-skid footwear while up.
    The bed was in the lowest position.
25. Placed the signal light and toilet tissue within reach. Reminded
    the person not to flush the toilet.
26. Discarded disposable items.
27. Removed the gloves. Decontaminated your hands.
28. Left the room if the person could be left alone.
29. Returned when the person signaled Or checked on the person
    every 5 minutes. Knocked before entering.
30. Decontaminated your hands. Put on gloves.
31. Lowered the bed rail if up.
32. Observed enema results for amount, color, consistency, shape,
    and odor. Called the nurse to observe results.
33. Provided perineal care as needed.
34. Removed the waterproof pad.
35. Emptied, cleaned, and disinfected equipment. Flushed the
    toilet after the nurse observed the results.
36. Returned equipment to its proper place.
37. Removed the gloves and practiced hand hygiene.
38. Assisted with hand washing. Wore gloves for this step.
39. Covered the person. Removed the bath blanket.

Post-Procedure

40. Provided for comfort.
41. Placed the signal light within reach.
42. Lowered the bed to its lowest position.
43. Raised or lowered bed rails. Followed the care plan.
44. Unscreened the person.
45. Completed a safety check of the room.
46. Followed center policy for dirty linen and used supplies.
47. Decontaminated your hands.
48. Reported and recorded your observations.

Date of Satisfactory Completion _____ Instructor's Initials _____

Giving an Oil-Retention Enema

Name: _____   Date: _____

Quality of Life	S	U	Comments
• Knocked before entering the person's room	___	___	___
• Addressed the person by name	___	___	___
• Introduced yourself by name and title	___	___	___
• Explained the procedure to the person before beginning and during the procedure	___	___	___
• Protected the person's rights during the procedure	___	___	___
• Handled the person gently during the procedure	___	___	___

Pre-Procedure

1. Followed *Delegation Guidelines:* Enemas. Saw *Promoting Safety and Comfort: Enemas*
2. Practiced hand hygiene.
3. Collected the following before going to the person's room:
   • Oil-retention enema
   • Waterproof pad
4. Arranged items in the person's room.
5. Decontaminated your hands.
6. Identified the person. Checked the ID bracelet against the assignment sheet. Called the person by name.
7. Put on gloves.
8. Collected the following:
   • Gloves
   • Bath blanket
9. Provided for privacy.
10. Raised the bed for body mechanics. Bed rails were up if used.

Procedure

11. Followed these steps:
    a. Lowered the bed rail near you if up.
    b. Removed the gloves and decontaminated your hands. Put on clean gloves.
    b. Covered the person with a bath blanket. Fan-folded top linens to the foot of the bed.
    c. Positioned the person in Sims' position or in left side-lying position.
    d. Placed a waterproof pad under the buttocks.
    e. Exposed the anal area.
    f. Placed the bedpan near the person.
    g. Removed the cap from the enema tip.
    h. Separated the buttocks to see the anus.
    i. Asked the person to take a deep breath through the mouth.
    j. Inserted the enema tip 2 inches into the rectum. Did this when the person was exhaling. Stopped if the person complained of pain, you felt resistance, or bleeding occurred.
    k. Squeezed and rolled the bottle gently. Released pressure on the bottle after you removed the tip from the rectum.
    l. Placed the bottle into the box, tip first.
12. Covered the person. Left the person in the Sims' or left side-lying position.
13. Encouraged the person to retain the enema for the time ordered.
14. Placed more waterproof pads on the bed if needed.
15. Removed the gloves. Decontaminated your hands.

Date of Satisfactory Completion _____ Instructor's Initials _____

Post-Procedure

		S	U	Comments
16.	Provided for comfort.			
17.	Placed the signal light within reach.			
18.	Lowered the bed to its lowest position.			
19.	Raised or lowered bed rails. Followed the care plan.			
20.	Unscreened the person.			
21.	Completed a safety check of the room.			
22.	Followed center policy for dirty linen and used supplies.			
23.	Decontaminated your hands.			
24.	Reported and recorded your observations.			
25.	Checked the person often.			

Date of Satisfactory Completion_____ Instructor's Initials _____

Changing an Ostomy Pouch

Name: _____   Date: _____

	S	U	Comments

Quality of Life
- Knocked before entering the person's room
- Addressed the person by name
- Introduced yourself by name and title
- Explained the procedure to the person before beginning and during the procedure
- Protected the person's rights during the procedure
- Handled the person gently during the procedure

Pre-Procedure
1. Followed *Delegation Guidelines:*
   Ostomy Pouches
   Saw *Promoting Safety and Comfort:*
   Ostomy Pouches
2. Practiced hand hygiene.
3. Collected the following before going to the person's room:
   - Clean pouch with skin barrier
   - Pouch clamp, clip, or wire closure
   - Clean ostomy belt (if used)
   - Gauze pads or washcloths
   - Adhesive remover wipes
   - Skin paste (optional)
   - Pouch deodorant
   - Disposable bag
4. Arranged your work area.
5. Decontaminated your hands.
6. Identified the person. Checked the ID bracelet against the assignment sheet. Called the person by name.
7. Put on gloves.
8. Collected the following:
   - Bedpan with cover
   - Waterproof pad
   - Bath blanket
   - Wash basin with warm water
   - Paper towels
   - Gloves
9. Provided for privacy.
10. Raised the bed for body mechanics. Bed rails were up if used.

Procedure
11. Lowered the bed rail near you if up.
12. Removed the gloves and decontaminated your hands. Put on clean gloves.
13. Covered the person with a bath blanket. Fan-folded top linens to the foot of the bed.
14. Placed a waterproof pad under the buttocks.
15. Disconnected the pouch from the belt if one was worn. Removed the belt.
16. Removed the pouch and skin barrier. Gently pushed the skin down and lifted up on the barrier. Used adhesive remover wipes if necessary.
17. Wiped the stoma and around it with a gauze pad. This removed excess stool and mucus. Discarded the gauze pad into the disposable bag.
18. Wet the gauze or the washcloth.
19. Washed the stoma and around it with a gauze pad or washcloth. Washed gently. Did not scrub or rub the skin.

Date of Satisfactory Completion_____   Instructor's Initials _____

Procedure—cont'd

	S	U	Comments
20. Patted dry with a gauze pad or towel.			
21. Observed the stoma and the skin around the stoma. Reported bleeding, skin irritation, or skin breakdown to the nurse.			
22. Removed the backing from the new pouch.			
23. Applied a thin layer of paste around the pouch opening. Allowed it to dry, following the manufacturer's instructions.			
24. Pulled the skin around the stoma taut. The skin was wrinkle-free.			
25. Centered the pouch over the stoma. The drain pointed downward.			
26. Pressed around the pouch and skin barrier so it sealed to the skin. Applied gentle pressure with your fingers. Started at the bottom and worked up around the sides to the top.			
27. Maintained the pressure for 1 to 2 minutes. Followed the manufacturer's instructions.			
28. Tugged down on the pouch gently.			
29. Added deodorant to the pouch.			
30. Closed the pouch at the bottom. Used a clamp, clip, or wire closure.			
31. Attached the ostomy belt if used. The belt was not too tight. You were able to slide 2 fingers under the belt.			
32. Removed the waterproof pad.			
33. Discarded disposable supplies into a disposable bag.			
34. Removed the gloves. Practiced hand hygiene.			
35. Covered the person. Removed the bath blanket.			

Post-Procedure

	S	U	Comments
36. Provided for comfort.			
37. Placed the signal light within reach.			
38. Lowered the bed to its lowest position.			
39. Raised or lowered bed rails. Followed the care plan.			
40. Unscreened the person.			
41. Decontaminated your hands. Put on gloves.			
42. Took the bedpan and disposable bag into the bathroom.			
43. Emptied the pouch and bedpan into the toilet. Observed the color, amount, consistency, and odor of stools. Flushed the toilet.			
44. Discarded the pouch into the disposable bag. Discarded the disposable bag.			
45. Emptied, cleaned, and disinfected equipment. Returned equipment to its proper place.			
46. Removed gloves. Practiced hand hygiene.			
47. Completed a safety check of the room.			
48. Followed center policy for dirty linens.			
49. Decontaminated your hands.			
50. Reported and recorded your observations.			

Date of Satisfactory Completion _____ Instructor's Initials _____

Measuring Intake and Output (NNAAP™)

Name: _____   Date: _____

Quality of Life	S	U	Comments
• Knocked before entering the person's room	___	___	_____
• Addressed the person by name	___	___	_____
• Introduced yourself by name and title	___	___	_____
• Explained the procedure to the person before beginning and during the procedure	___	___	_____
• Protected the person's rights during the procedure	___	___	_____
• Handled the person gently during the procedure	___	___	_____

Pre-Procedure

1. Followed *Delegation Guidelines:*
   Intake and Output
   Saw *Promoting Safety and Comfort:*
   Intake and Output   ___ ___ _____
2. Practiced hand hygiene.   ___ ___ _____
3. Collected the following:
   • Intake and output (I&O) record   ___ ___ _____
   • Graduates   ___ ___ _____
   • Gloves   ___ ___ _____

Procedure

4. Put on gloves.   ___ ___ _____
5. Measured intake as follows:
   a. Poured liquid remaining in the container into the graduate.   ___ ___ _____
   b. Measured the amount at eye level. Kept the container level.   ___ ___ _____
   c. Checked the serving amount on the I&O record.   ___ ___ _____
   d. Subtracted the remaining amount from the full serving amount. Noted the amount.   ___ ___ _____
   e. Poured fluid in the graduate back into the container.   ___ ___ _____
   f. Repeated steps for each liquid:
      (1) Poured liquid remaining in the container into the graduate.   ___ ___ _____
      (2) Measured the amount at eye level. Kept the container level.   ___ ___ _____
      (3) Checked the serving amount on the I&O record.   ___ ___ _____
      (4) Subtracted the remaining amount from the full serving amount. Noted the amount.   ___ ___ _____
      (5) Poured fluid in the graduate back into the container.   ___ ___ _____
   g. Added the amounts from each liquid together.   ___ ___ _____
   h. Recorded the time and amount on the I&O record.   ___ ___ _____
6. Measured output as follows:
   a. Poured fluid into the graduate used to measure output.   ___ ___ _____
   b. Measured the amount at eye level. Kept the container level.   ___ ___ _____
7. Disposed of fluid in the toilet. Avoided splashes.   ___ ___ _____
8. Cleaned and rinsed the graduates. Disposed of rinse into the toilet. Returned the graduates to their proper place.   ___ ___ _____
9. Cleaned and rinsed the bedpan, urinal, commode container, specimen pan, kidney basin, or other drainage container. Disposed of the rinse into the toilet. Returned item to its proper place.   ___ ___ _____
10. Removed the gloves. Decontaminated your hands.   ___ ___ _____
11. Recorded the output on the I&O record.   ___ ___ _____

Post-Procedure

12. Provided for comfort.   ___ ___ _____
13. Made sure the signal light was within reach.   ___ ___ _____
14. Completed a safety check of the room.   ___ ___ _____
15. Reported and recorded your observations.   ___ ___ _____

Date of Satisfactory Completion_____   Instructor's Initials _____

Preparing the Person for a Meal

Name: _____   Date: _____

Quality of Life	S	U	Comments
• Knocked before entering the person's room			
• Addressed the person by name			
• Introduced yourself by name and title			
• Explained the procedure to the person before beginning and during the procedure			
• Protected the person's rights during the procedure			
• Handled the person gently during the procedure			

Pre-Procedure

1. Followed *Delegation Guidelines:*
   Preparing for Meals
   Saw *Promoting Safety and Comfort:*
   Preparing for Meals
2. Practiced hand hygiene.
3. Collected the following:
   • Equipment for oral hygiene
   • Bedpan and cover, urinal, commode, or specimen pan
   • Toilet tissue
   • Wash basin
   • Soap
   • Washcloth
   • Towel
   • Gloves
4. Provided for privacy.

Procedure

5. Made sure eyeglasses and hearing aids were in place.
6. Assisted with oral hygiene. Made sure dentures were in place. Wore gloves, and decontaminated your hands after removing gloves.
7. Assisted with elimination. Made sure the incontinent person was clean and dry. Wore gloves, and practiced hand hygiene after removed gloves.
8. Assisted with hand washing. Wore gloves, and decontaminated your hands after removed gloves.
9. Did the following if the person was in bed:
   a. Raised the head of the bed to a comfortable position. (Fowler's position preferred.)
   b. Removed items from the overbed table. Cleaned the overbed table.
   c. Adjusted the overbed table in front of the person.
10. Did the following if the person was sitting in a chair:
    a. Positioned the person in a chair or wheelchair.
    b. Removed items from the overbed table. Cleaned the table.
    c. Adjusted the overbed table in front of the person.
11. Assisted the person to the dining area, if the person eats in dining area.

Post-Procedure

12. Provided for comfort.
13. Placed the signal light within reach.
14. Emptied, cleaned, and disinfected equipment. Returned equipment to its proper place. Wore gloves, and decontaminated your hands after removing gloves.
15. Straightened the room. Eliminated unpleasant noise, odors, or equipment.
16. Unscreened the person.
17. Completed a safety check of the room.
18. Decontaminated your hands.

Date of Satisfactory Completion _____   Instructor's Initials _____

Serving Meal Trays

Name: _____   Date: _____

	S	U	Comments

Quality of Life
- Knocked before entering the person's room
- Addressed the person by name
- Introduced yourself by name and title
- Explained the procedure to the person before beginning and during the procedure
- Protected the person's rights during the procedure
- Handle the person gently during the procedure

Pre-Procedure
1. Followed *Delegation Guidelines:*
   Serving Meal Trays
   Saw *Promoting Safety and Comfort:*
   Serving Meal Trays
2. Practiced hand hygiene.

Procedure
3. Made sure the tray was complete. Checked items on the tray with the dietary card. Made sure adaptive equipment was included.
4. Identified the person. Checked the ID bracelet against the assignment sheet. Called the person by name.
5. Placed the tray within the person's reach. Adjusted the overbed table as needed.
6. Removed food covers. Opened cartons, cut meat, buttered bread, and so on, as needed.
7. Placed the napkin, clothes protector, adaptive equipment, and eating utensils within reach.
8. Placed the signal light within reach.
9. Did the following when the person was done eating:
   a. Measured and recorded intake if ordered.
   b. Noted the amount and type of foods eaten.
   c. Checked for and removed any food in the mouth (pocketing). Wore gloves.
   d. Removed the tray.
   e. Cleaned spills. Changed soiled linen and clothing.
   f. Helped the person return to bed if needed.
   g. Assisted with oral hygiene and hand washing. Wore gloves. Decontaminated your hands after removing the gloves.

Post-Procedure
10. Provided for comfort.
11. Placed the signal light within reach.
12. Raised or lowered bed rails. Followed the care plan.
13. Completed a safety check of the room.
14. Followed center policy for soiled linen.
15. Decontaminated your hands.

Date of Satisfactory Completion_____   Instructor's Initials _____

Feeding the Person (NNAAP™)

Name: _____   Date: _____

	S	U	Comments

Quality of Life
- Knocked before entering the person's room
- Addressed the person by name
- Introduced yourself by name and title
- Explained the procedure to the person before beginning and during the procedure
- Protected the person's rights during the procedure
- Handled the person gently during the procedure

Pre-Procedure
1. Followed *Delegation Guidelines:*
   Feeding the Person
   Saw *Promoting Safety and Comfort:*
   Feeding the Person
2. Practiced hand hygiene.
3. Positioned the person in a comfortable position for eating (usually sitting or Fowler's).
4. Got the tray. Placed it on the overbed table or dining table.

Procedure
5. Identified the person. Checked the ID bracelet with the dietary card. Also called the person by name.
6. Draped a napkin across the person's chest and underneath the chin.
7. Told the person what foods and fluids were on the tray.
8. Prepared food for eating. Seasoned foods as the person preferred and was allowed on the care plan.
9. Served foods in the order the person preferred. Identified foods as you served them. Alternated between solid and liquid foods. Used a spoon for safety. Allowed enough time for chewing and swallowing. Did not rush the person.
10. Checked the person's mouth before offering more food or fluids. Made sure the person's mouth was empty between bites and swallows.
11. Used straws for liquids if person could not drink out of a glass or cup. Had one straw for each liquid. Provided short straws for weak persons.
12. Wiped the person's hands, face, and mouth as needed during the meal. Used a napkin.
13. Followed the care plan if the person had dysphagia; checked if the person could use a straw. Gave thickened liquids with a spoon.
14. Conversed with the person in a pleasant manner.
15. Encouraged the person to eat as much as possible.
16. Wiped the person's mouth with a napkin. Discarded the napkin.
17. Noted how much and which foods were eaten.
18. Measured and recorded intake if ordered.
19. Removed the tray.
20. Took the person back to his or her room, if in dining area.
21. Assisted with oral hygiene and hand washing. Provided for privacy, and put on gloves. Decontaminated your hands after removing the gloves.

Date of Satisfactory Completion_____   Instructor's Initials _____

Post-Procedure   S   U   **Comments**

22. Provided for comfort.   _____   _____   _____
23. Placed the signal light within reach.   _____   _____   _____
24. Raised or lowered bed rails. Followed the care plan.   _____   _____   _____
25. Completed a safety check of the room.   _____   _____   _____
26. Returned the food tray to the food cart.   _____   _____   _____
27. Decontaminated your hands.   _____   _____   _____
28. Reported and recorded your observations.   _____   _____   _____

Date of Satisfactory Completion _____   Instructor's Initials _____

Providing Drinking Water

Name: _____   Date: _____

Quality of Life	S	U	Comments
• Knocked before entering the person's room			
• Addressed the person by name			
• Introduced yourself by name and title			
• Explained the procedure to the person before beginning and during the procedure			
• Protected the person's rights during the procedure			
• Handled the person gently during the procedure			

Pre-Procedure
1. Followed *Delegation Guidelines: Providing Drinking Water* Saw *Promoting Safety and Comfort: Providing Drinking Water*
2. Obtained a list of persons who have special fluid orders from the nurse. Or used your assignment sheet.
3. Practiced hand hygiene.
4. Collected the following:
   • Cart
   • Ice chest filled with ice
   • Cover for ice chest
   • Scoop
   • Disposable cups
   • Straws
   • Paper towels
   • Water pitcher for resident use
   • Large water pitcher filled with cold water (optional, depended on center procedure)
   • Towel for the scoop
5. Covered the cart with paper towels. Arranged equipment on top of the paper towels.

Procedure
6. Took the cart to the person's room door. Did not take the cart into the room.
7. Checked the person's fluid orders. Used the list obtained from the nurse.
8. Identified the person. Checked the ID bracelet against the fluid order sheet or your assignment sheet. Also called the person by name.
9. Took the pitcher from the person's overbed table. Emptied it into the bathroom sink.
10. Determined if a new water pitcher was needed.
11. Used the scoop to fill the pitcher with ice. Did not let the scoop touch the rim or the inside of the pitcher.
12. Placed the scoop on the towel.
13. Filled the water pitcher with water. Got water from the bathroom, or used the larger water pitcher on the cart.
14. Placed the pitcher, disposable cup, and straw (if used) on the overbed table. Filled the cup with water. Did not let the water pitcher touch the rim or inside of the cup.
15. Made sure the pitcher, cup, and straw (if used) were within the person's reach.

Post-Procedure
16. Provided for comfort.
17. Placed the signal light within reach.
18. Completed a safety check of the room.

Date of Satisfactory Completion_____   Instructor's Initials _____

Post-Procedure—cont'd   S   U   **Comments**

19. Decontaminated your hands.   _____ _____ _____
20. Repeated for each resident:
    a. Took the cart to the person's room door. Did not take the
       cart into the room.   _____ _____ _____
    b. Checked the person's fluid orders. Used the list obtained
       from the nurse.   _____ _____ _____
    c. Identified the person. Checked the ID bracelet against
       the fluid order sheet or your assignment sheet. Also called
       the person by name.   _____ _____ _____
    d. Took the pitcher from the person's overbed table.
       Emptied it into the bathroom sink. _____ _____ _____
    e. Determined if a new water pitcher was needed. _____ _____ _____
    f. Used the scoop to fill the pitcher with ice. Did not let the
       scoop touch the rim or the inside of the pitcher. _____ _____ _____
    g. Placed the scoop on the towel.   _____ _____ _____
    h. Filled the water pitcher with water. Got water from the
       bathroom, or used the larger water pitcher on the cart. _____ _____ _____
    i. Placed the pitcher, disposable cup, and straw (if used) on
       the overbed table. Filled the cup with water. Did not let the
       water pitcher touch the rim or inside of the cup. _____ _____ _____
    j. Made sure the pitcher, cup, and straw (if used) were within
       the person's reach.
    k. Provided for comfort.   _____ _____ _____
    l. Placed the signal light within reach. _____ _____ _____
    m. Completed a safety check of the room. _____ _____ _____
    n. Decontaminated your hands.   _____ _____ _____

Date of Satisfactory Completion_____ Instructor's Initials _____

Performing Range-of-Motion Exercises (NNAAP™)

Name: _____   Date: _____

Quality of Life	S	U	Comments
• Knocked before entering the person's room	___	___	_____
• Addressed the person by name	___	___	_____
• Introduced yourself by name and title	___	___	_____
• Explained the procedure to the person before beginning and during the procedure	___	___	_____
• Protected the person's rights during the procedure	___	___	_____
• Handled the person gently during the procedure	___	___	_____

Pre-Procedure

1. Followed *Delegation Guidelines:*
   Range-of-Motion Exercises
   Saw *Promoting Safety and Comfort:*
   Range-of-Motion Exercises   ___ ___ _____
2. Practiced hand hygiene.   ___ ___ _____
3. Identified the person. Checked the ID bracelet against the assignment sheet. Called the person by name.   ___ ___ _____
4. Obtained a bath blanket.   ___ ___ _____
5. Provided for privacy.   ___ ___ _____
6. Raised the bed for body mechanics. Bed rails were up if used.   ___ ___ _____

Procedure

7. Lowered the bed rail near you if up.   ___ ___ _____
8. Positioned the person supine.   ___ ___ _____
9. Covered the person with a bath blanket. Fan-folded top linens to the foot of the bed.   ___ ___ _____
10. Exercised the neck *if allowed by the center and if the RN instructed you to do* so:
    a. Placed your hands over the person's ears to support the head. Supported the jaws with your fingers.   ___ ___ _____
    b. Flexionbrought the head forward. The chin touched the chest.   ___ ___ _____
    c. Extension—straightened the head.   ___ ___ _____
    d. Hyperextension—brought the head backward until the chin pointed up.   ___ ___ _____
    e. Rotation—turned the head from side to side.   ___ ___ _____
    f. Lateral flexion—moved the head to the right and to the left.   ___ ___ _____
    g. Repeated flexion, extension, hyperextension, rotation, and lateral flexion 5 times—or the number of times stated on the care plan.   ___ ___ _____
11. Exercised the shoulder:
    a. Grasped the wrist with one hand. Grasped the elbow with the other hand.   ___ ___ _____
    b. Flexion—raised the arm straight in front and over the head.   ___ ___ _____
    c. Extension—brought the arm down to the side.   ___ ___ _____
    d. Hyperextension—moved the arm behind the body. (Did this if the person was sitting in a straight-backed chair or was standing.)   ___ ___ _____
    e. Abduction—moved the straight arm away from the side of the body.   ___ ___ _____
    f. Adduction—moved the straight arm to the side of the body.   ___ ___ _____
    g. Internal rotation—bent the elbow. Placed it at the same level as the shoulder. Moved the forearm down toward the body.   ___ ___ _____
    h. External rotation—moved the forearm toward the head.   ___ ___ _____
    i. Repeated flexion, extension, hyperextension, abduction, adduction, and internal and external rotation 5 times—or the number of times stated on the care plan.   ___ ___ _____

Date of Satisfactory Completion_____   Instructor's Initials _____

Procedure—cont'd	S	U	Comments

12. Exercised the elbow:
   a. Grasped the person's wrist with one hand. Grasped the elbow with your other hand.
   b. Flexion—bent the arm so the same-side shoulder was touched. ___
   c. Extension—straightened the arm.
   d. Repeated flexion and extension 5 times—or the number of times stated on the care plan.
13. Exercised the forearm:
   a. Pronation—turned the hand so the palm was down.
   b. Supination—turned the hand so the palm was up.
   c. Repeated pronation and supination 5 times—or the number of times stated on the care plan.
14. Exercised the wrist:
   a. Held the wrist with both of your hands.
   b. Flexion—bent the hand down.
   c. Extension—straightened the hand.
   d. Hyperextension—bent the hand back.
   e. Radial flexion—turned the hand toward the thumb.
   f. Ulnar flexion—turned the hand toward the little finger.
   g. Repeated flexion, extension, hyperextension, and radial and ulnar flexion 5 times—or the number of times stated on the care plan.
15. Exercised the thumb:
   a. Held the person's hand with one hand. Held the thumb with your other hand.
   b. Abduction—moved the thumb out from the inner part of the index finger.
   c. Adduction—moved the thumb back next to the index finger.
   d. Oppositiontouched each finger with the thumb.
   e. Flexion—bent the thumb into the hand.
   f. Extension—moved the thumb out to the side of the fingers.
   g. Repeated abduction, adduction, opposition, flexion, and extension 5 times—or the number of times stated on the care plan.
16. Exercised the fingers:
   a. Abduction—spread the fingers and the thumb apart.
   b. Adduction—bought the fingers and thumb together.
   c. Extension—straightened the fingers so the fingers, hand, and arm were straight.
   d. Flexion—made a fist.
   e. Repeated abduction, adduction, extension, and flexion 5 times—or the number of times stated on the care plan.
17. Exercised the hip:
   a. Supported the leg. Placed one hand under the knee. Placed your other hand under the ankle.
   b. Flexion—raised the leg.
   c. Extension—straightened the leg.
   d. Abduction—moved the leg away from the body.
   e. Adduction—moved the leg toward the other leg.
   f. Internal rotation—turned the leg inward.
   g. External rotation—turned the leg outward.
   h. Repeated flexion, extension, abduction, adduction, and internal and external rotation 5 times—or the number of times stated on the care plan.

Date of Satisfactory Completion_____   Instructor's Initials _____

Procedure—cont'd   S   U   Comments

18. Exercised the knee:
   a. Supported the knee. Placed one hand under the knee.
      Placed your other hand under the ankle.
   b. Flexion—bent the leg.
   c. Extension—straightened the leg.
   d. Repeated flexion and extension of the knee 5 times—or the
      number of times stated on the care plan.
19. Exercised the ankle:
   a. Supported the foot and ankle. Placed one hand under
      the foot. Placed your other hand under the ankle.
   b. Dorsiflexion—pulled the foot forward. Pushed down on the
      heel at the same time.
   c. Plantar flexion—turned the foot down. Or pointed the toes.
   d. Repeated dorsiflexion and plantar flexion 5 times—or
      the number of time stated on the care plan.
20. Exercised the foot:
   a. Continued to support the foot and ankle.
   b. Pronation—turned the outside of the foot up and the
      inside down.
   c. Supination—turned the inside of the foot up and
      outside down.
   d. Repeated pronation and supination 5 times—or the number
      of times stated on the care plan.
21. Exercised the toes:
   a. Flexion—curled the toes.
   b. Extension—straightened the toes.
   c. Abduction—spread the toes apart.
   d. Adduction—pulled the toes together.
   e. Repeated flexion, extension, abduction, and adduction
      5 times—or the number of times stated on the care plan.
22. Covered the leg. Raised the bed rail if used.
23. Went to the other side. Lowered the bed rail near you if up.
24. Repeated exercises:
   a. Exercised the shoulder:
     (1) Grasped the wrist with one hand. Grasped the elbow
        with the other hand.
     (2) Flexion—raised the arm straight in front and over
        the head.
     (3) Extension—brought the arm down to the side.
     (4) Hyperextension—moved the arm behind the body.
        (Did this if the person was sitting in a straight-backed
        chair or was standing.)
     (5) Abduction—moved the straight arm away from the side
        of the body.
     (6) Adduction—moved the straight arm to the side of
        the body.
     (7) Internal rotation—bent the elbow. Placed it at the same
        level as the shoulder. Moved the forearm down toward
        the body.
     (8) External rotation—moved the forearm toward the head.
     (9) Repeated flexion, extension, hyperextension, abduction,
        adduction, and internal and external rotation 5 times—or
        the number of times stated on the care plan.

Date of Satisfactory Completion_____   Instructor's Initials _____

Procedure—cont'd	S	U	Comments
b. Exercised the elbow:			
(1) Grasped the person's wrist with one hand. Grasped the elbow with your other hand.	___	___	_____
(2) Flexion—bent the arm so the same-side shoulder was touched.	___	___	_____
(3) Extension—straightened the arm.	___	___	_____
(4) Repeated flexion and extension 5 times—or the number of times stated on the care plan.	___	___	_____
c. Exercised the forearm:			
(1) Pronation—turned the hand so the palm was down.	___	___	_____
(2) Supination—turned the hand so the palm was up.	___	___	_____
(3) Repeated pronation and supination 5 times—or the number of times stated on the care plan.	___	___	_____
d. Exercised the wrist:			
(1) Held the wrist with both of your hands.	___	___	_____
(2) Flexion—bent the hand down.	___	___	_____
(3) Extension—straightened the hand.	___	___	_____
(4) Hyperextension—bent the hand back.	___	___	_____
(5) Radial flexion—turned the hand toward the thumb.	___	___	_____
(6) Ulnar flexion—turned the hand toward the little finger.	___	___	_____
(7) Repeated flexion, extension, hyperextension, and radial and ulnar flexion 5 times—or the number of times stated on the care plan.	___	___	_____
e. Exercised the thumb:			
(1) Held the person's hand with one hand. Held the thumb with your other hand.	___	___	_____
(2) Abduction—moved the thumb out from the inner part of the index finger.	___	___	_____
(3) Adduction—moved the thumb back next to the index finger.	___	___	_____
(4) Opposition—touched each finger with the thumb.	___	___	_____
(5) Flexion—bent the thumb into the hand.	___	___	_____
(6) Extension—moved the thumb out to the side of the fingers.	___	___	_____
(7) Repeated abduction, adduction, opposition, flexion, and extension 5 times—or the number of times stated on the care plan.	___	___	_____
f. Exercised the fingers:			
(1) Abduction—spread the fingers and thumb apart.	___	___	_____
(2) Adduction—brought the fingers and thumb together.	___	___	_____
(3) Extension—straightened the fingers so the fingers, hand, and arm were straight.	___	___	_____
(4) Flexion—made a fist.	___	___	_____
(5) Repeated abduction, adduction, extension, and flexion 5 times—or the number of times stated on the care plan.	___	___	_____
g. Exercised the hip:			
(1) Supported the leg. Placed one hand under the knee. Placed your other hand under the ankle.	___	___	_____
(2) Flexion—raised the leg.	___	___	_____
(3) Extension—straightened the leg.	___	___	_____
(4) Abduction—moved the leg away from the body.	___	___	_____
(5) Adduction—moved the leg toward the other leg.	___	___	_____
(6) Internal rotation—turned the leg inward.	___	___	_____
(7) External rotation—turned the leg outward.	___	___	_____
(8) Repeated flexion, extension, abduction, adduction, and internal and external rotation 5 times—or the number of times stated on the care plan.	___	___	_____

Date of Satisfactory Completion_____ Instructor's Initials _____

Procedure—cont'd   S   U   Comments

h. Exercised the knee:
  (1) Supported the knee. Placed one hand under the knee.
    Placed your other hand under the ankle.
  (2) Flexion—bent the leg.
  (3) Extension—straightened the leg.
  (4) Repeated flexion and extension of the knee 5 times—or
    the number of times stated on the care plan.

i. Exercised the ankle:
  (1) Supported the foot and ankle. Placed one hand under
    the foot. Placed your other hand under the ankle.
  (2) Dorsiflexion—pulled the foot forward. Pushed down on
    the heel at the same time.
  (3) Plantar flexion—turned the foot down. Or pointed
    the toes.
  (4) Repeated dorsiflexion and plantar flexion 5 times—or
    the number of time stated on the care plan.

j. Exercised the foot:
  (1) Continued to support the foot and ankle.
  (2) Pronation—turned the outside of the foot up and the
    inside down.
  (3) Supination—turned the inside of the foot up and the
    outside down.
  (4) Repeated pronation and supination 5 times—or the
    number of times stated on the care plan.

k. Exercised the toes:
  (1) Flexion—curled the toes.
  (2) Extension—straightened the toes.
  (3) Abduction—spread the toes apart.
  (4) Adduction—pulled the toes together.
  (5) Repeated flexion, extension, abduction, and
    adduction 5 times—or the number of times stated
    on the care plan.

Post-Procedure
25. Provided for comfort.
26. Removed the bath blanket.
27. Placed the signal light within reach.
28. Lowered the bed to its lowest position.
29. Raised or lowered bed rails. Followed the care plan.
30. Returned the bath blanket its proper place.
31. Unscreened the person.
32. Completed a safety check of the room.
33. Decontaminated your hands.
34. Reported and recorded your observations.

Date of Satisfactory Completion _____   Instructor's Initials _____

Helping the Person Walk (NNAAP™)

Name: _____   Date: _____

Quality of Life	S	U	Comments

Quality of Life
- Knocked before entering the person's room
- Addressed the person by name
- Introduced yourself by name and title
- Explained the procedure to the person before beginning and during the procedure
- Protected the person's rights during the procedure
- Handled the person gently during the procedure

Pre-Procedure
1. Followed *Delegation Guidelines:*
   Ambulation
   Saw *Promoting Safety and Comfort:*
   Ambulation
2. Practiced hand hygiene.
3. Collected the following:
   - Robe and non-skid shoes
   - Paper or sheet to protect bottom linens
   - Gait (transfer) belt
4. Identified the person. Checked the ID bracelet against the assignment sheet. Also called the person by name.
5. Provided for privacy.

Procedure
6. Lowered the bed to its lowest position. Locked the bed wheels. Lowered the bed rail near you if up.
7. Fan-folded top linens to the foot of the bed.
8. Placed the paper or sheet under the person's feet. Put the shoes on the person. Fastened the shoes.
9. Helped the person dangle.
10. Helped the person put on the robe.
11. Applied the gait (transfer) belt.
12. Helped the person stand. Grasped the gait (transfer) belt at each side. If did not use a gait (transfer) belt, placed your arms under the person's arms around to the shoulder blades.
13. Stood at the person's weak side while the person gained balance. Held the belt at the side and back. If did not use a gait belt, had one arm around the back and the other at the elbow to support the person.
14. Encouraged the person to stand erect with the head up and back straight.
15. Helped the person walk. Walked to the side and slightly behind the person on the person's weak side. Provided support with the gait belt. If did not use a gait belt, had one arm around the back and the other at the elbow to support the person. Encouraged the person to use the hand rail on the person's strong side.
16. Encouraged the person to walk normally. The heel struck the floor first. Discouraged shuffling, sliding, or walking on tip-toes.
17. Walked the required distance if the person tolerated the activity. Did not rush the person.
18. Helped the person return to bed. Removed the gait belt.
19. Lowered the head of the bed. Helped the person to the center of the bed.
20. Removed the shoes. Removed the paper or sheet over the bottom sheet.

Date of Satisfactory Completion_____   Instructor's Initials _____

Post-Procedure

		S	U	Comments
21.	Provided for comfort.			
22.	Placed the signal light within reach.			
23.	Raised or lowered bed rails. Followed the care plan.			
24.	Returned the robe and shoes to their proper place.			
25.	Unscreened the person.			
26.	Completed a safety check of the room.			
27.	Decontaminated your hands.			
28.	Reported and recorded your observations.			

Date of Satisfactory Completion_____ Instructor's Initials _____

Using a Pulse Oximeter

Name: _____   Date: _____

Quality of Life	S	U	Comments
• Knocked before entering the person's room	___	___	_____
• Addressed the person by name	___	___	_____
• Introduced yourself by name and title	___	___	_____
• Explained the procedure to the person before beginning and during the procedure	___	___	_____
• Protected the person's rights during the procedure	___	___	_____
• Handled the person gently during the procedure	___	___	_____

Pre-Procedure
1. Followed *Delegation Guidelines: Pulse Oximetry* Saw *Promoting Safety and Comfort: Pulse Oximetry* ___ ___ _____
2. Practiced hand hygiene. ___ ___ _____
3. Collected the following:
   • Oximeter and sensor ___ ___ _____
   • Nail polish remover ___ ___ _____
   • Cotton balls ___ ___ _____
   • Tape ___ ___ _____
   • Towel ___ ___ _____
4. Arranged your work area. ___ ___ _____
5. Decontaminated your hands. ___ ___ _____
6. Identified the person. Checked the ID bracelet against the assignment sheet. Also called the person by name. ___ ___ _____
7. Provided for privacy. ___ ___ _____

Procedure
8. Provided for comfort. ___ ___ _____
9. Removed nail polish from the fingernail or toenail. Used nail polish remover and a cotton ball. ___ ___ _____
10. Dried the site with a towel. ___ ___ _____
11. Clipped or taped the sensor to the site. ___ ___ _____
12. Turned on the oximeter. ___ ___ _____
13. Set the high and low alarm limits for SpO_2 and pulse rate. Turned on audio and visual alarms. (This step for continuous monitoring.) ___ ___ _____
14. Checked the person's pulse (apical or radial) with the pulse on the display. If the pulses were not equal, told the nurse. ___ ___ _____
15. Read the SpO_2 on the display. Noted the value on the flow sheet and your assignment sheet. ___ ___ _____
16. Left the sensor in place for continuous monitoring. Otherwise, turned off the device and removed the sensor.

Post-Procedure
17. Provided for comfort. ___ ___ _____
18. Placed the signal light within reach. ___ ___ _____
19. Unscreened the person. ___ ___ _____
20. Completed a safety check of the room. ___ ___ _____
21. Returned the device to its proper place (unless monitoring was continuous). ___ ___ _____
22. Decontaminated your hands. ___ ___ _____
23. Reported and recorded the SpO_2, the pulse rate, and your other observations. ___ ___ _____

Date of Satisfactory Completion_____ Instructor's Initials _____

Assisting With Deep-Breathing and Coughing Exercises

Name: _____   Date: _____

	S	U	Comments
Quality of Life			
• Knocked before entering the person's room	___	___	_____
• Addressed the person by name	___	___	_____
• Introduced yourself by name and title	___	___	_____
• Explained the procedure to the person before beginning and during the procedure	___	___	_____
• Protected the person's rights during the procedure	___	___	_____
• Handled the person gently during the procedure	___	___	_____

Pre-Procedure

1. Followed *Delegation Guidelines:*
   Deep Breathing and Coughing
   Saw *Promoting Safety and Comfort*:
   Deep Breathing and Coughing
2. Practiced hand hygiene.
3. Identified the person. Checked the ID bracelet against the assignment sheet. Also called the person by name.
4. Provided for privacy.

Procedure

5. Lowered the bed rail if up.
6. Helped the person to a comfortable sitting position: dangling, semi-Fowler's, or Fowler's.
7. Had the person deep breathe:
   a. Had the person place the hands over the rib cage.
   b. Had the person take a deep breath. It should have been as deep as possible. Reminded the person to inhale through the nose.
   c. Asked the person to hold the breath for 2 to 3 seconds.
   d. Asked the person to exhale slowly through pursed lips. Asked the person to exhale until the ribs moved as far down as possible.
   e. Repeated 4 more times:
      (1) Deep breathed in through the nose.
      (2) Held 2 to 3 seconds.
      (3) Exhaled slowly with pursed lips until the ribs moved as far down as possible.
8. Asked the person to cough:
   a. Had the person place both hands over the incision, one hand on top of the other. The person could have held a pillow or folded towel over the incision.
   b. Had the person take a deep breath through the nose.
   c. Asked the person to cough strongly twice with the mouth open.

Post-Procedure

9. Provided for comfort.
10. Placed the signal light within reach.
11. Raised or lowered bed rails. Followed care plan.
12. Unscreened the person.
13. Completed a safety check of the room.
14. Decontaminated your hands.
15. Reported and recorded your observations.

Date of Satisfactory Completion_____   Instructor's Initials _____

Setting Up for Oxygen Administration

Name: _____   Date: _____

	S	U	Comments

Quality of Life
- Knocked before entering the person's room
- Addressed the person by name
- Introduced yourself by name and title
- Explained the procedure to the person before beginning and during the procedure
- Protected the person's rights during the procedure
- Handled the person gently during the procedure

Pre-Procedure
1. Followed *Delegation Guidelines:*
   Oxygen Administration Set-Up
   Saw *Promoting Safety and Comfort:*
   Oxygen Administration Set-Up
2. Practiced hand hygiene.
3. Collected the following before going to the person's room:
   - Oxygen device with connection tubing
   - Flowmeter
   - Humidifier (if ordered)
   - Distilled water (if used humidifier)
4. Arranged your work area.
5. Decontaminated your hands.
6. Identified the person. Checked the ID bracelet against the assignment sheet. Also called the person by name.

Procedure
7. Made sure the flowmeter was in the *OFF* position.
8. Attached the flowmeter to the wall outlet or to the tank.
9. Filled the humidifier with distilled water.
10. Attached the humidifier to the bottom of the flowmeter.
11. Attached the oxygen device and connecting tubing to the humidifier. *Did not set the flowmeter. Did not apply the oxygen device on the person.*
12. Placed the cap securely on the distilled water. Stored the water according to center policy.
13. Discarded the packaging from the oxygen device and connecting tubing.

Post-Procedure
14. Provided for comfort.
15. Placed the signal light within reach.
16. Decontaminated your hands.
17. Completed a safety check of the room.
18. Told the nurse when you were done.
    The nurse:
    a. *Turned on the oxygen and set the flow rate.*
    b. *Applied the oxygen device on the person.*

Date of Satisfactory Completion_____   Instructor's Initials _____

Taking a Temperature With a Glass Thermometer (NNAAP™)

Name: _____   Date: _____

	S	U	Comments

Quality of Life
- Knocked before entering the person's room
- Addressed the person by name
- Introduced yourself by name and title
- Explained the procedure to the person before beginning and during the procedure
- Protected the person's rights during the procedure
- Handled the person gently during the procedure

Pre-Procedure
1. Followed *Delegation Guidelines: Taking Temperatures*
   Saw *Promoting Safety and Comfort:*
   - *Glass Thermometers*
   - *Taking Temperatures*
2. For an *oral temperature*, asked the person not to eat, drink, smoke, or chew gum for at least 15 to 20 minutes or as required by center policy.
3. Practiced hand hygiene.
4. Collected the following:
   - Oral or rectal thermometer and holder
   - Tissues
   - Plastic covers if used
   - Gloves
   - Toilet tissue (rectal temperature)
   - Water-soluble lubricant (rectal temperature)
   - Towel (axillary temperature)
5. Decontaminated your hands.
6. Identified the person. Checked the ID bracelet against the assignment sheet. Also called the person by name.
7. Provided for privacy.

Procedure
8. Put on the gloves.
9. Rinsed the thermometer in cold water if it soaked in disinfectant. Dried it with tissues.
10. Checked for breaks, cracks, or chips.
11. Shook down the thermometer below the lowest number. Held the thermometer by the stem.
12. Inserted it into a plastic cover if used.
13. For an *oral temperature:*
    a. Asked the person to moisten his or her lips.
    b. Placed the bulb end of the thermometer under the tongue and to one side.
    c. Asked the person to close the lips around the thermometer to hold it in place.
    d. Asked the person not to talk. Reminded the person not to bite down on the thermometer.
    e. Left it in place for 2 to 3 minutes or as required by center policy. (*NOTE:* Some state competency tests require leaving the thermometer in place for 3 minutes.)
14. For a *rectal temperature:*
    a. Positioned the person in Sims' position.
    b. Put a small amount of lubricant on a tissue.
    c. Lubricated the bulb end of the thermometer.
    d. Folded back top linens; exposed the anal area.

Date of Satisfactory Completion_____   Instructor's Initials _____

Procedure—cont'd	S	U	Comments
e. Raised the upper buttock; exposed the anus.			
f. Inserted the thermometer 1 inch into the rectum. Did not force the thermometer. Remembered that glass thermometers can break.	___	___	_____
g. Held the thermometer in place for 2 minutes or as required by center policy. Did not let go of it while it was in the rectum.	___	___	_____
15. For an *axillary temperature:*			
a. Helped the person remove an arm from the gown. Did not expose the person.	___	___	_____
b. Dried the axilla with a towel.	___	___	_____
c. Placed the bulb end of the thermometer in the center of the axilla.	___	___	_____
d. Asked the person to place the arm over the chest to hold the thermometer in place. Held it and the arm in place if the person did not help.	___	___	_____
e. Left the thermometer in place for 5 to 10 minutes or as required by center policy.	___	___	_____
16. Removed the thermometer.	___	___	_____
17. Used tissues to remove plastic cover. Discarded the cover and tissues. Wiped the thermometer with a tissue if no cover was used. Wiped from the stem to the bulb end. Discarded the tissue.	___	___	_____
18. Read the thermometer.	___	___	_____
19. Noted the person's name and temperature on your notepad or assignment sheet. Wrote *R* for a rectal temperature. Wrote *A* for an axillary temperature.	___	___	_____
20. For a *rectal temperature*:			
a. Placed used toilet tissue on several thicknesses of toilet tissue.	___	___	_____
b. Placed the thermometer on clean toilet tissue.	___	___	_____
c. Wiped the anal area to remove excess lubricant and any feces.	___	___	_____
d. Covered the person.	___	___	_____
21. For an *axillary temperature:* Helped the person put the gown back on.	___	___	_____
22. Shook down the thermometer.	___	___	_____
23. Cleaned the thermometer according to center policy. Returned it to the holder.	___	___	_____
24. Discarded tissues and disposed of toilet tissue.	___	___	_____
25. Removed the gloves. Decontaminated your hands.	___	___	_____
Post-Procedure			
26. Provided for comfort.	___	___	_____
27. Placed the signal light within reach.	___	___	_____
28. Unscreened the person.	___	___	_____
29. Completed a safety check of the room.	___	___	_____
30. Decontaminated your hands.	___	___	_____
31. Reported and recorded the temperature. Noted the temperature site when reporting and recording. Reported any abnormal temperature at once.	___	___	_____

Date of Satisfactory Completion_____   Instructor's Initials _____

Taking a Temperature With an Electronic Thermometer

Name: _____   Date: _____

Quality of Life	S	U	Comments
• Knocked before entering the person's room	___	___	_____
• Addressed the person by name	___	___	_____
• Introduced yourself by name and title	___	___	_____
• Explained the procedure to the person before beginning and during the procedure	___	___	_____
• Protected the person's rights during the procedure	___	___	_____
• Handled the person gently during the procedure	___	___	_____

Pre-Procedure

1. Followed *Delegation Guidelines:*
   Taking Temperatures
   Saw *Promoting Safety and Comfort:*
   Taking Temperatures
2. For an *oral temperature,* asked the person not to eat, drink, smoke, or chew gum for at least 15 to 20 minutes or as required by center policy.
3. Practiced hand hygiene.
4. Collected the following:
   • Thermometer—electronic, tympanic membrane, temporal artery
   • Probe (blue for an oral or ancillary temperature; red for a rectal temperature)
   • Probe covers
   • Toilet tissue (rectal temperature)
   • Water-soluble lubricant (rectal temperature)
   • Gloves
   • Towel (axillary temperature)
5. Plugged the probe into the thermometer. (Did not do this for a tympanic membrane or temporal artery thermometer.)
6. Decontaminated your hands.
7. Identified the person. Checked the ID bracelet against the assignment sheet. Also called the person by name.

Procedure

8. Provided for privacy. Positioned the person for an oral, rectal, axillary, or tympanic membrane temperature.
9. Put on the gloves if contact with blood, body fluid, secretion, or excretion was likely.
10. Inserted the probe into the probe cover.
11. For an *oral temperature:*
    a. Asked the person to open the mouth and raise the tongue.
    b. Placed the covered probe at the base of the tongue and to one side.
    c. Asked the person to lower the tongue and close the mouth.
12. For a *rectal temperature:*
    a. Put some lubricant on a tissue.
    b. Lubricated the end of the covered probe.
    c. Exposed the anal area.
    d. Raised the upper buttock.
    e. Inserted the probe ½ inch into the rectum.
    f. Held the probe in place.

Date of Satisfactory Completion_____   Instructor's Initials _____

Procedure—cont'd   S   U   **Comments**

13. For *axillary temperature:*
   a. Helped the person remove an arm from the gown. Did not
      expose the person.   _____ _____ _____
   b. Dried the axilla with a towel.   _____ _____ _____
   c. Placed the covered probe in the axilla.   _____ _____ _____
   d. Placed the person's arm over the chest.   _____ _____ _____
   e. Held the probe in place.   _____ _____ _____
14. For a *tympanic membrane temperature:*
   a. Asked the person to turn his or her head so the ear was
      in front of you.   _____ _____ _____
   b. Pulled up and back on the ear to straighten the ear canal.   _____ _____ _____
   c. Inserted the thermometer.   _____ _____ _____
15. Started the thermometer.   _____ _____ _____
16. Held the probe in place until you heard a tone or saw a
   flashing or steady light.   _____ _____ _____
17. Read the temperature on the display.   _____ _____ _____
18. Removed the probe. Pressed the eject button to discard
   the cover.   _____ _____ _____
19. Noted the person's name and temperature on your notepad
   or assignment sheet. Wrote R for a rectal temperature.
   Wrote A for an axillary temperature.   _____ _____ _____
20. Returned it to the holder.   _____ _____ _____
21. Helped the person put the gown back on (axillary
   temperature). For a *rectal temperature:*
   a. Wiped the anal area with toilet tissue to remove lubricant.   _____ _____ _____
   b. Covered the person.   _____ _____ _____
   c. Disposed of used toilet tissue.   _____ _____ _____
   d. Removed the gloves. Decontaminated your hands.   _____ _____ _____

Post-Procedure

22. Provided for comfort.   _____ _____ _____
23. Placed the signal light within reach.   _____ _____ _____
24. Unscreened the person.   _____ _____ _____
25. Completed a safety check of the room.   _____ _____ _____
26. Returned the thermometer to the charging unit.   _____ _____ _____
27. Decontaminated your hands.   _____ _____ _____
28. Reported and recorded the temperature. Noted the
   temperature site when reporting and recording.
   Reported any abnormal temperature at once.   _____ _____ _____

Date of Satisfactory Completion _____ Instructor's Initials _____

Taking a Radial Pulse (NNAAP™)

Name: _____   Date: _____

	S	**U**	**Comments**

Quality of Life
- Knocked before entering the person's room
- Addressed the person by name
- Introduced yourself by name and title
- Explained the procedure to the person before beginning and during the procedure
- Protected the person's rights during the procedure
- Handled the person gently during the procedure

Pre-Procedure
1. Followed *Delegation Guidelines:*
   Taking Pulses
   Saw *Promoting Safety and Comfort:*
   Taking Pulses
2. Practiced hand hygiene.
3. Identified the person. Checked the ID bracelet against the assignment sheet. Called the person by name.
4. Provided for privacy.

Procedure
5. Had the person sit or lie down.
6. Located the radial pulse. Used your first 2 or 3 middle fingers.
7. Noted if the pulse was strong or weak, regular or irregular.
8. Counted the pulse for 30 seconds. Multiplied the number of beats by 2. Or counted the pulse for 1 minute if:
   a. Directed by the nurse and care plan.
   b. Required by center policy.
   c. The pulse was irregular.
   d. Required for your state competency test.
9. Noted the person's name and pulse on your notepad or assignment sheet. Noted the strength of the pulse. Noted if it was regular or irregular.

Post-Procedure
10. Provided for comfort.
11. Placed the signal light within reach.
12. Unscreened the person.
13. Completed a safety check of the room.
14. Decontaminated your hands.
15. Reported and recorded the pulse rate and your observations. Reported an abnormal pulse at once.

Date of Satisfactory Completion_____   Instructor's Initials _____

Taking an Apical Pulse

Name: _____   Date: _____

Quality of Life	S	U	Comments
• Knocked before entering the person's room	___	___	_____
• Addressed the person by name	___	___	_____
• Introduced yourself by name and title	___	___	_____
• Explained the procedure to the person before beginning and during the procedure	___	___	_____
• Protected the person's rights during the procedure	___	___	_____
• Handled the person gently during the procedure	___	___	_____

Pre-Procedure

	S	U	Comments
1. Followed *Delegation Guidelines:* *Taking Pulses* Saw *Promoting Safety and Comfort:* *Using a Stethoscope*	___	___	_____
2. Practiced hand hygiene.	___	___	_____
3. Collected a stethoscope and antiseptic wipes.	___	___	_____
4. Decontaminated your hands.	___	___	_____
5. Identified the person. Checked the ID bracelet against the assignment sheet. Also called the person by name.	___	___	_____
6. Provided for privacy.	___	___	_____

Procedure

	S	U	Comments
7. Cleaned the earpieces and diaphragm with the wipes.	___	___	_____
8. Had the person sit or lie down.	___	___	_____
9. Exposed the nipple area of the left chest. Did not expose a woman's breasts.	___	___	_____
10. Warmed the diaphragm in your palm.	___	___	_____
11. Placed the earpieces in your ears.	___	___	_____
12. Located the apical pulse. Placed the diaphragm 2 to 3 inches to the left of the breastbone and below the left nipple.	___	___	_____
13. Counted the pulse for 1 minute. Noted if the pulse was regular or irregular.	___	___	_____
14. Covered the person. Removed the earpieces.	___	___	_____
15. Noted the person's name and pulse on your notepad or assignment sheet. Noted if the pulse was regular or irregular.	___	___	_____

Post-Procedure

	S	U	Comments
16. Provided for comfort.	___	___	_____
17. Placed the signal light within reach.	___	___	_____
18. Unscreened the person.	___	___	_____
19. Completed a safety check of the room.	___	___	_____
20. Cleaned the earpieces and diaphragm with the wipes.	___	___	_____
21. Returned the stethoscope to its proper place.	___	___	_____
22. Decontaminated your hands.	___	___	_____
23. Reported and recorded your observations. Recorded the pulse rate with *Ap* for apical. Reported an abnormal pulse rate at once.	___	___	_____

Date of Satisfactory Completion _____   Instructor's Initials _____

Taking an Apical-Radial Pulse

Name: _____ Date: _____

	S	**U**	**Comments**

Quality of Life
- Knocked before entering the person's room
- Addressed the person by name
- Introduced yourself by name and title
- Explained the procedure to the person before beginning and during the procedure
- Protected the person's rights during the procedure
- Handled the person gently during the procedure

Pre-Procedure
1. Followed *Delegation Guidelines:*
   Taking Pulses
   Saw *Promoting Safety and Comfort:*
   - *Using a Stethoscope*
   - *Taking Pulses*
2. Asked a nursing team member to help you.
3. Practiced hand hygiene.
4. Collected a stethoscope and antiseptic wipes.
5. Decontaminated your hands.
6. Identified the person. Checked the ID bracelet against the assignment sheet. Also called the person by name.
7. Provided for privacy.

Procedure
8. Cleaned the earpieces and diaphragm with the wipes.
9. Had the person sit or lie down.
10. Exposed the nipple area of the left chest. Did not expose a woman's breasts.
11. Warmed the diaphragm in your palm.
12. Placed the earpieces in your ears.
13. Located the apical pulse. Your helper found the radial pulse.
14. Gave the signal to begin counting.
15. Counted the pulse for 1 minute.
16. Gave the signal to stop counting.
17. Covered the person. Removed the stethoscope earpieces.
18. Noted the person's name and apical and radial pulses on your notepad or assignment sheet. Subtracted the radial pulse from the apical pulse for the pulse deficit. Noted if the pulses were regular or irregular.

Post-Procedure
19. Provided for comfort.
20. Placed the signal light within reach.
21. Unscreened the person.
22. Completed a safety check of the room.
23. Cleaned the earpieces and diaphragm with the wipes.
24. Returned the stethoscope to its proper place.
25. Decontaminated your hands.
26. Reported and recorded your observations. (Reported an abnormal pulse at once.) Included:
    a. The apical and radial pulse rates.
    b. The pulse deficit.

Date of Satisfactory Completion_____ Instructor's Initials _____

Counting Respirations (NNAAP™)

Name: _____   Date: _____

Procedure	S	U	Comments
1. Followed *Delegation Guidelines: Respirations*			
2. Kept your fingers or stethoscope over the pulse site.	___	___	_____
3. Did not tell the person you were counting respirations.	___	___	_____
4. Began counting when the chest rose. Counted each rise and fall of the chest as 1 respiration.	___	___	_____
5. Noted the following:			
a. If respirations were regular.	___	___	_____
b. If both sides of the chest rose equally.	___	___	_____
c. The depth of the respirations.	___	___	_____
d. If the person had any pain or difficulty breathing.	___	___	_____
e. An abnormal respiratory pattern.	___	___	_____
6. Counted respirations for 30 seconds. Multiplied the number by 2. Counted respirations for 1 minute if:	___	___	_____
a. Directed by the nurse and care plan.	___	___	_____
b. Required by center policy.	___	___	_____
c. Respirations were abnormal or irregular.	___	___	_____
d. Required for your state competency test.	___	___	_____
7. Noted the person's name, respiratory rate, and any other observations on your notepad or assignment sheet.	___	___	_____

Post-Procedure

	S	U	Comments
8. Provided for comfort.	___	___	_____
9. Placed the signal light within reach.	___	___	_____
10. Unscreened the person.	___	___	_____
11. Completed a safety check of the room.	___	___	_____
12. Decontaminated your hands.	___	___	_____
13. Reported and recorded the respiratory rate and your observations. Reported abnormal respirations at once.	___	___	_____

Date of Satisfactory Completion _____   Instructor's Initials _____

Measuring Blood Pressure (NNAAP™)

Name: _____   Date: _____

	S	U	Comments

Quality of Life
- Knocked before entering the person's room
- Addressed the person by name
- Introduced yourself by name and title
- Explained the procedure to the person before beginning and during the procedure
- Protected the person's rights during the procedure
- Handled the person gently during the procedure

Pre-Procedure
1. Followed *Delegation Guidelines:*
   Measuring Blood Pressure
   Saw *Promoting Safety and Comfort:*
   - *Using a Stethoscope*
   - *Equipment*
2. Practiced hand hygiene.
3. Collected the following:
   - Sphygmomanometer
   - Stethoscope
   - Antiseptic wipes
4. Decontaminated your hands.
5. Identified the person. Checked the ID bracelet against the assignment sheet. Also called the person by name.
6. Provided for privacy.

Procedure
7. Cleaned the earpieces and diaphragm with the wipes. Warmed the diaphragm in your palm.
8. Had the person sit or lie down.
9. Positioned the person's arm level with the heart. The palm was up.
10. Stood no more than 3 feet away from the manometer. The mercury type was vertical, on a flat surface, and at eye level. The aneroid type was directly in front of you.
11. Exposed the upper arm.
12. Squeezed the cuff to expel any remaining air. Closed the valve on the bulb.
13. Found the brachial artery at the inner aspect of the elbow on the little finger side of the arm. Used your fingertips.
14. Placed the arrow on the cuff over the brachial artery. Wrapped the cuff around the upper arm at least 1 inch above the elbow. It was even and snug.
15. *One-step method:*
    a. Placed the stethoscope earpieces in your ears.
    b. Found the radial or brachial artery.
    c. Inflated the cuff until you could no longer feel the pulse. Noted this point.
    d. Inflated the cuff 30 mm Hg beyond the point where you last felt the pulse.
16. *Two-step method:*
    a. Found the radial or brachial artery.
    b. Inflated the cuff until you could no longer feel the pulse. Noted this point.
    c. Inflated the cuff 30 mm Hg beyond the point where you last felt the pulse.
    d. Deflated the cuff slowly. Noted the point where you felt the pulse.

Date of Satisfactory Completion_____   Instructor's Initials _____

Procedure—cont'd	S	U	Comments
e. Waited 30 seconds.	___	___	_____
f. Placed the stethoscope earpieces in your ears.	___	___	_____
g. Inflated the cuff 30 mm Hg beyond the point where you felt the pulse return.	___	___	_____
17. Placed the diaphragm of the stethoscope over the brachial artery. Did not place it under the cuff.	___	___	_____
18. Deflated the cuff at an even rate of 2 to 4 millimeters per second. Turned the valve counter-clockwise to deflate the cuff.	___	___	_____
19. Noted the point where you heard the first sound. This was the systolic reading. It was near the point where the radial pulse disappeared.	___	___	_____
20. Continued to deflate the cuff. Noted the point where the sound disappeared. This was the diastolic reading.	___	___	_____
21. Deflated the cuff completely. Removed it from the person's arm. Removed the stethoscope earpieces from your ears.	___	___	_____
22. Noted the person's name and blood pressure on your notepad or assignment sheet.	___	___	_____
23. Returned the cuff to the case or the wall holder.	___	___	_____
Post-Procedure			
24. Provided for comfort.	___	___	_____
25. Placed the signal light within reach.	___	___	_____
26. Unscreened the person.	___	___	_____
27. Completed a safety check of the room.	___	___	_____
28. Cleaned the earpieces and diaphragm with the wipes.	___	___	_____
29. Returned the equipment to its proper place.	___	___	_____
30. Decontaminated your hands.	___	___	_____
31. Reported and recorded the blood pressure. Reported an abnormal blood pressure at once.	___	___	_____

Date of Satisfactory Completion_____   Instructor's Initials _____

Preparing the Person for an Examination

Name: _____   Date: _____

	S	U	Comments

Quality of Life
- Knocked before entering the person's room
- Addressed the person by name
- Introduced yourself by name and title
- Explained the procedure to the person before beginning and during the procedure
- Protected the person's rights during the procedure
- Handled the person gently during the procedure

Pre-Procedure
1. Followed *Delegation Guidelines:*
   Preparing the Person
   Saw *Promoting Safety and Comfort:*
   Preparing the Person
2. Practiced hand hygiene.
3. Collected the following:
   - Flashlight
   - Sphygmomanometer
   - Stethoscope
   - Thermometer
   - Tongue depressors (blades)
   - Laryngeal mirror
   - Ophthalmoscope
   - Otoscope
   - Nasal speculum
   - Percussion (reflex) hammer
   - Tuning fork
   - Tape measure
   - Gloves
   - Water-soluble lubricant
   - Vaginal speculum
   - Cotton-tipped applicators
   - Specimen containers and labels
   - Disposable bag
   - Kidney basin
   - Towel
   - Bath blanket
   - Tissues
   - Drape (sheet, bath blanket, drawsheet, or paper drape)
   - Paper towels
   - Cotton balls
   - Waterproof pad
   - Eye chart (Snellen chart)
   - Slides
   - Gown
   - Alcohol wipes
   - Wastebasket
   - Container for soiled instruments
   - Marking pencils or pens
4. Decontaminated your hands.
5. Identified the person. Checked the ID bracelet against the assignment sheet. Also called the person by name.
6. Provided for privacy.

Date of Satisfactory Completion _____   Instructor's Initials _____

Procedure	**S**	**U**	**Comments**
7. Had the person put on the gown. Told the person to remove all clothes. Assisted as needed.	_____	_____	_____
8. Asked the person to void. Offered the bedpan, commode, or urinal if necessary. Provided for privacy.	_____	_____	_____
9. Transported the person to the exam room. (This was not done for an exam in the person's room.)	_____	_____	_____
10. Measured weight and height. Recorded the measurements on the exam form.	_____	_____	_____
11. Helped the person onto the exam table. Provided a step stool if necessary. (Omitted this step for an exam in person's room.)	_____	_____	_____
12. Raised the far bed rail (if used). Raised the bed to its highest level. (Omitted this step if using exam table.)	_____	_____	_____
13. Measured vital signs. Recorded them on the exam form.	_____	_____	_____
14. Positioned the person as directed.	_____	_____	_____
15. Draped the person.	_____	_____	_____
16. Placed a waterproof pad under the buttocks.	_____	_____	_____
17. Raised the bed rail near you if used.	_____	_____	_____
18. Provided adequate lighting.	_____	_____	_____
19. Put the signal light on for the examiner. Did not leave the person alone.	_____	_____	_____

Date of Satisfactory Completion_____ Instructor's Initials _____

Collecting a Random Urine Specimen

Name: _____   Date: _____

	S	U	Comments

Quality of Life
- Knocked before entering the person's room
- Addressed the person by name
- Introduced yourself by name and title
- Explained the procedure to the person before beginning and during the procedure
- Protected the person's rights during the procedure
- Handled the person gently during the procedure

Pre-Procedure
1. Followed *Delegation Guidelines:*
   Urine Specimens
   Saw *Promoting Safety and Comfort:*
   Urine Specimens
2. Practiced hand hygiene.
3. Collected the following:
   - Laboratory requisition slip
   - Specimen container and lid
   - Specimen label
   - Plastic bag
   - *BIOHAZARD* label (if needed)
4. Labeled the specimen container.
5. Arranged collected items in the person's bathroom.
6. Decontaminated your hands.
7. Identified the person. Checked the ID bracelet against the assignment sheet. Also called the person by name.
8. Put on gloves.
9. Collected the following:
   - Voiding receptacle—bedpan and cover, urinal, commode, or specimen pan
   - Graduate to measure output
   - Gloves
10. Provided for privacy.

Procedure
11. Asked the person to void into the receptacle. Reminded the person to put toilet tissue into the wastebasket or toilet. Toilet tissue was not put in the bedpan or specimen pan.
12. Took the receptacle to the bathroom.
13. Poured about 120 ml (4 ounces [4 oz]) into the specimen container.
14. Placed the lid on the specimen container. Put the container in the plastic bag. Did not let the container touch the outside of the bag. Applied a *BIOHAZARD* symbol according to center policy.
15. Measured urine output if ordered. Included the amount in the specimen container.
16. Emptied, cleaned, and disinfected equipment. Returned equipment to its proper place.
17. Removed the gloves, and practiced hand hygiene. Put on clean gloves.
18. Assisted with hand washing.
19. Removed the gloves. Decontaminated your hands.

Date of Satisfactory Completion_____   Instructor's Initials _____

Post-Procedure   S   U   **Comments**

20. Provided for comfort.   _____ _____ _____
21. Placed the signal light within reach.   _____ _____ _____
22. Raised or lowered bed rails. Followed the care plan. _____ _____ _____
23. Unscreened the person.   _____ _____ _____
24. Completed a safety check of the room.   _____ _____ _____
25. Decontaminated your hands.   _____ _____ _____
26. Reported and recorded your observations.   _____ _____ _____
27. Took the specimen and the requisition slip to the storage area. _____ _____ _____

Date of Satisfactory Completion_____ Instructor's Initials _____

Collecting a Midstream Specimen

Name: _____   Date: _____

	S	U	Comments
Quality of Life			
• Knocked before entering the person's room	___	___	_____
• Addressed the person by name	___	___	_____
• Introduced yourself by name and title	___	___	_____
• Explained the procedure to the person before beginning and during the procedure	___	___	_____
• Protected the person's rights during the procedure	___	___	_____
• Handled the person gently during the procedure	___	___	_____

Pre-Procedure
1. Followed *Delegation Guidelines:*
   Urine Specimens
   Saw *Promoting Safety and Comfort:*
   Urine Specimens   ___ ___ _____
2. Practiced hand hygiene.   ___ ___ _____
3. Collected the following:
   • Laboratory requisition slip   ___ ___ _____
   • Midstream specimen kit—includes specimen container, label, and towelettes and may have included sterile gloves   ___ ___ _____
   • Plastic bag   ___ ___ _____
   • Sterile gloves (if not part of kit)   ___ ___ _____
   • *BIOHAZARD* label (if needed)   ___ ___ _____
4. Arranged your work area.   ___ ___ _____
5. Decontaminated your hands.   ___ ___ _____
6. Identified the person. Checked the ID bracelet against the assignment sheet. Also called the person by name.   ___ ___ _____
7. Put on disposable gloves.   ___ ___ _____
8. Collected the following:
   • Voiding receptacle—bedpan and cover, urinal, commode, or specimen pan if needed   ___ ___ _____
   • Supplies for perineal care   ___ ___ _____
   • Graduate to measure output   ___ ___ _____
   • Disposable gloves   ___ ___ _____
   • Paper towel   ___ ___ _____
9. Provided for privacy.   ___ ___ _____

Procedure
10. Provided perineal care. (Wore gloves for this step. Decontaminated your hands after removing gloves.)   ___ ___ _____
11. Opened the sterile kit.   ___ ___ _____
12. Put on the sterile gloves.   ___ ___ _____
13. Opened the packet of towelettes inside the kit.   ___ ___ _____
14. Opened the sterile specimen container. Did not touch the inside of the container or the lid. Set the lid down so the inside faced up.   ___ ___ _____
15. *For a female*—cleaned the perineal area with the towelettes:
    a. Spread the labia with your thumb and index finger. Used your non-dominant hand. (This hand was contaminated and did not touch anything sterile).   ___ ___ _____
    b. Cleaned down the urethral area from front to back. Used a clean towelette for each stroke.   ___ ___ _____
    c. Kept the labia separated to collect the urine specimen.   ___ ___ _____
16. *For a male*—cleaned the penis with towelettes:
    a. Held the penis with your non-dominant hand.   ___ ___ _____
    b. Cleaned the penis starting at the meatus. Cleaned in a circular motion. Started at the center and worked outward.   ___ ___ _____
    c. Kept holding the penis until the specimen was collected.   ___ ___ _____

Date of Satisfactory Completion _____   Instructor's Initials _____

Procedure—cont'd   S   U   Comments

17. Asked the person to void into the receptacle.
18. Passed the specimen container into the stream of urine. (If female, kept the labia separated.)
19. Collected about 30-60 ml (1-2 ounces [1-2 oz]) of urine.
20. Removed the specimen container before the person stopped voiding.
21. Released the labia or penis. Allowed the person to finish voiding into the receptacle.
22. Put the lid on the specimen container. Touched only the outside of the container and lid.
23. Provided toilet tissue after the person was done voiding.
24. Took the receptacle to the bathroom.
25. Measured urine if intake and output (I&O) was ordered. Included the amount in the specimen container.
26. Emptied, cleaned, and disinfected equipment. Returned equipment to its proper place.
27. Removed the gloves and practiced hand hygiene. Put on clean disposable gloves.
28. Labeled the specimen container. Placed the container in the plastic bag. Did not let the container touch the outside of the bag. Applied a *BIOHAZARD* symbol according to center policy.
29. Assisted with hand washing.
30. Removed the gloves. Decontaminated your hands.

Post-Procedure

31. Provided for comfort.
32. Placed the signal light within reach.
33. Raised or lowered bed rails. Followed the care plan.
34. Unscreened the person.
35. Completed a safety check of the room.
36. Decontaminated your hands.
37. Reported and recorded your observations.
38. Took the specimen and the requisition slip to the storage area.

Date of Satisfactory Completion_____ Instructor's Initials_____

Collecting a 24-Hour Urine Specimen

Name: _____   Date: _____

Quality of Life

	S	**U**	**Comments**

- Knocked before entering the person's room
- Addressed the person by name
- Introduced yourself by name and title
- Explained the procedure to the person before beginning and during the procedure
- Protected the person's rights during the procedure
- Handled the person gently during the procedure

Pre-Procedure

1. Followed *Delegation Guidelines:*
   Urine Specimens
   Saw *Promoting Safety and Comfort:*
   - *Urine Specimens*
   - *The 24-Hour Urine Specimen*
2. Practiced hand hygiene.
3. Collected the following:
   - Laboratory requisition slip
   - Urine container for a 24-hour collection
   - Specimen label
   - Preservative if needed
   - Bucket with ice if needed
   - Two "24-hour Urine" labels
   - Funnel
   - *BIOHAZARD* label
4. Arranged collected items in the person's bathroom.
5. Labeled the urine container. Applied the *BIOHAZARD* label.
6. Placed one "24-hour Urine" label in the bathroom.
   Placed the other near the bed.
7. Decontaminated your hands.
8. Identified the person. Checked the ID bracelet against the assignment sheet. Also called the person by name.
9. Put on gloves.
10. Collected the following:
    - Voiding receptacle—bedpan and cover, urinal, commode, or specimen pan
    - Gloves
    - Graduate for output
11. Provided for privacy.

Procedure

12. Asked the person to void. Provided a voiding receptacle.
13. Measured and discarded the urine. Noted the time. This started the 24-hour collection period.
14. Marked the time on the collection container.
15. Emptied, cleaned, and disinfected equipment. Returned equipment to its proper place.
16. Removed the gloves and practiced hand hygiene. Put on clean gloves.
17. Assisted with hand washing.
18. Removed the gloves. Decontaminated your hands.
19. Marked the time the test began and the end time on the room and bathroom labels.
20. Reminded the person to:
    a. Use the voiding receptacle when voiding during the next 24 hours.
    b. Not have a bowel movement when voiding.

Date of Satisfactory Completion_____   Instructor's Initials _____

Procedure—cont'd	S	U	Comments
c. Put toilet tissue in the toilet or wastebasket.	___	___	_____
d. Put on the signal light after voiding.	___	___	_____
21. Returned to the room when the person signaled for you. Knocked before entering the room.	___	___	_____
22. Did the following after every voiding:			
a. Decontaminated your hands. Put on gloves.	___	___	_____
b. Measured urine if I&O was ordered.	___	___	_____
c. Poured urine into the container using the funnel. Did not spill any urine. Restarted the test if you spilled or discarded the urine.	___	___	_____
d. Emptied, cleaned, and disinfected equipment. Returned equipment to its proper place.	___	___	_____
e. Removed the gloves and practiced hand hygiene. Put on clean gloves.	___	___	_____
f. Assisted with hand washing.	___	___	_____
g. Removed the gloves. Decontaminated your hands.	___	___	_____
23. Asked the person to void at the end of the 24-hour period. Then you did the following:	___	___	_____
a. Decontaminated your hands. Put on gloves.	___	___	_____
b. Measured urine if I&O was ordered.	___	___	_____
c. Poured urine into the container using the funnel. Did not spill any urine. Restarted the test if you spilled or discarded the urine.	___	___	_____
d. Emptied, cleaned, and disinfected equipment. Returned equipment to its proper place.	___	___	_____
e. Removed the gloves and practiced hand hygiene. Put on clean gloves.	___	___	_____
f. Assisted with hand washing.	___	___	_____
g. Removed the gloves. Decontaminated your hands.	___	___	_____
Post-Procedure			
24. Provided for comfort.	___	___	_____
25. Placed the signal light within reach.	___	___	_____
26. Raised or lowered bed rails. Followed the care plan.	___	___	_____
27. Put on gloves.	___	___	_____
28. Removed the labels from the room and bathroom.	___	___	_____
29. Cleaned and returned equipment to its proper place. Discarded disposable items.	___	___	_____
30. Removed the gloves. Practiced hand hygiene.	___	___	_____
31. Unscreened the person.	___	___	_____
32. Completed a safety check of the room.	___	___	_____
33. Reported and recorded your observations.	___	___	_____
34. Took the specimen and the requisition slip to the storage area.	___	___	_____

Date of Satisfactory Completion _____   Instructor's Initials _____

Collecting a Double-Voided Specimen

Name: _____   Date: _____

	S	**U**	**Comments**

Quality of Life
- Knocked before entering the person's room
- Addressed the person by name
- Introduced yourself by name and title
- Explained the procedure to the person before beginning and during the procedure
- Protected the person's rights during the procedure
- Handled the person gently during the procedure

Pre-Procedure
1. Followed *Delegation Guidelines:*
   Urine Specimens
   Saw *Promoting Safety and Comfort:*
   Urine Specimens
2. Practiced hand hygiene. Put on gloves.
3. Collected the following:
   - Voiding receptacle—bedpan and cover, urinal, commode, or specimen pan
   - Two specimen containers
   - Urine testing equipment
   - Graduate to measure output
   - Gloves
4. Removed the gloves. Decontaminated your hands.
5. Identified the person. Checked the ID bracelet against the assignment sheet. Also called the person by name.
6. Provided for privacy.

Procedure
7. Put on gloves.
8. Asked the person to void into the receptacle. Reminded the person not to put toilet tissue in the receptacle.
9. Took the receptacle to the bathroom.
10. Measured urine if I&O was ordered.
11. Poured some urine into a specimen container.
12. Tested the specimen in case the person could not provide a second specimen. Discarded the urine. Noted the result on your assignment sheet.
13. Emptied, cleaned, and disinfected equipment. Returned equipment to its proper place.
14. Removed the gloves and practiced hand hygiene. Put on clean gloves.
15. Assisted with hand washing.
16. Removed the gloves. Decontaminated your hands.
17. Asked the person to drink an 8-ounce glass of water.
18. Did the following before leaving the room:
    a. Provided for comfort.
    b. Placed the signal light within reach.
    c. Raised or lowered the bed rails. Followed the care plan.
    d. Unscreened the person.
    e. Completed a safety check of the room.
    f. Decontaminated your hands.
19. Returned to room in 20-30 minutes. Decontaminated your hands.
20. Repeated the following steps:
    a. Practiced hand hygiene. Put on gloves.
    b. Collected the following:
       - Voiding receptacle—bedpan and cover, urinal, commode, or specimen pan

Date of Satisfactory Completion_____   Instructor's Initials _____

Procedure—cont'd   S   U   Comments

- • Two specimen containers
- • Urine testing equipment
- • Graduate to measure output
- • Gloves
- c. Removed the gloves. Decontaminated your hands.
- d. Identified the person. Checked the ID bracelet against the assignment sheet. Also called the person by name.
- e. Provided for privacy.
- f. Put on gloves.
- g. Asked the person to void into the receptacle. Reminded the person not to put toilet tissue in the receptacle.
- h. Took the receptacle to the bathroom.
- i. Measured urine if I&O was ordered.
- j. Poured some urine into a specimen container.
- k. Tested the specimen in case the person could not provide a second specimen. Discarded the urine. Noted the result on your assignment sheet.
- l. Emptied, cleaned, and disinfected equipment. Returned equipment to its proper place.
- m. Removed the gloves and practiced hand hygiene. Put on clean gloves.
- n. Assisted with hand washing.
- o. Removed the gloves. Decontaminated your hands.

Post-Procedure

21. Provided for comfort.
22. Placed the signal light within reach.
23. Raised or lowered bed rails. Followed the care plan.
24. Unscreened the person.
25. Completed a safety check of the room.
26. Decontaminated your hands.
27. Reported and recorded the results of the second test and any other observations.

Date of Satisfactory Completion _____ Instructor's Initials _____

Testing Urine With Reagent Strips

Name: _____   Date: _____

	S	U	Comments

Quality of Life
- Knocked before entering the person's room
- Addressed the person by name
- Introduced yourself by name and title
- Explained the procedure to the person before beginning and during the procedure
- Protected the person's rights during the procedure
- Handled the person gently during the procedure

Pre-Procedure
1. Followed *Delegation Guidelines:*
   Testing Urine
   Saw *Promoting Safety and Comfort:*
   - *Testing Urine*
   - *Using Reagent Strips*
2. Practiced hand hygiene. Put on gloves.
3. Collected the reagent strips ordered.
4. Decontaminated your hands.
5. Identified the person. Checked the ID bracelet against the assignment sheet. Also called the person by name.
6. Put on gloves.
7. Collected the following:
   - Equipment for collecting the urine specimen needed
   - Gloves
8. Provided for privacy.

Procedure
9. Collected the urine specimen, random or double-voided.
10. Removed the strip from the bottle. Put the cap on the bottle at once. It was on tight.
11. Dipped the test strip areas into the urine.
12. Removed the strip after the correct amount of time. Saw the manufacturer's instructions.
13. Tapped the strip gently against the container. This removed excess urine.
14. Waited the required amount of time. Saw the manufacturer's instructions.
15. Compared the strip with the color chart on the bottle. Read the results.
16. Discarded disposable items and the specimen.
17. Emptied, cleaned, and disinfected equipment. Returned equipment to its proper place.
18. Removed the gloves and practiced hand hygiene.

Post-Procedure
19. Provided for comfort.
20. Placed the signal light within reach.
21. Raised or lowered bed rails. Followed the care plan.
22. Unscreened the person.
23. Completed a safety check of the room.
24. Decontaminated your hands.
25. Reported and recorded the results and any other observations.

Date of Satisfactory Completion _____   Instructor's Initials _____

Straining Urine

Name: _____   Date: _____

Quality of Life	S	U	Comments

Quality of Life
- Knocked before entering the person's room
- Addressed the person by name
- Introduced yourself by name and title
- Explained the procedure to the person before beginning and during the procedure
- Protected the person's rights during the procedure
- Handled the person gently during the procedure

Pre-Procedure
1. Followed *Delegation Guidelines:*
   Testing Urine
   Saw *Promoting Safety and Comfort:*
   Testing Urine
2. Practiced hand hygiene. Put on gloves.
3. Collected the following before going to the person's room:
   - Laboratory requisition slip
   - Gauze or strainer
   - Specimen container
   - Specimen label
   - Two "Strain All Urine" labels
   - Plastic bag
   - *BIOHAZARD* label if needed
4. Labeled the specimen container.
5. Arranged collected items in the person's bathroom.
6. Placed one "Strain All Urine" label in the bathroom. Placed the other near the bed.
7. Decontaminated your hands.
8. Identified the person. Checked the ID bracelet against the assignment sheet. Also called the person by name.
9. Put on gloves.
10. Collected the following:
    - Voiding receptacle—bedpan and cover, urinal, commode, or specimen pan
    - Graduate
    - Gloves
11. Provided for privacy.

Procedure
12. Asked the person to use the voiding receptacle for urinating. Asked the person to put on the signal light after voiding.
13. Removed the gloves. Decontaminated your hands.
14. Returned to the room when the person signaled for you. Knocked before entering the room.
15. Decontaminated your hands. Put on gloves.
16. Placed the gauze or strainer into the graduate.
17. Poured urine into the graduate. Urine passed through the gauze or strainer.
18. Placed the gauze or strainer in the specimen container if any crystals, stones, or particles appeared.
19. Placed the specimen container in the plastic bag. Did not let the container touch the outside of the bag. Applied a *BIOHAZARD* symbol according to center policy.
20. Measured urine if intake and output was ordered.
21. Emptied, cleaned, and disinfected equipment. Returned equipment to its proper place.

Date of Satisfactory Completion_____   Instructor's Initials _____

Procedure—cont'd

	S	U	Comments
22. Removed the gloves and practiced hand hygiene. Put on clean gloves.			
23. Assisted with hand washing.	___	___	___
24. Removed the gloves. Decontaminated your hands.	___	___	___

Post-Procedure

	S	U	Comments
25. Provided for comfort.			
26. Placed the signal light within reach.	___	___	___
27. Raised or lowered bed rails. Followed the care plan.	___	___	___
28. Unscreened the person.	___	___	___
29. Completed a safety check of the room.	___	___	___
30. Decontaminated your hands.	___	___	___
31. Reported and recorded your observations.	___	___	___
32. Took the specimen container and requisition slip to the storage are.	___	___	___

Date of Satisfactory Completion_____   Instructor's Initials _____

Collecting a Stool Specimen

Name: _____   Date: _____

	S	U	Comments

Quality of Life
- Knocked before entering the person's room
- Addressed the person by name
- Introduced yourself by name and title
- Explained the procedure to the person before beginning and during the procedure
- Protected the person's rights during the procedure
- Handled the person gently during the procedure

Pre-Procedure
1. Followed *Delegation Guidelines:*
   Stool Specimens
   Saw *Promoting Safety and Comfort:*
   Stool Specimens
2. Practiced hand hygiene.
3. Collected the following before going to the person's room:
   - Laboratory requisition slip
   - Specimen pan for the toilet
   - Specimen container and lid
   - Specimen label
   - Tongue blade
   - Disposable bag
   - Plastic bag
   - *BIOHAZARD* label if needed
4. Labeled the specimen container.
5. Arranged collected items in the person's bathroom.
6. Decontaminated your hands.
7. Identified the person. Checked the ID bracelet against the assignment sheet. Also called the person by name.
8. Put on gloves.
9. Collected the following:
   - Voiding receptacle—bedpan and cover, urinal, commode, or specimen pan
   - Gloves
   - Toilet tissue
10. Provided for privacy.

Procedure
11. Asked the person to void. Provided the receptacle for voiding if the person did not use the bathroom. Emptied, cleaned, and disinfected the device. Returned it to its proper place.
12. Put the specimen pan on the toilet if the person used the bathroom. Placed it at the back of the toilet. Or provided a bedpan or commode.
13. Asked the person not to put toilet tissue into the bedpan, commode, or specimen pan. Provided a bag for toilet tissue.
14. Placed the signal light and toilet tissue within reach. Raised or lowered bed rails. Followed the care plan.
15. Removed the gloves. Decontaminated your hands.
16. Returned when the person signaled. Or checked on the person every 5 minutes. Knocked before entering.
17. Decontaminated your hands. Put on clean gloves.
18. Lowered the bed rail near you if up.
19. Removed the bedpan. Noted the color, amount, consistency, and odor of stools.
20. Provided perineal care if needed.

Date of Satisfactory Completion _____   Instructor's Initials _____

Procedure—cont'd   S   U   Comments

21. Collected the specimen:
    a. Used a tongue blade to take about 2 tablespoons of formed
       or liquid stool to the specimen container.
       Took the sample from the middle of a formed stool.
    b. Included pus, mucus, or blood present in the stool.
    c. Took stool from 2 different places in the bowel movement
       if required by center policy.
    d. Put the lid on the specimen container.
    e. Placed the container in the plastic bag. Did not let the
       container touch the outside of the bag. Applied a
       BIOHAZARD symbol according to center policy.
22. Wrapped the tongue blade in toilet tissue. Discarded it into
    the disposable bag.
23. Emptied, cleaned, and disinfected equipment.
    Returned equipment to its proper place.
24. Removed the gloves and practiced hand hygiene. Put on gloves.
25. Assisted with hand washing.
26. Removed the gloves. Decontaminated your hands.

Post-Procedure
27. Provided for comfort.
28. Placed the signal light within reach.
29. Raised or lowered bed rails. Followed the care plan.
30. Unscreened the person.
31. Completed a safety check of the room.
32. Took the specimen and requisition slip to the storage area.
33. Decontaminated your hands.
34. Reported and recorded your observations.

Date of Satisfactory Completion_____   Instructor's Initials _____

Testing a Stool Specimen for Blood

Name: _____   Date: _____

	S	U	Comments

Quality of Life
- Knocked before entering the person's room
- Addressed the person by name
- Introduced yourself by name and title
- Explained the procedure to the person before beginning and during the procedure
- Protected the person's rights during the procedure
- Handled the person gently during the procedure

Pre-Procedure
1. Followed *Delegation Guidelines: Testing Stool for Blood* Saw *Promoting Safety and Comfort: Testing Stool for Blood*
2. Practiced hand hygiene.
3. Collected the following before going to the person's room:
   - Hemoccult test kit
   - Tongue blades
4. Arranged collected items in the person's bathroom.
5. Decontaminated your hands.
6. Identified the person. Checked the ID bracelet against the assignment sheet. Also called the person by name.
7. Put on gloves.
8. Collected the following:
   - Equipment for collecting a stool specimen
   - Paper towels
   - Gloves
9. Provided for privacy.

Procedure
10. Collected a stool specimen.
11. Practiced hand hygiene. Put on gloves.
12. Opened the test kit.
13. Used a tongue blade to obtain a small amount of stool.
14. Applied a thin smear of stool on *box A* on the test paper.
15. Used another tongue blade to obtain stool from another part of the specimen.
16. Applied a thin smear of stool on *box B* on the test paper.
17. Closed the packet.
18. Turned the test packet to the other side. Opened the flap. Applied developer (from the kit) to *boxes A and B*. Followed manufacturer's instructions.
19. Waited the amount of time noted in the manufacturer's instructions. Time varied from 10 to 60 seconds.
20. Noted the color changes on your assignment sheet.
21. Disposed of test packet.
22. Wrapped the tongue blade in toilet tissue. Then discarded them.
23. Emptied, cleaned, and disinfected equipment. Returned equipment to its proper place.
24. Removed the gloves. Practiced hand hygiene.

Post-Procedure
25. Provided for comfort.
26. Placed the signal light within reach.
27. Raised or lowered bed rails. Followed the care plan.
28. Completed a safety check of the room.
29. Decontaminated your hands.
30. Reported and recorded the test results and your observations.

Date of Satisfactory Completion_____   Instructor's Initials _____

Collecting a Sputum Specimen

Name: _____   Date: _____

	S	U	Comments
Quality of Life			
• Knocked before entering the person's room			
• Addressed the person by name			
• Introduced yourself by name and title			
• Explained the procedure to the person before beginning and during the procedure			
• Protected the person's rights during the procedure			
• Handled the person gently during the procedure			

Pre-Procedure

1. Followed *Delegation Guidelines:*
   Sputum Specimens
   Saw *Promoting Safety and Comfort:*
   Sputum Specimens
2. Practiced hand hygiene.
3. Collected the following before going to the person's room:
   • Laboratory requisition slip
   • Sputum specimen container and lid
   • Specimen label
   • Plastic bag
   • *BIOHAZARD* label if needed
4. Labeled the container.
5. Arranged collected items in the person's bathroom.
6. Decontaminated your hands.
7. Identified the person. Checked the ID bracelet against the assignment sheet. Also called the person by name.
8. Collected gloves and tissues.
9. Provided for privacy. If able, the person used the bathroom for this procedure.

Procedure

10. Put on gloves.
11. Asked the person to rinse the mouth with clear water.
12. Had the person hold the container. Touched only the outside.
13. Asked the person to cover the mouth and nose with tissues when coughing. Followed center policy for used tissues.
14. Asked the person to take 2 or 3 deep breaths and cough up sputum.
15. Had the person expectorate directly into the container. Sputum did not touch the outside of the container.
16. Collected 1 to 2 tablespoons of sputum unless told to collect more.
17. Put the lid on the container.
18. Placed the container in the plastic bag. Did not let the container touch the outside of the bag. Applied a *BIOHAZARD* symbol according to center policy.
19. Removed gloves and decontaminated your hands. Put on clean gloves.
20. Assisted with hand washing.
21. Removed the gloves. Decontaminated your hands.

Date of Satisfactory Completion _____   Instructor's Initials _____

Post-Procedure   S   U   **Comments**

22. Provided for comfort.   _____ _____ _____
23. Placed the signal light within reach.   _____ _____ _____
24. Raised or lowered bed rails. Followed the care plan.   _____ _____ _____
25. Unscreened the person.   _____ _____ _____
26. Completed a safety check of the room.   _____ _____ _____
27. Decontaminated your hands.   _____ _____ _____
28. Took the specimen and requisition slip to the storage area.   _____ _____ _____
29. Decontaminated your hands.   _____ _____ _____
30. Reported and recorded your observations.   _____ _____ _____

Date of Satisfactory Completion_____ Instructor's Initials _____

Preparing the Person's Room

Name: _____   Date: _____

Procedure

	S	U	Comments

1. Followed *Delegation Guidelines:*
   Admitting, Transferring, and Discharging Residents
2. Practiced hand hygiene.
3. Collected the following:
   - Admission kit—wash basin, soap, toothpaste, toothbrush, water pitcher, and cup
   - Bedpan and urinal (if for a man)
   - Admission form
   - Thermometer
   - Sphygmomanometer
   - Stethoscope
   - Gown or pajamas (if needed)
   - Towels and washcloth
   - IV pole (if needed)
   - Other items requested by the nurse
4. Placed the following on the overbed table:
   - Thermometer
   - Sphygmomanometer
   - Stethoscope
   - Admission form
5. Placed the water pitcher and cup on the bedside stand or overbed table.
6. Placed the following in the bedside stand:
   - Admission kit
   - Bedpan and urinal
   - Gown or pajamas
   - Towels and washcloth
7. If the person arrived by stretcher:
   a. Made a surgical bed.
   b. Raised the bed to its highest level.
8. If the person was ambulatory or arrived by wheelchair:
   a. Left the bed closed.
   b. Lowered the bed to its lowest position.
9. Attached the signal light to the bed linens.
10. Decontaminated your hands.

Date of Satisfactory Completion_____   Instructor's Initials _____

Admitting a Person

Name: _____   Date: _____

	S	U	Comments

Quality of Life
- Knocked before entering the person's room
- Addressed the person by name
- Introduced yourself by name and title
- Explained the procedure to the person before beginning and during the procedure
- Protected the person's rights during the procedure
- Handled the person gently during the procedure

Pre-Procedure
1. Followed *Delegation Guidelines*:
   Admitting, Transferring, and Discharging Residents
   Saw *Promoting Safety and Comfort*:
   Admitting, Transferring, and Discharging Residents
2. Practiced hand hygiene.
3. Prepared the room.

Procedure
4. Checked the person's name on the admission form.
5. Greeted the person by name. Asked if he or she preferred a certain name.
6. Introduced yourself to the person and others present. Gave your name and title. Explained that you assist the nurse in giving care.
7. Introduced the roommate.
8. Provided for privacy. Asked family or friends to leave the room. Told them how much time you needed, and directed them to the waiting area. Allowed a family member or friend stay if the person preferred.
9. Allowed the person to stay dressed if his or her condition permitted. Or helped the person change into a gown or pajamas.
10. Provided for comfort. The person was in bed or in a chair as directed by the nurse.
11. Assisted the nurse with assessments:
    a. Measured vital signs.
    b. Measured weight and height.
    c. Collected information for the admission form as requested by the nurse.
12. Completed a clothing and personal belongings list.
13. Helped the person put away clothes and personal items. Put them in the closet, drawers, and bedside stand. (The family may have wanted to help with this step.)
14. Explained ordered activity limits.
15. Oriented the person to the area:
    a. Gave names of the nurses.
    b. Identified items in the bedside stand. Explained the purpose of each.
    c. Explained how to use the overbed table.
    d. Showed how to use the signal light.
    e. Showed how to use the bed, TV, and light controls.
    f. Explained how to make phone calls. Placed the phone within reach.
    g. Showed the person the bathroom. Also showed how to use the signal light in the bathroom.

Date of Satisfactory Completion_____   Instructor's Initials _____

Procedure—cont'd

	S	U	Comments
h. Explained visiting hours and policies.			
i. Explained where to find the nurses' station, lounge, chapel, dining room, and other areas.			
j. Identified staff—housekeeping, dietary, physical therapy, and others.			
k. Explained when meals and nourishments are served.			
16. Filled the water pitcher and cup if oral fluids were allowed.			
17. Placed the signal light within reach.			
18. Placed other controls and needed items within reach.			
19. Provided a denture container if needed. Labeled it with the person's name, room, and bed number.			
20. Labeled the person's property and personal care items with his or her name.			

Post-Procedure

	S	U	Comments
21. Provided for comfort.			
22. Lowered the bed to its lowest position.			
23. Raised or lowered bed rails. Followed the care plan.			
24. Completed a safety check of the room.			
25. Decontaminated your hands.			
26. Reported and recorded your observations.			

Date of Satisfactory Completion_____   Instructor's Initials _____

Measuring Weight and Height (NNAAP™)

Name: _____   Date: _____

Quality of Life	S	U	Comments
• Knocked before entering the person's room	___	___	_____
• Addressed the person by name	___	___	_____
• Introduced yourself by name and title	___	___	_____
• Explained the procedure to the person before beginning and during the procedure	___	___	_____
• Protected the person's rights during the procedure	___	___	_____
• Handled the person gently during the procedure	___	___	_____

Pre-Procedure

1. Followed *Delegation Guidelines: Measuring Weight and Height* Saw *Promoting Safety and Comfort: Measuring Weight and Height* ___ ___ _____
2. Asked the person to void. ___ ___ _____
3. Practiced hand hygiene. ___ ___ _____
4. Brought the scale and paper towels (for standing scale) to the person's room. ___ ___ _____
5. Decontaminated your hands. ___ ___ _____
6. Identified the person. Checked the ID bracelet against the assignment sheet. Also called the person by name. ___ ___ _____
7. Provided for privacy. ___ ___ _____

Procedure

8. Placed the paper towels on the scale platform. ___ ___ _____
9. Raised the height rod. ___ ___ _____
10. Moved the weights to zero (0). The pointer was in the middle. ___ ___ _____
11. Had the person remove the robe and footwear. Assisted as needed. ___ ___ _____
12. Helped the person stand on the scale. The person stood in the center of the scale. Arms were at the sides. ___ ___ _____
13. Moved the weights until the balance pointer was in the middle. ___ ___ _____
14. Noted the weight on your notepad or assignment sheet. ___ ___ _____
15. Asked the person to stand very straight. ___ ___ _____
16. Lowered the height rod until it rested on the person's head. ___ ___ _____
17. Noted the height on your notepad or assignment sheet. ___ ___ _____
18. Raised the height rod. Helped the person step off of the scale. ___ ___ _____
19. Helped the person put on a robe and non-skid footwear if he or she was to be up. Or helped the person back to bed. ___ ___ _____
20. Lowered the height rod. Adjusted the weights to zero (0) if this was center policy. ___ ___ _____

Post-Procedure

21. Provided for comfort. ___ ___ _____
22. Placed the signal light within reach. ___ ___ _____
23. Raised or lowered bed rails. Followed the care plan. ___ ___ _____
24. Unscreened the person. ___ ___ _____
25. Completed a safety check of the room. ___ ___ _____
26. Discarded the paper towels. ___ ___ _____
27. Returned the scale to its proper place. ___ ___ _____
28. Decontaminated your hands. ___ ___ _____
29. Reported and recorded the measurements. ___ ___ _____

Date of Satisfactory Completion_____   Instructor's Initials _____

Measuring Height—The Person Is in Bed

Name: _____   Date: _____

Quality of Life

	S	U	Comments

Quality of Life
- Knocked before entering the person's room
- Addressed the person by name
- Introduced yourself by name and title
- Explained the procedure to the person before beginning and during the procedure
- Protected the person's rights during the procedure
- Handled the person gently during the procedure

Pre-Procedure

1. Followed *Delegation Guidelines:*
   Measuring Weight and Height
   Saw *Promoting Safety and Comfort:*
   Measuring Weight and Height
2. Practiced hand hygiene.
3. Asked a co-worker to help you.
4. Collected a measuring tape and ruler.
5. Decontaminated your hands.
6. Identified the person. Checked the ID bracelet against the assignment sheet. Also called the person by name.
7. Provided for privacy.
8. Raised the bed for body mechanics. Bed rails were up if used.

Procedure

9. Lowered the bed rail near you.
10. Positioned the person supine if the position was allowed.
11. Had your co-worker hold the end of the measuring tape at the person's heel.
12. Pulled the measuring tape along the person's body. Pulled until it extended past the head.
13. Placed the ruler flat across the top of the person's head. It extended from the person's head to the measuring tape. Made sure the ruler was level.
14. Noted the height on your notepad or assignment sheet.

Post-Procedure

15. Provided for comfort.
16. Placed the signal light within reach.
17. Lowered the bed to its lowest position.
18. Raised or lowered bed rails. Followed the care plan.
19. Completed a safety check of the room.
20. Returned equipment to its proper place.
21. Decontaminated your hands.
22. Reported and recorded the height.

Date of Satisfactory Completion_____   Instructor's Initials _____

Transferring the Person to Another Nursing Unit

Name: _____   Date: _____

	S	U	Comments
Quality of Life			
• Knocked before entering the person's room	___	___	_____
• Addressed the person by name	___	___	_____
• Introduced yourself by name and title	___	___	_____
• Explained the procedure to the person before beginning and during the procedure	___	___	_____
• Protected the person's rights during the procedure	___	___	_____
• Handled the person gently during the procedure	___	___	_____

Pre-Procedure

1. Followed *Delegation Guidelines: Admitting, Transferring, and Discharging Residents* Saw *Promoting Safety and Comfort: Admitting, Transferring, and Discharging Residents* ___ ___ _____
2. Asked a co-worker to help you. ___ ___ _____
3. Practiced hand hygiene. ___ ___ _____
4. Collected the following:
   • Wheelchair or stretcher ___ ___ _____
   • Utility cart ___ ___ _____
   • Bath blanket ___ ___ _____
5. Decontaminated your hands. ___ ___ _____
6. Identified the person. Checked the ID bracelet against the assignment sheet. Also called the person by name. ___ ___ _____
7. Provided for privacy. ___ ___ _____

Procedure

8. Collected the person's belongings and care equipment. Placed them on the utility cart. ___ ___ _____
9. Transferred the person to a wheelchair or a stretcher. Covered the person with a blanket. ___ ___ _____
10. Transported the person to the new room. Your co-worker brought the utility cart. ___ ___ _____
11. Helped transfer the person to the bed or chair. Helped position the person. ___ ___ _____
12. Helped arrange the person's belongings and equipment. ___ ___ _____
13. Reported the following to the receiving nurse:
    a. How the person tolerated the transfer. ___ ___ _____
    b. Any observations made during the transfer. ___ ___ _____
    c. That the nurse will bring the medical record, care plan, Kardex, and drugs. ___ ___ _____

Post-Procedure

14. Returned the wheelchair or stretcher and the utility cart to the storage area. ___ ___ _____
15. Decontaminated your hands. ___ ___ _____
16. Reported and recorded the following:
    a. The time of the transfer. ___ ___ _____
    b. Who helped you with the transfer. ___ ___ _____
    c. Where the person was taken. ___ ___ _____
    d. How the person was transferred (bed, wheelchair, or stretcher). ___ ___ _____
    e. How the person tolerated the transfer. ___ ___ _____
    f. Who received the person. ___ ___ _____
    g. Any other observations. ___ ___ _____

Date of Satisfactory Completion_____   Instructor's Initials _____

Procedure Checklists

Chapter 31   357

Post-Procedure—cont'd

	S	U	Comments
17. Stripped the bed, and cleaned the unit. Decontaminated your hands, and put on gloves for this step. (The house-keeping staff may have done this step.)			
18. Removed the gloves. Decontaminated your hands.	___	___	_____
19. Followed center policy for dirty linen.	___	___	_____
20. Made a closed bed.	___	___	_____
21. Decontaminated your hands.	___	___	_____

Date of Satisfactory Completion_____ Instructor's Initials _____

Copyright © 2007, 2003 by Mosby, Inc., an affiliate of Elsevier Inc. All rights reserved.

Discharging the Person

Name: _____   Date: _____

	S	U	Comments

Quality of Life
- Knocked before entering the person's room
- Addressed the person by name
- Introduced yourself by name and title
- Explained the procedure to the person before beginning and during the procedure
- Protected the person's rights during the procedure
- Handled the person gently during the procedure

Pre-Procedure
1. Followed *Delegation Guidelines:*
   Admitting, Transferring, and Discharging Residents
   Saw *Promoting Safety and Comfort:*
   Admitting, Transferring, and Discharging Residents
2. Asked a co-worker to help you.
3. Practiced hand hygiene.
4. Identified the person. Checked the ID bracelet against the assignment sheet. Also called the person by name.
5. Provided for privacy.

Procedure
6. Helped the person dress as needed.
7. Helped the person pack. Checked all drawers and closets. Made sure all items were collected.
8. Checked off the clothing list and personal belongings list. Gave the lists to the nurse.
9. Told the nurse that the person was ready for the final visit. The nurse:
   a. Gave prescriptions written by the doctor.
   b. Provided discharge instructions.
   c. Got valuables from the safe.
   d. Had the person sign the clothing and personal belongings lists.
10. Got a wheelchair and a utility cart for the person's items. Asked a co-worker to help you.
11. Helped the person into the wheelchair.
12. Took the person to the exit area.
13. Locked the wheelchair wheels.
14. Helped the person out of the wheelchair and into the car.
15. Helped put the person's items into the car.

Post-Procedure
16. Returned the wheelchair and cart to the storage area.
17. Decontaminated your hands.
18. Reported and recorded the following:
    a. The time of the discharge.
    b. Who helped you with the discharge.
    c. How the person was transported.
    d. Who was with the person.
    e. The person's destination.
    f. Any other observations.

Date of Satisfactory Completion_____   Instructor's Initials _____

Post-Procedure—cont'd

	S	U	Comments
19. Stripped the bed, and cleaned the unit. Decontaminated your hands, and put on gloves for this step. (The house-keeping staff may have done this step.)			
20. Removed the gloves. Decontaminated your hands.	___	___	_____
21. Followed center policy for dirty linen.	___	___	_____
22. Made a closed bed.	___	___	_____
23. Decontaminated your hands.	___	___	_____

Date of Satisfactory Completion_____ Instructor's Initials _____

Applying Elastic Stockings (NNAAP™)

Name: _____   Date: _____

	S	U	Comments

Quality of Life
- Knocked before entering the person's room
- Addressed the person by name
- Introduced yourself by name and title
- Explained the procedure to the person before beginning and during the procedure
- Protected the person's rights during the procedure
- Handled the person gently during the procedure

Pre-Procedure
1. Followed *Delegation Guidelines:*
   Elastic Stockings
   Saw *Promoting Safety and Comfort:*
   Elastic Stockings
2. Practiced hand hygiene.
3. Obtained elastic stockings in the correct size and length.
4. Identified the person. Checked the ID bracelet against the assignment sheet. Also called the person by name.
5. Provided for privacy.
6. Raised the bed for body mechanics. Bed rail were up if used.

Procedure
7. Lowered the bed rail near you.
8. Positioned the person supine.
9. Exposed the legs. Fan-folded top linens toward the thighs.
10. Turned the stocking inside out down to the heel.
11. Slipped the foot of the stocking over the toes, foot, and heel.
12. Grasped the stocking top. Pulled the stocking up the leg. It turned right side out as it was pulled up. The stocking was even and snug.
13. Removed twists, creases, or wrinkles.
14. Repeated for the other leg:
    a. Turned the stocking inside out down to the heel.
    b. Slipped the foot of the stocking over the toes, foot, and heel.
    c. Grasped the stocking top. Pulled the stocking up the leg. It turned right side out as it was pulled up. The stocking was even and snug.
    d. Removed twists, creases, or wrinkles.

Post-Procedure
15. Covered the person.
16. Provided for comfort.
17. Placed the signal light within reach.
18. Lowered the bed to its lowest position.
19. Raised or lowered bed rails. Followed the care plan.
20. Unscreened the person.
21. Completed a safety check of the room.
22. Decontaminated your hands.
23. Reported and recorded your observations.

Date of Satisfactory Completion_____   Instructor's Initials _____

Applying Elastic Bandages

Name: _____   Date: _____

	S	U	Comments

Quality of Life
- Knocked before entering the person's room
- Addressed the person by name
- Introduced yourself by name and title
- Explained the procedure to the person before beginning and during the procedure
- Protected the person's rights during the procedure
- Handled the person gently during the procedure

Pre-Procedure
1. Followed *Delegation Guidelines:*
   Elastic Bandages
   Saw *Promoting Safety and Comfort:*
   Elastic Bandages
2. Practiced hand hygiene.
3. Collected the following:
   - Elastic bandage as directed by the nurse
   - Tape or clips (unless the bandage was Velcro)
4. Identified the person. Checked the ID bracelet against the assignment sheet. Also called the person by name.
5. Provided for privacy.
6. Raised the bed for body mechanics. Bed rails were up if used.

Procedure
7. Lowered the bed rail near you.
8. Helped the person to a comfortable position. Exposed the part you would bandage.
9. Made sure the area was clean and dry.
10. Held the bandage so the roll was up. The loose end was on the bottom.
11. Applied the bandage to the smallest part of the wrist, foot, ankle, or knee.
12. Made two circular turns around the part.
13. Made overlapping spiral turns in an upward direction. Each turn overlapped about ½ to ⅔ of the previous turn. Made sure the overlap was equal.
14. Applied the bandage smoothly with firm, even pressure. It was not tight.
15. Ended the bandage with two circular turns.
16. Secured the bandage in place with Velcro, tape, or clips. The clips were not under any body part.
17. Checked the fingers or toes for coldness or cyanosis (bluish color). Asked about pain, itching, numbness, or tingling. Removed the bandage if any were noted. Reported your observations to the nurse.

Post-Procedure
18. Provided for comfort.
19. Placed the signal light within reach.
20. Lowered the bed to its lowest position.
21. Raised or lowered bed rails. Followed the care plan.
22. Unscreened the person.
23. Completed a safety check of the room.
24. Decontaminated your hands.
25. Reported and recorded your observations.

Date of Satisfactory Completion_____   Instructor's Initials _____

Applying a Dry, Non-Sterile Dressing

Name: _____   Date: _____

Quality of Life	S	U	Comments
• Knocked before entering the person's room	___	___	___
• Addressed the person by name	___	___	___
• Introduced yourself by name and title	___	___	___
• Explained the procedure to the person before beginning and during the procedure	___	___	___
• Protected the person's rights during the procedure	___	___	___
• Handled the person gently during the procedure	___	___	___

Pre-Procedure

	S	U	Comments
1. Followed *Delegation Guidelines: Applying Dressings* Saw *Promoting Safety and Comfort: Applying Dressings*	___	___	___
2. Practiced hand hygiene.	___	___	___
3. Collected the following:			
• Gloves	___	___	___
• Personal protective equipment as needed	___	___	___
• Tape or Montgomery ties	___	___	___
• Dressings as directed by the nurse	___	___	___
• Saline solution as directed by the nurse	___	___	___
• Cleansing solution as directed by the nurse	___	___	___
• Adhesive remover	___	___	___
• Dressing set with scissors and forceps	___	___	___
• Plastic bag	___	___	___
• Bath blanket	___	___	___
4. Decontaminated your hands.	___	___	___
5. Identified the person. Checked the ID bracelet against the assignment sheet. Also called the person by name.	___	___	___
6. Provided for privacy.	___	___	___
7. Arranged your work area. You did not have to reach over or turn your back on your work area.	___	___	___
8. Raised the bed for body mechanics. Bed rails were up if used.	___	___	___

Procedure

	S	U	Comments
9. Lowered the bed rail near you.	___	___	___
10. Helped the person to a comfortable position.	___	___	___
11. Covered the person with a bath blanket. Fan-folded top linens to the foot of the bed.	___	___	___
12. Exposed the affected body part.	___	___	___
13. Made a cuff on the plastic bag. Placed it within reach.	___	___	___
14. Decontaminated your hands.	___	___	___
15. Put on needed personal protection equipment. Put on gloves.	___	___	___
16. Removed tape or undid Montgomery ties:			
a. *Tape:* Held the skin down. Gently pulled the tape toward the wound.			
b. *Montgomery ties:* Folded ties away from the wound.	___	___	___
17. Removed any adhesive from the skin. Wet a 4 × 4 gauze dressing with adhesive remover. Cleaned away from the wound.	___	___	___
18. Removed gauze dressings. Started with the top dressing and removed each layer. Kept the soiled side of each dressing away from the person's sight. Put dressings in the plastic bag. They did not touch the outside of the bag.	___	___	___
19. Removed the dressing over the wound very gently. If it stuck to the wound or drain site, moistened the dressing with saline.	___	___	___
20. Observed the wound, drain site, and wound drainage.	___	___	___

Date of Satisfactory Completion _____   Instructor's Initials _____

Procedure—cont'd   **S**   **U**   **Comments**

21. Removed the gloves and put them in a plastic bag. Decontaminated your hands.
22. Opened new dressings.
23. Cut the length of tape needed.
24. Put on clean gloves.
25. Cleaned the wound with saline as directed by the nurse.
26. Applied dressings as directed by the nurse.
27. Secured the dressings in place. Used tape or Montgomery ties.
28. Removed the gloves. Put them in the bag.
29. Removed and discarded personal protective equipment.
30. Decontaminated your hands.

Post-Procedure

31. Provided for comfort.
32. Placed the signal light within reach.
33. Lowered the bed to its lowest position.
34. Raised or lowered bed rails. Followed the care plan.
35. Returned equipment and supplies to the proper place. Left extra dressings and tape in the room.
36. Discarded used supplies into the bag. Tied the bag closed. Discarded the bag following center policy. (Wore gloves for this step.)
37. Cleaned your work area. Followed the Bloodborne Pathogen Standard.
38. Unscreened the person.
39. Completed a safety check of the room.
40. Decontaminated your hands.
41. Reported and recorded your observations.

Date of Satisfactory Completion _____ Instructor's Initials _____

Applying Heat and Cold Applications

Name: _____   Date: _____

Quality of Life	S	U	Comments
• Knocked before entering the person's room	___	___	___
• Addressed the person by name	___	___	___
• Introduced yourself by name and title	___	___	___
• Explained the procedure to the person before beginning and during the procedure	___	___	___
• Protected the person's rights during the procedure	___	___	___
• Handled the person gently during the procedure	___	___	___

Pre-Procedure

1. Followed *Delegation Guidelines: Heat and Cold Applications* Saw *Promoting Safety and Comfort: Heat and Cold Applications* ___ ___ ___
2. Practiced hand hygiene. ___ ___ ___
3. Collected the following:
   a. For a *hot compress:*
      • Basin ___ ___ ___
      • Bath thermometer ___ ___ ___
      • Small towel, washcloth, or gauze squares ___ ___ ___
      • Plastic wrap or aquathermia pad ___ ___ ___
      • Ties, tape, or rolled gauze ___ ___ ___
      • Bath towel ___ ___ ___
      • Waterproof pad ___ ___ ___
   b. For a *hot soak:*
      • Water basin or arm or foot bath ___ ___ ___
      • Bath thermometer ___ ___ ___
      • Waterproof pad ___ ___ ___
      • Bath blanket ___ ___ ___
   c. For a *sitz bath:*
      • Disposable sitz bath ___ ___ ___
      • Bath thermometer ___ ___ ___
      • Two bath blankets, bath towels, and a clean gown ___ ___ ___
   d. For a *hot or cold pack:*
      • Commercial pack ___ ___ ___
      • Towel ___ ___ ___
      • Pack cover ___ ___ ___
      • Ties, tape, or rolled gauze (if needed) ___ ___ ___
      • Waterproof pad ___ ___ ___
   e. For an *aquathermia pad:*
      • Aquathermia pad and heating unit ___ ___ ___
      • Distilled water ___ ___ ___
      • Flannel cover or other cover as directed by the nurse ___ ___ ___
      • Ties, tape, or rolled gauze ___ ___ ___
   f. For an *ice bag, ice collar, ice glove, or dry cold pack*:
      • Cold pack or ice bag, collar, or glove ___ ___ ___
      • Crushed ice ___ ___ ___
      • Flannel cover or other cover as directed by the nurse ___ ___ ___
      • Paper towels ___ ___ ___
   g. For a *cold compress:*
      • Large basin with ice ___ ___ ___
      • Small basin with cold water ___ ___ ___
      • Gauze squares, washcloths, or small towels ___ ___ ___
      • Waterproof pad ___ ___ ___

Date of Satisfactory Completion_____   Instructor's Initials _____

Pre-Procedure—cont'd

	S	U	Comments
4. Identified the person. Checked the ID bracelet against the assignment sheet. Also called the person by name.			
5. Provided for privacy.			

Procedure

6. Positioned the person for the procedure.
7. Placed the waterproof pad (if needed) under the body part.
8. For a *hot compress:*
   a. Filled the basin ½ to ⅔ full with hot water as directed by the nurse. Measured water temperature.
   b. Placed the compress in the water.
   c. Wrung out the compress.
   d. Applied the compress over the area. Noted the time.
   e. Covered the compress quickly. Used one of the following as directed by the nurse:
      (1) Applied plastic wrap and then a bath towel. Secured the towel in place with ties, tape, or rolled gauze.
      (2) Applied an aquathermia pad.
9. For a *hot soak:*
   a. Filled a container ½ full with hot water as directed by the nurse. Measured water temperature.
   b. Placed the part into the water. Padded the edge of the container with a towel. Noted the time.
   c. Covered the person with a bath blanket for warmth.
10. For a *sitz bath:*
    a. Placed the disposable sitz bath on the toilet seat.
    b. Filled the sitz bath ⅔ full with water as directed by the nurse. Measured water temperature.
    c. Secured the gown above the waist.
    d. Helped the person sit on the sitz bath. Noted the time.
    e. Provided for warmth. Placed a bath blanket around the shoulders. Placed another over the legs.
    f. Stayed with the person if he or she was weak or unsteady.
11. For a *hot or cold pack:*
    a. Squeezed, kneaded, or struck the pack as directed by the manufacturer's instructions.
    b. Placed the pack in the cover.
    c. Applied the pack. Noted the time.
    d. Secured the pack in place with ties, tape, or rolled gauze. Some packs are secured with Velcro straps.
12. For an *aquathermia pad:*
    a. Filled the heating unit to the fill line with distilled water.
    b. Removed the bubbles. Placed the pad and tubing below the heating unit. Tilted the heating unit from side to side.
    c. Set the temperature as the nurse directed (usually 105° F [40.5° C]). Removed the key. (Gave the key to the nurse after the procedure.)
    d. Placed the pad in the cover.
    e. Plugged in the unit. Allowed water to warm to the desired temperature.
    f. Set the heating unit on the bedside stand. Kept the pad and connecting hoses level with the unit. Hoses did not have kinks.
    g. Applied the pad to the part. Noted the time.
    h. Secured the pad in place with ties, tape, or rolled gauze. Did not use pins.

Date of Satisfactory Completion _____   Instructor's Initials _____

Procedure—cont'd	**S**	**U**	**Comments**

13. For an *ice bag, collar, or glove:*
   a. Filled the device with water. Put in the stopper.
     Turned the device upside down, checked for leaks. _____ _____ _____
   b. Emptied the device. _____ _____ _____
   c. Filled the device ½ to ⅔ full with crushed ice or ice chips. _____ _____ _____
   d. Removed excess air. Bent, twisted, or squeezed the device.
     Or pressed it against a firm surface. _____ _____ _____
   e. Placed the cap or stopper on securely. _____ _____ _____
   f. Dried the device with paper towels. _____ _____ _____
   g. Placed the device in the cover. _____ _____ _____
   h. Applied the device. Noted the time. _____ _____ _____
   i. Secured the device in place with ties, tape, or rolled gauze. _____ _____ _____
14. For a *cold compress:*
   a. Placed the small basin with cold water into the large basin with ice. _____ _____ _____
   b. Placed the compress into the cold water. _____ _____ _____
   c. Wrung out the compress. _____ _____ _____
   d. Applied the compress to the part. Noted the time. _____ _____ _____
15. Placed the signal light within reach. Unscreened the person. _____ _____ _____
16. Raised or lowered bed rails. Followed the care plan. _____ _____ _____
17. Checked the person every 5 minutes. Checked for signs and symptoms of complications. Removed the application if complications occurred. Told the nurse at once. _____ _____ _____
18. Checked the application every 5 minutes. Changed the application if cooling (hot applications) or warming (cold applications) occurred. _____ _____ _____
19. Removed the application at the specified time. Heat and cold applications usually left on for 15 to 20 minutes. (If bed rails were up, lowered the near one for this step.) _____ _____ _____

Post-Procedure
20. Provided for comfort. _____ _____ _____
21. Placed the signal light within reach. _____ _____ _____
22. Raised or lowered bed rails. Followed the care plan. _____ _____ _____
23. Unscreened the person. _____ _____ _____
24. Cleaned and returned re-usable items to the proper place. Followed center policy for soiled linen. Wore gloves. _____ _____ _____
25. Completed a safety check of the room. _____ _____ _____
26. Removed and discarded the gloves. Decontaminated your hands. _____ _____ _____
27. Reported and recorded your observations. _____ _____ _____

Date of Satisfactory Completion_____ Instructor's Initials _____

Caring for Eyeglasses

Name: _____   Date: _____

	S	U	Comments

Quality of Life
- Knocked before entering the person's room
- Addressed the person by name
- Introduced yourself by name and title
- Explained the procedure to the person before beginning and during the procedure
- Protected the person's rights during the procedure
- Handled the person gently during the procedure

Pre-Procedure
1. Followed *Delegation Guidelines:*
   Eyeglasses
   Saw *Promoting Safety and Comfort:*
   Eyeglasses
2. Practiced hand hygiene.
3. Collected the following:
   - Eyeglass case
   - Cleaning solution or warm water
   - Disposable lens cloth or cotton cloth

Procedure
4. Removed the eyeglasses:
   a. Held the frames in front of the ear on both sides.
   b. Lifted the frames from the ears. Brought the eyeglasses down away from the face.
5. Cleaned the lenses with cleaning solution or warm water. Cleaned in a circular motion. Dried the lenses with the cloth.
6. If the person did not wear the glasses:
   a. Opened the eyeglass case.
   b. Folded the glasses. Put them in the case. Did not touch the clean lenses.
   c. Placed the eyeglass case in the top drawer of the bedside stand. Or put it in the drawer of the overbed table.
7. If the person wore the eyeglasses:
   a. Unfolded the eyeglasses.
   b. Held the frames at each side. Placed them over the ears.
   c. Adjusted the eyeglasses so the nosepiece rested on the nose.
   d. Returned the eyeglass case to the top drawer in the bedside stand. Or put it in the drawer of the overbed table.

Post-Procedure
8. Provided for comfort.
9. Placed the signal light within reach.
10. Returned the cleaning solution to its proper place.
11. Discarded the disposable cloth.
12. Completed a safety check of the room.
13. Decontaminated your hands.
14. Reported and recorded your observations.

Date of Satisfactory Completion_____   Instructor's Initials _____

Adult CPR—One Rescuer

Name: _____   Date: _____

Procedure	S	U	Comments
1. Checked if the person was responding. Tapped or gently shook the person, called the person by name, and shouted "Are you OK?"	___	___	_____
2. Called for help. Activated the EMS system or center's emergency response system.	___	___	_____
3. Got the defibrillator (AED).	___	___	_____
4. Positioned the person supine on a hard, flat surface. Logrolled the person so there was no twisting of the spine. Placed the arms alongside the body.	___	___	_____
5. Opened the airway. Used the head tilt-chin lift method.	___	___	_____
6. Checked for adequate breathing. *Looked* to see if the chest rose and fell. *Listened* for the escape of air. *Felt* for the flow of air on your cheek.	___	___	_____
7. Gave 2 rescue breaths if the person was not breathing adequately. Each breath took only 1 second. Each breath made the chest rise. If the first breath did not make the chest rise, tried opening the airway again. Used the head tilt-chin lift method.	___	___	_____
8. Checked for a carotid pulse and for breathing, coughing, and moving. This should have taken 5 to 10 seconds. Used your other hand to keep the airway open with the head tilt-chin lift method. Started chest compressions if there were no signs of circulation.	___	___	_____
9. Gave chest compressions at a rate of 100 per minute. Gave 30 chest compressions followed by 2 rescue breaths. Established a regular rhythm, and counted out loud. (Tried "1 and, 2 and, 3 and, 4 and," and so on, to 30.)	___	___	_____
10. Checked for a carotid pulse every few minutes. Also checked for breathing, coughing, and moving.	___	___	_____
11. Continued CPR if the person had no signs of circulation. Continued the cycle of 30 compressions and 2 breaths. Checked for circulation every few minutes.	___	___	_____
12. Did the following if the person had signs of circulation:			
a. Checked for breathing.	___	___	_____
b. Positioned the person in the recovery position if the person was breathing.	___	___	_____
c. Monitored breathing and circulation.	___	___	_____
13. Did the following if the person had signs of circulation but breathing was absent:			
a. Gave 1 rescue breath every 5 to 6 seconds. This was at a rate of 10 to 12 breaths per minute.	___	___	_____
b. Monitored circulation.	___	___	_____

Date of Satisfactory Completion_____   Instructor's Initials _____

Adult CPR—Two Rescuers

Name: _____   Date: _____

Procedure	S	U	Comments
1. Checked if the person was responding. Tapped or gently shook the person, called the person by name, and shouted "Are you OK?"			
2. Called for help. Activated the EMS system or center's emergency response system.	_____	_____	_____
3. Got the defibrillator (AED). Had your partner ready the AED.	_____	_____	_____
4. Positioned the person supine on a hard, flat surface. Logrolled the person so there was no twisting of the spine. Placed the arms alongside the body.	_____	_____	_____
5. Opened the airway. Used the head tilt-chin lift method.	_____	_____	_____
6. Checked for adequate breathing. *Looked* to see if the chest rose and fell. *Listened* for the escape of air. *Felt* for the flow of air on your cheek.	_____	_____	_____
7. Checked for a carotid pulse and for breathing, coughing, and moving. This should have taken 5 to 10 seconds. Used your other hand to keep the airway open with the head tilt-chin lift method.	_____	_____	_____
8. Performed 2-person CPR if there were no signs of circulation:			
a. One rescuer gave chest compressions at a rate of 100 per minute—30 chest compressions followed by 2 rescue breaths. Established a regular rhythm, and counted out loud. (Tried "1 and, 2 and, 3 and, 4 and," and so on, to 30.)	_____	_____	_____
b. The other rescuer gave 2 rescue breaths after every 30 chest compressions.	_____	_____	_____
c. Changed positions every 2 minutes (after 5 cycles of 30 compressions and 2 breaths). The switch took no more than 5 seconds.	_____	_____	_____
9. Checked for a carotid pulse and for breathing, coughing, and moving every few minutes.	_____	_____	_____

Date of Satisfactory Completion_____   Instructor's Initials _____

Adult CPR With AED—Two Rescuers

Name: _____   Date: _____

Procedure	S	U	Comments

Procedure

1. Rescuer 1: Checked if the person was responding. Tapped or gently shook the person, called the person by name, and shouted "Are you OK?"   _____ _____ _____

2. Rescuer 2: Activated the EMS system or the center's emergency response system. Then got a defibrillaror (AED), and got it ready.   _____ _____ _____

3. Rescuer 1: Positioned the person supine on a hard, flat surface. Logrolled the person so there was no twisting of the spine. Placed the arms alongside the body.   _____ _____ _____

4. Rescuer 2:
   a. Opened the airway. Used the head tilt-chin lift method.   _____ _____ _____
   b. Checked for adequate breathing. *Looked* to see if the chest rises and falls. *Listened* for the escape of air. *Felt* for the flow of air on your cheek.   _____ _____ _____
   c. Gave 2 breaths if the person was not breathing adequately. Each breath took 1 second. Each breath made the chest rise. (If the first breath did not make the chest rise, tried to open the airway again. Used the head tilt-chin lift method.   _____ _____ _____
   d. Checked for a carotid pulse. This should have taken 5 to 10 seconds. Used your other hand to keep the airway open with the head tilt-chin lift method.   _____ _____ _____
   e. Exposed the person's chest.   _____ _____ _____
   f. Gave chest compressions at a rate of 100 per minute —30 chest compressions followed by 2 rescue breaths. Established a regular rhythm, and counted out loud—tried "1 and, 2 and 3, and 4," so on, to 30.   _____ _____ _____
   g. Gave 2 breaths.   _____ _____ _____

5. Rescuer 2:
   a. Opened the case with the AED   _____ _____ _____
   b. Turned on the AED   _____ _____ _____
   c. Attached adult electrode pads to the person's chest. Followed the instructions and diagram provided with the AED.   _____ _____ _____
   d. Attached the connecting cables to the AED.   _____ _____ _____
   e. Cleared away from the person. Made sure no one was touching the person.   _____ _____ _____
   f. Let the AED analyze the person's heart rhythm.   _____ _____ _____
   g. Made sure everyone was clear of the person if the AED advised a "shock."   _____ _____ _____
   h. Pressed the "SHOCK" button when the AED advised a "shock."   _____ _____ _____

6. Rescuers 1 and 2:
   a. Performed 2-person CPR: _____ _____ _____
   b. One rescuer gave chest compressions at the rate of 100 per minute—30 chest compressions followed by 2 breaths. Established a regular rhythm, and counted out loud—tried "1 and, 2 and, 3 and, 4 and," so on, to 30.   _____ _____ _____
   c. The other rescuer gave 2 breaths after every 30 chest compressions.   _____ _____ _____

Date of Satisfactory Completion_____   Instructor's Initials _____

Procedure—cont'd

	S	U	Comments
7. After 2 minutes (5 cycles of 30 compressions and 2 breaths). Rescuer 2:			
a. Cleared away from the person. Made sure no one was touching the person.			
b. Let the AED analyze the person's heart rhythm.	___	___	_____
	___	___	_____
c. Made sure everyone was clear of the person if the AED advised a "shock."			
	___	___	_____
d. Pressed the "SHOCK" button when the AED advised a "shock."			
e. Then continued CPR.	___	___	_____
	___	___	_____

Date of Satisfactory Completion_____   Instructor's Initials _____

Assisting With Postmortem Care

Name: _____   Date: _____

	S	U	Comments

Pre-Procedure

1. Followed *Delegation Guidelines:*
   Postmortem Care
   Saw *Promoting Safety and Comfort:*
   Postmortem Care
2. Practiced hand hygiene.
3. Collected the following:
   - Postmortem kit (shroud or body bag, gown, ID tags, gauze squares, safety pins)
   - Bed protectors
   - Wash basin
   - Bath towel and washcloths
   - Denture cup
   - Tape
   - Dressings
   - Gloves
   - Cotton balls
   - Valuables envelope
4. Provided for privacy.
5. Raised the bed for body mechanics.
6. Made sure the bed was flat.

Procedure

7. Put on gloves.
8. Positioned the body supine. Arms and legs were straight. A pillow was under the head and shoulders. Or raised the head of the bed 15 to 20 degrees if center policy.
9. Closed the eyes. Gently pulled the eyelids over the eyes. Applied moist cotton balls gently over the eyelids if the eyes did not stay closed.
10. Inserted dentures if it was center policy to do so. If not, placed them in a labeled denture cup.
11. Closed the mouth. If necessary, placed a rolled towel under the chin to keep the mouth closed.
12. Followed center policy for jewelry. Removed all jewelry, except for wedding rings if this is center policy. Listed the jewelry that you removed. Placed the jewelry and the list in a valuables envelope.
13. Placed cotton balls over the rings. Taped them in place.
14. Removed drainage containers.
15. Removed tubes and catheters as the nurse directed. Used the gauze squares as needed. Left tubes and catheters in place if there was to be an autopsy.
16. Bathed soiled areas with plain water. Dried thoroughly.
17. Placed a bed protector under the buttocks.
18. Removed soiled dressings. Replaced them with clean ones.
19. Put a clean gown on the body. Positioned the body supine. Arms and legs were straight. A pillow was under the head and shoulders. Or the head of the bed was raised 15 to 20 degrees if center policy.
20. Brushed and combed the hair if necessary.
21. Covered the body to the shoulders with a sheet if the family viewed the person.
22. Gathered the person's belongings. Put them in a bag labeled with the person's name. Made sure you included eyeglasses, hearing aids, and other valuables.

Date of Satisfactory Completion _____   Instructor's Initials _____

Procedure—cont'd

	S	U	Comments
23. Removed supplies, equipment, and linens. Straightened the room. Provided soft lighting.			
24. Removed the gloves. Decontaminated your hands.	___	___	_____
25. Let the family view the body. Provided for privacy. Returned to the room after they left.	___	___	_____
26. Decontaminated your hands. Put on gloves.	___	___	_____
27. Filled out the ID tags. Tied one to the ankle or to the right big toe.	___	___	_____
28. Placed the body in the body bag or covered it with a sheet. Or applied the shroud:			
a. Positioned the shroud under the person.	___	___	_____
b. Brought the top down over the head.	___	___	_____
c. Folded the bottom up over the feet.	___	___	_____
d. Folded the sides over the body.	___	___	_____
e. Pinned or taped the shroud in place.	___	___	_____
29. Attached the second ID tag to the shroud, sheet, or body bag.	___	___	_____
30. Left the denture cup with the body.	___	___	_____
31. Pulled the privacy curtain around the bed. Or closed the door.	___	___	_____

Post-Procedure

	S	U	Comments
32. Removed the gloves. Decontaminated your hands.	___	___	_____
33. Stripped the unit after the body had been removed. Wore gloves.			
34. Removed the gloves. Decontaminated your hands.	___	___	_____
35. Reported the following:			
a. The time the body was taken by the funeral director.	___	___	_____
b. What was done with jewelry, other valuables, and personal items.	___	___	_____
c. What was done with dentures.	___	___	_____

Date of Satisfactory Completion_____   Instructor's Initials _____

Competency Evaluation Review

PREPARING FOR THE COMPETENCY EVALUATION

After completing your state's training program, you need to pass the competency evaluation. The purpose of the competency evaluation is to make sure you can safely do your job. This section will help you prepare for the test.

COMPETENCY EVALUATION

The competency evaluation has a written test and a skills test. The number of questions varies with each state. Each question has four possible answers. Although some questions may appear to have more than one possible answer, there is only *one best* answer. You will have about 1 minute to read and answer each question. Some questions take less time to read and answer. Other questions take longer. You should have enough time to take the test without feeling rushed.

The content of the written test varies, depending on your state. Content may include:
- Activities of Daily Living—hygiene, dressing and grooming, nutrition and hydration, elimination, rest/sleep/comfort
- Basic Nursing Skills—infection control, safety/emergency, therapeutic/technical procedures (e.g., vital signs, bed making), data collection and reporting
- Restorative Skills—prevention, self care/independence
- Emotional and Mental Health Needs
- Spiritual and Cultural Needs
- Communication
- The Person's Rights
- Legal and Ethical Behavior
- Member of the Health Care Team
- Disease Process

The written test is given as a paper and pencil test in most states. Some test sites may use computers. You do not need computer experience to take the test on the computer. If you have difficulty reading English, you may request to take an oral test. Talk with your instructor or employer about details for computer testing or oral testing.

The skills test involves performing five nursing skills that you learned in your training program. These skills are randomly chosen—you do not select the skills. You are allowed about 30 minutes to do the skills. See p. 446 for more information about the skills test.

TAKING THE COMPETENCY EVALUATION

To register for the test, you need to complete an application. Your instructor or employer tells you when and where the tests are given. There is a fee for the evaluation. If you work in a nursing center, the employer pays this fee. If you pay the fee, you may need to purchase a money order or certified check. Make sure your name is on the money order or certified check. Cash and personal checks may not be accepted.

Plan to arrive at the test site about 15 to 30 minutes before the evaluation begins. Most centers do not admit you if you are late. Know the exact location of the test site and room. Actually drive or take transportation to the test site a few days or a week before the test. Making a "dry run" lets you know how much time you need to travel, park, and get to the test site. It will also help decrease your anxiety level.

To be admitted to the test, you need two pieces of identification (ID). The first form of ID is a government-issued document such as a driver's license or passport. It must have a current photo and your signature. The name on the ID must be the same as the name on your application form. If your name has changed and you have not been able to have the name changed on your identification documents, ask your instructor or employer what to do. The second form of ID must include your name and signature. Examples include a library card, hunting license, or credit card.

Take several sharpened Number 2 pencils to the test. For the skills test, you will need a watch with a second hand. You may need a person to play the role of the resident. Ask your instructor or employer how this is done in your state.

Taking the written test and skills test may take several hours. You may want to bring snacks or lunch and a beverage to the testing site. Eating and drinking are not allowed during the test. However, you may be told where you can eat while waiting for the test.

You cannot bring textbooks, study notes, or other materials into the testing room. The only exception may be a language translation dictionary that you show to the proctor (a person who monitors the test) before the test begins. Cell phones, beepers, calculators, or other electronic devices are not permitted during testing. Children and pets are not allowed in the testing areas.

STUDYING FOR THE COMPETENCY EVALUATION

You began to prepare for the written and skills test during your training program. You learned the basic nursing content and skills needed to provide safe, quality care. The following suggestions can help you study for the competency evaluation:
- Begin to study 2 to 3 weeks before the test. Plan to study for 1 to 2 hours each day.
- Decide on a specific time to study. Choose a study time that is best for you. This may be early in the morning before others are awake. It may be in the evening after others go to sleep. Try to choose a time when you are mentally alert.
- Pick a specific area to study in. This area should be quiet, well-lighted, and comfortable. You should have enough room to write and to spread out your books, notes, and other study aids—CD, DVD. The area does not need to be noise-free. The testing site is not absolutely quiet. You want to concentrate and not be distracted by the noise around you.
- Collect everything you need before settling down to study. This includes your textbook, notes, paper, highlighters, pens or pencils, CD, and DVD.

- Take short breaks when you need them. Take a break when your mind begins to wander or if you feel sleepy.
- Develop a study plan. Write your plan down so you can refer to it. Study one content area before going on to the next. For example, study personal hygiene before going on to vital signs. Do not jump from one subject to another.
- Use a variety of ways to study:
  - Use index cards to help you review abbreviations and terminology. Put the abbreviation or term on the front of the card and place the meaning on the back. Take the cards with you and review them whenever you have a break or are waiting.
  - Tape key points. You can listen to the tape while cooking or riding in the car.
  - Study groups are another way to prepare for a test. Group members can quiz each other.
- To remember what you are learning, try these ideas:
  - Relax when you study. When relaxed, you learn information quickly and recall it with greater ease.
  - Repeat what you are learning and say it out loud. This helps you remember the idea.
  - Make the information you are learning meaningful. Think about how the information will help you be a good nursing assistant.
  - Write down what you are learning. Writing helps you remember information. Prepare study sheets.
  - Be positive about what you are learning. You remember what you find interesting.
- Suggestions for studying if you have children:
  - When you first come home from work or school, spend time with your children. Then plan study time.
  - Select educational programs on TV that your children can watch as you study. Or get a CD-ROM from the library.
  - When you take your study breaks, spend time with your children.
  - Ask other adults to take care of the children while you study.
- Take the two 75-question practice tests in this section. Each question has the correct answer and the reason why an answer is correct or incorrect. If you practice taking tests, you are more likely to pass them. Take the practice tests under conditions similar to the real test. Work within time limits.
- If your state has a practice test and a candidate handbook, study the content. Some states have practice tests on-line.

MANAGING ANXIETY

Almost everyone dreads taking tests. It is common and normal to experience anxiety before taking a test. If used wisely, anxiety can actually help you do well. When you are anxious, that means you are concerned. You may be concerned about how prepared you are to take the test. Or you may be concerned about how you will feel about yourself if you do not pass the test. Being concerned usually results in some action. To overcome anxiety before the test:

- Study and prepare for the test. That helps increase your confidence as you recall or clarify what you have learned. Anxiety decreases as confidence increases.
  When you think you know the information, keep studying. This reinforces your learning.
- Develop a positive mental attitude. You can pass this test. You took tests in your training program and passed them. Praise yourself. Talk to yourself in a positive way. If a negative thought enters your mind, stop it at once. Challenge the mental thought and tell yourself you will pass the test.
- Visualize success. Think about how wonderful you will feel when you are notified that you have passed the test.
- Perform breathing exercises. Breathe slowly and deeply.
- Perform regular exercise. Exercise helps you stay physically fit. It also helps keep you calm.
- Good nourishment helps you think clearly. Eat a nourishing meal before the test. Do not skip breakfast. Vitamin C helps fight short-term stress. Protein and calcium help overcome the effects of long-term stress. Complex carbohydrates (pasta, nuts, yogurt) can help settle your nerves. Eat familiar foods the day before and the day of the test. Do not eat foods that could cause stomach or intestinal upset.
- Maintain a normal routine the day before the test.
- Get a good night's sleep before the test. Go to bed early enough so you do not oversleep or are too tired to get up. Set your alarm clock properly. You may want to set two alarm clocks.
- Do not "cram" the evening before or the day of the test. Last minute cramming increases your anxiety. Do something relaxing with family and friends.
- Avoid drinking large amounts of coffee, colas, water, or other beverages. You do not want to be uncomfortable with a full bladder when you take the test.
- Wear comfortable clothes. Dress in layers so that you are prepared for a cold or warm room.
- If you are a woman, remember that worry and anxiety can affect your menstrual cycle. Wear a panty liner, sanitary napkin, or tampon if you think your period may start. This eliminates worry about soiling your clothing during the test.
- Allow plenty of time for travel, traffic, and parking.
- Arrive early enough to use the restroom before the test begins.
- Do not talk about the test with others. Their panic or anxiety may affect your self-confidence.

TAKING THE TEST

Follow these guidelines for taking the test:
- Listen carefully, and follow all the instructions given by the proctor (person administering the test).
- When you receive the test, make certain you have all the test pages.
- Read and follow all directions carefully.
- You are not allowed to ask questions about the content of the test questions.
- Do deep-breathing and muscle-relaxation exercises as needed.
- Cheating of any kind is not allowed. If the proctor sees you giving or receiving any type of assistance, your test booklet is taken and you must leave the testing site.
- If using a computer answer sheet, completely fill in the bubble.

- If you make a mistake, erase the wrong answer completely. Do not make any stray marks on the paper. Not erasing completely or leaving stray marks could cause the computer to misread your answer.
- Do not worry or get anxious if people finish the test before you do. Persons who finish a test early do not necessarily have a better score than those who finish later.
- You cannot take any evaluation or materials or notes out of the testing room.

ANSWERING MULTIPLE CHOICE QUESTIONS

Pace yourself during the test. First, answer all the questions that you know. Then go back and answer skipped questions. Sometimes you will remember the answer later. Or another test question may give you a clue to the one you skipped. Spending too much time on a question can cost you valuable time later. To help you answer the questions or statements:

- Always read the questions or statements carefully. Do not scan or glance at questions. Scanning or glancing can cause you to miss important key words. Read each word of the question.
- Before reading the answers, decide what the answer is in your own words. Then read all four answers to the question. Select the one *best* answer.
- Do not read into a question. Take the question as it is asked. Do not add your own thoughts and ideas to the question. Do not assume or suppose "what if." Just respond to the information provided.
- Trust your common sense. If unsure of an answer, select your first choice. Do not change your answer unless you are absolutely sure of the correct answer. Your first reaction is usually correct.
- Look for key words in every question. Sometimes key words are in italics, highlighted, or underlined. Common key words are: always, never, first, except, best, not, correct, incorrect, true, or false.
- Know which words can make a statement correct (i.e., may, can, usually, most, at least, sometimes). The word "except" can make a question a false statement.
- Be careful of answers with these key words or phrases: always, never, every, only, all, none, at all times, or at no time. These words and phrases do not allow for exceptions. In nursing, exceptions are generally present. However, sometimes answers containing these words are correct. For example, which of the following is correct and which are incorrect:
  a. Always use a turning sheet.
  b. Never shake linens.
  c. Soap is used for all baths.
  d. The signal light must always be attached to the bed.

The correct answer is b. Incorrect answers are a, c, and d.

- Omit answers that are obviously wrong. Then choose the best of the remaining answers.
- Go back to the questions you skipped. Answer all questions by eliminating or narrowing your choices. Always mark an answer even if you are not sure.
- Review the test a second time for completeness and accuracy before turning it in.
- Make sure you have answered each question. Also check that you have given only *one* answer for each question.
- Remember that the test is not designed to trick or confuse you. The written competency evaluation tests what you know, not what you do not know. You know more than you are asked.

CHAPTER 1 INTRODUCTION TO LONG-TERM CARE

LONG-TERM CARE CENTERS

- Provide care to persons who need regular or continuous care.
- Promote physical and mental health. Residents are helped and encouraged to:
  - Understand and accept the limits of their health problems.
  - Understand and accept physical and mental changes.
  - Function within the limits of their health problems.
  - Focus on abilities, not disabilities.
  - Do as much for themselves as possible.
  - Change habits that make health problems worse.
  - Eat properly and exercise.

THE INTERDISCIPLINARY HEALTH CARE TEAM

- The **nursing team** involves those who provide nursing care—RNs, LPNs/LVNs, and nursing assistants. The roles and responsibilities of each member of the team differ.
- **Nursing assistants (nurse aide, health care assistant)** report to the nurse supervising their work. They give basic nursing care under the supervision of an RN or LPN/LVN.
- The **interdisciplinary health care team** involves the many health care workers whose skills and knowledge focus on the person's total care. The team works together to meet each person's needs. Coordinated care is needed. An RN leads this team.

RESIDENT RIGHTS

- Residents have rights relating to their everyday lives and care in a nursing center. Nursing centers must protect and promote the rights of residents. If a resident is incompetent and cannot exercise his or her rights, a responsible person (partner, adult child) or legal representative does so for them.
- Nursing centers must inform residents of their rights. It is given in the language the person understands. Resident rights are also posted throughout the center.
- Residents have the following rights:
  - The right to information about their care. This includes:
    - Access to medical records, incident reports, contracts, and financial records.
    - Information about his or her health condition.
    - Information about his or her doctor.
  - The right to refuse treatment. A person who does not give consent or refuses treatment cannot be given the treatment. Report any treatment refusal to the nurse.
  - The right to privacy and confidentiality. A person has the right to:
    - Personal privacy. The person's body is not exposed unnecessarily. Only staff directly involved in care and treatments are present. The person must give consent for others to be present.
    - Use the bathroom in private
    - Visit with others in private—in areas where others cannot see or hear them. This includes phone calls.
    - Send and receive mail without others interfering. No one can open mail the person sends or receives without his or her consent.
    - Confidentiality. Consent is needed to release information about the person's care, treatment, and condition. Consent is also needed to release medical and financial records.
  - The right to personal choice. A person may:
    - Choose his or her own doctor.
    - Take part in planning and deciding his or her care and treatment.
    - Choose activities, schedules, and care based on his or her preferences.
    - Choose when to get up and go to bed, what to wear, and what to eat.
    - Choose friends and visitors inside and outside the center.
  - The right to voice concerns, ask questions, and complain about treatment or care. The center must promptly try to correct the matter.
  - The right to not work for the center. However, the person can work or perform services if he or she wants to.
  - The right to form and take part in resident and family groups.
  - The right to keep and use personal items.
  - The right to be free from abuse, mistreatment, and neglect, including the right to be free from:
    - Verbal, sexual, physical, or mental abuse.
    - Involuntary seclusion.
  - The right to be free from restraints or to have body movements restricted.
- Nursing centers must care for residents in a manner that promotes dignity and self-esteem. It must promote physical, psychological, and mental well-being.
- Nursing centers must provide activity programs that allow personal choice. Many centers provide religious services for spiritual health. Assist residents to and from activity programs.

OMBUDSMAN PROGRAM

- The Older Americans Act requires an ombudsman program in every state. **Ombudsmen** protect the health, safety, welfare, and rights of residents. They also may

---

This review includes selected chapters only.

investigate and resolve complaints, provide support to resident and family groups, and help the center manage difficult problems.
- Because a family or resident may share a concern with you, you must know the policies and procedures for contacting an ombudsman.

REVIEW QUESTIONS

Circle the BEST answer.

1. Residents in long-term care are encouraged to
   a. Do as little for themselves as possible
   b. Focus on their disabilities
   c. Focus on their abilities
   d. Eat junk food and not exercise

2. Nursing assistants report to
   a. Other nursing assistants
   b. Licensed nurses
   c. The administrator
   d. The medical director

3. Residents have the right to the following *except*
   a. Refuse treatment they do not want
   b. Personal choice
   c. Privacy
   d. Be called "sweetie"

CHAPTER 2 THE NURSING ASSISTANT IN LONG-TERM CARE

ROLES AND RESPONSIBILITIES
- Rules for you to follow:
  - You are an assistant to the nurse.
  - A nurse assigns and supervises your work.
  - You report observations about the person's physical and mental status to the nurse.
  - Report changes in the person's condition or behavior at once.
  - The nurse decides what should be done for a person. You do not make these decisions.
  - Review directions and the care plan with the nurse before going to the person.
  - Perform no nursing task that you are not trained to do.
  - Perform no nursing task that you are not comfortable doing without a nurse's supervision.
  - Perform only the nursing tasks that your state and job description allow.
- Role limits for nursing assistants:
  - Never give medications.
  - Never insert tubes or objects into body openings. Do not remove tubes from the body.
  - Never take oral or telephone orders from doctors.
  - Never perform procedures that require sterile technique.
  - Never tell the person or family the person's diagnosis or treatment plans.
  - Never diagnose or prescribe treatments or drugs for anyone.
  - Never supervise others, including other nursing assistants.
  - Never ignore an order or request to do something.

DELEGATION
- RNs can delegate tasks to you. In some states, LPNs/LVNs can delegate tasks to you.
- You cannot delegate any task to other nursing assistants or to any other worker.
- When you agree to perform a task, you are responsible for your own actions. You must complete the task safely.
- You have the right to refuse a task when:
  - The task is beyond the legal limits of your role.
  - The task is not in your job description.
  - You were not prepared to perform the task.
  - The task could harm the person.
  - The person's condition has changed.
  - You do not know how to use the supplies or equipment.
  - Directions are not ethical or legal.
  - Directions are against center policies.
  - Directions are unclear or incomplete.
  - A nurse is not available for supervision.
- Never ignore an order or request to do something. Tell the nurse about your concerns.

ETHICAL ASPECTS
- **Ethics** is the knowledge of what is right conduct and wrong conduct. It also deals with choices or judgments about what should or should not be done. An ethical person does not cause a person harm.
- Ethical behavior involves not being prejudiced or biased—to make judgments and have views before knowing the facts. You should not judge a person by your values and standards. Also, do not avoid persons whose standards and values differ from your own.

LEGAL ASPECTS
- **Negligence** is an unintentional wrong. The negligent person did not act in a reasonable and careful manner. As a result, harm was caused to the person or property of another. The person did not mean to cause harm.
- **False imprisonment** is the unlawful restraint or restriction of a person's freedom of movement. It involves threatening to restrain a person, restraining a person, and preventing a person from leaving the center.
- **Invasion of privacy** is violating a person's right not to have his or her name, photo, or private affairs exposed or made public without giving consent.
- The Health Insurance Portability and Accountability Act (HIPAA) protects the privacy and security of a person's health information. Direct any questions about the person or the person's care to the nurse.
- **Assault** is intentionally attempting or threatening to touch a person's body without the person's consent. The person fears bodily harm.
- **Battery** is touching a person's body without his or her consent.

Informed Consent
- Consent is informed when the person clearly understands:
  - The reason for a treatment.
  - What will be done.
  - How it will be done.
  - Who will do it.
  - The expected outcomes.
  - Other treatment options.
  - The effects of not having the treatment.
- Persons who cannot give consent are persons who are under the legal age or mentally incompetent. Unconscious, sedated, or confused persons also do not give consent. Informed consent is given by a responsible party—wife, husband, daughter, son, legal representative.
- You are never responsible for obtaining written consent.

ELDER ABUSE
- **Abuse** is the intentional mistreatment or harm of another person.
- **Elder abuse** is any knowing, intentional, or negligent act by a person to an older adult. It may include physical harm, pain, neglect, involuntary seclusion, financial exploitation, emotional abuse, sexual abuse, or abandonment. Review Box 2-7, Signs of Elder Abuse, in the textbook.
- If you suspect a person is being abused, report your observations to the nurse.

REVIEW QUESTIONS

Circle the BEST answer.

1. You answer the telephone. The doctor starts to give you an order. You
   a. Take the order from the doctor
   b. Politely give your name and title, and ask the doctor to wait for the nurse. Promptly find the nurse
   c. Politely ask the doctor to call back later
   d. Ask the doctor if the nurse may call him back

2. To protect a person's privacy, you should do the following *except*
   a. Keep all information about the person confidential
   b. Discuss the person's treatment or diagnosis with the nurse supervising your work
   c. Open the person's mail
   d. Allow the person to visit with others in private

3. What should you do if you suspect an older person is being abused?
   a. Report the situation to the health department.
   b. Notify the nurse and discuss the observations with him or her.
   c. Notify the doctor about the suspected abuse.
   d. Ask the family why they were abusing the person.

4. When should you refuse a task?
   a. The task is not in your job description.
   b. The task is within the legal limits of your role.
   c. The directions for the task are clear.
   d. A nurse is available for questions and supervision.

5. A nurse delegates a task that you did not learn in your training. The task is in your job description. What is your appropriate response to the nurse?
   a. "I cannot do that task."
   b. "I did not learn that task in my training. Can you show me how to do it?"
   c. "I will ask the other nursing assistant to watch me do the task."
   d. "I will ask the other nursing assistant to do the task for me."

6. Which statement about ethics is *false*?
   a. An ethical person does not judge others by their values and standards.
   b. An ethical person avoids persons whose standards and values differ from their own.
   c. An ethical person is not prejudiced or biased.
   d. An ethical person does not cause harm to another person.

CHAPTER 3 WORK ETHICS
TEAMWORK ON THE JOB
- Practice good work ethics—work when scheduled, be cheerful and friendly, perform delegated tasks, be kind to others, be available to help others.
- Be ready to work when your shift starts. Arrive on your nursing unit a few minutes early.
- Stay the entire shift. When it is time to leave, report off-duty to the nurse.
- Gossiping is unprofessional and hurtful. To avoid being a part of **gossip**:
  - Remove yourself from a group or situation where gossip is occurring.
  - Do not make or repeat any comment that can hurt another person.
  - Do not make or repeat any comment that you do not know to be true.
  - Do not talk about residents, family members, visitors, co-workers, or the center at home or in social settings.
- **Confidentiality** means to trust others with personal and private information. The person's information is shared only among health team members involved in his or her care. Center and co-worker information also is confidential.
- Your speech and language must be professional:
  - Do not swear or use foul, vulgar, or abusive language.
  - Do not use slang.
  - Speak softly, gently, and clearly.
  - Do not shout or yell.
  - Do not fight or argue with a resident, family member, visitor, or co-worker.
- A courtesy is a polite, considerate, or helpful comment or act.
  - Address others by Miss, Mrs., Ms., Mr., or Doctor. Use a first name only if the person asks you to do so.
  - Say "please" and "thank you." Say "I'm sorry" when you make a mistake or hurt someone.
  - Let residents, families, and visitors enter elevators first.
  - Be thoughtful—compliment others, give praise.
  - Wish the person and family well when they leave the center.
  - Hold doors open for others.
  - Help others willingly when asked.
  - Do not take credit for another person's deeds. Give the person credit for the action.

- You must protect residents, visitors, co-workers, and yourself from harm. Know the contents in the employee handbook and the policy and procedure manuals. Follow center rules.
- Accept responsibility for your actions. Admit when you are wrong or make mistakes. Do not blame others. Do not make excuses for your actions. Learn from your mistakes.
- Handle the person's property carefully and prevent damage.

REVIEW QUESTIONS
Circle the BEST answer.
1. You believe you have good work ethics. This means you do the following *except*
   a. Work when scheduled
   b. Act cheerful and friendly
   c. Refuse to help others
   d. Perform tasks assigned by the nurse
2. A nursing assistant is gossiping about a co-worker. You should
   a. Stay with the group and listen to what is being said
   b. Repeat the comment to your family
   c. Remove yourself from the group where gossip is occurring
   d. Repeat the comment to another co-worker
3. You want to maintain confidentiality about others. You do the following *except*
   a. Avoid talking about co-workers and residents when others are present
   b. Avoid talking about a resident in the elevator, hallway, or dining area
   c. Share information about a resident with a nurse who is on another unit
   d. Avoid eavesdropping
4. When you are at work, you should do which of the following?
   a. Swear and use foul language.
   b. Use slang.
   c. Argue with a visitor.
   d. Speak clearly and softly.

CHAPTER 4 COMMUNICATING WITH THE HEALTH TEAM

COMMUNICATION

- For good communication:
  - Use words that mean the same thing to you and the receiver of the message.
  - Use familiar words.
  - Be brief and concise.
  - Give information in a logical and orderly manner.
  - Give facts, and be specific.
- The medical record is a way for the health team to share information about the person. If you know someone in the center but you do not give care to that person, you have no right to review the person's chart. To do so is an invasion of privacy.
- A person or legal representative may ask you for the chart. Report the request to the nurse.
- There are two types of resident care conferences—the interdisciplinary care planning conference and the problem-focused conference. The person has the right to take part in these planning conferences. Sometimes the family is involved. The person may refuse actions suggested by the health team. If you attend a conference, share your ideas and observations.

REPORTING

- You report care and observations to the nurse. Follow these rules:
  - Be prompt, thorough, and accurate.
  - Give the person's name, and room and bed number.
  - Give the time your observations were made or the care was given.
  - Report only what you observed or did yourself.
  - Give reports as often as the person's condition requires or when the nurse asks you to.
  - Report any changes from normal or changes in the person's condition at once.
  - Use your written notes to give a specific, concise, and clear report.

RECORDING

- Rules for recording are:
  - Always use ink. Use the color required by the center.
  - Include the date and time for every recording.
  - Make sure writing is readable and neat.
  - Use only center-approved abbreviations.
  - Use correct spelling, grammar, and punctuation.
  - Do not use ditto marks.
  - Never erase or use correction fluid. Follow the center's procedure for correcting errors.
  - Sign all entries with your name and title as required by center policy.
  - Do not skip lines.
  - Make sure each form is stamped with the person's name and other identifying information.
  - Record only what you observed and did yourself.
  - Never chart a procedure, treatment, or care measure until after it is completed.
  - Be accurate, concise, and factual. Do not record judgments or interpretations.
  - Record in a logical and sequential manner.
  - Be descriptive. Avoid terms with more than one meaning.
  - Use the person's exact words whenever possible. Use quotation marks to show that the statement is a direct quote.
  - Chart any changes from normal or changes in the person's condition. Also chart that you informed the nurse (include the nurse's name), what you told the nurse, and the time you made the report.
  - Do not omit information.
  - Record safety measures. Example: Reminding a person not to get out of bed.

MEDICAL TERMINOLOGY AND ABBREVIATIONS

- Medical terminology and abbreviations are used in health care. Someone may use a word or phrase that you do not understand. If so, ask the nurse to explain its meaning.
- Use only the abbreviations accepted by the center. Review Box 4-3, Medical Terminology, in the textbook.

PHONE COMMUNICATION

- Guidelines for answering phones:
  - Answer the call after the first ring if possible.
  - Do not answer the phone in a rushed or hasty manner.
  - Give a courteous greeting. Identify the nursing unit and your name and title.
  - When taking a message, write down the caller's name, phone number, date and time, and message.
  - Repeat the message and phone number back to the caller.
  - Ask the caller to "Please hold" if necessary.
  - Do not lay the phone down or cover the receiver with your hand when not speaking to the caller. The caller may hear confidential information.
  - Return to a caller on hold within 30 seconds.
  - Do not give confidential information to any caller.
  - Transfer a call if appropriate. Tell the caller you are going to transfer the call; give the name and phone number in case the call gets disconnected.
  - End the conversation politely.
  - Give the message to the appropriate person.

REVIEW QUESTIONS

Circle the BEST answer.

1. For good communication, you should do the following *except*
   a. Use words with more than one meaning
   b. Use familiar words to the person or family
   c. Give facts in a brief and concise manner
   d. Give information in a logical and orderly manner

2. When reporting care and observations to the nurse, you do the following *except*
   a. Give the person's name and room and bed number
   b. Report only what you observed or did yourself
   c. Report any changes from normal or changes in the person's condition at once
   d. Report any changes from normal or changes in the person's condition at the end of the shift

3. When you record in a person's chart, you do the following *except*
   a. Record what you observed and did
   b. Record the person's response to the treatment or procedure
   c. Use abbreviations that are not on the accepted list for the center
   d. Record the time the observation was made or the treatment performed

CHAPTER 5 ASSISTING WITH THE NURSING PROCESS
NURSING PROCESS

- The **nursing process** is the method nurses use to plan and deliver nursing care.
- You play a key role by making observations as you care and talk with the person.
- **Observation** is using the senses of sight, hearing, touch, and smell to collect information. Box 5-1, Basic Observations, in your textbook lists the basic observations you need to make and report to the nurse. Examples are:
  - Can the person give his name, the time, and location when asked?
  - Can the person move the arms and legs?
  - Is the skin pale or flushed?
  - Is there drainage from the eyes? What color is the drainage?
  - Does the person like the food served?
  - Can the person bathe without help?
- Observations you need to report to the nurse at once are:
  - A change in the person's ability to respond.
  - A change in the person's mobility.
  - Complaints of sudden, severe pain.
  - A sore or reddened area on the person's skin.
  - Complaints of a sudden change in vision.
  - Complaints of pain or difficulty breathing.
  - Abnormal respirations.
  - Complaints of or signs of difficulty swallowing.
  - Vomiting.
  - Bleeding.
  - Vital signs outside their normal ranges.
- **Objective data (signs)** are seen, heard, felt, or smelled.
- **Subjective data (symptoms)** are things a person tells you about that you cannot observe through your senses.

REVIEW QUESTIONS
Circle the BEST answer.

1. Which statement about observations is *false*?
   a. Observation is part of the assessment step in the nursing process.
   b. Observation uses the senses of smell, sight, and hearing, but not touch.
   c. You make many observations as you care and talk with people.
   d. You report observations to the nurse.
2. Objective data include all the following *except*
   a. The person has pain in his abdomen
   b. The person's pulse is 76
   c. The person's urine is dark amber
   d. The person's breath has an odor

CHAPTER 6 UNDERSTANDING THE RESIDENT

CARING FOR THE PERSON

- The whole person needs to be considered when you provide care—physical, social, psychological, and spiritual parts. These parts are woven together and cannot be separated.
- Follow these rules to address them with dignity and respect:
  - Call residents by their titles—Mr. Jones, Mrs. Smith, Miss Turner, Dr. Gonzalez.
  - Do not call residents by their first names unless they ask you to.
  - Do not call residents by any other name unless they ask you to.
  - Do not call residents Grandma, Papa, Sweetheart, Honey, or other name.

BASIC NEEDS

- According to Maslow, **basic needs** must be met for a person to survive and function.
- Physiological or physical needs—are required for life. They are oxygen, food, water, elimination, rest, and shelter.
- Safety and security needs—relate to feeling safe from harm, danger, and fear.
- Love and belonging needs—relate to love, closeness, affection, and meaningful relationships with others. Family, friends, and the health team can meet love and belonging needs.
- **Self-esteem** needs—relate to thinking well of oneself and to seeing oneself as useful and having value. People often lack self-esteem when ill, injured, older, or disabled.
- The need for **self-actualization**—involves learning, understanding, and creating to the limit of a person's capacity. Rarely, if ever, is it totally met.

CULTURE AND RELIGION

- People come from many **cultures**, races, and nationalities. Family practices, food choices, hygiene habits, clothing styles, and language are part of their culture. The person's culture also influences health beliefs and practices.
- **Religion** relates to spiritual beliefs, needs, and practices. A person's religion influences health and illness practices. Many may want to pray and observe religious practices. Assist residents to attend religious services as needed. If a person wants to see a spiritual leader or advisor, tell the nurse. Provide privacy during the visit.
- A person may not follow all the beliefs and practices of his or her culture or religion. Some people do not practice a religion.
- Respect and accept the person's culture and religion. Learn about practices and beliefs different from your own. Do not judge a person by your standards.

BEHAVIOR ISSUES

- Many people accept illness and disability as part of aging. Their behavior is pleasant.
- Some people are angry. Anger may be communicated verbally and nonverbally. You might have problems dealing with the person's anger. If so, ask the nurse for help.
- A person with demanding behavior is critical of others. Nothing seems to please the person.
- The person with self-centered behavior cares only about his or her own needs. The person demands the time and attention of others.
- A person with aggressive behavior may swear, bite, hit, pinch, scratch, or kick. Protect the person, others, and yourself from harm.
- The withdrawn person has little or no contact with family, friends, and staff. He or she spends time alone and does not take part in social or group events. Some people are generally not social and prefer to be alone.
- Some people may have inappropriate sexual behaviors. The behaviors may be on purpose or caused by disease, confusion, dementia, or drug side effects.
- You cannot avoid persons with unpleasant behaviors or who lose control. Review Box 6-1, Dealing With Behavior Issues, in the textbook.

COMMUNICATING WITH THE PERSON

- Respect the person's rights, culture, and religion.
- Give the person time to process the information that you give.
- Ask questions to see if the person understood you.
- Include the person in conversations when others are present.
- When talking with a person follow these rules:
  - Face the person.
  - Position yourself at the person's eye level.
  - Control the loudness and tone of your voice.
  - Speak clearly, slowly, and distinctly.
  - Do not use slang or vulgar words.
  - Repeat information as needed.
  - Ask one question at a time, and wait for an answer.
  - Do not shout, whisper, or mumble.
  - Be kind, courteous, and friendly.
- Keep written messages brief and concise. Use a black felt pen on white paper, and print in large letters.
- Some persons cannot speak or read. Ask questions that have "yes" and "no" answers. A picture board may be helpful.
- **Nonverbal communication** does not use words. Messages are sent with gestures, facial expressions, posture, body movements, touch, and smell. Nonverbal messages more accurately reflect a person's feelings than words do. A person may say one thing but act another way. Watch the person's eyes, hand movements, gestures, posture, and other actions.
- Touch is a very important form of nonverbal communication. It conveys comfort, caring, love, affection, interest, trust, concern, and reassurance. Touch should be gentle. Touch means different things to different people. Some people do not like to be touched.

- People send messages through their **body language**—facial expressions, gestures, posture, hand and body movements, gait, eye contact, and appearance. Your body language should show interest, enthusiasm, caring, and respect for the person. Often you need to control your body language. Control reactions to odors from body fluids, secretions, or excretions.

Communication Methods
- **Listening** means to focus on verbal and nonverbal communication. You use sight, hearing, touch, and smell. To be a good listener:
  - Face the person.
  - Have good eye contact with the person.
  - Lean toward the person. Do not sit back with your arms crossed.
  - Respond to the person. Nod your head, and ask questions.
  - Avoid the communication barriers.
- **Paraphrasing** is restating the person's message in your own words.
- *Direct questions* focus on certain information. You ask the person something you need to know.
- *Open-ended questions* lead or invite the person to share thoughts, feelings, or ideas. The person chooses what to talk about.
- *Clarifying* lets you make sure that you understand the message. You can ask the person to repeat the message, say you do not understand, or restate the message.
- *Focusing* deals with a certain topic. It is useful when a person rambles or wanders in thought.
- *Silence* is a very powerful way to communicate. Silence on your part shows caring and respect for the person's situation and feelings.

Communication Barriers
- *Using unfamiliar language.* You and the person must use and understand the same language.
- *Cultural differences.* A person from another country may attach different meanings to verbal and nonverbal communication from what you intended.
- *Changing the subject.* Avoid changing the subject whenever possible.
- *Giving your opinions.* Opinions involve judging values, behavior, or feelings. Let others express feelings and concerns. Do not make judgments or jump to conclusions.
- *Talking a lot when others are silent.* Talking too much is usually because of nervousness and discomfort with silence.
- *Failure to listen.* Do not pretend to listen. It shows lack of caring and interest. You may miss complaints of pain, discomfort, or other symptoms that you must report to the nurse.
- *Pat answers.* "Don't worry." "Everything will be okay." These make the person feel that you do not care about his or her concerns, feelings, and fears.
- *Illness and disability.* Speech, hearing, vision, cognitive function, and body movements may be affected. Verbal and nonverbal communication are affected.
- *Age.* Values and communication styles vary among age-groups.

RESIDENTS WITH DISABILITIES
- Common courtesies and manners apply to any person with a disability. Review Box 6-2, Disability Etiquette, in the textbook.
- The person who is comatose is unconscious and cannot respond to others. Often the person can feel touch and pain. Assume that the person hears and understands you. Use touch, and give care gently. Practice these measures:
  - Knock before entering the person's room.
  - Tell the person your name, the time, and the place every time you enter the room.
  - Give care on the same schedule every day.
  - Explain what you are going to do.
  - Tell the person when you are finishing care.
  - Use touch to communicate care, concern, and comfort.
  - Tell the person what time you will be back to check on him or her.
  - Tell the person when you are leaving the room.

FAMILY AND FRIENDS
- If you need to give care when visitors are there, protect the right to privacy. Politely ask the visitors to leave the room when you give care. A partner or family member may help you if the resident consents.
- Treat family and visitors with courtesy and respect.
- Do not discuss the person's condition with family and friends. Refer their questions to the nurse. A visitor may upset or tire a person. Report your observations to the nurse.

REVIEW QUESTIONS
Circle the BEST answer.
1. While caring for a person, you need to
   a. Consider the person's physical and social needs
   b. Consider the person's physical, social, psychological, and spiritual needs
   c. Consider only the person's cultural needs
   d. Ignore the person's spiritual needs
2. When referring to residents, you should
   a. Refer to them by their room number
   b. Call them "Honey"
   c. Call them by their first name
   d. Call them by their name and title
3. Based on Maslow's theory of basic needs, which person's needs must be met first?
   a. The person who wants to talk about her granddaughter's wedding
   b. The person who is uncomfortable in the dining room
   c. The person who wants mail opened
   d. The person who asks for more water
4. Which statement about culture is *false*?
   a. A person's culture influences health beliefs and practices.
   b. You must respect and accept a person's culture.
   c. You should learn about another person's culture that is different from yours.
   d. You should ignore the person's culture while you give his or her care.

5. Which statement about religion and spiritual beliefs is *false*?
   a. A person's religion influences health and illness practices.
   b. You should assist a person to attend services in the nursing center.
   c. Many people find comfort and strength from religion during illness.
   d. A person must follow all beliefs of his or her religion.

6. A person is angry and is shouting at you. You should do the following *except*
   a. Stay calm and professional
   b. Yell at the person so he will listen to you
   c. Listen to what the person is saying
   d. Report the person's behavior to the nurse

7. A person tries to scratch and kick you. You should
   a. Protect yourself from harm
   b. Argue with the person
   c. Become angry with the person
   d. Refuse to care for the person

8. When speaking with another person, you do the following *except*
   a. Position yourself at the person's eye level
   b. Speak slowly, clearly, and distinctly
   c. Shout, mumble, and whisper
   d. Ask one question at a time

9. Which statement about listening is *false*?
   a. You use sight, hearing, touch, and smell when you listen.
   b. You observe nonverbal cues.
   c. You have good eye contact with the person.
   d. You sit back with your arms crossed.

10. Which statement about silence is *false*?
    a. Silence is a powerful way to communicate.
    b. Silence gives people time to think.
    c. You should talk a lot when the other person is silent.
    d. Silence helps when the person is upset and needs to gain control.

11. A person speaks a foreign language. You should do the following *except*
    a. Keep messages short and simple
    b. Use gestures and pictures
    c. Shout or speak loudly
    d. Repeat the message in other words

12. When caring for a person who is comatose, you do the following *except*
    a. Tell the person your name when you enter the room
    b. Explain what you are doing
    c. Use touch to communicate care and comfort
    d. Make jokes about how sick the person is

CHAPTER 8 THE OLDER PERSON
LATE ADULTHOOD

- Aging is normal. It is not a disease. Normal aging does not mean loss of health.
- Physical, psychological, and social changes occur.
- The **developmental tasks** for Late Adulthood are:
  - Adjusting to decreased strength and loss of health.
  - Adjusting to retirement and reduced income.
  - Coping with a partner's death.
  - Developing new friends and relationships.
  - Preparing for one's own death.
- Some myths about aging are:
  - All old people are the same.
  - Aging means illness and disability.
  - Older persons lose interest in sex.
  - Older people are lonely and isolated.
  - Mental function declines with age.
  - Most older persons live in nursing centers.
  - Old people are crabby and rude.
- Some facts about aging are:
  - Each person is unique. People age in different ways.
  - Although older persons are at risk for health problems, most are healthy.
  - Many older people enjoy a fulfilling sex life. Sexuality is important throughout life.
  - Most older people have contact with their children and regular contact with sisters and brothers. Many older persons have jobs, do volunteer work, and enjoy hobbies.
  - Older persons may receive and process information more slowly than younger people. However, people learn until very late in life.
  - In 2000, 4.5% of the people 65 years and older lived in nursing centers.
  - Although some old people are crabby and rude, so are people of all ages.

PHYSICAL CHANGES

- Body processes slow down. Energy level and body efficiency decline.
- *The integumentary system.* The skin thins and sags. Wrinkles appear. Dry skin occurs and may cause itching. Brown spots appear on the skin. The person is more sensitive to cold. Nails become thick and tough. Feet may have poor circulation. White or gray hair is common. Hair thins. There is hair loss in men. Facial hair may occur in women. Hair is dryer.
- *The musculoskeletal system.* Muscle and bone strength are lost. Bones become brittle and break easily. Vertebrae shorten. Joints become stiff and painful. Mobility decreases. There is a gradual loss of height.
- *The nervous system.* Confusion, dizziness, and fatigue may occur. Responses are slower. The risk for falls increases. Forgetfulness increases. Memory is shorter. Events from long ago are remembered better than recent ones. Older persons have a harder time falling asleep. Sleep periods are shorter. Older persons wake often during the night and have less deep sleep. Less sleep is needed. They may rest or nap during the day. They may go to bed early and get up early.

- *Touch.* Touch and sensitivity to pain and pressure are reduced. So is sensing heat and cold.
- *The eye.* Eyelids thin and wrinkle. Tear secretion is less. The pupil becomes smaller and responds less to light. Vision is poor at night or in dark rooms. The eye takes longer to adjust to lighting changes. Clear vision is reduced. Greens and blues are harder to see.
- *The ear.* High-pitched sounds are hard to hear. Hearing loss may occur. Wax secretion decreases. Wax becomes harder and thicker. It is easily impacted.
- *The circulatory system.* The heart muscle weakens. Arteries narrow and are less elastic. Poor circulation occurs in many body parts.
- *The respiratory system.* Respiratory muscles weaken. Lung tissue becomes less elastic. Difficult, labored, or painful breathing may occur with activity. The person may lack strength to cough and clear the airway of secretions. Respiratory infections and diseases may develop.
- *The digestive system.* Less saliva is produced. The person may have difficulty swallowing (**dysphagia**). Indigestion may occur. Loss of teeth and ill-fitting dentures cause chewing problems and digestion problems. Flatulence and constipation can occur. Fewer calories are needed as energy and activity levels decline. More fluids are needed.
- *The urinary system.* Urine is more concentrated. Bladder muscles weaken. Bladder size decreases. Urinary frequency or urgency may occur. Many older persons have to urinate at night. Urinary incontinence may occur. In men, the prostate gland enlarges. This may cause difficulty urinating or frequent urination.
- *The reproductive system.* In men, testosterone decreases. An erection takes longer. Orgasm is less forceful. Women experience menopause. Female hormones of estrogen and progesterone decrease. The uterus, vagina, and genitalia shrink (atrophy). Vaginal walls thin. There is vaginal dryness. Arousal takes longer. Orgasm is less intense.

REVIEW QUESTIONS
Circle the BEST answer.

1. Which statement is *false*?
   a. Physical changes occur with aging.
   b. Energy level and body efficiency decline with age.
   c. Some people age faster than others.
   d. Normal aging means loss of health.
2. As a person ages, the integumentary system changes. Which statement is *false*?
   a. Dry skin and itching occur.
   b. Nails become thick and tough.
   c. There is an increased sensitivity to pain.
   d. Skin is injured more easily.
3. Which statement is *false* about the musculoskeletal system and aging?
   a. Strength decreases.
   b. Vertebrae shorten.
   c. Mobility increases.
   d. Bone mass decreases.

4. Which statement about the nervous system and aging is *false*?
   a. Reflexes slow.
   b. Memory may be shorter.
   c. Sleep patterns change.
   d. Forgetfulness decreases.

5. Which statement about the digestive system and aging is *false*?
   a. Appetite decreases.
   b. Less saliva is produced.
   c. Flatulence and constipation may decrease.
   d. Teeth may be lost.

6. Which statement about the urinary system and aging is *false* ?
   a. Urine becomes more concentrated.
   b. Urinary frequency may occur.
   c. Urinary urgency may occur.
   d. Bladder muscles become stronger.

7. Which statement about aging is a *myth*?
   a. People age in different ways.
   b. All old people are crabby and rude.
   c. Many older people enjoy a fulfilling sex life.
   d. Most older persons are healthy.

CHAPTER 9 SEXUALITY
SEXUALITY AND SEX
- **Sexuality** is important throughout life. Illness, injury, and aging can affect sexuality.
- Changes in sexual function greatly affect the person. Fear, worry, anger, and depression are common. The person's feelings are normal and expected.

SEXUALITY AND OLDER PERSONS
- Older persons love, fall in love, hold hands, and embrace. Many have intercourse.
- The nursing team promotes the meeting of sexual needs. Married couples in nursing centers share the same room. They can share the same bed if their conditions permit.
- Single persons may develop relationships. They are allowed time together, not kept apart.

THE SEXUALLY AGGRESSIVE PERSON
- Some people flirt or make sexual advances or comments. Some expose themselves, masturbate, or touch the staff.
- If the purpose of touch is sexual, be a professional about the matter. Ask the person not to touch you. Tell the person what behaviors make you uncomfortable. Politely ask the person not to act that way. Allow privacy if the person is becoming aroused. Provide for safety. Discuss the matter with the nurse. The nurse can help you understand the behavior.

- Not all touch is sexual. Sometimes touch serves to gain attention or to signal a health problem.
- People in nursing centers must be protected from unwanted sexual comments and advances. This is sexual abuse. Tell the nurse right away if anyone makes an unwanted sexual comment or advance.

REVIEW QUESTIONS
Circle the BEST answer.
1. A husband and wife may share the same bed in the nursing center.
   a True
   b. False
2. Sometimes a person uses touch to gain attention, not to be sexually aggressive.
   a. True
   b. False
3. A resident touches you in a sexual way. You should do the following *except*
   a. Ask the person not to touch you
   b. Discuss the matter with the nurse
   c. Tell the person what behaviors make you uncomfortable
   d. Ask the person if you should call a dating service for him
4. Two single persons may "cuddle" in the same bed if both consent.
   a. True
   b. False

CHAPTER 10 SAFETY
THE SAFE ENVIRONMENT
- The health care team must provide for a safe environment. The goal is to decrease the person's risk of accidents and injuries without limiting mobility and independence.
- If you see something unsafe, correct the matter right away if you can. You cannot correct some safety issues. Follow center policy for reporting them.

ACCIDENT RISK FACTORS
- Older persons are at risk for accidents.
- People need to know their surroundings to protect themselves from injury.
- People who are agitated and have aggressive behaviors are prone to accidents.
- Persons with poor vision may be prone to accidents.
- Persons with hearing loss are at risk for accidents.
- Persons with impaired smell and touch may be prone to accidents.
- Some diseases and injuries affect mobility. A person may be aware of danger but is unable to move to safety.
- Drugs have side effects. Report behavior changes and the person's complaints.

IDENTIFYING THE PERSON
- Always identify the person before you begin a task or procedure.
- Most persons receive identification (ID) bracelets when admitted to the nursing center. Some nursing centers have photo ID systems.
- Alert and oriented persons may choose not to wear ID bracelets. Follow center policy and the care plan to identify the person.

PREVENTING BURNS
- Have residents smoke only in smoking areas.
- Do not allow residents to use space heaters, a heating pad, or an electric blanket.
- Turn on cold water first. Turn off hot water first. Check for "hot spots" in bath water. Measure bath or shower water temperature.
- Assist with eating and drinking so hot foods or fluids are not spilled.
- Refer to Box 10-1, Safety Measures to Prevent Burns, in the textbook.

PREVENTING POISONING
- Poor vision and confusion are major risk factors. Make sure the person cannot reach hazardous materials. Follow center procedures for storing personal care items. They can cause harm when swallowed.

PREVENTING SUFFOCATION
- Cut food into small, bite-sized pieces.
- Make sure dentures fit properly and are in place.
- Make sure the person can chew and swallow the food served.
- Report loose teeth and dentures.
- Check the care plan for swallowing problems before serving snacks or fluids.
- Tell the nurse at once if the person has swallowing problems.
- Do not give oral food or fluids to persons with feeding tubes.
- Follow aspiration procedures.
- Do not leave a person unattended in a bathtub or shower.
- Move all persons from the area if you smell smoke.
- Position the person in bed properly.
- Use bed rails and restraints correctly.
- Use restraints correctly.

Choking
- Choking or foreign-body airway obstruction (FBAO) occurs when foreign bodies obstruct the airway. Air cannot pass through the air passages to the lungs. The body does not get enough oxygen. This can lead to cardiac arrest.
- Choking often occurs during eating. A large, poorly chewed piece of meat is the most common cause. Other common causes include laughing and talking while eating.
- Older persons are at risk for choking.
- With mild airway obstruction, some air moves in and out of the lungs. The person is conscious. Usually the person can speak. Often forceful coughing can remove the object.
- With severe airway obstruction, the conscious person clutches at the throat—the "universal sign of choking." The person has difficulty breathing. Some persons cannot breathe, speak, or cough. The person appears pale and cyanotic. Air does not move in and out of the lungs. If the obstruction is not removed, the person will die. Severe airway obstruction is an emergency.
- Use the Heimlich maneuver to relieve FBAO. It involves abdominal thrusts. The maneuver is performed with the person standing, sitting, or lying down.
- Chest thrusts are used for very obese persons and pregnant women.
- Call for help when a person has an obstructed airway. Report and record what happened, what you did, and the person's response.

PREVENTING EQUIPMENT ACCIDENTS
- All equipment is unsafe if broken, not used correctly, or not working properly.
- Inspect all equipment before use. Three-pronged plugs are used on all electrical items.
- Review Box 10-4, Safety Measures to Prevent Equipment Accidents, in the textbook.

WHEELCHAIR SAFETY
- Check the wheel locks to be sure you can lock and unlock them.
- Check for flat or loose tires.
- Make sure the wheel spokes are intact.

- Make sure the casters point forward.
- Position the person's feet on the footplates.
- Push the chair forward when transporting the person.
- Lock both wheels before you transfer a person to or from the wheelchair.
- Do not let the person stand on the footplates.
- Do not let the footplates fall back onto the person's legs.
- Clean the wheelchair according to center policy.
- Refer to Box 10-5, Wheelchair and Stretcher Safety, in the textbook.

HANDLING HAZARDOUS SUBSTANCES

- Hazardous substances include oxygen, mercury, disinfectants, and cleaning agents.
- A container must have a warning label. If a label is removed or damaged, do not use the substance. Take the container to the nurse. Do not leave the container unattended.
- Check the material safety data sheet (MSDS) before using a hazardous substance, cleaning up a leak or spill, or disposing of the substance.
- Tell the nurse about a leak or spill right away. Do not leave a leak or spill unattended.
- Review Box 10–6, Safety Measures for Hazardous Substances, in the textbook.

FIRE SAFETY

- Safety measures are needed where oxygen is used and stored:
- "No Smoking" signs are placed on the door and near the person's bed.
- The person and visitors are reminded not to smoke in the room.
- Smoking materials are removed from the room.
- Electrical items are turned off before being unplugged.
- Wool blankets and fabrics that cause static electricity are not used.
- The person wears a cotton gown or pajamas.
- Electrical items are in good working order.
- Lit candles and other open flames are not allowed.
- Materials that ignite easily are removed from the room.
- Review Box 10–7, Fire Prevention Measures, in the textbook
- Know your center's policies and procedures for fire emergencies. Know where to find fire alarms, fire extinguishers, and emergency exits. Remember the word RACE:
- R—rescue. Rescue persons in immediate danger. Move them to a safe place.
- A—alarm. Sound the nearest fire alarm. Notify the telephone operator.
- C—confine. Close doors and windows. Turn off oxygen or electrical items.
- E—extinguish. Use a fire extinguisher on a small fire.

- To promote safety during a fire:
- Clear equipment from all normal and emergency exits.
- Do not use elevators.
- Touch doors before opening them. Do not open a hot door.
- If your clothing is on fire, drop to the floor, cover your face, and roll to smother flames.
- If another person's clothing is on fire, get the person to the ground, roll the person, or cover the person with a blanket, bedspread, or coat.
- Remember the word PASS for using a fire extinguisher:
- P—pull the safety pin.
- A—aim low. Aim at the base of the fire.
- S—squeeze the lever. This starts the stream of water.
- S—sweep back and forth. Sweep side to side at the base of the fire.

REVIEW QUESTIONS
Circle the BEST answer.
1. You see a water spill in the hallway. What will you do?
   a. Ask housekeeping to wipe up the spill right away.
   b. Wipe up the spill right away.
   c. Report the spill to the nurse.
   d. Ask the resident to walk around the spill.
2. An electrical outlet in a person's room does not work. What will you do?
   a. Tell the administrator about the problem.
   b. Tell another nursing assistant about the problem.
   c. Try to repair the electrical outlet.
   d. Follow the center's policy for reporting the problem.
3. Accident risk factors include all of the following *except*
   a. Poor vision
   b. Hearing problems
   c. Dulled sense of smell
   d. Walking without difficulty
4. To prevent a person from being burned, you should do the following *except*
   a. Supervise the smoking of persons who are confused
   b. Turn cold water on first; turn hot water off first
   c. Do not let the person sleep with a heating pad
   d. Allow smoking in bed
5. To prevent suffocation, you should do the following *except*
   a. Make sure dentures fit properly
   b. Check the care plan for swallowing problems before serving food or liquids
   c. Leave a person alone in a bathtub or shower
   d. Position the person in bed properly
6. Which statement about mild airway obstruction is *false*?
   a. Some air moves in and out of the lungs.
   b. The person is conscious.
   c. Usually the person cannot speak.
   d. Forceful coughing will often remove the object.

7. The "universal sign of choking" is
   a. Clutching at the chest
   b. Clutching at the throat
   c. Not being able to talk
   d. Not being able to breathe
8. Which statement about wheelchair safety is *false*?
   a. Lock the wheels before transferring a resident to or from a wheelchair.
   b. The person's feet should rest on the footplate when you are pushing the wheelchair.
   c. Let the footplates fall back onto a person's legs.
   d. Check for flat or loose tires.
9. Which of the following is *not* a safety measure with oxygen?
   a. "No Smoking" signs are placed on the resident's door and near the bed.
   b. Lit candles and other open flames are permitted in the room.
   c. Electrical items are turned off before being unplugged.
   d. The person wears a cotton gown or pajamas.
10. You have discovered a fire in the nursing center. You should do the following *except*
    a. Rescue persons in immediate danger
    b. Sound the nearest fire alarm
    c. Open doors and windows, and keep oxygen on
    d. Use a fire extinguisher on a small fire that has not spread to a larger area
11. When using a fire extinguisher, you do the following *except*
    a. Pull the safety pin on the fire extinguisher
    b. Aim at the top of the flames
    c. Squeeze the lever to start the stream of water
    d. Sweep the stream of water back and forth

CHAPTER 11 PREVENTING FALLS

FALLS

- Falls are the most common accidents in centers. Persons older than 65 years and those who have fallen in the past are more at risk. Most falls occur in resident rooms and bathrooms. Most occur between 6:00 PM and 9:00 PM. Falls are more likely during shift changes.
- Causes for falls are poor lighting, cluttered floors, and out-of-place furniture. So are wet and slippery floors, bathtubs, and showers. Waxed floors, throw rugs, and improper shoes may cause falls. Other factors that may cause falls are weakness, vision problems, confusion, and balance problems. Review Box 11-1, Factors Increasing the Risk of Falls, in the textbook.
- Review Box 11-2, Safety Measures to Prevent Falls, in the textbook.

BEDRAILS

- **Bed rails** are needed by persons who are unconscious or sedated with drugs. Some confused and disoriented people need them. If a person needs bed rails, keep them up at all times except when giving bedside nursing care.
- Bed rails present hazards. The person can fall when trying to get out of bed. Or the person can get caught, trapped, entangled, or strangled.
- Because bed rails prevent the person from getting out of bed, they are considered restraints. Bed rails cannot be used unless they are needed to treat a person's medical symptoms. The person or legal representative must give consent for raised bed rails. The need for bed rails is carefully noted in the person's medical record and the care plan. If a person uses bed rails, check the person often. Record when you checked the person and your observations.
- To prevent falls:
  - Never leave the person alone when the bed is raised.
  - Always lower the bed to its lowest position when you are done giving care.
  - If a person does not use bed rails and you need to raise the bed, ask a co-worker to stand on the far side of the bed to protect the person from falling.
  - If you raise the bed to give care, always raise the far bed rail if you are working alone.
  - Be sure the person who uses raised bed rails has access to items on the bedside stand and overbed table. The signal light, water pitcher and cup, tissues, phone, and TV and light controls should be within the person's reach.

FALL PREVENTION

- Hand rails and grab bars give support to persons who are weak or unsteady.
- Bed wheels are locked at all times except when moving the bed. Wheelchair and stretcher wheels are locked when transferring a person.

- Use a **transfer belt (gait belt)** to support a person who is unsteady or disabled. Always follow the manufacturer's instructions. Apply the belt over clothing and under the breasts. The belt buckle is never positioned over the person's spine. Tighten the belt so it is snug. You should be able to slide 4 fingers under the belt.
- If a person starts to fall, do not try to prevent the fall. You could injure yourself and the person. Ease the person to the floor, and protect the person's head. Do not let the person get up before the nurse checks for injuries. An incident report is completed after all falls.

REVIEW QUESTIONS
Circle the BEST answer.

1. Falls are the most common accidents in nursing centers.
   a. True
   b. False
2. Most falls occur in
   a. Resident rooms and bathrooms
   b. Dining rooms
   c. Hallways
   d. Activity rooms
3. Which statement about falls is *false*?
   a. Poor lighting, cluttered floors, and throw rugs may cause falls.
   b. Improper shoes and needing to use the bathroom may cause falls.
   c. Most falls occur between 6:00 PM and 9:00 PM.
   d. Falls are less likely to occur during shift changes.
4. Which statement about bed rails is *false*?
   a. The nurse and care plan tell you when to raise bed rails.
   b. Bedrails are considered restraints.
   c. You may leave a person alone when the bed is raised and the bed rails are down.
   d. Bed rails can present hazards because people try to climb over them.
5. Which statement about transfer/gait belts is *false*?
   a. To use the belt safely, follow manufacturer's instructions.
   b. Always apply the belt over clothing.
   c. Tighten the belt so it is very snug and breathing is impaired.
   d. Place the belt buckle off center so it is not over the spine.
6. A person becomes faint in the hallway and begins to fall. You should do the following *except*
   a. Ease the person to the floor
   b. Protect the person's head
   c. Let the person get up before the nurse checks him or her
   d. Help the nurse complete the incident report

CHAPTER 12 RESTRAINT ALTERNATIVES AND SAFE RESTRAINT USE
RESTRAINTS

- A **restraint** is any item, object, device, garment, material, or drug that limits or restricts a person's freedom of movement or access to one's body.
- Some furniture or barriers prevent free movement:
  - Geriatric chairs.
  - Any chair placed so close to the wall that the person cannot move.
  - Sheets tucked in so tightly that they restrict movement.
  - Bed rails.
- OBRA, state laws, and accrediting agencies have guidelines about restraint use. They do not forbid restraint use. They require trying all other appropriate alternatives first.
- Knowing and treating the cause for harmful behaviors can prevent restraint use. There are many alternatives to restraints, such as answering the signal light promptly or giving a back massage. For other alternatives see Box 12-2, Alternatives to Restraint Use, in the textbook.
- Restraints can cause serious harm and even death. Injuries may occur from using the wrong restraint, applying it wrong, or keeping it on too long. Cuts, bruises, and fractures are common. The most serious risk is death from strangulation.
- The person may have mental effects from restraints. The person may experience depression, anger, agitation, embarrassment, humiliation, and mistrust. Self-esteem may be affected.
- Refer to Box 12-1, Risks of Restraint Use, in the textbook.

LEGAL ASPECTS

- Restraints are used only as a last resort to protect persons from harming themselves or others. They are not used for staff convenience or to discipline a person.
- A written doctor's order is required to use a restraint.
- The least restrictive restraint is used. It allows the greatest amount of movement or body access possible.
- Informed consent, by the person or his or her legal representative, is required before a restraint is used. The doctor or nurse obtains consent.
- If you apply an unneeded restraint, you could face false imprisonment charges.

SAFETY GUIDELINES

- Review Box 12-3, Safety Measures for Using Restraints, in the textbook.
- Restraints can increase confusion and agitation. Restrained persons need repeated explanations and reassurance. Spending time with them has a calming effect.
- Follow the manufacturer's instructions when applying and securing the restraint. The restraint must be snug and firm, but not tight. You could be negligent if you do not apply or secure a restraint properly.
- Make sure the signal light is within reach. Ask the person to use it at the first sign of problems or discomfort.
- Check the person and the restraint at least every 15 minutes or more often as required by the care plan. Report and record your observations.

- Check the person's circulation at least every 15 minutes if wrist, mitt, or ankle restraints are applied. A pulse should be felt at a pulse site below the restraint. Fingers or toes should be warm and pink. Tell the nurse at once if:
  - You cannot feel a pulse.
  - Fingers or toes are cold, pale, or blue in color.
  - The person complains of pain, numbness, or tingling in the restrained part.
  - The skin is red or damaged.
- Check the person at least every 15 minutes if a vest, jacket, or belt restraint is used. The person should be able to breathe easily. Call the nurse at once if the person is not breathing or is having difficulty breathing.
- At least every 2 hours you need to:
  - Remove the restraint.
  - Reposition the person.
  - Help the person meet food, fluid, hygiene, and elimination needs.
  - Give skin care.
  - Perform range-of-motion exercises or help the person walk.
  - Provide for comfort.
- Report and record the following:
  - Type of restraint applied.
  - Body part or parts restrained.
  - Reason for the restraint.
  - Safety measures taken.
  - Time you applied the restraint.
  - Time you removed the restraint.
  - Care given when restraint was removed.
  - Skin color and condition.
  - Pulse felt in the restrained part.
  - Changes in the person's behavior.
  - Complaints of a tight restraint; difficulty breathing; and pain, numbness, or tingling in the restrained part. Report these complaints to the nurse at once.

REVIEW QUESTIONS
Circle the BEST answer.

1. A geriatric chair or a bedrail may be considered a restraint if free movement is restricted.
   a. True
   b. False
2. Which statement about the use of restraints is *false*?
   a. Restraints can be used for staff convenience.
   b. A person may experience depression, anger, and agitation when restraints are on.
   c. A person may be embarrassed and humiliated when restraints are on.
   d. Restraints can cause serious injury and death.
3. Restraints can increase a person's confusion and agitation.
   a. True
   b. False

4. The person with a restraint should be observed at least every
   a. 15 minutes
   b. 30 minutes
   c. Hour
   d. 2 hours
5. Restraints need to be removed at least every
   a. Hour
   b. 2 hours
   c. 3 hours
   d. 4 hours

6. You should record all the following *except*
   a. The type of restraint used
   b. The consent for the restraint
   c. The time you removed the restraint
   d. The care you gave when the restraint was removed

CHAPTER 13 PREVENTING INFECTION
INFECTION
- Older persons are at risk for infection. An infection can become life-threatening before the older person has obvious signs and symptoms. Be alert to minor changes in the person's behavior or condition.
- Review Box 13-1, Signs and Symptoms of Infection, in the textbook.
- A **healthcare–associated infection (HAI)** is an infection acquired in a health care agency. Hospitals, nursing centers, clinics, and home care settings are examples. HAIs also are called *nosocomial infections*.
- The health team prevents the spread of HAIs by medical asepsis and **surgical asepsis (sterile technique).** Isolation Precautions and the Bloodborne Pathogen Standard also prevent HAIs.

MEDICAL ASEPSIS
- **Medical asepsis (clean technique)** refers to the practices used to remove or destroy pathogens. Medical asepsis also prevents pathogens from spreading from one person or place to another person or place.
- Hand hygiene is the easiest and most important way to prevent the spread of infection. Wash your hands with soap and water:
  - Before and after giving care to residents.
  - When they are visibly dirty or soiled with blood, saliva, vomitus, urine, feces, vaginal discharge, mucus, semen, wound drainage, pus, and other body fluids.
  - After removing gloves.
  - Before eating and after using the restroom.
  - When moving from a contaminated body site to a clean body site when giving care.
  - After contact with objects and equipment in the person's setting.
- Use an alcohol-based hand rub to decontaminate your hands if they are not visibly soiled. Review Box 13-2, Rules for Hand Hygiene, in the textbook.
- Most health care equipment is disposable. Multi-use items, such as bedpans, urinals, wash basins, and water pitchers and cups, are used many times. Multi-use items are intended for one person. Do not borrow these items from one person to use for another person.

ISOLATION PRECAUTIONS
- Isolation Precautions prevent the spread of communicable or contagious diseases.
- Standard Precautions are part of the CDC's Isolation Precautions. They reduce the risk of spreading pathogens. They also reduce the risk of spreading known and unknown infections. Standard Precautions are for all residents whenever care is given. They prevent the spread of infection from:
  - Blood.
  - All body fluids, secretions, and excretions (except sweat) even if blood is not visible.
  - Non-intact skin.
  - Mucous membranes.

- Review Box 13-4, Standard Precautions, in the textbook.
- Review Box 13-5, Transmission-Based Precautions, in the textbook.
- Isolation Precautions involve wearing personal protective equipment (PPE). This includes gloves, gown, mask, and goggles or a face shield. PPE also includes shoes, boots, and leg coverings. The nurse tells you what PPE to use.
- Wear gloves whenever contact with blood, body fluids, secretions, excretions, mucous membranes, and non-intact skin is likely. Wearing gloves is the most common protective measure used with Isolation Precautions.
- Remember the following when wearing gloves:
  - The outside of gloves are contaminated.
  - Gloves are easier to put on when your hands are dry.
  - You need a new pair for every person.
  - Remove and discard torn, cut, or punctured gloves at once. Practice hand hygiene. Then put on a new pair.
  - Wear gloves once. Discard them after use.
  - Put on clean gloves just before touching mucous membranes or non-intact skin.
  - Put on new gloves whenever gloves become contaminated with blood, body fluids, secretions, or excretions.
  - Change gloves whenever moving from a contaminated body site to a clean body site.
  - Make sure gloves cover your wrists. If you wear a gown, gloves cover the cuffs.
  - Remove gloves so the inside part is on the outside.
  - Decontaminate your hands after removing gloves.
- Latex allergies are common and can cause skin rashes. Asthma and shock are more serious problems. Report skin rashes and breathing problems at once. If you or a resident has a latex allergy, wear latex-free gloves.
- Gowns must completely cover your neck to your knees. The gown front and sleeves are considered contaminated. A wet gown is contaminated. Gowns are used once. When removing a gown, roll it away from you. Keep it inside out.
- Masks protect the spread of microbes from the respiratory tract. They are disposable. A wet or moist mask is contaminated. When removing a mask, touch only the ties or elastic bands.
- The outside of goggles or a face shield is contaminated. Use the headband or ear pieces to remove the device.
- Contaminated items, linens, and trash are bagged to remove them from the person's room. Follow center policy for bagging and transporting contaminated items. All bags have the *BIOHAZARD* symbol. Double bagging is not needed unless the outside of the bag is soiled.
- Specimens are transported to the laboratory in biohazard specimen bags.

REVIEW QUESTIONS
Circle the BEST answer.

1. A healthcare–associated infection (nosocomial infection) is
   a. An infection free of disease-producing microbes
   b. An infection that develops in a person cared for in any setting where health care is given
   c. An infection acquired by health care workers
   d. An infection acquired only by older persons

2. Which statement about hand hygiene is *false*?
   a. Hand hygiene is the easiest way to prevent the spread of infection.
   b. Hand hygiene is the most important way to prevent the spread of infection.
   c. Hand hygiene is practiced before and after giving care to a person.
   d. If hands are visibly soiled, hand hygiene can be done with an alcohol-based hand rub.

3. When washing your hands, you should do the following *except*
   a. Stand away from the sink so your clothes do not touch the sink
   b. Keep your hands lower than your elbows
   c. Wash your hands for at least 15 seconds
   d. Dry your arms from the forearms to the fingertips

4. Which statement about wearing gloves is *false*?
   a. The insides of gloves are contaminated.
   b. You need a new pair of gloves for each person you care for.
   c. Change gloves when moving from a contaminated body site to a clean body site.
   d. Gloves need to cover your wrists.

5. Which statement is *false*?
   a. Gowns must cover you from your neck to your waist.
   b. A moist mask is contaminated.
   c. The outside of goggles is contaminated.
   d. You should wash your hands after removing a gown, mask, or goggles.

6. Which statement about PPE is *false*?
   a. Remove PPE when a garment becomes contaminated.
   b. Wear gloves when handling or touching contaminated items or surfaces.
   c. Wash or decontaminate disposable gloves for reuse.
   d. Remove PPE before leaving the work area.

CHAPTER 14 BODY MECHANICS
PRINCIPLES OF BODY MECHANICS
- Your strongest and largest muscles are in the shoulders, upper arms, hips, and thighs. Use these muscles to lift and move residents and heavy objects.
- For good body mechanics:
  - Bend your knees and squat to lift a heavy object. Do not bend from your waist.
  - Hold items close to your body and base of support.
- To safely and efficiently handle and move persons and heavy objects, follow these rules:
  - Keep your body in good alignment with a wide base of support.
  - Use an upright working posture. Bend your legs. Do not bend your back.
  - Avoid unnecessary bending and reaching. Raise the bed so it is close to your waist.
  - Face your work area. This prevents unnecessary twisting.
  - Push, pull, or slide heavy objects whenever you can rather than lifting them.
  - Do not lean over a person to give care.
  - Widen your base of support when pushing or pulling. Move your front leg forward when pushing. Move your rear leg back when pulling.
  - Use both hands and arms to lift, move, or carry objects.
  - Turn your whole body when changing the direction of your movement. Move and turn your feet in the direction of the turn instead of twisting your body.
  - Work with smooth and even movements.
  - Get help from a co-worker to move heavy objects.
  - Do not lift objects higher than chest level.
- You are at risk for a musculoskeletal disorder. Always report a work-related injury as soon as possible. Early attention can help prevent the problem from becoming worse.

POSITIONING THE PERSON
- The person must be properly positioned at all times. Regular position changes and good alignment promote comfort and well-being. Breathing is easier. Circulation is promoted. Pressure ulcers and contractures are prevented.
- Whether in bed or in a chair, the person is repositioned at least every 2 hours. To safely position a person, use good body mechanics. Ask a co-worker to help you if needed.
- Pillows and positioning devices support body parts and keep the person in good alignment.
- **Fowler's position** is a semi-sitting position. The head of the bed is raised 45 to 60 degrees.

- **Supine (dorsal recumbent) position** is the back-lying position.
- In the **prone position**, a person lies on the abdomen with the head turned to one side.
- In the **lateral position**, a person lies on one side or the other.
- The **Sims' position (semi-prone side position)** is a left side-lying position. The upper leg is sharply flexed so it is not on the lower leg. The lower arm is behind the person.
- Persons who sit in chairs must hold their upper bodies and heads erect. For good alignment:
  - The person's back and buttocks are against the back of the chair.
  - Feet are flat on the floor or wheelchair footplates. Never leave feet unsupported.
  - Backs of the knees and calves are slightly away from the edge of the seat.
  - The nurse may ask you to put a pillow between the person's lower back and the chair.

REVIEW QUESTIONS
Circle the BEST answer.
1. To lift and move residents and heavy objects you should
   a. Use the muscles in your lower arms
   b. Use the muscles in your legs
   c. Use the muscles in your shoulders, upper arms, hips, and thighs
   d. Use the muscles in your abdomen
2. For good body mechanics, you should do all of the following *except*
   a. Bend your knees and squat to lift a heavy object
   b. Bend from your waist to lift a heavy object
   c. Hold items close to your body and base of support
   d. Bend your legs, do not bend your back
3. Which statement is *false*?
   a. A person must be properly positioned at all times.
   b. Regular position changes and good alignment promote comfort and well-being.
   c. Regular position changes and good alignment promote pressure ulcers and contractures.
   d. When a person is in good alignment, breathing is easier and circulation is promoted.
4. In Fowler's position
   a. The head of the bed is flat
   b. The head of the bed is raised to 90 degrees
   c. The head of the bed is raised between 45 and 60 degrees
   d. The head of the bed is raised between 30 and 35 degrees

CHAPTER 15 SAFE RESIDENT HANDLING, MOVING, AND TRANSFERS

PREVENTING WORK-RELATED INJURIES

- To prevent work-related injuries:
  - Wear shoes that provide good traction.
  - Use assistive equipment and devices whenever possible.
  - Get help from other staff.
  - Plan and prepare for the task. Know what equipment you will need and on what side of the bed to place the chair or wheelchair.
  - Schedule harder tasks early in your shift.
  - Balance easier and harder tasks.
  - Tell the resident what he or she can do to help. Give clear, simple instructions.
  - Do not hold or grab the person under the arms.
- For additional guidelines, review Box 15-2, Preventing Work-Related Injuries, in the textbook.

MOVING PERSONS UP IN BED

- Protect the person's skin from tears. Friction and shearing injure the skin and cause infection and pressure ulcers.
- Reduce friction and shearing by:
  - Rolling the person.
  - Using a lift sheet (turning sheet).
  - Using a turning pad, slide board, slide sheet, or a large incontinence product.
- You can sometimes move lightweight adults up in bed alone if they can assist and use a trapeze.
- Lower the head of the bed to a level appropriate for the person.

TURNING PERSONS

- Turning persons onto their sides helps prevent complications from bedrest. Certain procedures and care measures also require the side-lying position. After the person is turned, position him or her in good alignment. Support the person in the side-lying position.

SITTING ON THE SIDE OF THE BED (DANGLING)

- Many older persons become dizzy or faint when getting out of bed too fast. They need to sit on the side of the bed before walking or transferring. Some persons increase activity in stages—bedrest, to sitting on the side of the bed, to sitting in a chair, to walking.
- While dangling, the person coughs and deep breathes. He or she moves the legs back and forth in circles to stimulate circulation. Provide for warmth during the dangling procedure.
- Observations to report and record:
  - Pulse and respiratory rates.
  - Pale or bluish skin color (cyanosis).
  - Complaints of light-headedness, dizziness, or difficulty breathing.
  - How well the activity was tolerated.
  - The length of time the person dangled.
  - The amount of help needed.
  - Other observations and complaints.

TRANSFERRING PERSONS

- Correctly place the chair, wheelchair, or other device for a safe transfer.
- Have the person wear non-skid footwear for transfers.
- Lock wheels of bed, wheelchair, stretcher, or other assist device.
- After the transfer, position the person in good alignment.
- Transfer/gait belts are used to support residents during transfers. They are also used to reposition persons in chairs and wheelchairs.
- Safety is important for transfers. Help the person out of bed on his or her strong side. Help the person from the wheelchair to the bed on his or her strong side. In transferring, the strong side moves first.
- The person must not put his or her arms around your neck.

MECHANICAL LIFTS

- Persons who cannot help themselves are transferred with mechanical lifts. So are persons who are too heavy for the staff to transfer.
- Before using a mechanical lift, you must be trained in its use. The sling, straps, hooks, and chains must be in good repair. The person's weight must not exceed the lift's capacity. At least two staff members are needed. Always follow the manufacturer's instructions for using the lift.
- Falling from the lift is a common fear. To promote the person's mental comfort, always explain the procedure before you begin. Also show the person how the lift works.

REVIEW QUESTIONS

Circle the BEST answer.

1. Friction and shearing are reduced by doing the following *except*
   a. Rolling the person
   b. Using a lift sheet or turning pad
   c. Using a pillow
   d. Using a slide board or slide sheet
2. After a person is turned, you must position him or her in good alignment.
   a. True
   b. False
3. Which statement about dangling is *false*?
   a. Many older persons become dizzy or faint when they first dangle.
   b. The person should cough and deep breathe while dangling.
   c. The person moves his or her legs before dangling.
   d. You should cover the person's shoulders with a robe or blanket while dangling.

4. You are transferring a person from the bed to a wheelchair. Which statement is *false*?
   a. The person should wear non-skid footwear.
   b. The person may put his or her arm around your neck.
   c. You should use a gait/transfer belt.
   d. You should lock the wheelchair wheels.

5. A person has a weak left side and a strong right side. In transferring the person from the bed to the wheelchair, his or her strong (right) side moves first.
   a. True
   b. False

CHAPTER 16 THE RESIDENT'S UNIT
COMFORT
- To protect older and chronically ill persons from drafts:
  - Make sure they wear correct clothing.
  - Make sure they wear enough clothing.
  - Offer lap robes to cover their legs.
  - Provide enough blankets for warmth.
  - Cover them with bath blankets when giving care.
  - Move them from drafty areas.
- To reduce odors in nursing centers:
  - Empty, clean, and disinfect bedpans, urinals, commodes, and kidney basins promptly.
  - Check to make sure toilets are flushed.
  - Check incontinent people often.
  - Clean persons who are wet or soiled from urine, feces, or wound drainage.
  - Change wet or soiled linens and clothing promptly.
  - Keep laundry containers closed.
  - Follow center policy for wet or soiled clothing.
  - Dispose of incontinence and ostomy products promptly.
  - Use room deodorizers as needed.
- To decrease noise:
  - Control your voice.
  - Handle equipment carefully.
  - Keep equipment in good working order.
  - Answer phones, signal lights, and intercoms promptly.
- Adjust lighting to meet the person's changing needs. Glares, shadows, and dull lighting can cause falls, headaches, and eyestrain. A bright room is cheerful. Dim light is better for relaxing and rest. Always keep light controls within the person's reach.

ROOM FURNITURE AND EQUIPMENT
- Beds are raised to give care. They are positioned at the lowest level when not giving care.
- Bed wheels are locked at all times except when moving the bed.
- Use bed rails as the nurse and care plan direct.
- Basic bed positions:
  - Flat is the usual sleeping position.
  - **Fowler's position**—a semi-sitting position. The head of the bed is raised between 45 and 60 degrees.
  - **Semi-Fowler's position**—the head of the bed is raised 30 degrees. In some centers, semi-Fowler's position is defined as the head of the bed is raised 30 degrees and the knee portion is raised 15 degrees. This position is comfortable and prevents sliding down in bed. However, raising the knee portion can interfere with circulation in the legs. To give safe care, check with the nurse before raising the knee portion of the bed.
- *Entrapment* means the person can get caught, trapped, or entangled in spaces created by bed rails, the mattress, the bed frame, or the head and foot boards. Serious injuries and deaths have occurred from entrapment. If a person is at risk for entrapment, report your concerns to the nurse at once. If a person is caught, trapped, or entangled, try to release the person. Call for the nurse at once.

- Never place bedpans, urinals, or soiled linen on the overbed table or on top of the bedside stand. Clean the table and bedside stand after using them for a work surface.
- Always pull the curtain completely around the bed before giving care. Privacy curtains do not block sound or conversations.
- The signal light must always be kept within the person's reach—in the room, bathroom, and shower or tub room. You must:
  - Place the signal light on the person's strong side.
  - Remind the person to signal when help is needed.
  - Answer signal lights promptly.
  - Answer bathroom and shower or tub room signal lights at once.
- Persons with limited hand mobility may need special communication measures.
- Nursing centers must provide each person with closet space. The person must have free access to the closet and its contents. Center staff can inspect a person's closet or drawers if hoarding is suspected. The person is informed of the inspection and is present when it takes place. Have a co-worker present when you inspect a person's closet.
- Keep the person's room clean, neat, safe, and comfortable.

REVIEW QUESTIONS
Circle T if the statement is true or F if the statement is false.
1. T F Serious injuries and death have occurred from entrapment.
2. T F You should never place bedpans, urinals, or soiled linen on the overbed table.
3. T F You should clean the bedside stand if you use it for a work surface.

Circle the BEST answer.
4. The following protect a person from drafts *except*
   a. Wearing enough clothing
   b. Lap robes
   c. Using a sheet when giving care
   d. Providing blankets
5. To reduce odors, you do the following *except*
   a. Empty bedpans and commodes promptly
   b. Keep laundry containers open
   c. Check to make sure toilets are flushed
   d. Clean persons who are wet or soiled from urine or feces
6. Which statement about the signal light is *false*?
   a. The signal light must always be within the person's reach.
   b. Place the signal light on the person's strong side.
   c. You have to answer the signal lights only for residents assigned to you.
   d. Answer signal lights promptly.
7. You suspect a person is hoarding food in her closet. What do you do first?
   a. Tell another nursing assistant what you suspect.
   b. Inspect the closet without telling the resident.
   c. Tell the nurse.
   d. Tell the resident you are going to inspect the closet.

CHAPTER 17 BEDMAKING
BEDS
- Clean, dry, and wrinkle-free linens are important. Comfort is promoted. Skin breakdown and pressure ulcers are prevented. Do the following to keep beds neat and clean:
  - Straighten linens whenever loose or wrinkled and at bedtime.
  - Check for and remove food and crumbs after meals.
  - Check linens for dentures, eyeglasses, hearing aids, sharp objects, and other items.
  - Change linens whenever they become wet, soiled, or damp.
  - Follow Standard Precautions and the Bloodborne Pathogen Standard.
- Linens are usually changed weekly on the person's bath day. Pillowcases, top and bottom sheets, and draw sheets may be changed twice a week. Linens are always changed if wet, damp, soiled, or very wrinkled.

HANDLING LINENS
- When handling linen:
  - Practice medical asepsis.
  - Always hold linen away from your body and uniform. Your uniform is considered dirty.
  - Never shake linen.
  - Never put clean or dirty linen on the floor.
  - Do not bring unneeded linens into the person's room. Once in the room, extra linen is considered contaminated. It cannot be used for another person.
  - Roll each piece of dirty linen away from you. The side that touched the person is inside the roll and away from you.

MAKING BEDS
- Use good body mechanics.
- Follow the rules of medical asepsis.
- Follow Standard Precautions and the Bloodborne Pathogen Standard.
- Follow the rules for safe resident handling, moving, and transfers.
- Practice hand hygiene before handling clean linen.

- Practice hand hygiene after handling dirty linen.
- Bring enough linen into the person's room.
- Do not use torn or frayed linen.
- Cover a plastic drawsheet with a cotton drawsheet.
- Make as much of one side of the bed as possible before going to the other side.
- Face hem-stitching outward, away from the person.
- To save time and energy, make beds with a co-worker.

The Occupied Bed
- You make an occupied bed when the person stays in bed. Keep the person in good alignment. Follow restrictions or limits in the person's movement or position.

REVIEW QUESTIONS
Circle the BEST answer.
1. To keep beds neat and clean, do the following *except*
   a. Straighten linens whenever loose or wrinkled
   b. Check for and remove food and crumbs after meals
   c. Check linens for dentures, eyeglasses, and hearing aids
   d. Change linen monthly
2. Which statement is *false*?
   a. Practice medical asepsis when handling linen.
   b. Always hold linens away from your body and uniform.
   c. Shake linens to remove crumbs.
   d. Put dirty linens in the dirty laundry bin.
3. Once in the person's room, extra linen is considered contaminated. It can be used for another person.
   a. True
   b. False
4. Roll each piece of dirty linen away from you. The side that touched the person is inside the roll.
   a. True
   b. False
5. Wear gloves when removing linen from the person's bed.
   a. True
   b. False

CHAPTER 18 HYGIENE

ORAL HYGIENE

- Oral hygiene keeps the mouth and teeth clean. It prevents mouth odors and infections, increases comfort, and makes food taste better.
- Flossing removes plaque and tartar from the teeth as well as food from between the teeth. Flossing is usually done after brushing. If done once a day, bedtime is the best time to floss.
- Sponge swabs are used for persons with sore, tender mouths and for persons who are unconscious. Check the foam on the sponge swab to be sure it is tight on the stick.
- Report and record:
  - Dry, cracked, swollen, or blistered lips.
  - Mouth or breath odor.
  - Redness, swelling, irritation, sores, or white patches in the mouth or on the tongue.
  - Bleeding, swelling, or redness of the gums.
  - Loose teeth.
  - Rough, sharp, or chipped areas on dentures.
- Assist with oral hygiene after sleep, after meals, and at bedtime. Always follow the care plan.
- Follow Standard Precautions and the Bloodborne Pathogen Standard.

Mouth Care for the Unconscious Person

- Unconscious persons have dry mouths. They also have crusting on the tongue and mucous membranes. Use sponge swabs to apply the cleaning agent. To prevent cracking of the lips, apply a lubricant to the lips.
- To prevent **aspiration** on the unconscious person:
  - Position the person on one side with the head turned well to the side.
  - Use only a small amount of fluid to clean the mouth.
  - Do not insert dentures. Dentures are not worn when the person is unconscious.
- When giving oral hygiene, keep the person's mouth open with a padded tongue blade.
- Mouth care is given at least every 2 hours. Follow the nurse's direction and the care plan.

Denture Care

- Mouth care is given and dentures are cleaned as often as natural teeth. Dentures are usually removed at bedtime. Remind people not to wrap dentures in tissues or napkins.
- Dentures are slippery when wet. During cleaning, firmly hold them over a basin of water lined with a towel. Use a cleaning agent, and follow the manufacturer's instructions.
- Hot water causes dentures to lose their shape. If dentures are not worn after cleaning, store them in a container with cool water or a denture soaking solution.
- Label the denture cup with the person's name, room number, and bed number. Report lost or damaged dentures to the nurse at once. Losing or damaging dentures is negligent conduct.

- Many people do not like being seen without their dentures. If you clean dentures, return them to the person as quickly as possible.
- Persons with partial dentures have some natural teeth. They need to brush and floss the natural teeth.

BATHING

- Bathing cleans the skin and the mucous membranes of the genital and anal areas. A bath is refreshing and relaxing. Circulation is stimulated and body parts exercised. You have time to talk to the person. You also can make observations.
- Soap dries the skin. Therefore older persons usually need a complete bath or shower twice a week. Partial baths are taken the other days. Some bathe daily but not with soap. Thorough rinsing is needed when using soap. Lotions and oils keep the skin soft. Review Box 18-1, Rules for Bathing, in the textbook.
- Water temperature for complete bed baths and partial bed baths is between 110° F and 115° F. Older persons have fragile skin and need lower water temperatures. Measure water temperature with a bath thermometer or by dipping your elbow or inner wrist into the basin.
- Report and record:
  - The color of the skin, lips, nail beds, and sclera.
  - The location and description of rashes.
  - Dry skin.
  - Bruises or open areas.
  - Pale or reddened areas, particularly over bony parts.
  - Drainage or bleeding from wounds or body openings.
  - Swelling of the feet and legs.
  - Corns or calluses on the feet.
  - Skin temperature.
  - Complaints of pain or discomfort.
- Before bathing, assist the person with elimination needs.
- Provide for warmth. Cover the person with a bath blanket.
- Follow Standard Precautions and the Bloodborne Pathogen Standard.
- Use caution when applying powders. Do not use powders near persons with respiratory disorders. Do not sprinkle or shake powder onto the person. To safely apply powder:
  - Turn away from the person.
  - Sprinkle a small amount onto your hands or a cloth.
  - Apply the powder in a thin layer.
  - Make sure powder does not get on the floor. Powder is slippery and can cause falls.
- The complete bed bath involves washing the person's entire body in bed. Wash around the person's eyes with water. Do not use soap. Gently wipe from the inner to the outer aspect of the eye. Use a clean part of the washcloth for each stroke. Ask the person if you should use soap to wash the face. Let the person wash the genital area if he or she is able.
- Give a back massage after the bath. Apply deodorant or antiperspirant, lotion, and powder as requested. Comb and brush the hair. Empty and clean the wash basin.

- The partial bath involves bathing the face, hands, axillae (underarms), back, buttocks, and perineal area. You assist the person as needed. Most need help washing the back.
- A tub bath can cause a person to feel faint, weak, or tired. The person may need a transfer bench, a tub with a side entry door, a wheelchair or stretcher lift, or a mechanical lift to get in and out of the tub.
- Some people can use a regular shower. Have the person use the grab bars for support during the shower. Use a bath mat if the shower does not have non-skid surfaces. Never let weak or unsteady persons stand in the shower. They may need to use shower chairs, shower stalls or cabinets, or shower trolleys. Some shower rooms have two or more stations. Protect the person's privacy. Properly screen and cover the person.
- Water temperature for tub baths and showers is usually 105° F. Report and record dizziness and light-headedness.

THE BACK MASSAGE
- The back massage relaxes muscles and stimulates circulation.
- Massages are given after the bath and with evening care. You also can give back massages at other times, such as after repositioning a person.
- Observe the skin for breaks, bruises, reddened areas, and other signs of skin breakdown.
- Lotion reduces friction during the massage. It is warmed before applying.
- Use firm strokes. Keep your hands in contact with the person's skin.
- After the massage, apply some lotion to the elbows, knees, and heels.
- Back massages are dangerous for some persons. Check with the nurse and the care plan before giving a person a back massage.
- Do not massage reddened bony areas. Reddened areas signal skin breakdown and pressure ulcers. Massage can lead to more tissue damage.
- Wear gloves if the person's skin is not intact. Always follow Standard Precautions and the Bloodborne Pathogen Standard.

PERINEAL CARE
- Perineal care involves cleaning the genital and anal areas. It is done daily during the bath and whenever the area is soiled with urine or feces. The person does perineal care if able.
- *Perineal* and *perineum* are not common terms. Most people understand *privates*, *private parts*, *crotch*, *genitals*, or the *area between the legs*. Use terms the person understands.
- Standard Precautions, medical asepsis, and the Bloodborne Pathogen Standard are followed.
- Work from the cleanest area to the dirtiest—commonly called cleaning from "front to back." On a woman, clean from the urethra (cleanest) to the anal (dirtiest) area. On a male, start at the meatus of the urethra and work outward.

- Use warm water. Use washcloths, towelettes, cotton balls, or swabs according to center policy. Rinse thoroughly. Pat dry. Water temperature is usually 105° F to 109° F.
- Report and record:
  - Odors.
  - Redness, swelling, discharge, bleeding, or irritation.
  - Complaints of pain, burning, or other discomfort.
  - Signs of urinary or fecal incontinence.

REVIEW QUESTIONS
Circle the BEST answer.
1. Oral hygiene does the following *except*
   a. Keeps the mouth and teeth clean
   b. Prevents mouth odors and infections
   c. Decreases comfort
   d. Makes food taste better
2. When giving oral hygiene, you should report and record the following *except*
   a. Dry, cracked, swollen, or blistered lips
   b. Redness, sores, or white patches in the mouth
   c. Bleeding, swelling, or redness of the gums
   d. The number of fillings a person has
3. A person is unconscious. When you do his mouth care, you do the following *except*
   a. Use only a small amount of fluid to clean his mouth
   b. Use your fingers to keep his mouth open
   c. Explain what you are doing
   d. Give mouth care at least every 2 hours
4. Which statement about dentures is *false*?
   a. Dentures are slippery when wet.
   b. During cleaning, hold dentures over a basin of water lined with a towel.
   c. Store dentures in cool water.
   d. Remind people to wrap their dentures in tissues or napkins.
5. Bathing does the following *except*
   a. Cleanses the skin
   b. Stimulates circulation
   c. Makes a person tense
   d. Permits you to observe the person's skin
6. The water temperature for a complete bed bath is
   a. 102° F to 108° F
   b. 110° F to 115° F
   c. 115° F to 120° F
   d. 120° F to 125° F
7. Which statement is *false*?
   a. Use powder near persons with respiratory disorders.
   b. Before applying powder, check with the nurse and the care plan.
   c. Before applying powder, sprinkle a small amount of powder onto your hands.
   d. Apply powder in a thin layer.
8. To test water temperature, you can do the following *except*
   a. Use a bath thermometer
   b. Dip your elbow into the basin
   c. Ask the person to dip his finger into the basin
   d. Dip your inner wrist into the basin

9. When washing a person's eyes, you should do the following *except*
   a. Use only water
   b. Gently wipe from the inner to the outer aspect of the eye
   c. Gently wipe from the outer to the inner aspect of the eye
   d. Use a clean part of the washcloth for each stroke

10. Which statement is *false*?
    a. A back massage relaxes and stimulates circulation.
    b. Massages are given after the bath and with evening care.
    c. You can observe the person's skin before beginning the massage.
    d. You should use cold lotion for the massage.

11. When giving female perineal care, you should work from the urethra to the anal area.
    a. True
    b. False

12. When giving male perineal care, start at the meatus and work outward.
    a. True
    b. False

CHAPTER 19 GROOMING
GROOMING
- Hair care, shaving, and nail and foot care prevent infection and promote comfort. They also affect love, belonging, and self-esteem. To perform grooming measures, the person may use adaptive devices. This promotes the person's independence and quality of life.

HAIR CARE
- Brushing and combing prevent tangled and matted hair.
- When brushing and combing hair, start at the scalp and brush or comb to the hair ends.
- When giving hair care, place a towel across the person's back and shoulders to protect garments from falling hair. If the person is in bed, give hair care before changing the linens and pillowcase.
- Never cut hair for any reason. Tell the nurse if you think the person's hair needs to be cut.
- Special measures are needed for curly, coarse, and dry hair. Check the care plan.
- Tell the nurse if you have concerns about the person's brush or comb.
- Shampooing frequency depends on the person's needs and preferences. Usually shampooing is done weekly on the person's bath or shower day.
- Hair is dried and styled as quickly as possible after the shampoo.
- During shampooing, report and record:
  - Scalp sores.
  - Flaking.
  - Itching.
  - Presence of nits or lice.
  - Patches of hair loss.
  - Very dry or very oily hair.
  - Matted or tangled hair.
  - How the person tolerated the procedure.
- Keep shampoo away from and out of eyes. Have the person hold a washcloth over the eyes.
- Wear gloves if the person has scalp sores.
- Follow Standard Precautions and the Bloodborne Pathogen Standard.

SHAVING
- Rules for shaving:
  - Use electric razors for persons who take anticoagulant drugs.
  - Protect bed linens.
  - Soften the skin before shaving.
  - Hold the skin taut as needed.
  - Shave in the correct direction. If shaving the face with a safety razor, shave in the direction of hair growth.
  - If using an electric shaver, shave against the direction of hair growth.
  - Do not nick, cut, or irritate the skin.
  - Rinse the body part thoroughly.
  - Apply direct pressure to nicks and cuts.
  - Report nicks, cuts, or irritation to the nurse at once.
  - Clean the shaver after use.
- When using a safety razor, follow Standard Precautions and the Bloodborne Pathogen Standard.

- Wash and comb mustaches and beards daily and as needed. Ask the person how to groom his mustache or beard. Never trim a mustache or beard without the person's consent.
- Many women shave their legs and underarms. This practice varies among cultures. Legs and underarms are shaved after bathing when the skin is soft.

NAIL AND FOOT CARE
- Nail and foot care prevent infection, injury, and odors.
- Nails are easier to trim and clean right after soaking or bathing.
- Use nail clippers to cut fingernails. Never use scissors. Use extreme caution to prevent damage to nearby tissues.
- Follow Standard Precautions and the Bloodborne Pathogen Standard.
- Report and record:
  - Reddened, irritated, or callused areas.
  - Breaks in the skin.
  - Corns on top of and between the toes.
  - Very thick nails.
  - Loose nails.
- You do not cut or trim toenails if a person has diabetes or poor circulation to the legs and feet or takes drugs that affect blood clotting. Also, do not cut or trim toenails if the person has very thick nails or ingrown toenails. The RN or podiatrist cuts toenails and provides foot care for these persons.
- When doing foot care, check between the toes for cracks and sores. If left untreated, a serious infection could occur.
- The feet of persons with decreased sensation or circulatory problems may easily burn because they do not feel hot temperatures.
- After soaking, apply lotion to the feet. Because the lotion can cause slippery feet, help the person put on non-skid footwear before you transfer the person or let the person walk.

CHANGING CLOTHING AND HOSPITAL GOWNS
- When changing clothing:
  - Provide for privacy.
  - Encourage the person to do as much as possible.
  - Let the person choose what to wear. Make sure the right undergarments are chosen.
  - Remove clothing from the strong or "good" (unaffected) side first.
  - Put clothing on the weak (affected) side first.
  - Support the arm or leg when removing or putting on a garment.

REVIEW QUESTIONS
Circle T if the statement is true or F if the statement is false.
1. T   F   Hair care, shaving, and nail and foot care prevent infection and promote comfort.
2. T   F   If a person's hair is matted, you may cut the hair.

3. T F When giving hair care, place a towel across the person's back and shoulders to protect garments from falling hair.
4. T F You should wear gloves when shampooing a person who has scalp sores.
5. T F A person takes an anticoagulant. Therefore he shaves with an electric razor.
6. T F You should wear gloves when shaving a person.
7. T F Never trim a mustache or beard without the person's consent.
8. T F Mustaches and beards need daily care.
9. T F You do not cut toenails if the person has diabetes.

Circle the BEST answer.
10. Fingernails are cut with
    a. Scissors
    b. Nail clippers
    c. An emery board
    d. A nail file
11. Which statement is *false*?
    a. Provide privacy when a person is changing clothes.
    b. Most residents wear street clothes during the day.
    c. Let the person choose what to wear.
    d. You may tear a person's clothing.

CHAPTER 20 URINARY ELIMINATION
NORMAL URINATION
- Observe urine for color, clarity, odor, amount, and particles. Normal urine is pale yellow, straw-colored, or amber. It is clear with no particles. A faint odor is normal. Some foods and drugs affect urine color. Ask the nurse to observe urine that looks or smells abnormal. Report complaints of urgency or painful or difficult urination.
- Follow Standard Precautions and the Bloodborne Pathogen Standard when handling bedpans urinals, commodes, and their contents. Thoroughly clean and disinfect bedpans, urinals, and commodes after use.
- Review Box 20-1, Rules for Normal Urination, in the textbook.

URINARY INCONTINENCE
- If **urinary incontinence** is a new problem, tell the nurse at once.
- Incontinence is embarrassing. Garments are wet, and odors develop. Skin irritation, infection, and pressure ulcers are risks. The person's pride, dignity, and self-esteem are affected. Social isolation, loss of independence, and depression are common.
- Good skin care and dry garments and linens are essential. Promoting normal urinary elimination prevents incontinence in some people. Other people may need bladder training. Review Box 20-2, Nursing Measures for Persons With Urinary Incontinence, in the textbook.
- Caring for persons with incontinence is stressful. Remember, the person does not choose to be incontinent. If you find yourself becoming short-tempered and impatient, talk to the nurse at once. Kindness, empathy, understanding, and patience are needed.

CATHETERS
- The catheter must not pull at the insertion site. Hold the catheter securely during catheter care. Then properly secure the catheter. Also make sure the tubing is not under the person. Besides obstructing urine flow, lying on the tubing is uncomfortable. It can also cause skin breakdown.
- Follow Standard Precautions and the Bloodborne Pathogen Standard. Review Box 20-3, Caring for Persons With Indwelling Catheters, in the textbook.
- Report and record:
  - Complaints of pain, burning, irritation, or the need to void.
  - Crusting, abnormal drainage, or secretions.
  - The color, clarity, and odor of urine.
  - Particles in the urine.
  - Drainage system leaks.

Drainage Systems
- A closed drainage system is used for indwelling catheters. The drainage bag hangs from the bed frame, chair, or wheelchair. It must not touch the floor. The bag is always kept lower than the person's bladder. Do not hang the drainage bag on a bed rail.
- Drainage bags are emptied and measured at the end of every shift and when the bag is full. Follow Standard Precautions and the Bloodborne Pathogen Standard.
- Empty and measure a leg bag when it is half full.
- Report and record:
  - The amount of urine measured.
  - The color, clarity, and odor of urine.
  - Particles in the urine.
  - Complaints of pain, burning, irritation, or the need to urinate.
  - Urinary system leaks.
- If the drainage system is disconnected accidentally, tell the nurse at once. Do not touch the ends of the catheter or tubing. Do the following:
  - Practice hand hygiene. Put on gloves.
  - Wipe the end of the tube with an antiseptic wipe.
  - Wipe the end of the catheter with another antiseptic wipe.
  - Do not put the ends down. Do not touch the ends after you clean them.
  - Connect the tubing to the catheter.
  - Discard the wipes into a biohazard bag.
  - Remove gloves. Practice hand hygiene.

Condom Catheters
- Condom catheters are also called *external catheters*, *Texas catheters*, and *urinary sheaths*.
- Condom catheters are changed daily after perineal care.
- To apply a condom catheter, follow the manufacturer's instructions. Follow Standard Precautions and the Bloodborne Pathogen Standard.
- Some condom catheters are self-adhering. Other catheters are secured in place with elastic tape in a spiral manner. Never use adhesive tape to secure catheters. It does not expand. Blood flow to the penis is cut off, injuring the penis.
- When removing or applying a condom catheter, report and record the following observations:
  - Reddened or open areas on the penis.
  - Swelling of the penis.
  - Color, clarity, and odor of urine.
  - Particles in the urine.
  - Do not apply a condom catheter if the penis is red, irritated, or shows signs of skin breakdown. Report your observations to the nurse at once.

BLADDER TRAINING
- Bladder training helps some persons with urinary incontinence. Control of urination is the goal. Bladder control promotes comfort and quality of life. It also increases self-esteem. You assist with bladder training as directed by the nurse and the care plan.

REVIEW QUESTIONS
Circle the BEST answer.
1. Which statement is *false*?
   a. Normal urine is yellow, straw-colored, or amber.
   b. Urine with a strong odor is normal.
   c. Some foods and drugs affect urine color.
   d. Observe urine for color, clarity, odor, amount, and particles.

2. Which observation does *not* need to be reported to the nurse promptly?
   a. Complaints of urgency
   b. Burning on urination
   c. Painful or difficult urination
   d. Clear amber urine
3. Which statement is *false*?
   a. Incontinence is embarrassing.
   b. Caring for persons with incontinence may be stressful.
   c. Incontinence is a personal choice.
   d. Be kind and patient to persons who are incontinent.
4. A person with a catheter complains of pain. You should notify the nurse at once.
   a. True
   b. False
5. Which statement is *false*?
   a. The urine drainage system should hang from the bed frame or chair.
   b. The urine drainage system should hang on a bed rail.
   c. The urine drainage system must be off the floor.
   d. The urine drainage system must be kept lower than the person's bladder.

6. Which statement is *false*?
   a. Condom catheters are changed daily.
   b. Follow manufacturer's instructions when applying a condom catheter.
   c. Use adhesive tape to secure a condom catheter in place.
   d. Report and record open or reddened areas on the penis at once.
7. The goal of bladder training is to
   a. Allow the person to use the toilet
   b. Keep the catheter
   c. Gain control of urination
   d. Decrease self-esteem

CHAPTER 21 BOWEL ELIMINATION
NORMAL BOWEL ELIMINATION

- Stools are normally brown, soft, formed, moist, and shaped like the rectum. They have a normal odor caused by bacterial action in the intestines. Certain foods and drugs cause odors.
- Carefully observe stools before disposing of them. Observe and report the color, amount, consistency, odor, and shape of stools. Also, observe and report the presence of blood or mucus, frequency of defecation, and any complaints of pain or discomfort.
- Follow Standard Precautions and the Bloodborne Pathogen Standard when in contact with stools.

FACTORS AFFECTING BOWEL ELIMINATION

- *Privacy.* Bowel elimination is a private act.
- *Habits.* Many people have a bowel movement after breakfast. Some read. Defecation is easier when a person is relaxed.
- *Diet—high-fiber foods.* Fiber helps prevent constipation.
- *Diet—other foods.* Some foods cause constipation. Other foods cause frequent stools or diarrhea.
- *Fluids.* Drinking 6 to 8 glasses of water daily promotes normal bowel elimination. Warm fluids—coffee, tea, hot cider, warm water—increase peristalsis.
- *Activity.* Exercise and activity maintain muscle tone and stimulate peristalsis.
- *Drugs.* Drugs can prevent constipation or control diarrhea. Some have diarrhea or constipation as side effects.
- *Aging.* Older persons may have constipation. Some lose bowel control. They may not completely empty the rectum. They often need to defecate about 30 to 45 minutes after the first bowel movement.
- *Disability.* Some people cannot control bowel movements. A bowel training program is needed.
- To provide comfort and safety during bowel elimination:
  - Provide for privacy.
  - Help the person to the toilet or commode. Or provide the bedpan as soon as requested.
  - Make sure the bedpan is warm.
  - Position the person in a normal sitting or squatting position.
  - Cover the person for warmth and privacy.
  - Allow enough time for defecation.
  - Place the signal light and the toilet tissue within reach.
  - Leave the room if the person can be alone. Check on the person every 5 minutes.
  - Stay nearby if the person is weak or unsteady.
  - Provide perineal care.
  - Dispose of stools promptly. This reduces odor and prevents the spread of microbes.
  - Assist the person with hand washing after elimination.
  - Follow the care plan if the person has fecal incontinence.

CONSTIPATION

- Common causes of **constipation** are a low-fiber diet and ignoring the urge to defecate. Other causes include decreased fluid intake, inactivity, drugs, aging, and certain diseases.
- Dietary changes, fluids, and activity prevent or relieve constipation. So do drugs and enemas.

FECAL IMPACTION

- **Fecal impaction** results if constipation is not relieved. The person cannot defecate. Liquid feces pass around the hardened fecal mass in the rectum. The liquid feces seep from the anus.
- Abdominal discomfort, abdominal distention, nausea, cramping, and rectal pain are common. Older persons have poor appetite or confusion. Some persons have an elevated temperature. Report these signs and symptoms to the nurse.
- The nurse does a digital exam to check for an impaction. Drugs and enemas may be ordered by the doctor. Sometimes the nurse removes the fecal mass with a gloved finger.

DIARRHEA

- The need to defecate is urgent. Some people cannot get to a bathroom in time. Abdominal cramping, nausea, and vomiting occur.
- Assist with elimination needs promptly, dispose of stools promptly, and give good skin care. Liquid stools irritate the skin. So does frequent wiping with toilet paper. Skin breakdown and pressure ulcers are risks.
- Fluid lost through diarrhea is replaced. Otherwise **dehydration** occurs.

FECAL INCONTINENCE

- **Fecal incontinence** is the inability to control the passage of feces and gas through the anus.
- Fecal incontinence affects the person emotionally. Frustration, embarrassment, anger, and humiliation are common. The person may need:
  - Bowel training.
  - Help with elimination after meals and every 2 to 3 hours.
  - Incontinence products to keep garments and linens clean.
  - Good skin care.

FLATULENCE

- Causes include swallowing air while eating and drinking and bacterial action in the intestines. Other causes may be gas-forming foods, constipation, bowel and abdominal surgeries, and drugs that decrease peristalsis.
- If flatus is not expelled, the intestines distend. Abdominal cramping or pain, shortness of breath, and a swollen abdomen occur. "Bloating" is a common complaint. Exercise, walking, moving in bed, and the left side-lying position often produce flatus. Enemas and drugs may be ordered.

BOWEL TRAINING

- Bowel training has two goals:
  - To gain control of bowel movements.
  - To develop a regular pattern of elimination. Fecal impactions, constipation, and fecal incontinence are prevented.
- Factors that promote elimination are part of the care plan and bowel training program.

REVIEW QUESTIONS

Choose the BEST answer.

1. Which statement is *false*?
   a. Lack of privacy can prevent defecation.
   b. Low-fiber foods promote defecation.
   c. Drinking 6 to 8 glasses of water daily promotes normal bowel elimination.
   d. Exercise stimulates peristalsis.

2. Which of the following *does not* prevent constipation?
   a. A high-fiber diet
   b. Increased fluid intake
   c. Exercise
   d. Ignoring the urge to defecate

3. A person has fecal incontinence. You should do the following *except*
   a. Be patient
   b. Help with elimination after meals
   c. Provide good skin care
   d. Scold the person for being incontinent

CHAPTER 22 NUTRITION AND FLUIDS
FACTORS AFFECTING EATING AND NUTRITION

- *Culture.* Dietary practices, food choices, and food preparation vary among cultural groups.
- *Religion.* Selecting, preparing, and eating food often involve religious practices. Review Box 22-3, Religion and Dietary Practices, in the textbook.
- *Finances.* People with limited incomes often buy the cheaper carbohydrate foods. Their diets often lack protein and certain vitamins and minerals.
- *Appetite.* Illness, drugs, anxiety, pain, and depression can cause lack of appetite. Unpleasant sights, thoughts, and smells are other causes.
- *Personal choice.* Food choices depend on how food looks, how it is prepared, its smell, and ingredients.
- *Body reactions.* People usually avoid foods that cause allergic reactions. They also avoid foods that cause nausea, vomiting, diarrhea, indigestion, gas, or headaches.
- *Illness.* Appetite usually decreases during illness and recovery from injuries. However, nutritional needs are increased.
- *Age.* With aging, changes occur in the gastrointestinal system. Taste and smell dull. Appetite decreases. Secretion of digestive juices decreases.

THE SODIUM-CONTROLLED DIET

- A sodium-controlled diet decreases the amount of sodium in the body. The diet involves:
  - Omitting high-sodium foods. Review Box 22-4, High-Sodium Foods, in the textbook.
  - Not adding salt to food at the table.
  - Limiting the amount of salt used in cooking.
  - Diet planning.

DIABETES MEAL PLANNING

- Diabetes meal planning is for people with diabetes. It involves the resident's food preferences and calories needed. It also involves eating meals and snacks at regular times.
- Serve the resident's meals and snacks on time to maintain a certain blood sugar level.
- Always check the tray to see what was eaten. Tell the nurse what the person did and did not eat. If not all the food was eaten, a between-meal nourishment is needed. The nurse tells you what to give. Tell the nurse about changes in the person's eating habits.

THE DYSPHAGIA DIET

- **Dysphagia** means difficulty swallowing. Food thickness is changed to meet the person's needs. Review Box 22-5, Dysphagia Diet, in the textbook.
- You may need to feed a person with dysphagia. To promote the person's comfort:
  - Know the signs and symptoms of dysphagia. Review Box 22-6 in the textbook.
    - The person avoids food that needs chewing.
    - The person avoids food with certain textures and temperatures.

- The person tires during a meal.
- Food spills out of the person's mouth while eating.
- Food "pockets" or is "squirreled" in the person's cheeks.
- The person eats slowly, especially solid foods.
- The person complains that food will not go down or that food is stuck.
- The person frequently coughs or chokes before, during, or after swallowing.
- The person regurgitates food after eating.
- The person spits out food suddenly and almost violently.
- Food comes up through the person's nose.
- The person is hoarse—especially after eating.
- After swallowing, the person makes gargling sounds while talking or breathing.
- The person has a runny nose, sneezes, or has excessive drooling of saliva.
- The person complains of heartburn.
- Appetite is decreased.
- Feed the person according to the care plan and swallow guide.
- Follow aspiration precautions. Review Box 22-7 in the textbook.
  - Help the person with meals and snacks. Follow the care plan.
  - Position the person in Fowler's position or upright in a chair for meals and snacks.
  - Support the upper back, shoulders, and neck with a pillow. Follow the care plan.
  - Observe for signs and symptoms of aspiration during meals and snacks.
  - Check the person's mouth after eating for pocketing. Check inside the cheeks, under the tongue, and on the roof of the mouth. Remove any food.
  - Position the person in a chair or in semi-Fowler's position after eating. The person maintains this position for at least 1 hour after eating. Follow the care plan.
  - Provide mouth care after eating.
  - Report and record your observations.
- Report changes in how the person eats.
- Report choking, coughing, or difficulty breathing during or after meals. Also report abnormal breathing or respiratory sounds. Report these observations at once.

FLUID BALANCE

- Fluid balance is needed for health. The amount of fluid taken in (**input**) and the amount of fluid lost (**output**) must be equal. If fluid intake exceeds fluid output, body tissues swell with water (**edema**).
- **Dehydration** is a decrease in the amount of water in body tissues. Fluid output exceeds intake. Common causes are poor fluid intake, vomiting, diarrhea, bleeding, excess sweating, and increased urine production.

Normal Fluid Requirements
- An adult needs 1500 ml of water daily to survive. About 2000 to 2500 ml of fluid per day is needed for normal fluid balance. The water requirement increases with hot weather, exercise, fever, illness, and excess fluid loss.
- Older persons may have a decreased sense of thirst. Their bodies need water, but they may not feel thirsty. Offer water often.

Special Orders for Fluids
- The doctor may order the amount and kind of fluid a person can have every day:
  - *Encourage fluids.* The person drinks an increased amount of fluid. I&O records are kept.
  - *Restrict fluids.* Fluids are limited to a certain amount. I&O records are kept.
  - *Nothing by mouth (NPO).* The person cannot eat or drink.
  - *Thickened liquids.* All liquids are thickened, including water.

Intake and Output Records
- All fluids taken by mouth are measured and recorded—water, milk, and so forth. So are foods that melt at room temperature—ice cream, sherbet, pudding, gelatin, and Popsicles.
- Output includes urine, vomitus, diarrhea, and wound drainage.
- To measure intake and output, you need to know:
  - 1 ounce (oz) equals 30 ml.
  - A pint is about 500 ml.
  - A quart is about 1000 ml.
  - The serving sizes of bowls, dishes, cups, pitchers, glasses, and other containers.
- An I&O record is kept at the bedside. Record I&O measurements in the correct column. Amounts are totaled at the end of the shift. The totals are recorded in the person's chart.
- The urinal, commode, bedpan, or specimen pan is used for voiding. Remind the person not to void in the toilet. Also remind the person not to put toilet tissue into the receptacle.
- Measure output at eye level.

MEETING FOOD AND FLUID NEEDS
- Tell the nurse when a person's appetite or the ability to eat changes.
- Preparing residents for meals promotes their comfort:
  - Assist with elimination needs.
  - Provide oral hygiene. Make sure dentures are in place.
  - Make sure eyeglasses and hearing aids are in place.
  - Make sure incontinent persons are clean and dry.
  - Position the person in a comfortable position. Assist with hand washing.
- Prompt serving keeps food at the correct temperature.

Feeding the Person
- Serve food and fluid in the order the person prefers. Offer fluids during the meal.

- Use teaspoons to feed the person.
- Persons who need to be fed are often angry, humiliated, and embarrassed. Some are depressed or refuse to eat. Let them do as much as possible. If strong enough, let them hold milk or juice glasses. Never let them hold hot drinks.
- Tell the visually impaired person what is on the tray. Describe what you are offering. For persons who feed themselves, use the numbers on the clock for the location of foods.
- Many people pray before eating. Allow time and privacy for prayer.
- Meals provide social contact with others. Engage the person in pleasant conversations. Also, sit facing the person.
- Report and record:
  - The amount and kind of food eaten.
  - Complaints of nausea or dysphagia.
  - Signs and symptoms of dysphagia.
  - Signs and symptoms of aspiration.
- The person will eat better if not rushed.
- Wipe the person's hands, face, and mouth as needed during the meal.

Providing Drinking Water
- Residents need fresh drinking water. Follow the center's procedure for providing fresh water.
- Water glasses and pitchers can spread microbes. To prevent the spread of microbes:
  - Label the water pitcher with the person's name and room and bed number.
  - Do not touch the rim or inside of the water glass, cup, or pitcher.
  - Do not let the ice scoop touch the rim or inside of the water glass, cup, or pitcher.
  - Place the ice scoop in the holder or on a towel, not in the ice container or dispenser.
  - Make sure the person's water pitcher and cup are clean and free of cracks and chips.

Calorie Counts
- Calorie records are kept for some people. On a flow sheet, note what the person ate and how much. A nurse or dietitian converts these portions into calories.

REVIEW QUESTIONS
Circle the BEST answer.
1. A person is on a sodium-controlled diet. Which statement is *true*?
   a. High-sodium foods are allowed.
   b. Salt is added at the table.
   c. Pretzels and potato chips are a good snack.
   d. The amount of salt used in cooking is limited.
2. A person is a diabetic. You should do the following *except*
   a. Serve his meals and snacks late
   b. Always check his tray to see what he ate
   c. Tell the nurse what he ate and did not eat
   d. Provide a between-meal nourishment as the nurse directs

3. A person has dysphagia. You should do the following *except*
   a. Report choking and coughing during a meal at once
   b. Report difficulty in breathing during a meal at the end of the shift
   c. Report changes in how the person eats
   d. Follow aspiration precautions

4. Older persons have a decreased sense of thirst.
   a. True
   b. False

5. A person is on intake and output. He just ate ice cream. This is recorded as intake.
   a. True
   b. False

6. A person drank a pint of milk at lunch. You know he drank
   a. 250 ml of milk
   b. 350 ml of milk
   c. 500 ml of milk
   d. 750 ml of milk

7. The soup bowl holds 6 ounces. A person ate all of the soup. You record his intake as
   a. 50 ml
   b. 120 ml
   c. 180 ml
   d. 200 ml

8. When feeding a person, you do the following *except*
   a. Use a teaspoon to feed the person
   b. Offer fluids during the meal
   c. Let the person do as much as possible
   d. Stand so you can feed 2 people at once

9. A person is visually impaired. You do the following *except*
   a. Tell the person what is on the tray
   b. Use the numbers on a clock to tell the person the location of food
   c. If feeding the person, describe what you are offering
   d. Let the person guess what is served

CHAPTER 24 EXERCISE AND ACTIVITY
COMPLICATIONS OF BEDREST
- Pressure ulcers, constipation, and fecal impactions can result. Urinary tract infections and renal calculi can occur. So can blood clots and pneumonia.
- A **contracture** is the lack of joint mobility caused by abnormal shortening of a muscle. Common sites are the fingers, wrists, elbows, toes, ankles, knees, and hips. The person is permanently deformed and disabled.
- **Atrophy** is the decrease in size or the wasting away of tissue. Tissues shrink in size.
- **Orthostatic hypotension (postural hypotension)** is abnormally low blood pressure when the person suddenly stands up. The person is dizzy and weak and has spots before the eyes. **Syncope** (fainting) can occur. To prevent orthostatic hypotension, have the person change slowly from a lying or sitting position to a standing position. Review Box 24-1, Preventing Orthostatic Hypotension, in the textbook.

POSITIONING
- Supportive devices are often used to support and maintain the person in a certain position:
  - Bed boards—are placed under the mattress to prevent the mattress from sagging.
  - Foot boards—are placed at the foot of mattresses.
  - Trochanter rolls—prevent the hips and legs from turning outward (external rotation). Pillows or sandbags also keep the hips and knees in alignment.
  - Hip abduction wedges—keep the hips abducted.
  - Hand rolls or hand grips—prevent contractures of the thumb, fingers, and wrist.
  - Splints—keep the elbows, wrists, thumbs, fingers, ankles, and knees in normal position.
  - Bed cradles—keep the weight of top linens off the feet and toes.

EXERCISE
- Exercise helps prevent contractures, muscle atrophy, and other complications of bedrest.
- A trapeze is used for exercises to strengthen arm muscles. The trapeze is also used to move up and turn in bed.
- During rehabilitation, the person works to improve strength and endurance. The goal may be to improve the person's independence to attain the highest level of function possible.

RANGE-OF-MOTION EXERCISES
- **Range-of-motion (ROM)** exercises involve moving the joints through their complete range of motion. They are usually done at least 2 times a day. Joint movements:
  - Abduction—moving a body part away from the midline of the body.
  - Adduction—moving a body part toward the midline of the body.
  - Extension—straightening a body part.
  - Flexion—bending a body part.

- Hyperextension—excessive straightening of a body part.
- Dorsiflexion—bending the toes and foot up at the ankle.
- Rotation—turning the joint.
- Internal rotation—turning the joint inward.
- External rotation—turning the joint outward.
- Plantar flexion—bending the foot down at the ankle.
- Pronation—turning the joint downward.
- Supination—turning the joint upward.
- Range-of-motion exercises can cause injury if not done properly. Practice these rules:
  - Exercise only the joints the nurse tells you to exercise.
  - Expose only the body part being exercised.
  - Use good body mechanics.
  - Support the part being exercised.
  - Move the joint slowly, smoothly, and gently.
  - Do not force a joint beyond its present range of motion.
  - Do not force a joint to the point of pain.
  - Perform ROM exercises to the neck only if allowed by center policy.

AMBULATION
- Walking regularly helps prevent muscle loss. Follow the care plan when helping a person walk. Use a gait (transfer) belt if the person is weak or unsteady. The person uses hand rails along the wall. Always check the person for orthostatic hypotension.
- When you help the person walk, walk to the side and slightly behind the person on the person's weak side. Encourage the person to use the hand rail on his or her strong side.
- A cane is held on the strong side of the body. The cane tip is about 6 to 10 inches to the side of the foot. It is about 6 to 10 inches in front of the foot on the strong side. The grip is level with the hip. To walk:
  - *Step A:* The cane is moved forward 6 to 10 inches.
  - *Step B:* The weak leg (opposite the cane) is moved forward even with the cane.
  - *Step C:* The strong leg is moved forward and ahead of the cane and the weak leg.
- A walker gives more support than a cane. To use the standard walker:
  - The walker is picked up and moved about 6 to 8 inches in front of the person.
  - The person moves the weak leg and foot up to the walker.
  - The person moves the strong leg and foot up to the walker.
- Braces support weak body parts, prevent or correct deformities, or prevent joint movement. A brace is applied over the ankle, knee, or back. Skin and bony points under braces are kept clean and dry. Report redness or signs of skin breakdown at once. Also report complaints of pain or discomfort.

REVIEW QUESTIONS

Choose the BEST answer.

1. To prevent orthostatic hypotension, you should
    a. Move a person from the lying position to the sitting position quickly
    b. Move a person from the sitting position to the standing position quickly
    c. Move a person from the lying or sitting position to a standing position slowly
    d. Keep the person in bed
2. Exercise helps prevent contractures and muscle atrophy.
    a. True
    b. False
3. When performing ROM exercises, you should force a joint to the point of pain.
    a. True
    b. False
4. A person's left leg is weaker than his right. The person holds the cane on his right side.
    a. True
    b. False

CHAPTER 25 COMFORT, REST, AND SLEEP
COMFORT
- **Comfort** is a state of well-being. The person has no physical or emotional pain.
- Age, illness, activity, temperature, ventilation, noise, odors, and lighting affect comfort.
- Do not assume that a person is comfortable. Ask the person.

FACTORS AFFECTING PAIN
- *Past experience.* The severity of pain, its cause, how long it lasted, and if relief occurred all affect the person's current response to pain.
- *Anxiety.* Pain and anxiety are related. Pain can cause anxiety. Anxiety increases how much pain the person feels. Reducing anxiety helps lessen pain.
- *Rest and sleep.* Pain seems worse when a person is tired or restless.
- *Attention.* The more a person thinks about pain, the worse it seems.
- *Personal and family duties.* Often pain is ignored when there are children to care for. Some deny pain if a serious illness is feared.
- *The value or meaning of pain.* To some people, pain is a weakness. For some persons, pain means avoiding daily routines and people. Some people like doting and pampering by others. The person values pain and wants such attention.
- *Support from others.* Dealing with pain is often easier when family and friends offer comfort and support. Just being nearby helps. Facing pain alone is hard for persons.
- *Culture.* In some cultures, the person in pain shows no reaction to it. Strong verbal and nonverbal reactions to pain are seen in other cultures. Non–English-speaking persons may have problems describing pain.
- *Illness.* Some diseases cause decreased pain sensations.
- *Age.* Chronic pain may mask new pain. Older persons may ignore or deny new pain. They may think it relates to a known health problem. Some older persons cannot verbally communicate pain. Changes in behavior may signal that the person has pain. Always report changes in the person's behavior to the nurse.

SIGNS AND SYMPTOMS
- You cannot see, hear, touch, or smell the person's pain. Rely on what the person tells you. Promptly report any information you collect about pain. Use the person's exact words when reporting and recording pain. The nurse needs the following information:
  - *Location.* Where is the pain?
  - *Onset and duration.* When did the pain start? How long has it lasted?
  - *Intensity.* Ask the person to rate the pain. Use a pain scale.
  - *Description.* Ask the person to describe the pain.
  - *Factors causing pain.* Ask when the pain started and what the person was doing.
  - *Factors affecting pain.* Ask what makes the pain better and what makes it worse.
- *Vital signs.* Increases often occur with acute pain. They may be normal with chronic pain.
- *Other signs and symptoms.* Dizziness, nausea, vomiting, weakness, numbness, and tingling. Review Box 25-2, Signs and Symptoms of Pain, in the textbook.

NURSING MEASURES
- Measures to promote comfort and relieve pain include:
  - Position the person in good alignment. Use pillows for support.
  - Keep bed linens tight and wrinkle-free.
  - Make sure the person is not lying on drainage tubes.
  - Assist with elimination needs.
  - Provide blankets for warmth and to prevent chilling.
  - Use correct handling, moving, and turning procedures.
  - Wait 30 minutes after pain drugs are given before giving care or starting activities.
  - Give a back massage.
  - Provide soft music to distract the person.
  - Talk softly and gently.
  - Use touch to provide comfort.
  - Allow family and friends at the bedside as requested by the person.
  - Avoid sudden or jarring movements of the bed or chair.
  - Handle the person gently.
  - Practice safety measures if the person takes strong pain drugs or sedatives.
  - Apply warm or cold applications as directed by the nurse.
  - Provide a calm, quiet, darkened setting.

REST
- Basic needs must be met for a person to rest.
- Promote rest by meeting safety and security needs.
- Many persons have rituals or routines before resting. Follow them whenever possible.
- Love and belonging are important for rest.
- Meet self-esteem needs.
- Some persons are refreshed after a 15- or 20-minute rest. Others need more time.
- Ill or injured persons need to rest more often.

FACTORS AFFECTING SLEEP
- *Illness.* Illness increases the need for sleep.
- *Nutrition.* Sleep needs increase with weight gain. Foods with caffeine prevent sleep.
- *Exercise.* People tire after exercise. Being tired helps people sleep well. Exercise before bedtime interferes with sleep. Exercise is avoided 2 hours before bedtime.
- *Environment.* People adjust to their usual sleep settings.
- *Drugs and other substances.* Sleeping pills promote sleep. Drugs for anxiety, depression, and pain may cause the person to sleep.
- *Life-style changes.* Travel, vacation, and social events often affect sleep and wake times.
- *Emotional problems.* Fear, worry, depression, and anxiety affect sleep.

PROMOTING SLEEP

- Organize care for uninterrupted rest.
- Avoid physical activity before bedtime.
- Encourage the person to avoid business or family matters before bedtime.
- Allow a flexible bedtime.
- Provide a comfortable room temperature.
- Let the person take a warm bath or shower.
- Provide a bedtime snack.
- Avoid caffeine and alcoholic beverages.
- Have the person void before going to bed.
- Make sure incontinent persons are clean and dry.
- Follow bedtime routines.
- Have the person wear loose-fitting sleepwear.
- Provide for warmth for those who tend to be cold.
- Reduce noise.
- Darken the room—close shades, blinds, and the privacy curtain.
- Dim lights in the hallways and the nursing unit.
- Make sure linens are clean, dry, and wrinkle-free.
- Position the person in good alignment and in a comfortable position.
- Support body parts.
- Give a back massage.
- Assist with relaxation exercises as ordered.
- Provide measures to relieve pain.
- Let the person read, listen to music, or watch TV.
- Assist with relaxation exercises as ordered.
- Sit and talk with the person.
- Distraction, relaxation, and guided imagery also promote rest.
- Report your observations about how the person slept.

REVIEW QUESTIONS
Circle the BEST answer.

1. Which statement is *false*?
   a. Pain can cause anxiety.
   b. Reducing anxiety may help lessen pain.
   c. Pain seems less when a person is tired.
   d. A person tends to focus on pain when unable to sleep.

2. A person complains of pain. You will do the following *except*
   a. Ask where the pain is
   b. Ask when the pain started
   c. Ask what the intensity of the pain is on a scale of 1 to 10
   d. Ask why he or she is complaining about pain

3. You can promote rest for a person by doing the following *except*
   a. Asking the person if he or she would like coffee or tea
   b. Placing the signal light within reach
   c. Providing clean, dry, and wrinkle-free linens
   d. Following the person's routines and rituals before rest

4. To promote sleep for a person, you should do the following *except*
   a. Follow the person's wishes
   b. Follow the care plan
   c. Follow the person's rituals and routines before bedtime
   d. Tell the person when to go to bed

CHAPTER 26 OXYGEN NEEDS
FACTORS AFFECTING OXYGEN NEEDS
- The respiratory and circulatory systems must function properly for cells to get enough oxygen. Altered function of any body system affects oxygen needs.
- **Respiratory depression** means slow, weak respirations at a rate of fewer than 12 per minute. Respirations are too shallow to bring enough oxygen into the lungs.
- **Respiratory arrest** is when breathing stops.

ALTERED RESPIRATORY FUNCTION
- Restlessness, dizziness, disorientation, and confusion are signs of **hypoxia**. So are behavior and personality changes, problems concentrating and following directions, apprehension, and anxiety. The person may also be cyanotic or in a sitting position, leaning forward. Report signs and symptoms of hypoxia to the nurse at once. Hypoxia is life-threatening.
- Adults normally have 12 to 20 respirations per minute. They are quiet, effortless, and regular. Both sides of the chest rise and fall equally. Report these observations promptly:
  - **Tachypnea**—rapid breathing. Respirations are 24 or more per minute.
  - **Bradypnea**—slow breathing. Respirations are fewer than 12 per minute.
  - **Apnea**—lack or absence of breathing.
  - **Dyspnea**—difficult, labored, painful breathing.
  - **Cheyne-Stokes respirations**—respirations gradually increase in rate and depth. Then they become shallow and slow. Breathing may stop for 10 to 20 seconds.
  - **Orthopnea**—breathing deeply and comfortably only when sitting.
  - Complaints of shortness of breath or being "winded" or "short-winded."
  - Cough—dry and hacking, harsh and barking, productive or non-productive.
  - Sputum:
    - Color: yellow, green, brown, or red.
    - Odor: foul odor.
    - Consistency: thick, frothy (with bubbles or foam).
    - **Hemoptysis:** bloody sputum.
  - Noisy respirations—wheezing, crowing sounds, or wet-sounding respirations.
  - Chest pain.
  - Cyanosis (bluish color)—skin, lips, nail beds, mucous membranes.
  - Changes in vital signs.

PROMOTING OXYGENATION
- *Positioning.* Breathing is usually easier in semi-Fowler's and Fowler's positions. Persons with difficulty breathing often prefer the **orthopneic position.**
- *Deep breathing and coughing.* Deep breathing moves air into most parts of the lungs. Coughing removes mucus. Deep breathing and coughing are usually done every 2 hours while the person is awake.

ASSISTING WITH OXYGEN THERAPY
- You do not give oxygen. You assist the nurse in providing safe care.
- Always check the oxygen level when you are with or near persons using these oxygen sources. Report a low oxygen level to the nurse at once.
- The person usually receives oxygen through a nasal cannula or a simple face mask.
- When giving care and checking the person, always check the flow rate. Tell the nurse at once if it is too high or too low. A nurse or respiratory therapist will adjust the flow rate.

Oxygen Safety
- Follow the rules for fire and the use of oxygen in Chapter 10.
- Never remove the oxygen device.
- Make sure the oxygen device is secure but not tight.
- Check for signs of irritation from the oxygen device—behind the ears, under the nose, around the face, and cheekbones.
- Keep the face clean and dry when a mask is used.
- Never shut off the oxygen flow.
- Do not adjust the flow rate unless allowed by your state and center.
- Tell the nurse at once if the humidifier is not bubbling.
- Secure tubing in place. Tape or pin it to the person's garment following center policy.
- Make sure there are no kinks in the tubing.
- Give oral hygiene as directed.
- Make sure the oxygen device is clean and free of mucus.
- Maintain an adequate water level in the humidifier.

REVIEW QUESTIONS
Circle the BEST answer.
1. Which statement is *false*?
   a. Restlessness, dizziness, and disorientation are signs of hypoxia.
   b. Hypoxia is life-threatening.
   c. Report signs and symptoms of hypoxia at the end of the shift.
   d. Anything that affects respiratory function can cause hypoxia.
2. Adults normally have
   a. 8 to 10 respirations per minute
   b. 10 to 12 respirations per minute
   c. 12 to 20 respirations per minute
   d. 20 to 24 respirations per minute
3. Dyspnea is
   a. Rapid breathing with 24 or more respirations per minute
   b. Slow breathing with fewer than 12 respirations per minute
   c. Difficult, labored, or painful breathing
   d. Lack or absence of breathing

4. Which statement about positioning is *false*?
   a. Breathing is usually easier in semi-Fowler's or Fowler's position.
   b. Persons with difficulty breathing often prefer the orthopneic position.
   c. Position changes are needed at least every 4 hours.
   d. Follow the person's care plan for positioning preferences.

5. A person has a nasal cannula. Which statement is *false*?
   a. The nasal cannula is kept on while eating.
   b. You will watch his nose area for irritation.
   c. You will watch his ears and cheekbones for skin breakdown.
   d. You will take the cannula off when he is eating.

CHAPTER 28 MEASURING VITAL SIGNS

VITAL SIGNS

- Accuracy is essential when you measure, record, and report vital signs. If unsure of your measurements, promptly ask the nurse to take them again.
- Report the following at once:
  - Any vital sign that is changed from a prior measurement.
  - Vital signs above the normal range.
  - Vital signs below the normal range.

BODY TEMPERATURE

- Normal body temperatures depend on the site:
  - Oral 98.6° F (37° C).
  - Rectal 99.6° F (37.5° C).
  - Axillary 97.6° F (36.5° C).
  - Tympanic 98.6° F (37° C).
  - Temporal 99.6° F (37.5° C).
- Older persons have lower body temperatures than younger persons.
- If a mercury-glass thermometer breaks, tell the nurse at once. Do not touch the mercury. The center must follow special procedures for handling all hazardous materials.
- When using a glass thermometer:
  - Use the person's thermometer.
  - Use a rectal thermometer only for rectal temperatures.
  - Rinse the thermometer under cold, running water if it was soaking in a disinfectant. Dry it from the stem to the bulb end with tissues.
  - Discard a thermometer if it is broken, cracked, or chipped.
  - Shake down the thermometer to below 94° F or 34° C before using it.
  - Clean and store the thermometer following center policy.
  - Use plastic covers following center policy.
  - Practice medical asepsis.
  - Follow Standard Precautions and the Bloodborne Pathogen Standard.
- *The oral site.* The glass thermometer remains in place 2 to 3 minutes or as required by center policy. Remind the person not to talk.
- *The rectal site.* Lubricate the bulb end of the rectal thermometer. Insert the glass thermometer 1 inch into the rectum. Hold the thermometer in place for 2 minutes or as required by center policy. Privacy is important.
- *The axillary site.* The axilla must be dry. The glass thermometer stays in place for 5 to 10 minutes or as required by center policy.
- Electronic thermometers measure temperature in a few seconds.
- Tympanic membrane thermometers are gently inserted into the ear. The temperature is measured in 1 to 3 seconds. These thermometers are not used if there is ear drainage.

PULSE

- The adult pulse rate is between 60 and 100 beats per minute. Report these abnormal rates to the nurse at once:
  - **Tachycardia**—the heart rate is more than 100 beats per minute.
  - **Bradycardia**—the heart rate is less than 60 beats per minute.
- The rhythm of the pulse should be regular. Report and record an irregular pulse rhythm.
- Report and record if the pulse force is strong, full, bounding, weak, thready, or feeble.
- The radial pulse is used for routine vital signs. Do not use your thumb to take a pulse.
- Count the pulse for 30 seconds and multiply by 2 if the center policy permits. If the pulse is irregular, count it for 1 minute. Report and record if the pulse is regular or irregular.

RESPIRATIONS

- Count respirations when the person is at rest. Count respirations right after taking a pulse.
- Count respirations for 30 seconds and multiply the number by 2 if the center policy permits. If an abnormal pattern is noted, count the respirations for 1 minute.
- Report and record:
  - The respiratory rate.
  - If both sides of the chest rise equally.
  - The depth of the respirations.
  - If the person has any pain or difficulty breathing.
  - Any respiratory noises.
  - An abnormal respiratory pattern.

BLOOD PRESSURE

- Factors affecting blood pressure are age, gender, blood volume, stress, and pain. Review Box 28-2, Factors Affecting Blood Pressure, in the textbook.
- Blood pressure has normal ranges:
  - Systolic pressure (upper number)—less than 120 mm Hg.
  - Diastolic pressure (lower number)—less than 80 mm Hg.
- Hypertension—blood pressure measurements that remain above a systolic pressure of 140 mm Hg or a diastolic pressure of 90 mm Hg. Report any systolic measurement above 120 mm Hg. Also report a diastolic pressure above 80 mm Hg.
- Hypotension—when the systolic blood pressure is below 90 mm Hg and the diastolic pressure is below 60 mm Hg. Report a systolic pressure below 90 mm Hg. Also report a diastolic pressure below 60 mm Hg.
- Systolic and diastolic pressures are normally higher in older persons.
- Guidelines for measuring blood pressure:
  - Do not take a blood pressure on an arm with an IV infusion, a cast, or a dialysis access site. If a person had breast surgery, do not take a blood pressure on that side. Avoid taking a blood pressure on an injured arm.

- Let the person rest for 10 to 20 minutes before measuring blood pressure.
- Measure blood pressure with the person sitting or lying.
- Apply the cuff to the bare upper arm. Clothing can affect the measurement.
- Make sure the cuff is snug. Loose cuffs can cause inaccurate readings.
- Use the correct cuff size—a larger cuff if the person is obese or has a large arm and a small cuff if the person has a very small arm.
- Place the diaphragm of the stethoscope firmly over the brachial artery.
- Make sure the room is quiet.
- Have the sphygmomanometer where you can clearly see it.
- Measure the systolic and diastolic pressures. The first sound is the systolic pressure. The point where the sound disappears is the diastolic pressure.
- Take the blood pressure again if you are not sure of an accurate measurement. Wait 30 to 60 seconds before repeating the measurement.
- Tell the nurse at once if you cannot hear the blood pressure.

REVIEW QUESTIONS
Circle the BEST answer.

1. Which statement about taking a rectal temperature is *false*?
   a. The bulb end of the thermometer needs to be lubricated.
   b. The thermometer is held in place for 5 minutes.
   c. Privacy is important.
   d. The normal baseline temperature is 99.6° F (37.5° C).

2. Which pulse rate should you report at once?
   a. A pulse rate of 56 beats per minute
   b. A pulse rate of 60 beats per minute
   c. A pulse rate of 80 beats per minute
   d. A pulse rate of 100 beats per minute

3. Which statement is *false*?
   a. An irregular pulse is counted for 1 minute.
   b. You may use your thumb to take a radial pulse rate.
   c. The radial pulse is usually used to count a pulse rate.
   d. Tachycardia is a fast pulse rate.

4. Which blood pressure should you report?
   a. 120/80 mm Hg
   b. 130/70 mm Hg
   c. 110/68 mm Hg
   d. 98/68 mm Hg

CHAPTER 31 ADMITTING, TRANSFERRING, AND DISCHARGING RESIDENTS

ADMISSIONS

- **Admission** is the official entry of a person into the nursing center. During the admission process:
  - Identifying information is obtained from the person or family.
  - Either a nurse or you will take the person to his or her room.
  - A nurse or social worker explains the resident's rights to the person and family.
  - The person signs admitting papers and a general consent form. If the person is not mentally competent to give consent, the legal representative does so. The nurse or admission coordinator obtains the needed signatures.
  - The person's photo is taken. Then the person receives an ID bracelet.
- You prepare the person's room before the person arrives.
- Admission is your first chance to make a good impression. You must:
  - Greet the person by name and title.
  - Introduce yourself by name and title.
  - Make roommate introductions.
  - Act in a professional manner.
  - Treat the person with dignity and respect.
- Do not rush the admission process.
- Help the person unpack. The person may want to hang pictures or display photos.
- During the admission process, you will:
  - Collect some information for the admission form.
  - Measure the person's weight and height.
  - Measure the person's vital signs.
  - Complete a clothing and personal belongings list.
  - Orient the person to the room, the nursing unit, and the center.
- When weighing a person, follow the manufacturer's instructions and center procedures for using the scales. Follow these guidelines when measuring weight and height:
  - The person wears only a gown or pajamas. No footwear is worn.
  - The person voids before being weighed.
  - Weigh the person at the same time of day. Before breakfast is the best time.
  - Use the same scale for daily, weekly, and monthly weights.
  - Balance the scale at zero before weighing the person.

TRANSFERS

- The doctor, nurse, or social worker explains the reasons for the transfer. You assist with the transfer or perform the entire procedure. The person is transported by wheelchair, stretcher, or the bed. Support and reassure the person. Use good communication skills:
  - Avoid pat answers—"It will be OK."
  - Use touch to provide comfort.
  - Introduce the person to the staff and roommate.
  - Wish the person well as you leave him or her.

DISCHARGES

- The doctor must write a discharge order before the person can leave. The nurse tells you when the person may leave and how to transport him or her.
- If a person wants to leave the center without the doctor's permission, tell the nurse at once. The nurse or social worker handles the matter.

REVIEW QUESTIONS

Circle the BEST answer.

1. When admitted, you explain the resident's rights to the person and family.
   a. True
   b. False
2. When a person is admitted, you do the following *except*
   a. Greet the person by name and title
   b. Treat the person with dignity and respect
   c. Introduce the person to his or her roommate
   d. Rush the admission procedure
3. Which statement is *false*?
   a. Have the person void before being weighed.
   b. Weigh the person at the same time of day.
   c. Balance the scale at zero before weighing the person.
   d. Have the person wear shoes when being weighed.
4. A person wants to leave the nursing center without the doctor's permission, you should tell the nurse at once.
   a. True
   b. False

CHAPTER 32 WOUND CARE

- Prevent skin injury and give good skin care to help prevent skin breakdown. Common causes of skin breakdown include:
  - Age-related changes in the skin.
  - Dryness.
  - Fragile and weak capillaries.
  - General thinning of the skin.
  - Loss of fatty layer under the skin.
  - Decreased sensation to touch, heat, and cold.
  - Poor nutrition and poor hydration.
  - Decreased mobility.
  - Sitting in a chair or lying in bed most or all of the day.
  - Chronic diseases (diabetes, high blood pressure).
  - Diseases that decrease circulation.
  - Incontinence.
  - Moisture in dark areas (skin folds, under the breasts, perineal area).
  - Pressure on bony parts.
  - Poor fingernail and toenail care.
  - Friction and shearing.
  - Edema.
- Older and disabled persons are at great risk. Their skin is easily injured.

SKIN TEARS

- The hands, arms, and lower legs are common sites for **skin tears**.
- Tell the nurse at once if you cause or find a skin tear.
- Measures to prevent skin tears include:
  - Keep your fingernails short and smoothly filed.
  - Keep the person's fingernails short and smoothly filed. Report long and tough toenails.
  - Do not wear rings with large or raised stones. Do not wear bracelets.
  - Be patient and calm when the person is confused or agitated or resists care.
  - Follow the care plan and safety rules to move, turn, position, or transfer the person.
  - Pad bed rails and wheelchair arms, footplates, and leg supports. Follow the care plan.
  - Follow the care plan and safety rules to bathe the person.
  - Dress and undress the person carefully.
  - Dress the person in soft clothes with long sleeves and long pants.
  - Provide good lighting so the person can see.
  - Provide a safe area for wandering.
  - Keep the skin moisturized. Apply lotion according to the care plan.
  - Offer fluids. Follow the care plan.

PRESSURE ULCERS

- *Decubitus ulcer, bedsore,* and *pressure sore* are other terms for pressure ulcer.
- A pressure ulcer usually occurs over a bony prominence—the back of the head, shoulder blades, elbows, hips, spine, sacrum, knees, ankles, heels, toes, and ears. In obese people, they can occur in abdominal folds, the legs, the buttocks, the thighs, and under the breasts.

- Persons at risk for pressure ulcers are those who:
  - Are bedfast or confined to a chair.
  - Need some or total help in moving.
  - Are agitated or have involuntary muscle movements.
  - Have loss of bowel or bladder control.
  - Are exposed to moisture.
  - Have poor nutrition.
  - Have poor fluid balance.
  - Have lowered mental awareness.
  - Have problems sensing pain or pressure.
  - Have circulatory problems.
  - Are older.
  - Are obese or very thin.
- In persons with light skin, a reddened bony area is the first sign of a pressure ulcer. In persons with dark skin, a bony area may appear red, blue, or purple. The area may feel warm or cool. The person may complain of pain, burning, tingling, or itching in the area.
- Preventing pressure ulcers is much easier than trying to heal them. Review Box 32-5, Measures to Prevent Pressure Ulcers, in the textbook.
- The person at risk for pressure ulcers may be placed on foam, air, alternating air, gel, or water mattress.
- Protective devices are often used to prevent and treat pressure ulcers and skin breakdown. Protective devices include a bed cradle, heel and elbow protectors, and heel and foot elevators. Gel or fluid-filled pads and cushions, eggcrate-type pads, and special beds are common devices. Other equipment may include pillows, trochanter rolls, and footboards.
- Report and record any signs of skin breakdown or pressure ulcers at once.

CIRCULATORY ULCERS

- **Circulatory ulcers (vascular ulcers)** are open sores on the lower legs or feet. To prevent circulatory ulcers:
  - Remind the person not to sit with the legs crossed.
  - Reposition the person at least every 2 hours or according to the care plan.
  - Do not use elastic or rubber band–type garters to hold socks or hose in place.
  - Do not dress the person in tight clothes.
  - Provide good skin care daily. Keep the feet clean and dry.
  - Do not scrub or rub the skin during bathing and drying.
  - Keep linens clean, dry, and wrinkle-free.
  - Make sure shoes fit well.
  - Keep pressure off the heels and other bony areas.
  - Check the person's legs and feet. Report skin breaks or changes in skin color.
  - Do not massage over pressure points. Never rub or massage reddened areas.
  - Use protective devices as the nurse directs. Follow the care plan.
  - Follow the care plan for walking and exercise.

- **Venous ulcers (stasis ulcers)** are open sores on the lower legs or feet. The heels and inner aspect of the ankles are common sites for venous ulcers. To prevent venous ulcers:
  - Follow the person's care plan to prevent skin breakdown. Review the measures to prevent circulatory ulcers.
  - Prevent injury. Do not bump the legs and feet.
  - Handle, move, and transfer the person carefully and gently.
- You do not cut the toenails of persons with diseases affecting the circulation.

Elastic Stockings

- Elastic stockings also are called *anti-embolism or anti-embolic (AE) stockings, TED hose.*
- The person usually has two pairs of stockings. One pair is washed; the other pair is worn.
- Stockings should not have twists, creases, or wrinkles after you apply them.
- Stockings are applied before the person gets out of bed.

OTHER TYPES OF ULCERS

- **Arterial ulcers** are open wounds on the lower legs or feet caused by poor arterial blood flow. They are found between the toes, on top of the toes, and on the outer side of the ankle. Professional foot care is important. Follow the care plan, and prevent further injury. Review the measures to prevent circulatory ulcers.
- A **diabetic foot ulcer** is an open wound on the foot caused by complications from diabetes.
  - When nerves are affected, the person can lose sensation in a foot or leg. The person may not feel pain, heat, or cold. Therefore the person may not feel a cut, blister, burn, or other trauma to the foot. Infection and a large sore can develop.
  - When blood flow to the foot decreases, tissues and cells do not get needed oxygen and nutrients. A sore does not heal properly. Tissue death (gangrene) can occur.

- Check the diabetic person's feet every day. Report signs of foot problems to the nurse.

REVIEW QUESTIONS
Circle the BEST answer.

1. The following can cause a skin tear *except*
   a. Friction and shearing
   b. Holding a person's arm or leg too tight
   c. Rings, watches, bracelets
   d. Trimmed, short nails
2. You may expect to find a pressure ulcer at all of the following sites *except*
   a. Back of the head
   b. Ears
   c. Top of the thigh
   d. Toes
3. In obese people, pressure ulcers can occur between abdominal folds.
   a. True
   b. False
4. Which statement about elastic stockings is *false*?
   a. Elastic stockings are also called anti-embolic stockings.
   b. Elastic stockings should be wrinkle-free after being applied.
   c. A person usually has two pairs of elastic stockings.
   d. Elastic stockings are applied after a person gets out of bed.
5. A person is diabetic. Which statement is *false*?
   a. The person may not feel pain in her feet.
   b. The person may not feel heat or cold in her feet.
   c. You need to check his feet weekly for foot problems.
   d. The person is at risk for diabetic foot ulcers.

CHAPTER 34 HEARING, SPEECH, AND VISION DISORDERS

EAR DISORDERS

- Temporary hearing loss can occur from earwax (**cerumen**). You do not try to remove earwax. Do not insert anything, including cotton swabs, into the ear.
- Obvious signs and symptoms of hearing loss include:
  - Speaking too loudly.
  - Leaning forward to hear.
  - Turning and cupping the better ear toward the speaker.
  - Answering questions or responding inappropriately.
  - Asking for words to be repeated.
  - Asking others to speak louder or to speak more slowly and clearly.
  - Having trouble hearing on the phone.
  - Finding it hard to follow conversations when two or more people are talking.
  - Turning up the TV, radio, or music volume so loud that others complain.
  - Thinking that others are mumbling or slurring words.
  - Having problems understanding women and children.
- To promote communication:
  - Reduce or eliminate background noises.
  - Provide a quiet place to talk.
  - Have the person sit in small groups or where he or she can hear best.
  - Have the person wear his or her hearing aid. It must be turned on and working.
  - Have the person wear needed eyeglasses or contact lenses.
  - Alert the person to your presence. Do not startle or approach the person from behind.
  - Position yourself at the person's level.
  - Face the person when speaking.
  - Stand or sit in good light. Stand or sit on the side of the better ear.
  - Speak clearly, distinctly, and slowly.
  - Speak in a normal tone of voice. Do not shout.
  - Adjust the pitch of your voice as needed.
  - Do not cover your mouth, smoke, eat, or chew gum while talking.
  - Keep your hands away from your face.
  - State the topic of the conversation first.
  - Tell the person when you are changing the subject.
  - Use short sentences and simple words.
  - Use gestures and facial expressions to give useful clues.
  - Write out important names and words.
  - Say things in another way if the person does not seem to understand.
  - Keep conversations and discussions short.
  - Repeat and rephrase statements as needed.
  - Be alert to messages sent by your facial expressions, gestures, and body language.
- Hearing aids are battery-operated. If they do not seem to work properly:
  - Check if the hearing aid is on. It has an *on and off* switch.
  - Check the battery position.
  - Insert a new battery if needed.
- Clean the hearing aid. Follow the nurse's direction and the manufacturer's instructions.
- Hearing aids are turned off when not in use. The battery is removed. Hair spray or other hair care products should not be used when a person is wearing a hearing aid.
- Handle and care for hearing aids properly. If lost or damaged, report it to the nurse at once.

SPEECH DISORDERS

- **Aphasia** means the inability to speak.
- The person with aphasia may be frustrated, depressed, and angry.

IMPAIRED VISION AND BLINDNESS

- Follow these guidelines when caring for blind and visually impaired persons:
  - Report worn carpeting and other flooring.
  - Keep furniture, equipment, and electrical cords out of areas where the person will walk.
  - Keep table and desk chairs pushed in under the table or desk.
  - Keep doors fully open or fully closed.
  - Keep drawers fully closed.
  - Report burnt out bulbs in the room, lounges, dining areas, hallways, and other areas.
  - Provide lighting as the person prefers. Tell the person when the lights are on or off.
  - Adjust window coverings to prevent glares.
  - Provide a consistent mealtime setting.
  - Keep the signal light and the TV, light, and other controls within the person's reach.
  - Turn on night-lights in the person's room and bathroom.
  - Practice safety measures to prevent falls.
  - Orient the person to the room.
  - Let the person move about. Let him or her touch and find furniture and equipment.
  - Do not leave the person in the middle of a room.
  - Do not rearrange furniture and equipment.
  - Tell the person when you are coming to a curb or steps.
  - Inform the person of doors, turns, furniture, and other obstructions when walking.
  - Complete a safety check before leaving the room.
  - Have the person use railings when climbing stairs.
  - Make sure the person wears comfortable shoes that fit correctly.
  - Assist with walking as needed. Have the person lightly hold onto your arm just above the elbow. Have the person walk about a half step behind you. Never push, pull, or guide the person in front of you. Walk at a normal pace.
  - Let the person do as much for himself or herself as possible.
  - Provide visual and adaptive devices. Follow the care plan.
  - Face the person when speaking. Speak slowly and clearly.
  - Use a normal tone of voice. Do not shout.

- Identify yourself when you enter the room. Do not touch the person until you have indicated your presence.
- Ask the person how much he or she can see.
- Identify others. Explain where each person is located and what the person is doing.
- Address the person by name.
- Speak directly to the person.
- Feel free to use words such as "see," "look," "read," or "watch TV."
- Feel free to refer to colors, shapes, patterns, designs, and so forth.
- Describe people, places, and things thoroughly.
- Offer to help.
- Warn the person of dangers.
- Leave the person's belongings in the same place that you found them. Do not move or rearrange things.
- Listen to the person. Give the person verbal cues that you are listening.
- Answer the person's questions.
- Give step-by-step explanations of procedures as you perform them.
- Give specific directions.
- Tell the person when you are leaving the room or area.
- Tell the person when you are ending a conversation.
- Guide the person to a seat by placing your guiding arm on the seat.
- Blind and visually impaired persons learn to move about using a long cane with a red tip or using a dog guide. Do not pet, feed, or distract a dog guide.

Corrective Lenses

- Clean eyeglasses daily and as needed.
- Protect eyeglasses from loss or damage. When not worn, put them in their case.
- Contact lenses are cleaned, removed, and stored according to the manufacturer's instructions.
- Report and record:
  - Eye redness or irritation.
  - Eye drainage.
  - Complaints of eye pain, blurred or fuzzy vision, uncomfortable lenses.

REVIEW QUESTIONS
Circle the BEST answer.

1. A person has taken his hearing aid out for the evening. You do the following *except*
   a. Make sure the hearing aid is turned off
   b. Keep the battery in the hearing aid
   c. Place the hearing aid in a safe place
   d. Handle the hearing aid carefully
2. A person is blind. You do the following *except*
   a. Identify yourself when you enter his room
   b. Describe people, places, and things thoroughly
   c. Rearrange his furniture without telling him
   d. Encourage him to do as much for himself as possible
3. A person is hard-of-hearing. You do the following *except*
   a. Face the person when speaking
   b. Speak clearly, distinctly, and slowly
   c. Use facial expressions and gestures to give clues
   d. Use long sentences
4. A person is blind. When talking, you do the following *except*
   a. Use a normal voice tone
   b. Use words such as "see," "look," or "read"
   c. Speak to the person
   d. Speak loudly

CHAPTER 36 MENTAL HEALTH PROBLEMS
BASIC CONCEPTS
- **Mental health** means the person copes with and adjusts to everyday stresses in ways accepted by society.
- **Mental illness** is a disturbance in the ability to cope with or adjust to stress. Behavior and function are impaired. **Mental disorder, emotional illness,** and **psychiatric disorder** also mean mental illness.

ANXIETY DISORDERS
- **Anxiety** is a vague, uneasy feeling in response to stress. The person may not know why or the cause. The person senses danger or harm—real or imagined. Refer to Box 36-1, Signs and Symptoms of Anxiety, in the textbook.
- Some anxiety is normal. Coping and defense mechanisms are used to relieve anxiety. Review Box 36-2, Defense Mechanisms, in the textbook.
- *Panic disorder.* **Panic** is an intense and sudden feeling of fear, anxiety, terror, or dread. Onset is sudden with no obvious reason. The person cannot function. Many people avoid places where panic attacks occur.
- *Phobia.* **Phobia** means fear, panic, or dread. The person has an intense fear of an object, situation, or activity that has little or no actual danger. The person avoids what is feared. When faced with the fear, the person has high anxiety and cannot function.
- *Obsessive-compulsive disorder (OCD).* An **obsession** is a recurrent, unwanted thought, idea, or image. **Compulsion** is repeating an act over and over again. The act may not make sense, but the person has much anxiety if the act is not done. Some persons with OCD also have depression, eating disorders, substance abuse, and other anxiety disorders.

SCHIZOPHRENIA
- *Schizophrenia* means split mind. The person with schizophrenia has severe mental impairment:
  - Thinking and behavior are disturbed.
  - The person has problems relating to others.
  - The person may have difficulty organizing thoughts. His or her responses are inappropriate.
  - The person has false beliefs *(delusions).*
  - The person has *hallucinations* (sees, hears, smells, or feels things that are not real).
  - Communication is disturbed. The person may ramble or repeat what another says. Sometimes speech cannot be understood. He or she may make up words.
  - The person may withdraw or lack interest in others.
  - Some people regress or move back to an earlier time of their life.
  - Some persons with schizophrenia attempt suicide. If a person talks about or tries to commit suicide, call the nurse at once. Do not leave the person alone.

MOOD DISORDERS
- Mood (or affective) disorders involve feelings, emotions, and moods.

- *Bipolar disorder.* The person with bipolar disorder has severe extremes in mood, energy, and ability to function. There are emotional lows (depression) and emotional highs (mania). This disorder is also called *manic-depressive illness.* The disorder is chronic and must be managed throughout life. Review Box 36-3, Signs and Symptoms of Bipolar Disorder, in the textbook. Bipolar disorder can damage relationships and affect school or work performance. Some people are suicidal. If a person talks about or tries to commit suicide, call the nurse at once. Do not leave the person alone.
- *Major depression.* Depression involves the body, mood, and thoughts. Review Box 36-3, Signs and Symptoms of Bipolar Disorder, in the textbook for symptoms. Symptoms affect work, study, sleep, eating, and other activities. The person is very sad.
- Depression is common in older persons. They have many losses—death of family and friends, loss of health, loss of body functions, loss of independence. Loneliness and the side effects of some drugs also are causes. Review Box 36-4, Signs and Symptoms of Depression in Older Persons, in the textbook.

CARE AND TREATMENT
- Treatment of mental health problems involves having the person explore his or her thoughts and feelings. This is done through psychotherapy and behavior, group, occupational, art, and family therapies. Often drugs are ordered.
- The care plan reflects the person's needs. The physical, safety and security, and emotional needs of the person must be met.
- Communication is important. Be alert to nonverbal communication.

REVIEW QUESTIONS
Circle the BEST answer.
1. A person may not know why anxiety occurs.
   a. True
   b. False
2. Panic is an intense and sudden feeling of fear, anxiety, terror, or dread.
   a. True
   b. False
3. A person with an obsessive-compulsive disorder has a ritual that is repeated over and over again.
   a. True
   b. False
4. A person talks about suicide. You must do the following *except*
   a. Call the nurse at once
   b. Stay with the person
   c. Leave the person alone
   d. Stay calm

5. Which statement about depression in older persons is *false*?
   a. Depression rarely occurs in older persons.
   b. Depression is often overlooked in older persons.
   c. Loneliness may be a cause of depression in older persons.
   d. Side effects of some drugs may cause depression in older persons.

6. Which statement is *false*?
   a. Communication is important when caring for a person with a mental health problem.
   b. You should be alert to nonverbal communication when caring for a person with a mental health problem.
   c. The care plan reflects the needs of the person.
   d. The focus is only on the person's emotional needs.

CHAPTER 37 CONFUSION AND DEMENTIA

- Certain diseases affect the brain. Changes in the brain can affect cognitive function.
- Cognitive function relates to memory, thinking, reasoning, ability to understand, judgment, and behavior.

CONFUSION

- When caring for the confused person:
  - Follow the person's care plan.
  - Provide for safety.
  - Face the person and speak clearly.
  - Call the person by name every time you are in contact with him or her.
  - State your name and show your name tag.
  - Give the date and time each morning. Repeat as needed during the day and evening.
  - Explain what you are going to do and why.
  - Give clear, simple directions and answers to questions.
  - Ask clear, simple questions. Give the person time to respond.
  - Keep calendars and clocks with large numbers in the person's room.
  - Have the person wear eyeglasses and hearing aids as needed.
  - Use touch to communicate.
  - Place familiar objects and pictures within the person's view.
  - Provide newspapers, magazines, TV, and radio. Read to the person if appropriate.
  - Maintain the day-night cycle.
  - Provide a calm, relaxed, and peaceful setting.
  - Follow the person's routine.
  - Break tasks into small steps when helping the person.
  - Do not rearrange furniture or the person's belongings.
  - Encourage the person to take part in self-care.
  - Be consistent.

DEMENTIA

- Dementia is not a normal part of aging. Most older people do not have dementia.
- Some early warning signs include problems with dressing, cooking, and driving. Also, getting lost in familiar places and misplacing items.
- Alzheimer's disease is the most common type of permanent dementia.

ALZHEIMER'S DISEASE

- Alzheimer's disease (AD) is a brain disease. Memory, thinking, reasoning, judgment, language, behavior, mood, and personality are affected.
- The classic sign of AD is gradual loss of short-term memory. Warning signs include:
  - Asking the same questions over and over again.
  - Repeating the same story—word for word, again and again.
  - The person forgets activities that were once done regularly with ease.
  - Losing the ability to pay bills or balance a checkbook.
  - Getting lost in familiar places. Or misplacing household objects.
  - Neglecting to bathe or wearing the same clothes over and over again. Meanwhile, the person insists that a bath was taken or that clothes were changed.
  - Relying on someone else to make decisions or answer questions that he or she would have handled.
  - Review Box 37-4, Signs of AD, in the textbook for other signs of AD.
- The following behaviors are common with AD:
  - *Wandering*. Persons with AD are not oriented to person, place, and time. They may wander away from home and not find their way back.
  - *Sundowning*. With **sundowning,** signs, symptoms, and behaviors of AD increase during hours of darkness. As daylight ends, confusion, restlessness, anxiety, agitation, and other symptoms increase.
  - *Hallucinations*. A **hallucination** is seeing, hearing, or feeling something that is not real.
  - *Delusions*. People with AD may think they are some other person. A person may believe that the caregiver is someone else.
  - *Catastrophic reactions*. The person reacts as if there is a disaster or tragedy.
  - *Agitation and restlessness*. The person may pace, hit, or yell.
  - *Aggression and combativeness*. These behaviors include hitting, pinching, grabbing, biting, or swearing.
  - *Screaming*. Persons with AD scream to communicate.
  - *Abnormal sexual behaviors*. Sexual behaviors may involve the wrong person, the wrong time, and the wrong place. Persons with AD cannot control behavior.
  - *Repetitive behaviors*. Persons with AD repeat the same motions over and over again.

CARE OF PERSONS WITH AD AND OTHER DEMENTIAS

- Safety, hygiene, nutrition and fluids, elimination, and activity needs must be met. So must comfort and sleep needs. Review Box 37-6, Care of Persons With AD and Other Dementias, in the textbook.
- Treat persons with AD with dignity and respect. They have the same rights as persons who are alert and active.
- The person can have other health problems and injuries. However, the person may not recognize pain, fever, constipation, incontinence, or other signs and symptoms. Carefully observe the person. Report any change in the person's usual behavior to the nurse.
- Infection is a risk. Provide good skin care, oral hygiene, and perineal care after bowel and bladder elimination.
- Supervised activities meet the person's needs and cognitive abilities.
- Impaired communication is a common problem. Avoid giving orders, wanting the truth, and correcting the person's errors.
- Always look for dangers in the person's room and in the hallways, lounges, dining areas, and other areas on the nursing unit. Remove the danger if you can.
- Every staff member must be alert to persons who wander. Such persons are allowed to wander in safe areas.

REVIEW QUESTIONS

Circle the BEST answer.

1. Cognitive function involves all of the following *except*
   a. Memory and thinking
   b. Reasoning and understanding
   c. Judgment and behavior
   d. Personality and mood
2. When caring for a confused person, you do the following *except*
   a. Provide for safety
   b. Maintain the day-night schedule
   c. Keep calendars and clocks in the person's room
   d. Ask difficult-to-understand questions, complex directions
3. Which statement about dementia is *false*?
   a. The person may have changes in personality.
   b. Dementia is a normal part of aging.
   c. Alzheimer's disease is the most common type of dementia.
   d. The person may have changes in behavior.
4. When caring for persons with AD, you do following *except*
   a. Provide good skin care
   b. Talk to them in a calm voice
   c. Observe them closely for unusual behavior
   d. Allow personal choice in wandering.

CHAPTER 39 REHABILITATION AND RESTORATIVE CARE

- A **disability** is any lost, absent, or impaired physical or mental function.
- **Rehabilitation** is the process of restoring the person to his or her highest possible level of physical, psychological, social, and economic function. The focus is on improving abilities. This promotes function at the highest level of independence.

REHABILITATION AND THE WHOLE PERSON

- Rehabilitation takes longer in older persons. Changes from aging affect healing, mobility, vision, hearing, and other functions. Chronic health problems can slow recovery.
- There are various aspects to rehabilitation:
  - *Physical.* Rehabilitation starts when the person first seeks health care. Complications, such as contractures and pressure ulcers, are prevented.
  - *Elimination.* Bowel or bladder training may be needed. Fecal impaction, constipation, and fecal incontinence are prevented.
  - *Self-care.* Self-care for **activities of daily living (ADL)** is a major goal. Self-help devices are often needed.
  - *Mobility.* The person may need crutches, a walker, a cane, a brace, or a wheelchair.
  - *Nutrition.* The person may need a special diet or enteral nutrition.
  - *Communication.* Speech therapy and communication devices may be helpful.
- A disability also has psychological and social aspects:
  - A disability can affect function and appearance. Self-esteem and relationships may suffer. The person may feel unwhole, useless, unattractive, unclean, or undesirable. The person may deny the disability. The person may expect therapy to correct the problem. He or she may be depressed, angry, and hostile.
  - Successful rehabilitation depends on the person's attitude. The person must accept his or her limits and be motivated. The focus is on abilities and strengths. Despair and frustration are common. Progress may be slow. Remind persons of their progress. They need help accepting disabilities and limits. Give support, reassurance, and encouragement. Spiritual support helps some people.
- Economic aspects also affect a disability. Some persons cannot return to their jobs. The person is assessed for work skills, work history, interests, and talents. The goal is for the person to become gainfully employed.

REHABILITATION

- Rehabilitation is a team effort. The person is the key member. The health team helps the person set goals and plan care. All help the person regain function and independence.
- Every part of your job focuses on promoting the person's independence. Preventing decline in function is a goal. Review Box 39-2, Assisting With Rehabilitation and Restorative Care, in the textbook.

QUALITY OF LIFE

- *Protect his or her right to privacy.* The person relearns old or practices new skills in private. Others do not need to see mistakes, falls, spills, or clumsiness.
- *Encourage personal choice.* This gives the person control.
- *Protect the right to be free from abuse and mistreatment.* Sometimes improvement is not seen for weeks. Repeated explanations and demonstrations may have little or no results. You and other staff and family may become upset and short-tempered. However, no one can shout, scream, or yell at the person. You cannot call the person names or hit or strike the person. Unkind remarks are not allowed. Report signs of abuse or mistreatment.
- *Learn to deal with your anger.* The person does not choose loss of function. If the process upsets you, discuss your feelings with the nurse.
- *Encourage activities.* Provide support and reassurance to the person with the disability. Remind the person that others with disabilities can give support and understanding.
- *Provide a safe setting.* The setting must meet the person's needs. The overbed table, bedside stand, and signal light are moved to the person's strong side.
- *Show patience, understanding, and sensitivity.* The person may be upset and discouraged. Give support, encouragement, and praise when needed. Stress the person's abilities and strengths. Do not give pity or sympathy.

REVIEW QUESTIONS
Circle the BEST answer.

1. Successful rehabilitation depends on the person's attitude.
   a. True
   b. False
2. A person with a disability may be depressed, angry, and hostile.
   a. True
   b. False
3. A person needs rehabilitation. You should do the following *except*
   a. Let the person relearn old skills in private
   b. Let the person practice new skills in private
   c. Encourage the person to make choices
   d. Shout at the person
4. You saw a family member hit and scream at a person. You need to report your observations to the nurse.
   a. True
   b. False
5. A person has a weak left arm. You will
   a. Place the signal light on his left side
   b. Place the signal light on his right side
   c. Give him sympathy
   d. Give him pity

CHAPTER 40 BASIC EMERGENCY CARE
EMERGENCY CARE
- A nurse decides when to activate the Emergency Medical System.
- Some centers allow nursing assistants to start CPR. Others do not. Know your center's policy.
- Rules for emergency care include:
  - Know your limits. Do not do more than you are able.
  - Stay calm.
  - Know where to find emergency supplies.
  - Follow Standard Precautions and the Bloodborne Pathogen Standard to the extent possible.
  - Check for breathing, a pulse, and bleeding.
  - Keep the person lying down or as you found him or her.
  - Perform necessary emergency measures.
  - Call for help.
  - Do not remove clothes unless you have to.
  - Keep the person warm. Cover the person with a blanket, coats, or sweaters.
  - Reassure the person. Explain what is happening.
  - Do not give the person food or fluids.
  - Keep onlookers away. They invade privacy.
  - Review the rules in Box 40-1, Rules of Emergency Care, in the textbook for more information.

SEIZURES
- You cannot stop a seizure. However, you can protect the person from injury:
  - Follow the rules for emergency care listed previously.
  - Do not leave the person alone.
  - Lower the person to the floor.
  - Note the time the seizure started.
  - Place something soft under the person's head.
  - Loosen tight jewelry and clothing around the person's neck.
  - Turn the person onto his or her side. Make sure the head is turned to the side.
  - Do not put any object or your fingers between the person's teeth.
  - Move furniture, equipment, and sharp objects away from the person.
  - Note the time when the seizure ends.
  - Make sure the mouth is clear of food, fluids, and saliva after the seizure.
  - Provide Basic Life Support if the person is not breathing after the seizure.

FAINTING
- Warning signals are dizziness, perspiration, and blackness before the eyes. The person looks pale. The pulse is weak. Respirations are shallow if consciousness is lost. Emergency care includes:
  - Have the person sit or lie down before fainting occurs.
  - If sitting, the person bends forward and places the head between the knees.
  - If the person is lying down, raise the legs.
  - Loosen tight clothing.
  - Keep the person lying down if fainting has occurred.
  - Do not let the person get up until symptoms have subsided for about 5 minutes.
  - Help the person to a sitting position after recovery from fainting.

REVIEW QUESTIONS
Circle the BEST answer.
1. During an emergency, you do all of the following *except*
   a. Perform only procedures you have been trained to do
   b. Keep the person lying down or as you found him or her
   c. Let the person become cold
   d. Reassure the person and explain what is happening
2. During an emergency, you keep onlookers away.
   a. True
   b. False
3. During a seizure, you do the following *except*
   a. Turn the person's body to the side
   b. Note the time the seizure started and ended
   c. Place your fingers in the person's mouth
   d. Turn the person's head to the side
4. Which statement about fainting is *false*?
   a. If standing, have the person sit down before fainting.
   b. If sitting, have the person bend forward and place his head between his knees before fainting occurs.
   c. Tighten the person's clothing.
   d. Raise the legs if the person is lying down.

CHAPTER 41 THE DYING PERSON
ATTITUDES ABOUT DEATH
- Practices and attitudes about death differ among cultures. Also, attitudes about death are closely related to religion.
- Adults fear pain and suffering, dying alone, and the invasion of privacy. They also fear loneliness and separation from loved ones. Adults often resent death because it affects plans, hopes, dreams, and ambitions.
- Older persons usually have fewer fears than younger adults. They have more experience with dying and death. Some welcome death as freedom from pain and suffering.

THE STAGES OF DYING
- Dr. Kübler-Ross described five stages of dying. They are:
  - Denial—the person refuses to believe he or she is going to die.
  - Anger—there is anger and rage, often at family, friends, and the health team.
  - Bargaining—often the person bargains with God for more time.
  - Depression—the person is sad and mourns things that were lost.
  - Acceptance—the person is calm and at peace. The person accepts death.
- Dying persons do not always pass through all five stages. A person may never get beyond a certain stage. Some move back and forth between stages.

PSYCHOLOGICAL, SOCIAL, AND SPIRITUAL NEEDS
- Let the person express feelings and emotions in his or her own way. Do not worry about saying the wrong thing or finding the right words. You do not need to say anything.
- Touch shows caring and concern. Sometimes the person does not want to talk but needs you nearby. Silence, along with touch, is a meaningful way to communicate.
- Some people may want to see a spiritual leader. Or they may want to take part in religious practices.

PHYSICAL NEEDS
- Body processes slow. The person is weak. Changes occur in levels of consciousness.
- Vision blurs and gradually fails. Explain what you are doing to the person or in the room. Provide good eye care.
- Hearing is one of the last functions lost. Always assume that the person can hear.
- Speech becomes difficult. Anticipate the person's needs. Do not ask questions that need long answers.
- Frequent oral hygiene is given as death nears.
- Crusting and irritation of the nostrils can occur. Carefully clean the nose.
- Skin care and bathing are necessary. Change linens and gowns whenever needed.

- Urinary and fecal incontinence may occur. Give perineal care as needed.
- Promote comfort. Semi-Fowler's position is usually best for breathing problems.
- The person's room should be comfortable and pleasant.

THE FAMILY
- This is a difficult time for family. The family goes through stages like the dying person. Be available, courteous, and considerate.
- The person and family need time together. However, you cannot neglect care because the family is present. Most centers let family members help give care.

SIGNS OF DEATH
- There are signs that death is near:
  - Movement, muscle tone, and sensation are lost.
  - Abdominal distention, fecal incontinence, nausea, and vomiting are common.
  - The skin feels cool, pale, or mottled. The person perspires heavily.
  - The pulse is fast, weak, and irregular. Blood pressure starts to fall.
  - Slow or rapid respirations are observed. Mucus collects in the airway. This causes the death rattle that is heard.
  - Pain decreases as the person loses consciousness.
- The signs of death include no pulse, no respirations, and no blood pressure. The pupils are dilated and fixed.

CARE OF THE BODY AFTER DEATH
- Postmortem care is done to maintain a good appearance of the body.
- Moving the body when giving postmortem care can cause remaining air in the lungs, stomach, and intestines to be expelled. When air is expelled, sounds are produced.
- When giving postmortem care, follow Standard Precautions and the Bloodborne Pathogen Standard.

QUALITY OF LIFE
- A person has the right to die in peace and with dignity. Review Box 41-1, A Dying Patient's Bill of Last Rights, in the textbook.
- The dying person also has these rights:
  - The right to privacy before and after death. Do not expose the person unnecessarily.
  - The right to visit others in private.
  - The right to confidentiality before and after death.
  - The right to be free from abuse, mistreatment, and neglect.
  - Freedom from restraint.
  - The right to have personal possessions.
  - The right to a safe and home-like setting.
  - The right to personal choice. The dying person may refuse treatment. The health team must respect choices to refuse treatment and not prolong life.

REVIEW QUESTIONS

Circle the BEST answer.

1. Which statement is *false*?
   a. Adults fear dying alone.
   b. Older persons usually have fewer fears about dying than younger adults.
   c. Adults often resent death.
   d. All adults welcome death.

2. Persons in the denial stage of dying
   a. Are angry
   b. Bargain with God
   c. Are calm and at peace
   d. Refuse to believe that they are dying

3. When caring for a person who is dying, you should do the following *except*
   a. Listen to the person
   b. Use touch to show care and concern
   c. Provide privacy during spiritual moments
   d. Talk about your feelings about death

4. When caring for a dying person, you provide all of the following *except*
   a. Eye care
   b. Oral hygiene
   c. Good skin care
   d. Physical exercise

5. The dying person has the right to accept or refuse medical treatment.
   a. True
   b. False

6. When giving postmortem care, you should wear gloves.
   a. True
   b. False

Practice Examination 1

This test contains 75 questions. For each question, circle the BEST answer.

1. A nurse asks you to give a person his drug when he is done in the bathroom. Your response to the nurse is
   A. "I will give the drug for you."
   B. "I will ask the other nursing assistant to give the drug."
   C. "I am sorry, but I cannot give that drug. I will let you know when he is out of the bathroom."
   D. "I refuse to give that drug."

2. An ethical person
   A. Does not judge others
   B. Avoids persons whose standards and values are different from his or hers
   C. Is prejudiced and biased
   D. Causes harm to another person

3. You smell alcohol on the breath of a co-worker. You
   A. Ignore the situation
   B. Tell the co-worker to get counseling
   C. Take a break and drink some alcohol too
   D. Tell the nurse at once

4. A person's signal light goes unanswered. He gets out of bed and falls. His leg is broken. This is
   A. Neglect
   B. Emotional abuse
   C. Physical abuse
   D. Malpractice

5. Your mom asks you about a person on your unit. Your response is
   A. "She is walking better now that she is receiving physical therapy."
   B. "I'm sorry, but I cannot talk about her. It is unprofessional, and violates the person's privacy and confidentiality."
   C. "Don't tell anyone I told you, but she is getting worse."
   D. "She has been very sad recently and needs visitors."

6. You are going off duty. The nursing assistant coming on duty is on the unit with you. A person puts her light on. Your response is
   A. "I'm ready to go. I will let you answer that light."
   B. "I've been here all day so I am not answering that light."
   C. "No one helped me answer lights when I came on duty."
   D. "I will answer that light so you can get organized for the shift."

7. When recording in the medical record, you
   A. Write in pencil
   B. Spell words incorrectly
   C. Use only center-approved abbreviations
   D. Record what your co-worker did

8. You are answering the phone in the nurses' station. You
   A. Answer in a rushed manner
   B. Give a courteous greeting
   C. End the conversation and hang-up without saying good-bye
   D. Give confidential information about a resident to the caller

9. A person who was admitted to the nursing center yesterday does not feel safe. You
   A. Are rude as you care for the person
   B. Ignore the person's request for information
   C. Show the person around the nursing center
   D. Act rushed as you care for the person

10. A person is angry and is shouting at you. You should
    A. Yell back at the person
    B. Stay calm and professional
    C. Put the person in a room away from others
    D. Call the family

11. When speaking with another person, you
    A. Use medical terms that may not be familiar to the person
    B. Mumble your words as you talk
    C. Ask several questions at a time
    D. Speak clearly and distinctly

12. To use a transfer or gait belt safely, you should
    A. Ignore the manufacturer's instructions
    B. Leave the excess strap dangling
    C. Apply the belt over bare skin
    D. Apply the belt under the breasts

13. When you are listening to a person, you
    A. Look around the room
    B. Sit with your arms crossed
    C. Act rushed and not interested in what the person is saying
    D. Have good eye contact with the person

14. When caring for a person who is comatose, you
    A. Make jokes about how sick the person is
    B. Care for the person without talking to him or her
    C. Explain what you are doing to him or her
    D. Discuss your problems with the other nursing assistant in the room with you

15. You need to give care to a person when a visitor is present. You
    A. Politely ask the visitor to leave the room
    B. Do the care in the presence of the visitor
    C. Expose the person's body in front of the visitor
    D. Rudely tell the visitor where to wait while you care for the person

16. A person tells you he wants to talk with a minister. You
    A. Ignore the request
    B. Tell the nurse
    C. Ask what the person wants to discuss with the minister
    D. Tell the person there is no need to talk with a minister

17. When you care for a person who has a restraint, you
    A. Observe the person every 15 minutes
    B. Remove the restraint and reposition the person every 4 hours
    C. Apply the restraint tightly
    D. Apply the restraint incorrectly
18. As a person ages
    A. The skin becomes less dry
    B. Muscle strength increases
    C. Reflexes are faster
    D. Bladder muscles weaken
19. A person you are caring for touches your buttocks several times. You
    A. Tell the person you like being touched
    B. Ask the person not to touch you again
    C. Tell the person's daughter
    D. Tell the person's girlfriend
20. You see a person sliding out of a wheelchair. You
    A. Ignore the person
    B. Tell the nursing assistant assigned to the person
    C. Position the person correctly in the wheelchair
    D. Tell the nurse the person needs repositioning
21. You cannot read the person's name on the ID bracelet. You
    A. Tell the nurse so a new bracelet can be made
    B. Ignore the fact that you cannot read the name
    C. Ask another nursing assistant to identify the person
    D. Tell the family the person needs a new ID bracelet
22. The universal sign of choking is
    A. Holding your breath
    B. Clutching at the throat
    C. Having difficulty breathing
    D. Coughing
23. A person is on a diabetic diet. You
    A. Serve the person's meals late
    B. Let the person eat whenever he or she is hungry
    C. Sometimes check the tray to see what was eaten
    D. Tell the nurse about changes in the person's eating habits
24. With mild airway obstruction
    A. The person is usually unconscious
    B. The person cannot speak
    C. Forceful coughing often does not remove the object
    D. Forceful coughing often can remove the object
25. The Heimlich maneuver involves
    A. Abdominal thrusts
    B. Chest thrusts
    C. Spine thrusts
    D. A finger sweep when the person is conscious
26. Faulty electrical equipment
    A. Can be used in a nursing center
    B. Should be given to the nurse
    C. Should be taken home by you for repair
    D. Should be used only with alert persons

27. A warning label has been removed from a hazardous substance container. You
    A. May use the substance if you know what is in the container
    B. Leave the container where it is
    C. Take the container to the nurse and explain the problem
    D. Tell another nursing assistant about the missing label
28. A person's beliefs and values are different from your views. What should you do?
    A. Refuse to care for the person.
    B. Delegate care to another nursing assistant.
    C. Tell the nurse about your concerns.
    D. Tell the person how you feel.
29. You find a person smoking in the nursing center. You should
    A. Ignore the situation
    B. Tell the person to leave
    C. Tell another nursing assistant
    D. Ask the person to put the cigarette out and show him or her where smoking is permitted
30. During a fire, the first thing you do is
    A. Rescue persons in immediate danger
    B. Sound the nearest fire alarm
    C. Close doors and windows to confine the fire
    D. Extinguish the fire
31. A person with Alzheimer's disease has increased restlessness and confusion as daylight ends. You
    A. Try to reason with the person
    B. Ask the person to tell you what is bothering him or her
    C. Provide a calm, quiet setting late in the day
    D. Complete his or her treatments and activities late in the day
32. To prevent suffocation, you should
    A. Make sure dentures fit loosely
    B. Cut food into large pieces
    C. Make sure the person can chew and swallow the food served
    D. Ignore loose teeth or dentures
33. When using a wheelchair, you should
    A. Lock both wheels before you transfer a person to and from the wheelchair
    B. Lock only one wheel before you transfer a person to and from the wheelchair
    C. Let the person's feet touch the floor when the chair is moving
    D. Let the person stand on the footplates
34. A person begins to fall while you are walking him or her. You should
    A. Try to prevent the fall
    B. Ease the person to the floor
    C. Yell at the person for falling
    D. Tell the nurse at the end of the shift
35. A person has a restraint on. You know that
    A. Restraints are used for staff convenience
    B. Death from strangulation is a risk factor to using a restraint
    C. Restraints may be used to punish a person
    D. A written nurse's order is required for a restraint

36. Before feeding a person, you
    A. Tell the other nursing assistant
    B. Go to the restroom
    C. Wash your hands
    D. Tell the nurse
37. When wearing gloves, you remember to
    A. Wear them several times before discarding them
    B. Wear the same ones from room to room
    C. Wear gloves with a tear or puncture
    D. Change gloves when they become contaminated with urine
38. When washing your hands, you
    A. Use hot water
    B. Let your uniform touch the sink
    C. Keep your watch at your wrist
    D. Keep your hands and forearms lower than your elbows
39. You need to move a box from the floor to the counter in the utility room. You
    A. Bend from your waist to pick up the box
    B. Hold the box away from your body as you pick it up
    C. Bend your knees and squat to lift the box
    D. Stand with your feet close together as you pick up the box
40. The nurse asks you to place a person in Fowler's position. You
    A. Put the bed flat
    B. Raise the head of the bed between 45 and 60 degrees
    C. Raise the head of the bed between 80 and 90 degrees
    D. Raise the head of the bed 15 degrees
41. You accidentally scratch a person. This is
    A. Neglect
    B. Negligence
    C. Malpractice
    D. Physical abuse
42. You positioned a person in a chair. For good body alignment, you
    A. Have the person's back and buttocks against the back of the chair
    B. Leave the person's feet unsupported
    C. Have the backs of the person's knees touch the edge of the chair
    D. Have the person sit on the edge of the chair
43. You need to transfer a person with a weak left leg from the bed to the wheelchair. You
    A. Get the person out of bed on the left side
    B. Get the person out of bed on the right side
    C. Keep the person in bed
    D. Ask the person what side moves first
44. A person tries to scratch and kick you. You should
    A. Protect yourself from harm
    B. Argue with the person
    C. Become angry with the person
    D. Ignore the person

45. When moving a person up in bed
    A. Window coverings may be left open so people can look in
    B. Body parts may be exposed
    C. Ask the person to help
    D. Ask the person to lie still
46. For comfort, most older persons prefer
    A. Rooms that are cold
    B. Restrooms that smell of urine
    C. Loud talking and laughter in the nurses' station
    D. Lighting that meets their needs
47. Signal lights are
    A. Placed on the person's strong side
    B. Answered when time permits
    C. Kept on the bedside table
    D. Kept on the person's weak side
48. A nurse asks you to inspect a person's closet. You
    A. Tell the nurse you cannot do this
    B. Inspect the closet when the person is in the dining room
    C. Ask the person if you can inspect his or her closet
    D. Ask the nurse to inspect the closet
49. When changing bed linens, you
    A. Hold the linen close to your uniform
    B. Shake the sheet when putting it on the bed
    C. Take only needed linen into the person's room
    D. Put dirty linen on the floor
50. To use a fire extinguisher, you
    A. Keep the safety pin in the extinguisher
    B. Direct the hose or nozzle at the top of the fire
    C. Squeeze the lever to start the stream of water
    D. Sweep the stream of water at the top of the fire
51. When doing mouth care for an unconscious person, you
    A. Do not need to wear gloves
    B. Give mouth care at least every 2 hours
    C. Place the person in a supine position
    D. Keep the mouth open with your fingers
52. A person is angry because he did not get to the activity room on time because a co-worker did not come to work. How should you respond to him?
    A. "It's not my fault. A co-worker called off today and we are short-staffed."
    B. "I'm sorry you were late for activities. I will try to plan better."
    C. "I am doing the best I can."
    D. "I'm just too busy."
53. You are asked to clean a person's dentures. You
    A. Use hot water
    B. Hold the dentures firmly and line the basin with a towel
    C. Wrap the dentures in tissues after cleaning
    D. Store the dentures in a denture cup with the person's name on it
54. When bathing a person, you notice a rash that was not there before. You
    A. Do nothing
    B. Tell the person
    C. Tell the nurse and record it in the medical record
    D. Tell the person's daughter

55. When washing a person's eyes, you
  A. Use soap
  B. Clean the eye near you first
  C. Wipe from the inner to the outer aspect of the eye
  D. Wipe from the outer aspect to the inner aspect of the eye
56. When giving a back massage, you
  A. Use cold lotion
  B. Use light strokes
  C. Massage reddened bony areas
  D. Look for bruises and breaks in the skin
57. You need to give perineal care to a female. You
  A. Separate the labia and clean downward from front to back
  B. Separate the labia and clean upward from back to front
  C. Wear gloves only if there is drainage
  D. Only use water
58. When giving a person a tub bath or shower, you
  A. Do not give the person a signal light
  B. Turn the hot water on first, then the cold water
  C. Stay within hearing distance if the person can be left alone
  D. Direct water toward the person while adjusting the water temperature
59. A person is on an anticoagulant. You
  A. Use a safety razor
  B. Use an electric razor
  C. Let him grow a beard
  D. Let him choose which type of razor to use
60. A person with a weak left arm wants to remove his or her sweater. You
  A. Let the person do it without any assistance
  B. Help the person remove the sweater from his or her right arm first
  C. Help the person remove the sweater from his or her left arm first
  D. Tell the person to keep the sweater on
61. When talking with a person, you should call the person
  A. "Honey"
  B. By his or her first name
  C. By his or her title—Mr. or Mrs. or Miss
  D. "Grandpa" or "Grandma"
62. A person has an indwelling catheter. You
  A. Let the person lie on the tubing
  B. Disconnect the catheter from the drainage tubing every 8 hours
  C. Secure the catheter to the lower leg
  D. Measure and record the amount of urine in the drainage bag
63. A person needs to eat a diet that contains carbohydrates. Carbohydrates
  A. Are needed for tissue repair and growth
  B. Provide energy and fiber for bowel elimination
  C. Provide energy
  D. Are needed for nerve and muscle function

64. You are taking a rectal temperature with a glass thermometer. You
  A. Insert the thermometer before lubricating it
  B. Leave the privacy curtain open
  C. Leave the thermometer in place for 10 minutes
  D. Hold the thermometer in place
65. A person has a blood pressure of 86/58. You
  A. Report the BP to the nurse at once
  B. Record the BP but do not tell the nurse
  C. Ask the unit secretary to tell the nurse
  D. Retake the BP in 30 minutes before telling the nurse
66. On which person would you take an oral temperature?
  A. An unconscious person
  B. The person receiving oxygen
  C. The person who breathes through his or her mouth
  D. A conscious person
67. When caring for a person who is blind or visually impaired, you
  A. Offer the person your arm and have the person walk a half step behind you
  B. Do as much for the person as possible
  C. Shout at the person when talking with him or her
  D. Touch the person before indicating your presence
68. You are caring for a person with dementia. You
  A. Misplace the person's clothes
  B. Choose the activities the person attends
  C. Send personal items home
  D. Let the family make choices if the person cannot
69. When caring for a person with a disability, you
  A. Can shout or scream at the person
  B. Can hit or strike the person
  C. Can call the person names
  D. Discuss your anger with the nurse
70. While bathing a person, you
  A. Keep doors and windows open
  B. Wash from the dirtiest areas to cleanest areas
  C. Encourage the person to help as much as possible
  D. Rub the skin dry
71. When a person is dying
  A. Assume that the person can hear you
  B. Oral care is done every 5 hours
  C. Skin care is done weekly
  D. Reposition the person every 3 hours
72. A person is on intake and output. You
  A. Measure only liquids such as water and juice
  B. Measure ice cream and gelatin as part of intake
  C. Measure IV fluids
  D. Measure tube feedings
73. A person has been on bedrest. You need to have the person walk. What will you do first?
  A. Help the person move quickly.
  B. Have the person dangle before getting out of bed.
  C. Have the person sit in a chair.
  D. Walk with the person as soon as he or she gets out of bed.

74. Your ring accidentally causes a skin tear on an elderly person. You
    A. Tell yourself to be more careful the next time
    B. Tell the nurse at once
    C. Do nothing
    D. Hope no one finds out

75. To protect a person's privacy, you should
    A. Keep all information about the person confidential
    B. Discuss the person's treatment with another nursing assistant in the lunch room
    C. Open the person's mail
    D. Keep the privacy curtain open when providing care to the person

Practice Examination 2

This test contains 75 questions. For each question, circle the BEST answer.

1. You can refuse to do a delegated task when
   A. You are too busy
   B. You do not like the task
   C. The task is not in your job description
   D. It is the end of the shift

2. Mr. Smith does not want lifesaving measures. You
   A. Explain to Mr. Smith why he should have lifesaving measures
   B. Respect his decision
   C. Explain to Mr. Smith's family why lifesaving measures are needed
   D. Tell your friend about Mr. Smith's decision

3. You are walking by a resident's room. You hear a nurse shouting at a person. This is
   A Battery
   B. Malpractice
   C. Verbal abuse
   D. Neglect

4. When communicating with a foreign-speaking person, you
   A. Speak loudly or shout
   B. Use medical terms the person may not understand
   C. Use words the person seems to understand
   D. Speak quickly and mumble

5. To protect a person from getting burned, you
   A. Allow smoking in bed
   B. Turn hot water on first, then cold water
   C. Assist the person with drinking or eating hot food
   D. Let the person sleep with a heating pad

6. To prevent equipment accidents, you should
   A. Use two-pronged plugs on all electrical devices
   B. Follow the manufacturer's instructions
   C. Wipe up spills when you have time
   D. Use unfamiliar equipment without training

7. To prevent a person from falling, you should
   A. Ignore signal lights
   B. Use throw rugs on the floor
   C. Keep the bed in a high position
   D. Use grab bars in showers

8. You need to wash your hands
   A. Before you document a procedure
   B. After you remove gloves
   C. After you talk with a person
   D. After you talk with a co-worker

9. You need to turn a heavy person in bed. You
   A. Do the procedure alone
   B. Keep the privacy curtain open
   C. Ask the person to lie still
   D. Use good body mechanics

10. When transferring a person from a wheelchair to bed, you *never*
    A. Ask a co-worker to help you
    B. Use a transfer or gait belt
    C. Have the person put his or her arms around your neck
    D. Lock the wheels on the wheelchair

11. When making a bed, you
    A. Keep the bed in the low position
    B. Wear gloves when removing linen
    C. Raise the head of the bed
    D. Raise the foot of the bed

12. To give perineal care to a male, you
    A. Use a circular motion and work toward the meatus
    B. Use a circular motion and start at the meatus and work outward
    C. Wear gloves only if there is drainage
    D. Use only water

13. A person with a left weak arm wants to put his or her sweater on. You
    A. Let the person do it without any assistance
    B. Help the person put the sweater on his or her right arm first
    C. Help the person put the sweater on his or her left arm first
    D. Tell the person to keep the sweater on

14. A person has an indwelling catheter. You
    A. Let the drainage bag touch the floor
    B. Keep the drainage bag higher than the bladder
    C. Hang the drainage bag on a bed rail
    D. Have the drainage bag hang from the bed frame or chair

15. A person needs to eat a diet that contains protein. Protein
    A. Is needed for tissue repair and growth
    B. Provides energy and fiber for bowel elimination
    C. Provides energy
    D. Is needed for nerve and muscle function

16. Older persons
    A. Have an increased sense of thirst
    B. Need less water than younger persons
    C. May not feel thirsty
    D. Seldom need to have water offered to them

17. A person is NPO. You
    A. Post a sign in the bathroom
    B. Keep the water pitcher filled at the bed side
    C. Remove the water pitcher and glass from the room
    D. Provide oral hygiene every day

18. A person drank 3 oz of milk at lunch. He or she drank
    A. 30 ml
    B. 60 ml
    C. 90 ml
    D. 120 ml

442

19. When feeding a person, you
    A. Offer fluids at the end of the meal
    B. Use forks
    C. Do not talk to the person
    D. Allow time for chewing and swallowing
20. You need to do ROM to a person's right shoulder. You
    A. Force the joint beyond its present ROM
    B. Move the joint quickly
    C. Force the joint to the point of pain
    D. Support the part being exercised
21. A person has a weak left leg. The person should
    A. Hold the cane in his or her left hand
    B. Hold the cane in his or her right hand
    C. Hold the cane in either hand
    D. Use a walker
22. To promote comfort and relieve pain, you
    A. Keep wrinkles in the bed linens
    B. Position the person in good alignment
    C. Talk loudly to the person
    D. Use sudden and jarring movements of the bed or chair
23. A person is receiving oxygen through a nasal cannula. You
    A. Turn the oxygen higher when he or she is short of breath
    B. Fill the humidifier when it is not bubbling
    C. Check behind the ears and under the nose for signs of irritation
    D. Remove the cannula when the person goes to the dining room
24. You accidentally dropped a mercury-glass thermometer. You
    A. Tell the nurse at once
    B. Put the mercury in your pocket
    C. Pick up the pieces of glass with your hands
    D. Touch the mercury
25. When taking a person's pulse, you
    A. Use the brachial pulse
    B. Take the pulse for 30 seconds if it is irregular
    C. Tell the nurse if the pulse is less than 60
    D. Use your thumb to take a pulse
26. You are counting respirations on a person. You
    A. Tell the person you are counting his or her respirations
    B. Count for 1 minute if an abnormal breathing pattern is noted
    C. Report a rate of 16 to the nurse at once
    D. Count for 30 seconds if an abnormal breathing pattern is noted
27. You are taking blood pressures on people assigned to you. An older person has a blood pressure of 188/96. You
    A. Report the BP to the nurse at once
    B. Finish taking all the blood pressures before telling the nurse
    C. Retake the BP in 30 minutes before telling the nurse
    D. Ask the unit secretary to tell the nurse about the BP

28. When would you take a rectal temperature?
    A. The person has diarrhea.
    B. The person is confused.
    C. The person is unconscious.
    D. The person is agitated.
29. A person has been admitted to the nursing center recently. You
    A. Encourage the person to stay in his or her room
    B. Ignore his or her questions
    C. Introduce the person to other residents
    D. Let the social worker repeat information to him or her
30. When taking a person's height and weight, you
    A. Let the person wear shoes
    B. Have the person void before being weighed
    C. Weigh the person at different times of the day
    D. Balance the scale every 6 months
31. A person is bedfast. To prevent pressure ulcers, you
    A. Reposition the person at least every 3 hours
    B. Massage reddened areas
    C. Let heels and ankles touch the bed
    D. Keep the skin free of moisture from urine, stools, or perspiration
32. A person has a hearing problem. When talking with the person, you
    A. Keep the TV or radio on
    B. Shout
    C. Face the person
    D. Speak quickly
33. When caring for a person who is blind or visually impaired, you
    A. Place furniture and equipment where the person walks
    B. Keep the lights off
    C. Explain the location of food and beverages
    D. Rearrange furniture and equipment
34. You are caring for a person with dementia. You
    A. Share information about the person's care
    B. Share information about the person's condition
    C. Protect confidential information
    D. Expose the person's body when you provide care
35. When caring for a confused person, you
    A. Call the person "Honey"
    B. Do not need to explain what you are doing
    C. Ask clear, simple questions
    D. Remove the calendar from the person's room
36. A person with Alzheimer's disease likes to wander. You
    A. Keep the person in his or her room
    B. Restrain the person
    C. Argue with the person who wants to leave
    D. Exercise the person as ordered
37. Restorative nursing programs
    A. Help maintain the lowest level of function
    B. Promote self-care measures
    C. Focus on the disability, not the person
    D. Help the person lose strength and independence

38. When caring for a person with a disability, you
    A. Focus on his or her limitations
    B. Expect progress to a rehabilitation program to be fast
    C. Remind the person of his or her progress in the rehabilitation program
    D. Deny the disability
39. After a person dies, you
    A. Can expose his or her body unnecessarily
    B. Can discuss the person's diagnosis with your family
    C. Can talk about the family's reactions to your friends
    D. Respect the person's right to privacy
40. You enter a person's room and find a fire in the wastebasket. Your first action is to
    A. Remove the person from the room
    B. Close the door
    C. Call for help
    D. Activate the fire alarm
41. You leave a person lying in urine and he or she develops a bedsore. This is
    A. Fraud
    B. Neglect
    C. Assault
    D. Battery
42. A nurse asks you to place a drug and a sterile dressing on a small foot wound. You
    A. Agree to do the task
    B. Ask another nursing assistant to do the task
    C. Politely tell the nurse you cannot do that task
    D. Report the nurse to the director of nursing
43. You observe a person's urine is foul-smelling and dark amber. Your first action is to
    A. Tell the other nursing assistant
    B. Tell the person
    C. Tell the nurse
    D. Record the observation
44. A daughter asks you for water for her mom. Your response is
    A. "I am not caring for your mom. I will get her nursing assistant for you."
    B. "I do not have time to do that."
    C. "That's not my job."
    D. "I will be happy to do that."
45. A person has a restraint on. You
    A. Observe the person for breathing and circulation complications every 30 minutes
    B. Know that unnecessary restraint is false imprisonment
    C. Use the most restrictive type of restraint
    D. Know that restraints decrease confusion and agitation
46. The nurse asks you to place a person in the supine position. You
    A. Elevate the head of the bed 45 degrees
    B. Elevate the foot of the bed 15 degrees
    C. Place the person on his or her back with the bed flat
    D. Place the person on his or her abdomen
47. The most important way to prevent or avoid spreading infection is to
    A. Wash hands
    B. Cover your nose when coughing
    C. Use disposable gloves
    D. Wear a mask
48. You are eating lunch and a nursing assistant begins to gossip about another person. You
    A. Join the conversation and talk about the person
    B. Remove yourself from the group
    C. Tell your roommate about the gossip you heard at lunch
    D. Tell another nursing assistant about the gossip you heard
49. When moving a person up in bed, you should
    A. Raise the head of the bed
    B. Ask the person to keep his or her legs straight
    C. Cause friction and shearing
    D. Ask a co-worker to help you
50. A person is on a sodium-controlled diet. This means
    A. Canned vegetables are omitted from his or her diet
    B. Salt may be added to food at the table
    C. Large amounts of salt are used in cooking
    D. Ham is eaten regularly
51. Elastic stockings
    A. Are applied after a person gets out of bed
    B. Should not have wrinkles or creases after being applied
    C. Come in one size only
    D. Are forced on the person
52. While walking, the person begins to fall. You
    A. Call for help
    B. Reach for a chair
    C. Ease the person to the floor
    D. Ask a visitor to help
53. Before bathing a person, you should
    A. Offer the bedpan or urinal
    B. Partially undress the person
    C. Raise the head of the bed
    D. Open the privacy curtain
54. When taking a rectal temperature, you insert the thermometer
    A. 1 inch
    B. 1.5 inches
    C. 2 inches
    D. 2.5 inches
55. Touch
    A. Is a form of nonverbal communication
    B. Is a form of verbal communication
    C. Means the same thing to everyone
    D. Should be used for all persons
56. You may share information about a person's care and condition to
    A. The staff caring for the person
    B. The person's daughter
    C. Your family members
    D. The volunteer in the gift shop

57. A person tells you he or she has pain upon urination. You
    A. Tell the nurse
    B. Let the nurse document this information
    C. Ask the person to tell you if it happens again
    D. Tell the person's son
58. A person's culture and religion are different from yours. You
    A. Laugh about the person's customs
    B. Tell your family about the person's customs
    C. Ask the person to explain his or her beliefs and practices to you
    D. Tell the person his or her beliefs and customs are silly
59. You need to wear gloves when you
    A. Do range-of-motion exercises
    B. Feed a person
    C. Give perineal care
    D. Walk a person
60. An older person is normally alert. Today he or she is confused. What should you do?
    A. Ask the person why he or she is confused.
    B. Ignore the confusion.
    C. Check to see if the person is confused later in the day.
    D. Tell the nurse.
61. While walking with a person, he or she tells you he feels faint. What do you do first?
    A. Have the person sit down.
    B. Call for the nurse.
    C. Open the window.
    D. Ask the person to take a deep breath.
62. You are asked to encourage fluids for a person. You
    A. Increase the person's fluid intake
    B. Decrease the person's fluid intake
    C. Limit fluids to meal times
    D. Keep fluids where the person cannot reach them
63. Communication fails when you
    A. Use words the other person understands
    B. Talk too much
    C. Let others express their feelings and concerns
    D. Talk about a topic that is uncomfortable
64. During bathing, a person may
    A. Decide what products to use
    B. Be exposed in the shower room
    C. Have visitors present without his or her permission
    D. Have no personal choices
65. People in late adulthood need to
    A. Adjust to increased income
    B. Adjust to their health being better
    C. Develop new friends and relationships
    D. Adjust to increased strength
66. One myth about aging is that
    A. People develop throughout life
    B. Many older people enjoy a fulfilling sex life
    C. Mental function declines with age
    D. Most older people are healthy

67. You find clean linen on the floor in a person's room. You
    A. Use the linen to make the bed
    B. Return the linen to the linen cart
    C. Put the linen in the laundry
    D. Tell the nurse
68. When doing mouth care on an unconscious person, you
    A. Use a large amount of fluid
    B. Position the person on his or her side
    C. Do the task without telling the person what you are doing
    D. Insert his or her dentures when done
69. When brushing or combing a person's hair, you
    A. Cut matted or tangled hair
    B. Encourage the person to do as much as possible
    C. Style the hair as you want
    D. Perform the task weekly
70. When providing nail and foot care, you
    A. Cut fingernails with scissors
    B. Trim toenails for a diabetic person
    C. Trim toenails for a person with poor circulation
    D. Check between the toes for cracks and sores
71. An indwelling catheter becomes disconnected from the drainage system. You
    A. Reconnect the tubing to the catheter quickly without gloves
    B. Tell the nurse at once
    C. Get a new drainage system
    D. Touch the ends of the catheter
72. Urinary drainage bags are
    A. Emptied and measured every day
    B. Emptied and measured at the end of each shift
    C. Kept on the floor
    D. Kept higher than the person's bladder
73. A person needs a condom catheter applied. You remember to
    A. Apply it to a penis that is red and irritated
    B. Use adhesive tape to secure the catheter
    C. Use elastic tape to secure the catheter
    D. Act in an unprofessional manner
74. For comfort during bowel elimination
    A. Have the person use the bedpan rather than the bathroom or commode if possible
    B. Permit visitors to stay
    C. Keep the door and privacy curtain open
    D. Leave the person alone if possible
75. You are transferring a person with a weak right side from the wheelchair to the bed. You
    A. Place the wheelchair on the left side of the bed
    B. Place the wheelchair on the right side of the bed
    C. Keep the person in the wheelchair
    D. Ask the person what side moves first

Skills Evaluation

Each state has its own policies and procedures for the skills test. The following information is an overview of what to expect:

- To pass the skills evaluation, you will need to perform all 5 skills correctly.
- A nurse evaluates your performance of certain skills. Having someone watch as you work is not a new experience. Your instructor evaluated your performance during your training program. While you are working, your supervisor evaluates your skills.
- Mannequins and people are used as "residents," depending on the skills you are performing.
- If you make a mistake, tell the evaluator what you did wrong. Then perform the skill correctly. Do not panic.
- Take whatever equipment you normally take or use at work. Wear a watch with a second hand. You may need it to measure vital signs and check how much time you have left.
- Evaluators assess other things besides correct skills performance:
  - Hand washing is evaluated at the beginning of the skills test. You are expected to know when to wash your hands. Therefore you may not be told to do so. Follow the rules for hand hygiene during the test.
  - Always follow the rules of medical asepsis. For example, remove gloves and dispose of them properly. Keep clean linen separated from dirty linen.
  - Before entering a person's room, knock on the door. Greet the person by name and introduce yourself before beginning a procedure. Check the ID or the photo ID to make certain you are giving care to the right person.
  - Always protect the person's rights throughout the skills test.
  - Explain what you are going to do before beginning the procedure and as needed throughout the procedure.
  - Communicate with the person as you give care. Focus on the person's needs and interests. Always treat the person with respect. Do not talk about yourself or your personal problems.
  - Provide privacy. This involves pulling the privacy curtain around the bed, closing doors, and asking visitors to leave the room.
  - Promote safety for the person. For example, lock the wheelchair when you transfer a person to and from it. Place the bed in the lowest horizontal position when the person must get out of bed or when you are done giving care.
  - Make sure the signal light is within the person's reach. Attaching it to the bed or bed rail does not mean the person can reach it.
  - Use good body mechanics. Raise the bed and overbed table to a good working height.

- Provide for comfort:
  - Make sure the person and linens are clean and dry. Change or straighten bed linens as needed.
  - Position the person for comfort and in good alignment.
  - Provide pillows as directed by the nurse and the care plan.
  - Raise the head of the bed as the person prefers and allowed by the nurse and the care plan.
  - Provide for warmth. The person may need an extra blanket, a lap blanket, a sweater, socks, and so on.
  - Adjust lighting to meet the person's needs.
  - Make sure eyeglasses and hearing aids are in place as needed.
  - Ask the person if he or she is comfortable.
  - Ask the person if there is anything else you can do for him or her.

SKILLS

Ask your instructor to tell you which of the following skills are tested in your state. The skills marked with an asterisk (*) are used with permission of Promissor. These skills are offered as a study guide to you. The word "client" refers to the resident or person receiving care. You are responsible for following the most current standards, practices, and guidelines of your state.

The steps in **bold** are *critical element steps*. If you miss a critical element step, you will automatically fail the test. For example, you are to transfer a client from the bed to a wheelchair. You will fail if you do not lock the wheels on the wheelchair before transferring the person. An automatic failure is one that could potentially cause harm to a person. Your state may mark critical element steps in another way—underline or *italics*. If your state has one, review the candidate's handbook.

❑ *WASHES HANDS   CHAPTER 13

1. Turns on water at sink
2. Wets hands and wrists thoroughly
3. Applies skin cleanser or soap to hands
4. **Lathers all surfaces of fingers and hands, including above the wrists, producing friction, for at least 10 (ten) seconds**
5. Rinses all surfaces of hands and wrists without contaminating hands
6. Uses clean, dry paper towel to dry all surfaces of hands, wrists, and fingers without contaminating hands
7. Uses clean, dry paper towel; clean, dry area of paper towel; or knee to turn off faucet without contaminating hands
8. Disposes of used paper towel(s) in wastebasket immediately after shutting off faucet

*From the candidate handbook and the Promissor Website, Copyright © 2005, used with the permission of Promissor, Inc.

❑ *MEASURES AND RECORDS WEIGHT OF AMBULATORY CLIENT   CHAPTER 31
1. Washes hands before contact with client
2. Identifies self to client by name and addresses client by name
3. Explains procedure to client, speaking clearly, slowly, and directly, maintaining face-to-face contact whenever possible
4. Starts with scale balanced at zero before weighing client
5. Assists client to step up onto center of scale
6. Determines client's weight
7. Assists client off scale before recording weight
8. Before leaving client, places signaling device within client's reach
9. **Records weight within +/– (plus or minus) 2 lbs of evaluator's reading**
10. Washes hands as final step

❑ *PROVIDES MOUTH CARE   CHAPTER 18
1. Washes hands before contact with client
2. Identifies self to client by name and addresses client by name
3. Explains procedure to client, speaking clearly, slowly, and directly, maintaining face-to-face contact whenever possible
4. Provides for client's privacy throughout procedure with curtain, screen, or door
5. Before providing mouth care, ensures client is in upright sitting position
6. Puts on gloves before cleaning client's mouth
7. Places towel across client's chest before providing mouth care
8. Moistens toothbrush or toothette
9. Applies toothpaste to toothbrush or toothette
10. **Cleans entire mouth (including tongue and all surfaces of teeth), using gentle motions**
11. Assists client to rinse his or her mouth
12. Holds emesis basin to client's chin
13. Wipes client's mouth and removes towel
14. Disposes of soiled linen in soiled linen container
15. Maintains clean technique with placement of toothbrush or toothette throughout procedure
16. Cleans and returns implements to proper storage
17. After completing procedure, removes gloves without contaminating self and disposes of gloves appropriately
18. Repositions head of bed to client's choice
19. Before leaving client, places signaling device within client's reach
20. Leaves bed in lowest position
21. Washes hands as final step

❑ *DRESSES CLIENT WITH AFFECTED RIGHT ARM   CHAPTER 19
1. Washes hands before contact with client
2. Identifies self to client by name and addresses client by name
3. Explains procedure to client, speaking clearly, slowly, and directly, maintaining face-to-face contact whenever possible
4. Provides for client's privacy during procedure with curtain, screen, or door
5. Asks client which outfit he or she would like to wear and dresses client in outfit of choice
6. Removes client's gown without completely exposing client
7. **Assists client to put right (affected) arm through right sleeve of shirt, sweater, or slip before placing garment on left (unaffected) arm**
8. Assists client to put on skirt, pants, or dress
9. Before standing client, places bed at safe and appropriate level for client
10. Before standing client, applies non-skid footwear
11. Puts on all items, moving client's body gently and naturally, avoiding force and over-extension of limbs and joints
12. Finishes with client dressed appropriately (clothing right side out, zippers/buttons fastened, etc.) and seated
13. Places gown in soiled linen container
14. Before leaving client, places signaling device within client's reach
15. Washes hands as final step

❑ *TRANSFERS CLIENT FROM BED TO WHEELCHAIR   CHAPTER 15
1. Washes hands before contact with client
2. Identifies self to client by name and addresses client by name
3. Explains procedure to client, speaking clearly, slowly, and directly, maintaining face-to-face contact whenever possible
4. Provides for client's privacy during procedure with curtain, screen, or door
5. Positions wheelchair close to bed with arm of wheelchair almost touching bed
6. Before transferring client, folds up footrests
7. Before transferring client, places bed at safe and appropriate level for client
8. **Before transferring client, locks wheels on wheelchair**
9. Before transferring client, supports client's back and hips and assists client to sitting position with feet flat on floor
10. Before transferring client, puts non-skid footwear on client and securely fastens

11. *With transfer (gait) belt:* Stands in front of client, positioning self to ensure safety of candidate and client during transfer (for example, knees bent, feet apart, back straight), places belt around client's waist, and grasps belt
    Without transfer belt: Stands in front of client, positioning self to ensure safety of candidate and client during transfer (for example, knees bent, feet apart, back straight, arms around client's torso under arms)
12. Provides instructions to enable client to assist in transfer
13. Braces client's lower extremities to prevent slipping
14. Counts to three (or says other prearranged signal) to alert client to begin transfer
15. On signal, gradually assists client to stand
16. Assists client to pivot to front of wheelchair with back of client's legs against wheelchair
17. Lowers client into wheelchair
18. Repositions client with hips touching back of wheelchair and removes transfer belt, if used
19. Positions client's feet on footrests
20. Before leaving client, places signaling device within client's reach
21. Washes hands as final step

❑ *ASSISTS CLIENT TO AMBULATE   CHAPTER 24

1. Washes hands before contact with client
2. Identifies self to client by name and addresses client by name
3. Explains procedure to client, speaking clearly, slowly, and directly, maintaining face-to-face contact whenever possible
4. **Before ambulating, puts on and properly fastens non-skid footwear**
5. Before standing client, places bed at safe and appropriate level for client
6. Stands in front of and facing client
7. Braces client's lower extremities
8. *With transfer (gait) belt:* Places belt around client's waist and grasps belt, while assisting client to stand
   Without transfer belt: Places arms around client's torso under client's armpits, while assisting client to stand
9. *With transfer belt:* Walks slightly behind and to one side of client for full distance, while holding onto belt
   Without transfer belt: Walks slightly behind and to one side of client for full distance, with arm supporting client's back
10. After ambulation, assists client to position of comfort and safety in bed and removes transfer belt, if used
11. Before leaving client, places signaling device within client's reach
12. Washes hands as final step

❑ *CLEANS AND STORES DENTURES   CHAPTER 18

1. Washes hands before beginning procedure
2. Puts on gloves before handling dentures
3. Before handling dentures, protects dentures from possible breakage (for example, by lining sink/basin with a towel/washcloth or by filling it with water)
4. Rinses dentures in cool, running water before brushing them
5. Applies toothpaste or denture cleanser to toothbrush
6. Brushes dentures on all surfaces
7. Rinses all surfaces of dentures under cool, running water
8. Rinses denture cup before placing clean dentures in it
9. Places dentures in clean denture cup with solution or cool water
10. Cleans and returns implements to proper storage
11. Places dentures in denture cup; then returns denture cup to proper storage
12. Maintains clean techniques with placement of dentures and toothbrush throughout procedure
13. Disposes of sink liner in appropriate container or drains sink
14. After completing procedure, removes gloves without contaminating self and disposes of gloves appropriately
15. Washes hands as final step

❑ *PERFORMS PASSIVE RANGE OF MOTION (ROM) FOR ONE SHOULDER   CHAPTER 24

1. Washes hands before contact with client
2. Identifies self to client by name and addresses client by name
3. Explains procedure to client, speaking clearly, slowly, and directly, maintaining face-to-face contact whenever possible
4. Provides for client's privacy throughout procedure with curtain, screen, or door
5. Supports client's arm at elbow and wrist while performing range of motion for shoulder
6. Raises client's straightened arm toward ceiling and back toward head of bed and returns to flat position (flexion/extension) (REPEAT AT LEAST 3 TIMES)
7. Moves client's straightened arm away from client's side of body toward head of bed, and returns client's straightened arm to midline of client's body (abduction/adduction) (REPEAT AT LEAST 3 TIMES)
8. Places client's flexed elbow at client's shoulder level, rotates forearm toward head of bed, and rotates forearm down toward bottom hip (rotation) (REPEAT AT LEAST 3 TIMES)
9. **While supporting the limb, moves joint gently, slowly, and smoothly through range of motion to the point of resistance, discontinuing exercise if pain occurs**
10. Leaves bed in lowest position

11. Before leaving client, places signaling device within client's reach
12. Washes hands as final step

❑ *PERFORMS PASSIVE RANGE OF MOTION (ROM) FOR ONE KNEE AND ONE ANKLE   CHAPTER 24

1. Washes hands before contact with client
2. Identifies self to client by name and addresses client by name
3. Explains procedure to client, speaking clearly, slowly, and directly, maintaining face-to-face contact whenever possible
4. Provides for client's privacy throughout procedure with curtain, screen, or door
5. Supports client's leg at knee and ankle while performing range of motion for knee
6. Bends knee to point of resistance and then returns leg flat to bed (extension/flexion) (REPEAT AT LEAST 3 TIMES)
7. Supports foot and ankle while performing range of motion for ankle
8. Keeping foot on bed, pushes/pulls foot toward head (dorsiflexion) and pushes/pulls foot down, toes point down (plantar flexion) (REPEAT AT LEAST 3 TIMES)
9. **While supporting limb, moves joints gently, slowly, and smoothly through range of motion to point of resistance, discontinuing if pain occurs**
10. Leaves bed in lowest position
11. Before leaving client, places signaling device within client's reach
12. Washes hands as final step

❑ *MEASURES AND RECORDS URINARY OUTPUT   CHAPTER 22

1. Washes hands as first step
2. Puts on gloves before handling bedpan
3. Pours contents of bedpan into measuring container without spilling or splashing any urine
4. Measures amount of urine while keeping container level
5. After measuring urine, empties contents of measuring container into toilet without splashing
6. Rinses measuring container and pours rinse water into toilet
7. Rinses bedpan and pours rinse water into toilet
8. Returns bedpan and measuring container to proper storage
9. After storing bedpan and measuring container, removes and disposes of gloves without contaminating self
10. Washes hands before recording output
11. **Records contents of container in output column within +/− (plus or minus) 25 cc/ml of evaluator's reading**

❑ *ASSISTS CLIENT WITH USE OF BEDPAN   CHAPTER 20

1. Washes hands before contact with client
2. Identifies self to client by name and addresses client by name
3. Explains procedure to client, speaking clearly, slowly, and directly, maintaining face-to-face contact whenever possible
4. Provides for client's privacy throughout procedure with curtain, screen, or door
5. Before placing bedpan, lowers head of bed
6. **Places bedpan correctly under client's buttocks (Standard bedpan: position bedpan so wider end of pan is aligned with client's buttocks; Fracture pan: position bedpan with handle toward foot of bed)**
7. Raises head of bed after placing bedpan under client
8. Puts toilet tissue within client's reach
9. Leaves signaling device within client's reach while client is using bedpan
10. Asks client to signal when finished
11. Lowers head of bed before removing bedpan
12. Puts on gloves before removing bedpan
13. Removes bedpan and empties contents into toilet
14. Rinses bedpan, pouring rinse water into toilet, and returns to proper storage
15. After storing bedpan, removes and disposes of gloves without contaminating self
16. Assists client to wash hands after using bedpan and disposes of soiled washcloth or wipes in proper container
17. Leaves bed in lowest position
18. Before leaving client, places signaling device within client's reach
19. Avoids unnecessary exposure of client throughout procedure
20. Washes hands as final step

❑ *PROVIDES PERINEAL CARE FOR INCONTINENT CLIENT   CHAPTER 18
Steps 9 through 13 are order-dependent

1. Washes hands before contact with client
2. Identifies self to client by name and addresses client by name
3. Explains procedure to client, speaking clearly, slowly, and directly, maintaining face-to-face contact whenever possible
4. Provides for client's privacy throughout procedure with curtain, screen, or door
5. Tests water temperature and ensures it is safe and comfortable before washing, and adjusts if necessary
6. Puts on gloves before contact with linen, incontinence pad, and/or client
7. Protects client from wet incontinence pad while keeping bed clean and dry (for example, rolls pad into itself with wet side in/dry side out or removes pad and uses clean, dry pad or protective linen)
8. Exposes perineal area

9. Washes entire perineal area with soapy washcloth, moving from front to back, while using clean area of washcloth or clean washcloth for each stroke
10. Rinses entire perineal area, moving from front to back, while using clean area of washcloth or clean washcloth for each stroke
11. Dries entire perineal area, moving from front to back, using a blotting motion with towel
12. Turns client on side
13. Washes, rinses, and dries buttocks and perineal area without contaminating perineal area
14. Removes wet incontinence pad or protective linen after drying buttocks
15. Places a dry incontinence pad under client
16. Repositions client
17. Disposes of linen and incontinence pad in proper containers
18. Empties, rinses, and wipes basin and returns to proper storage
19. Removes and disposes of gloves without contaminating self after returning basin to storage
20. Before leaving client, places signaling device within client's reach
21. Leaves bed in lowest position
22. Avoids unnecessary exposure of client throughout procedure
23. Washes hands as final step

❑ *PROVIDES CATHETER
   CARE   CHAPTER 20
1. Washes hands before contact with client
2. Identifies self to client by name and addresses client by name
3. Explains procedure to client, speaking clearly, slowly, and directly, maintaining face-to-face contact when possible
4. Provides for client's privacy throughout procedure with curtain, screen, or door
5. Tests water in basin to determine if it is safe and comfortable before washing, and adjusts if necessary
6. Puts on gloves before contact with linen and/or client
7. Exposes area surrounding catheter only
8. Places towel or pad under catheter tubing before washing
9. Applies soap to wet washcloth
10. Holds catheter near meatus to avoid tugging catheter
11. Cleans at least 4 inches of catheter nearest meatus, moving in only one direction (that is, away from meatus), using clean area of cloth for each stroke
12. Rinses at least 4 inches of catheter nearest meatus, moving in only one direction (that is, away from meatus), using clean area of cloth for each stroke
13. Disposes of linen in proper containers
14. Empties, rinses, and wipes basin and returns to proper storage
15. Removes and disposes of gloves without contaminating self after returning basin to storage

16. Before leaving client, places signaling device within client's reach
17. Leaves bed in lowest position
18. Avoids unnecessary exposure of client throughout procedure
19. Washes hands as final step

❑ *TAKES AND RECORDS
   ORAL TEMPERATURE   CHAPTER 28
1. Washes hands before contact with client
2. Identifies self to client by name and addresses client by name
3. Explains procedure to client, speaking clearly, slowly, and directly, maintaining face-to-face contact whenever possible
4. Holds oral thermometer by stem
5. Before inserting oral thermometer in client's mouth, shakes oral thermometer down to 96° F or lower
6. Inserts bulb end of oral thermometer into client's mouth, under tongue and to one side
7. Tells client to hold oral thermometer in mouth with lips closed and assists as necessary
8. Leaves oral thermometer in place for at least 3 minutes
9. Reads oral thermometer before cleaning thermometer
10. Cleans oral thermometer and/or returns it to container for used thermometers
11. Before leaving client, places signaling device within client's reach
12. Washes hands after cleaning oral thermometer and/or returning it to container for used thermometers
13. Records oral temperature within +/- (plus or minus) 0.2° of evaluator's reading

❑ *TAKES AND RECORDS RADIAL
   PULSE, AND COUNTS AND
   RECORDS RESPIRATIONS   CHAPTER 28
1. Washes hands before contact with client
2. Identifies self to client by name and addresses client by name
3. Explains procedure to client, speaking clearly, slowly, and directly, maintaining face-to-face contact whenever possible
4. Places fingertips on thumb side of client's wrist to locate pulse
5. Counts beats for 1 full minute
6. Records pulse rate within +/- (plus or minus) 4 beats of evaluator's reading
7. Counts respirations for 1 full minute
8. Records respiration rate within +/- (plus or minus) 2 breaths of evaluator's reading
9. Before leaving client, places signaling device within client's reach
10. Washes hands as final step

❏ *TAKES AND RECORDS
CLIENT'S BLOOD PRESSURE
(TWO-STEP PROCEDURE)   CHAPTER 28

1. Washes hands before contact with client
2. Identifies self to client by name and addresses client by name
3. Explains procedure to client, speaking clearly, slowly, and directly, maintaining face-to-face contact whenever possible
4. Before using stethoscope, wipes diaphragm and earpieces of stethoscope with alcohol
5. Positions client's arm with palm up
6. Places blood pressure cuff snugly on client's upper arm, with sensor placed over artery
7. Locates radial pulse with fingertips
8. Inflates cuff to no more than 30 mm Hg above point where pulse is last felt
9. Deflates cuff
10. Locates brachial pulse
11. Places diaphragm over brachial artery
12. Places earpieces of stethoscope in ears
13. Inflates cuff to no more than 30 mm Hg above point at which pulse was last felt
14. Deflates cuff slowly
15. Before leaving client, places signaling device within client's reach
16. **Records both systolic and diastolic pressures each within +/– (plus or minus) 4 mm of evaluator's reading**
17. Washes hands as final step

❏ *PUTS ONE KNEE-HIGH ELASTIC
STOCKING ON CLIENT   CHAPTER 32

1. Washes hands before contact with client
2. Identifies self to client by name and addresses client by name
3. Explains procedure to client, speaking clearly, slowly, and directly, maintaining face-to-face contact whenever possible
4. Provides for client's privacy during procedure with curtain, screen, or door
5. Turns stocking inside-out at least to heel area
6. Places foot of stocking over toes, foot, and heel
7. Pulls top of stocking over foot, heel, and leg
8. Moves client's foot and leg gently and naturally, avoiding force and over-extension of limb and joints throughout procedure
9. **Finishes procedure with no twists or wrinkles and stocking properly placed**
10. Before leaving client, places signaling device within client's reach
11. Washes hands as final step

❏ *MAKES AN OCCUPIED
BED   CHAPTER 17

1. Washes hands before contact with client
2. Identifies self to client by name and addresses client by name

3. Explains procedure to client, speaking clearly, slowly, and directly, maintaining face-to-face contact whenever possible
4. Places clean linen on clean surface within candidate's reach (for example, bedside stand, overbed table, or chair)
5. Provides for client's privacy throughout procedure with curtain, screen, or door
6. Lowers head of bed before moving client
7. Loosens top linen from end of bed on working side
8. After raising side rail, assists client to turn onto side, moving away from candidate toward raised side rail
9. Loosens bottom soiled linen on working side
10. Moves bottom soiled linen toward center of bed
11. Places and tucks in clean bottom linen or fitted bottom sheet on working side (if flat sheet is used, tucks in at top and working side)
12. After raising side rail, assists client to turn onto clean bottom sheet
13. Removes soiled bottom linen, avoiding contact with clothes, and places it in an appropriate location within room
14. Pulls and tucks in clean bottom linen, finishing with bottom sheet free of wrinkles
15. Covers client with clean top sheet and appropriately removes soiled top sheet
16. Finishes with clean linen anchored and centered
17. Replaces pillowcase
18. Before leaving client, places signaling device within client's reach
19. Leaves bed in lowest position
20. Disposes of soiled linen in soiled linen container
21. Avoids contamination of clean linen throughout procedure
22. Avoids unnecessary exposure of client throughout procedure
23. Washes hands as final step

❏ *PROVIDES FOOT CARE   CHAPTER 19

1. Washes hands before contact with client
2. Identifies self to client by name and addresses client by name
3. Explains procedure to client, speaking clearly, slowly, and directly, maintaining face-to-face contact whenever possible
4. Provides for client's privacy during procedure with curtain, screen, or door
5. Tests water temperature and ensures it is safe and comfortable before placing client's foot in water, and adjusts if necessary
6. Completely submerges foot in water
7. Removes foot from water, washing entire foot, including between toes, with soapy washcloth
8. Rinses entire foot, including between toes
9. Dries entire foot, including between toes
10. Puts lotion in hand
11. Warms lotion by rubbing hands together

* From the candidate handbook and the Promissor Website, Copyright © 2005, used with the permission of Promissor, Inc.

* From the candidate handbook and the Promissor Website, Copyright © 2005, used with the permission of Promissor, Inc.

12. Massages lotion into entire foot (top and bottom), removing excess (if any) with towel
13. Assists client to replace sock
14. Supports foot and ankle properly throughout procedure
15. Before leaving client, places signal device within client's reach
16. Empties, rinses, and wipes bath basin, and returns to proper storage
17. Disposes of soiled linen in soiled linen container
18. Washes hands as final step

❑ *PROVIDES FINGERNAIL CARE   CHAPTER 19
1. Washes hands before contact with client
2. Identifies self to client by name and addresses client by name
3. Explains procedure to client, speaking clearly, slowly, and directly, maintaining face-to-face contact whenever possible
4. Tests water temperature and ensures it is safe and comfortable before immersing client's fingers in water, and adjusts if necessary
5. Immerses client's fingers in basin of water, which is placed at comfortable level for client
6. Dries client's hand, including between fingers
7. Cleans under nails with orangewood stick
8. Wipes orangewood stick on towel after each nail
9. Grooms nails with file or emery board
10. Finishes with nails smooth and free of rough edges
11. Before leaving client, places signaling device within client's reach
12. Empties, rinses, and wipes basin, and returns to proper storage
13. Disposes of soiled linen in soiled linen container
14. Washes hands as final step

❑ *FEEDS CLIENT WHO CANNOT FEED SELF   CHAPTER 22
1. Washes hands before feeding client
2. Identifies self to client by name and addresses client by name
3. Explains procedure to client, speaking clearly, slowly, and directly, maintaining face-to-face contact whenever possible
4. Before feeding client, ensures client is in an upright sitting position
5. Before feeding, picks up name card and verifies that client has received the tray prepared for him or her
6. Before feeding client, assists client to put on clothing protector
7. Sits at client's eye level
8. Alternate types of food offered, allowing for client preferences (that is, does not feed all of one type before offering another type)
9. Offers the food in bite-size pieces
10. Makes sure client's mouth is empty before next bite of food or sip of beverage

11. Offers beverage to client throughout meal
12. Talks with client during meal
13. Wipes food from client's mouth and hands as necessary and at end of meal
14. Removes clothing protector and disposes in proper container
15. Before leaving client, places signaling device within client's reach
16. Removes food tray
17. Washes hands as final step

❑ *POSITIONS CLIENT ON SIDE   CHAPTER 15
1. Washes hands before contact with client
2. Identifies self to client by name and addresses client by name
3. Explains procedure to client, speaking clearly, slowly, and directly, maintaining face-to-face contact whenever possible
4. Provides for client's privacy throughout procedure with curtain, screen, or door
5. Before turning client, lowers head of bed
6. Before turning client, moves client's body toward self
7. After raising side rail, slowly rolls client onto side toward raised side rail while supporting client's body
8. **Positions client in proper body alignment Proper body alignment requires:**
   - **Head supported by pillow**
   - **Shoulder adjusted so client is not lying on arm**
   - **Top arm supported**
   - **Back supported by supportive device**
   - **Top knee flexed**
   - **Top leg supported by supportive device with hip in proper alignment**
9. Covers client with top linen
10. Before leaving client, places signaling device within client's reach
11. Washes hands as final step

❑ *GIVES MODIFIED BED BATH (FACE AND ONE ARM, HAND, AND UNDERARM)   CHAPTER 18
1. Washes hands before contact with client
2. Identifies self to client by name and addresses client by name
3. Explains procedure to client, speaking clearly, slowly, and directly, maintaining face-to-face contact whenever possible
4. Provides for client's privacy throughout procedure with curtain, screen, or door
5. Removes or folds back top bedding, keeping client covered with bath blanket (or top sheet)
6. Removes client's gown
7. Tests water temperature and ensures it is safe and comfortable before bathing client, and adjusts if necessary

8. Washes face with wet washcloth (no soap) beginning with eyes, using a different area of washcloth for each eye, washing inner aspect to outer aspect
9. Dries face with towel, using blotting motion
10. Exposes one arm
11. Places towel under arm
12. Using washcloth and towel, washes with soap, rinses, and dries arm, hand, and underarm
13. Moves client's body gently and naturally, avoiding force and over-extension of limbs and joints throughout procedure
14. Puts clean gown on client
15. Removes bath blanket and pulls up bedcovers
16. Before leaving client, places signaling device within client's reach
17. Empties, rinses, and wipes bath basin and returns to proper storage
18. Places soiled clothing and linen in soiled linen container
19. Leaves bed in lowest position
20. Avoids unnecessary exposure of client throughout procedure
21. Washes hands as final step

NOTE: The skills that follow are not Promissor skills. However, they are written close to Promissor language.

❑ ABDOMINAL THRUST   CHAPTER 10
1. Asks client if he or she is choking
2. Stands behind client
3. Wraps arms around client's waist
4. Makes fist with one hand
5. Places thumb side of fist against abdomen
6. Positions fist in middle above naval and below sternum (breastbone)
7. Grasps fist with your other hand
8. Presses fist and hand into client's abdomen with quick, upward thrust 3 to 5 times
9. Repeats thrusts until object is expelled or person loses consciousness

❑ AMBULATION WITH CANE OR WALKER   CHAPTER 24
1. Washes hands before contact with client
2. Identifies self to client by name and addresses client by name
3. Explains procedure to client, speaking clearly, slowly, and directly, maintaining face-to-face contact whenever possible
4. Locks bed wheels or wheelchair brakes
5. Assists client to sitting position
6. **Before ambulating, puts on and properly fastens non-skid footwear**
7. Positions cane or walker correctly
8. Assists client to stand, using correct body mechanics
9. Stabilizes cane or walker and ensures client stabilizes cane or walker
10. Stands behind and slightly to side of client
11. Ambulates client
12. Assists client to pivot and sit, using correct body mechanics

13. Before leaving client, places signaling device within client's reach
14. Washes hands as final step

❑ BACKRUB   CHAPTER 18
1. Washes hands before contact with client
2. Identifies self to client by name and addresses client by name
3. Explains procedure to client, speaking clearly, slowly, and directly, maintaining face-to-face contact whenever possible
4. Provides for client's privacy during procedure with curtain, screen, or door
5. Ensures client safety by placing bed rail up on opposite side of bed, as appropriate
6. Positions client in side-lying position with his or her back toward you
7. Exposes back
8. Places small amount of lotion onto hands and rubs together to warm
9. Rubs entire back in upward, outward motion for approximately 2 to 3 minutes; does not massage reddened bony areas
10. Provides for comfort
11. Before leaving client, places signaling device within client's reach
12. Washes hands as final step

❑ FLUID INTAKE   CHAPTER 22
1. Observes dinner tray
2. Uses pad and pencil, or calculator, to estimate number of milliliters (ml) of fluid consumed from each container
3. Obtains total fluids consumed in milliliters (ml)
4. Records total fluid consumed on I&O sheet
5. Calculated total is within required range

❑ GOWN AND GLOVES   CHAPTER 13
1. Washes hands
2. Holds gown and lets it unfold
3. Places hands and arms through sleeves
4. Ties strings at back of neck
5. Ties waist strings at back, making sure gown covers uniform
6. Puts on gloves, making sure gloves overlap gown at wrist
7. Provides care
8. Removes and discards gloves in appropriate container
9. Removes gown—unties waist strings and neck strings
10. Turns gown inside out as it is removed
11. Discards gown in appropriate container
12. Washes hands as final step

❑ HAIR CARE   CHAPTER 19
1. Washes hands before contact with client
2. Identifies self to client by name and addresses client by name
3. Explains procedure to client, speaking clearly, slowly, and directly, maintaining face-to-face contact whenever possible
4. Collects comb or brush and bath towel

5. Places towel across client's back and shoulders
6. Asks client how to style hair
7. Combs or brushes hair gently and completely
8. Leaves hair neatly brushed, combed, and styled
9. Removes towel
10. Before leaving client, places signaling device within client's reach
11. Washes hands as final step

❏ MEASURE AND RECORD CONTENT OF URINARY DRAINAGE BAG   CHAPTER 20

1. Washes hands
2. Identifies self to client by name and addresses client by name
3. Explains procedure to client, speaking clearly, slowly, and directly, maintaining face-to-face contact whenever possible
4. Puts on gloves
5. Empties urine from drainage bag into measuring container without touching tubing against container
6. Clamps drain and places it into bag pocket
7. Ensures that drainage bag is on non-movable part of bed, not touching floor
8. Measures amount of urine at eye level while keeping container level
9. After measuring urine, empties contents of measuring container into toilet without splashing
10. Rinses measuring container and disposes of rinse
11. Removes and disposes of gloves without contaminating self
12. Washes hands before recording urine output
13. **Records contents of container in output column**
14. **Recorded amount of urinary output is within required range**

❏ MOUTH CARE OF A COMATOSE CLIENT   CHAPTER 18

1. Washes hands before contact with client
2. Identifies self to client by name and addresses client by name
3. Explains procedure to client, speaking clearly, slowly, and directly, maintaining face-to-face contact whenever possible
4. Provides for client's privacy during procedure with curtain, screen, or door
5. Positions client on side with head turned well to one side
6. Protects client's chest and bed from soiling
7. Puts on gloves before cleaning client's mouth
8. Uses swabs or toothbrush and toothpaste or other cleaning solutions
9. **Cleans entire mouth (including tongue and all surfaces of teeth), using gentle motions**
10. Cleans and dries face
11. Provides for comfort
12. Cleans and returns implements to proper storage
13. After completing procedure, removes gloves without contaminating self and disposes of gloves appropriately
14. Washes hands as final step

❏ PASSING FRESH WATER   CHAPTER 22

1. Washes hands before contact with client
2. Assembles equipment—ice, scoop, pitcher
3. Identifies self to client by name and addresses client by name
4. Explains procedure to client, speaking clearly, slowly, and directly, maintaining face-to-face contact whenever possible
5. Scoops ice into water pitcher
6. Properly uses and stores ice scoop:
   a. Ice does not touch hand
   b. Scoop placed in appropriate receptacle after each use
7. Adds water to pitcher
8. Returns pitcher to client
9. Before leaving client, places signaling device within client's reach
10. Washes hands as final step

❏ RANGE OF MOTION HIP AND KNEE   CHAPTER 24

1. Washes hands before contact with client
2. Identifies self to client by name and addresses client by name
3. Explains procedure to client, speaking clearly, slowly, and directly, maintaining face-to-face contact whenever possible
4. Provides for client's privacy during procedure with curtain, screen, or door
5. Positions client supine and in good body alignment
6. Supports client's leg by placing one hand under knee and other hand under heel
7. Moves entire leg away from body (REPEAT AT LEAST 3 TIMES)
8. Moves entire leg toward body (REPEAT AT LEAST 3 TIMES)
9. Bends client's knee and hip toward client's trunk (REPEAT AT LEAST 3 TIMES)
10. Straightens knee and hip (REPEAT AT LEAST 3 TIMES)
11. **While supporting limb, moves joints gently, slowly, and smoothly through range of motion to point of resistance, discontinuing exercise if pain occurs**
12. Provides for comfort
13. Before leaving client, places signaling device within client's reach
14. Washes hands as final step

❏ RANGE OF MOTION LOWER EXTREMITY (HIP, KNEE, ANKLE)   CHAPTER 24

1. Washes hands before contact with client
2. Identifies self to client by name and addresses client by name
3. Explains procedure to client, speaking clearly, slowly, and directly, maintaining face-to-face contact whenever possible
4. Provides for client's privacy during procedure with curtain, screen, or door
5. Positions client supine and in good body alignment
6. Supports client's leg by placing one hand under knee and other hand under heel

7. Moves entire leg away from body (REPEAT AT LEAST 3 TIMES)
8. Moves entire leg toward body (REPEAT AT LEAST 3 TIMES)
9. Bends client's knee hip toward client's trunk (REPEAT AT LEAST 3 TIMES)
10. Straightens knee and hip (REPEAT AT LEAST 3 TIMES)
11. Flexes and extends ankle through range-of-motion exercises (REPEAT AT LEAST 3 TIMES)
12. Rotates ankle through range-of-motion exercises (REPEAT AT LEAST 3 TIMES)
13. **While supporting limb, moves joints gently, slowly, and smoothly through range of motion to point of resistance, discontinuing exercise if pain occurs**
14. Provides for comfort
15. Before leaving client, places signaling device within client's reach
16. Washes hands as final step

❑ RANGE OF MOTION UPPER EXTREMITY (SHOULDER, ELBOW, WRIST, FINGER)   CHAPTER 24
1. Washes hands before contact with client
2. Identifies self to client by name and addresses client by name
3. Explains procedure to client, speaking clearly, slowly, and directly, maintaining face-to-face contact whenever possible
4. Provides for client's privacy during procedure with curtain, screen, or door
5. Supports client's extremity above and below joints while performing range of motion
6. Raises client's straightened arm toward ceiling and back toward head of bed and returns to flat position (flexion/extension) (REPEAT AT LEAST 3 TIMES)
7. Moves client's straightened arm away from client's side of body toward head of bed, and returns client's straightened arm to midline of client's body (abduction/adduction) (REPEAT AT LEAST 3 TIMES)
8. Moves client's shoulder through rotation range-of-motion exercises (REPEAT AT LEAST 3 TIMES)
9. Flex and extend elbow through range-of-motion exercises (REPEAT AT LEAST 3 TIMES)
10. Provide range-of-motion exercises to wrist (REPEAT AT LEAST 3 TIMES)
11. Move finger and thumb joints through range-of-motion exercises (REPEAT AT LEAST 3 TIMES)
12. **While supporting body part, moves joint gently, slowly, and smoothly through range of motion to point of resistance, discontinuing exercise if pain occurs**
13. Before leaving client, places signaling device within client's reach
14. Washes hands as final step

❑ TAKES AND RECORDS AXILLARY TEMPERATURE, PULSE, AND RESPIRATIONS   CHAPTER 28
1. Washes hands before contact with client
2. Identifies self to client by name and addresses client by name

3. Explains procedure to client, speaking clearly, slowly, and directly, maintaining face-to-face contact whenever possible
4. Provides for client's privacy during procedure with curtain, screen, or door
5. Turns on digital oral thermometer
6. Dries axilla and places thermometer in the center of the axilla
7. Holds thermometer in place for appropriate length of time
8. Removes and reads thermometer
9. Records temperature on pad of paper
10. **Recorded temperature is within required range**
11. Discards sheath from thermometer
12. Places fingertips on thumb side of client's wrist to locate radial pulse
13. Counts beats for 1 full minute
14. Records pulse rate on pad of paper
15. **Recorded pulse is within required range**
16. Counts respirations for 1 full minute
17. Records respirations on pad of paper
18. **Recorded respirations are within required range**
19. Before leaving client, places signaling device within client's reach
20. Washes hands as final step

❑ TRANSFERS CLIENT FROM WHEELCHAIR TO BED   CHAPTER 15
1. Washes hands before contact with client
2. Identifies self to client by name and addresses client by name
3. Explains procedure to client, speaking clearly, slowly, and directly, maintaining face-to-face contact whenever possible
4. Provides for client's privacy during procedure with curtain, screen, or door
5. Positions wheelchair close to bed with arm of wheelchair almost touching bed
6. Before transferring client, folds up footrests
7. Before transferring client, places bed at safe and appropriate level for client
8. **Before transferring client, locks wheels on wheelchair and locks bed brakes**
9. *With transfer (gait) belt:* Stands in front of client, positioning self to ensure safety of candidate and client during transfer (for example, knees bent, feet apart, back straight), places belt around client's waist, and grasps belt. Tightens belt so that fingers of candidate's hand can be slipped between transfer/gait belt and client
   Without transfer belt: Stands in front of client, positioning self to ensure safety of candidate and client during transfer (for example, knees bent, feet apart, back straight, arms around client's torso under arms)
10. Provides instructions to enable client to assist in transfer
11. Braces client's lower extremities to prevent slipping
12. Counts to three (or says other prearranged signal) to alert client to begin transfer
13. On signal, gradually assists client to stand

14. Assists client to pivot and sit on bed in manner that ensures safety
15. Removes transfer belt, if used
16. Assists client to remove non-skid footwear
17. Assists client to move to center of bed
18. Provides for comfort and good body alignment
19. Before leaving client, places signaling device within client's reach
20. Washes hands as final step

❑ WEIGHING AND MEASURING HEIGHT OF AN AMBULATORY CLIENT   CHAPTER 31

1. Washes hands before contact with client
2. Identifies self to client by name and addresses client by name
3. Explains procedure to client, speaking clearly, slowly, and directly, maintaining face-to-face contact whenever possible
4. Starts with scale balanced at zero before weighing client
5. Assists client to step up onto center of scale
6. Determines client's weight and height
7. Assists client off scale before recording weight and height
8. Before leaving client, places signaling device within client's reach
9. **Records weight and height within required range**
10. Washes hands as final step

AFTER THE PROCEDURE
After you demonstrate a skill, complete a safety check of the room:
- The person is wearing eyeglasses and hearing aids as needed. They are stored inside the case and in the bedside stand if not worn.
- The signal light is plugged in and within reach.
- Bed rails are up or down, according to the care plan.
- The bed is in the lowest horizontal position.
- The bed position is locked if needed.
- Manual bed cranks are in the down position.
- Bed wheels are locked.
- Assistive devices are within reach. Walker, cane, and wheelchair are examples.
- The overbed table, filled water pitcher and cup, tissues, phone, TV controls, and other needed items are within reach.
- Unneeded equipment is unplugged or turned off.
- Harmful substances are stored properly. Lotion, mouthwash, shampoo, after-shave, and other personal care products are examples.
- Food and other items brought by the family and visitors are safe for the person.
- Floors are free of spills and clutter.

AFTER THE TEST
Celebrate—you have completed the competency evaluation. The length of time for you to get your test results varies with each state. In the meantime, try to relax. Continue your daily routine, and be the best nursing assistant you can be.

Answers to Competency Review Questions

Chapter 1
1. c
2. b
3. d

Chapter 2
1. b
2. c
3. b
4. a
5. b
6. b

Chapter 3
1. c
2. c
3. c
4. d

Chapter 4
1. a
2. d
3. c

Chapter 5
1. b
2. a

Chapter 6
1. b
2. d
3. d
4. d
5. d
6. b
7. a
8. c
9. d
10. c
11. c
12. d

Chapter 8
1. d
2. c
3. c
4. d
5. c
6. d
7. b

Chapter 9
1. a
2. a
3. d
4. a

Chapter 10
1. b
2. d
3. d
4. d
5. c
6. c
7. b
8. c
9. b
10. c
11. b

Chapter 11
1. a
2. a
3. d
4. c
5. c
6. c

Chapter 12
1. a
2. a
3. a
4. a
5. b
6. b

Chapter 13
1. b
2. d
3. d
4. a
5. a
6. c

Chapter 14
1. c
2. b
3. c
4. c

Chapter 15
1. c
2. a
3. c
4. b
5. a

Chapter 16
1. T
2. T
3. T
4. c
5. b
6. c
7. c

Chapter 17
1. d
2. c
3. b
4. a
5. a

Chapter 18
1. c
2. d
3. b
4. d
5. c
6. b
7. a
8. c
9. c
10. d
11. a
12. a

Chapter 19
1. T
2. F
3. T
4. T
5. T
6. T
7. T
8. T
9. T
10. b
11. d

Chapter 20
1. b
2. d
3. c
4. a
5. b
6. c
7. c

Chapter 21
1. a
2. d
3. d

Chapter 22
1. d
2. a
3. b
4. a
5. a
6. c
7. c
8. d
9. d

Chapter 24
1. c
2. a
3. b
4. a

Chapter 25
1. c
2. d
3. a
4. d

Chapter 26
1. c
2. c
3. c
4. c
5. d

Chapter 28
1. b
2. a
3. b
4. b

Chapter 31
1. b
2. d
3. d
4. a

Chapter 32
1. d
2. c
3. a
4. d
5. c

Chapter 34
1. b
2. c
3. d
4. d

Chapter 36
1. a
2. a
3. a
4. c
5. a
6. d

Chapter 37
1. d
2. d
3. b
4. d

Chapter 39
1. a
2. a
3. d
4. a
5. b

Chapter 40
1. c
2. a
3. c
4. c

Chapter 41
1. d
2. d
3. d
4. d
5. a
6. a

Answers to Practice Examination 1

1. **C** You never give drugs. You may politely refuse to do a task that you have not been trained to do. However, you need to tell the nurse. Do not ignore a request to do something. Page 20, Chapter 2.
2. **A** An ethical person does not judge others or cause harm to another person. Ethical behavior involves not being prejudiced or biased. Ethical behavior also involves not avoiding persons whose standards and values are different from your own. Page 26, Chapter 2.
3. **D** An ethical person is knowledgeable of what is right conduct and wrong conduct. Health care workers do not drink alcohol before coming to work and do not drink alcohol while working. Page 27, Chapter 2.
4. **A** Neglect is failure to provide a person with the goods or services needed to avoid physical harm, mental anguish, or mental illness. Page 27, Chapter 2.
5. **B** The resident's information is confidential. Information about the resident is shared only among health team members involved in his or her care. Page 28, Chapter 2.
6. **D** End-of-shift is a time for good teamwork. Continue to do your job. Your attitude is important. Page 44, Chapter 3.
7. **C** Write in ink, spell words correctly, and use only center-approved abbreviations. Page 59, Chapter 4.
8. **B** Give a courteous greeting. End the conversation politely and say good-bye. Confidential information about a resident or employee is not given to any caller. Page 65, Chapter 4.
9. **C** Many persons do not feel safe and secure when admitted to a nursing center. You need to be kind and understanding. Show the person the nursing center, listen to his or her concerns, explain routines and procedures, and repeat information as needed. Page 78, Chapter 6.
10. **B** When a person is angry or hostile, stay calm and professional. The person is usually not angry with you. He or she may be angry at another person or situation. Page 82, Chapter 6.
11. **D** Use words that are familiar to the person. Speak clearly, slowly, and distinctly. Also, ask one question at a time and wait for an answer. Page 82, Chapter 6.
12. **D** Follow the manufacturer's instructions. The excess strap should be tucked under the belt. The belt is applied over clothing and under the breasts. Page 157, Chapter 11.
13. **D** Listening requires that you care and have interest in the other person. Have good eye contact with the person. Focus on what the person is saying. Page 84, Chapter 6.
14. **C** Assume that a comatose person hears and understands you. Talk to the person and tell him or her what you are going to do. Page 87, Chapter 6.
15. **A** Protect a person's right to privacy when giving care. Politely ask visitors to leave the room. Do not expose the person's body in front of them. Show visitors where to wait. Page 87, Chapter 6.
16. **B** If a person wants to talk with a minister or spiritual leader, tell the nurse. Many people find comfort and strength from prayer and religious practices. Page 79, Chapter 6.
17. **A** Observe the person with a restraint at least every 15 minutes. Remove the restraint and reposition the person every 2 hours. Apply a restraint so it is snug and firm, but not tight. You could be negligent if the restraint is not applied properly. Page 166, Chapter 12.
18. **D** The skin becomes more dry, muscle strength decreases, reflexes are slower, and bladder muscles weaken. Page 113, Chapter 8.
19. **B** Always act in a professional manner. Page 125, Chapter 9.
20. **C** If you see something unsafe, correct the matter right away. Page 128, Chapter 10.
21. **A** Tell the nurse at once. It is important to do the correct procedure on the right person. You have to be able to read the person's name on the ID bracelet or use the photo ID to identify the person. Page 130, Chapter 10.
22. **B** Clutching at the throat is the "universal sign of choking." Page 131, Chapter 10.
23. **D** When a person is on a diabetic diet, tell the nurse about changes in the person's eating habits The person's meals and snacks need to be served on time. The person needs to eat at regular intervals to maintain a certain blood sugar. Always check the tray to see what was eaten. Page 382, Chapter 22.
24. **D** With mild airway obstruction, the person is conscious and can speak. Often forceful coughing can remove the object. Page 131, Chapter 10.
25. **A** The Heimlich maneuver involves abdominal thrusts. Page 132, Chapter 10.
26. **B** Do not use for or give faulty electrical equipment to persons in nursing centers. Take the item to the nurse. Page 134, Chapter 10.
27. **C** If a warning label is removed or damaged, do not use the substance. Take the container to the nurse and explain the problem. Page 137, Chapter 10.
28. **C** An ethical person realizes a person's values and standards may be different from his or hers. Page 26, Chapter 2.
29. **D** Remind a person not to smoke inside the center. Page 138, Chapter 10.
30. **A** During a fire, remember the word RACE. Page 139, Chapter 10.
31. **C** If a person with Alzheimer's disease has sundowning (increased restlessness and confusion as daylight ends), provide a calm, quiet setting late in

the day. Do not try to reason with the person because he or she cannot understand what you are saying. Do not ask the person to tell you what is bothering him or her. Communication is impaired. Complete treatments and activities early in the day. Page 628, Chapter 37.

32. **C** Make sure dentures fit properly. Cut food into small pieces, and make sure the person can chew and swallow the food served. Report loose teeth or dentures to the nurse. Page 131, Chapter 10.

33. **A** Lock both wheels before you transfer a person to and from the wheelchair. The person's feet are on the footplates before moving the chair. Do not let the person stand on the footplates. Page 136, Chapter 10.

34. **B** Ease the person to the floor. Do not try to prevent the fall or yell at the person. The person should not get up before the nurse checks for injuries. Therefore the nurse needs to be told as soon as the fall occurs. Page 158, Chapter 11.

35. **B** Death from strangulation is the most serious risk factor to using a restraint. Restraints are not used for staff convenience or to punish a person. A written doctor's order is required before a restraint can be applied. Page 165, Chapter 12.

36. **C** Wash your hands before and after giving care to a person. Page 182, Chapter 13.

37. **D** Gloves need to be changed when they become contaminated with blood, body fluids, secretions, and excretions. Page 190, Chapter 13.

38. **D** When washing your hands, keep your hands and forearms lower than your elbows. Do not use hot water or let your uniform touch the sink. Push your watch up your arm so you can wash past your wrist. Page 183, Chapter 13.

39. **C** Bend your knees and squat to lift a heavy object. Hold items close to your body when lifting a heavy object. For a wider base of support and more balance, stand with your feet apart. Do not bend from your waist when lifting objects. Page 204, Chapter 14.

40. **B** The head of the bed is raised between 45 and 60 degrees for Fowler's position. Page 207, Chapter 14.

41. **B** Negligence—an unintentional wrong in which a person did not act in a reasonable and careful manner and causes harm to a person or the person's property. Page 27, Chapter 2.

42. **A** Have the person's back and buttocks against the back of the chair. Feet are flat on the floor or the wheelchair plates. Backs of the person's knees and calves are slightly away from the edge of the seat. Page 209, Chapter 14.

43. **B** Help the person out of bed on his or her strong side. In transferring, the strong side moves first. It pulls the weaker side along. Page 232, Chapter 15.

44. **A** When a person tries to bite, scratch, pinch, or kick you, you need to protect the person, others, and yourself from harm. Page 82, Chapter 6.

45. **C** Protect the person's right to privacy at all times. Screen the person properly, and do not expose body parts. Page 244, Chapter 15.

46. **D** For comfort, adjust lighting to meet the person's changing needs. Nursing centers maintain a temperature range of 71° F to 81° F. Unpleasant odors may be offensive or embarrassing to people. Many older persons are sensitive to noise. Page 248, Chapter 16.

47. **A** Signal lights are placed on the person's strong side and kept within the person's reach. Signal lights are answered promptly. Page 254, Chapter 16.

48. **C** You must have the person's permission to open or search closets or drawers. Page 255, Chapter 16.

49. **C** When handling linens, do not take unneeded linen to a person's room. Once in the room, extra linen is considered contaminated. Because your uniform is considered dirty, always hold linen away from your body. To prevent the spread of microbes, never shake linen. Never put clean or dirty linens on the floor. Page 261, Chapter 17.

50. **C** To use a fire extinguisher, remember the word PASS. P—pull the safety pin, A—aim low, S—squeeze the lever, S—sweep back and forth. Page 140, Chapter 10.

51. **B** Mouth care is given at least every 2 hours for an unconscious person. To prevent aspiration, you position the person on one side with the head turned well to the side. Use a padded tongue blade to keep the person's mouth open. Wear gloves. Page 282, Chapter 18.

52. **B** A good attitude is needed at work. Be willing to help others. Be pleasant and respectful of others. Page 44, Chapter 3.

53. **B** During cleaning, firmly hold dentures over a basin of water lined with a towel. This prevents them from falling onto a hard surface and breaking. Clean and store dentures in cool water. Hot water causes dentures to lose their shape. To prevent losing dentures, label the denture cup with the person's name. Page 283, Chapter 18.

54. **C** Report and record the location and description of the rash. Page 288, Chapter 18.

55. **C** Gently wipe the eye from the inner aspect to the outer aspect of the eye. Clean the far eye first. Do not use soap. Page 289, Chapter 18.

56. **D** When giving a back massage, wear gloves if the person's skin has open areas. Warm the lotion before applying it to the person. Use firm strokes. Do not massage reddened bony areas. This can lead to more tissue damage. Page 298, Chapter 18.

57. **A** Separate the labia and clean downward from front to back. Wear gloves and use soap. Page 300, Chapter 18.

58. **C** Stay within hearing distance if the person can be left alone. Place the signal light within the person's reach. Cold water is turned on first, then hot water. Direct water away from the person while adjusting the water temperature. Page 294, Chapter 18.

59. **B** Electric razors are used when a person is on an anticoagulant. An anticoagulant prevents or slows down blood clotting. Bleeding occurs easily. A nick or cut from a safety razor can cause bleeding. Page 313, Chapter 19.

60. **B** Remove clothing from the strong or "good" (unaffected) side first. Page 319, Chapter 19.

61. **C** Address a person with dignity and respect. Call the person by his or her title—Mr., or Mrs., or Miss. Address a person by his or her first name, or another name, if the person asks you to. Page 77, Chapter 6.

62. **D** Measure and record the amount of urine in the drainage bag. The catheter is secured to the person's thigh or abdomen. Do not disconnect the catheter from the drainage tubing. Do not let the person lie on the tubing. Page 340, Chapter 20.

63. **B** Carbohydrates provide energy and fiber for bowel elimination. Page 375, Chapter 22.

64. **D** When taking a rectal temperature, the thermometer is held in place so it is not lost into the rectum or broken. Lubricate the bulb end of the thermometer for easy insertion and to prevent tissue damage. Provide for privacy. A glass thermometer remains in place for 2 minutes or as required by policy. Page 473, Chapter 28.

65. **A** Report any systolic pressure below 90 mm Hg and any diastolic pressure below 60 mm Hg at once. Record the BP. Retake the BP in 30 minutes if the nurse asks you to. It is your responsibility to tell the nurse, not the unit secretary's. Page 485, Chapter 28.

66. **D** Oral temperatures are not taken on unconscious persons, persons receiving oxygen, or persons who breathe through their mouth. Page 471, Chapter 28.

67. **A** To assist with walking, offer the person your arm and have the person walk a half step behind you. When caring for a person who is blind or visually impaired, let the person do as much for himself or herself as possible. Use a normal voice tone. Do not shout at the person. Identify yourself when you enter the room. Do not touch the person until you have indicated your presence. Page 572, Chapter 34.

68. **D** The person with confusion and dementia has the right to personal choice. He or she also has the right to keep and use personal items. The family makes choices if the person cannot. Page 632, Chapter 37.

69. **D** No one can shout, scream, or hit the person. Nor can they call the person names. The person did not choose loss of function. Discuss your feelings with the nurse. Page 649, Chapter 39.

70. **C** Encourage the person to help as much as possible. Doors and windows are closed to reduce drafts. You wash from the cleanest areas to the dirtiest areas. Pat the skin dry to avoid irritating or breaking the skin. Page 286, Chapter 18.

71. **A** When a person is dying, always assume that the person can hear you. Reposition the person every 2 hours to promote comfort. Skin care, personal hygiene, back massages, oral hygiene, and good body alignment promote comfort. Page 670, Chapter 41.

72. **B** Foods that melt at room temperature—ice cream, sherbet, custard, pudding, gelatin, and Popsicles—are measured and recorded as intake. The nurse measures ands records IV fluids and tube feedings. Page 386, Chapter 22.

73. **B** After bedrest, activity increases slowly and in steps. First the person dangles. Sitting in a chair follows. Next the person walks in the room and then in the hallway. Page 419, Chapter 24.

74. **B** Tell the nurse at once if you find or cause a skin tear. Page 534, Chapter 32.

75. **A** Treat the resident with respect and ensure privacy. The resident has a right not to have his or her private affairs exposed or made public without giving consent. Only staff involved in the resident's care should see, handle, or examine his or her body. Page 28, Chapter 2.

Answers to Practice Examination 2

1. **C** You may politely refuse to do a task that is not in your job description. Page 25, Chapter 2.
2. **B** An ethical person realizes a person's values and standards may be different from his or hers. Page 26, Chapter 2.
3. **C** Verbal abuse is using oral or written words or statements that speak badly of, sneer at, criticize, or condemn a person. Page 29, Chapter 2.
4. **C** Speak in a normal tone. Use words the person seems to understand, and speak slowly and distinctly. Page 82, Chapter 6.
5. **C** Do not allow smoking in bed. Turn cold water on first, then hot water. Assist the person with drinking or eating hot food. Do not let the person sleep with a heating pad. Page 131, Chapter 10.
6. **B** Use three-pronged plugs on all electrical devices, and follow the manufacturer's instructions on equipment. Wipe up spills right away. Do not use unfamiliar equipment. Ask for training if you are unfamiliar with something. Page 135, Chapter 10.
7. **D** Answer signal lights promptly. Throw rugs, scatter rugs, and area rugs are not used. The person's bed should be in the lowest horizontal position, except when giving care. Grab bars should be used when the person showers. Page 153, Chapter 11.
8. **B** Decontaminate your hands after removing gloves. Page 184, Chapter 13.
9. **D** Use good body mechanics, provide for privacy, and use pillows as directed by the nurse. The signal light should be placed within the person's reach after positioning. Page 207, Chapter 14.
10. **C** A person must not put his or her arms around your neck. He or she can pull you forward or cause you to lose your balance. Neck, back, and other injuries from falls are possible. Ask a co-worker to help you, and you should use a transfer or gait belt. Lock the wheels on the wheelchair. Page 214, Chapter 15.
11. **B** Wear gloves when removing linen. Linens may contain blood, body fluids, secretions, or excretions. Raise the bed for good body mechanics. The bed is flat when you place clean linens on it. Page 264, Chapter 17.
12. **B** Use a circular motion, start at the meatus, and work outward. Gloves are worn. Soap is used. Page 303, Chapter 18.
13. **C** Put clothing on the weak (affected) side first. Page 319, Chapter 20.
14. **D** The drainage bag hangs from the bed frame or chair. It must not touch the floor. The bag is always kept lower than the person's bladder. The drainage bag does not hang on the bed rail. Page 340, Chapter 20.
15. **A** Protein is needed for tissue repair and growth. Page 375, Chapter 22.
16. **C** Older persons may not feel thirsty (decreased sense of thirst). Offer water often. Page 385, Chapter 22.
17. **C** NPO means nothing by mouth. An NPO sign is posted above the bed. The water pitcher and glass are removed from the room. Oral hygiene is performed frequently. Page 386, Chapter 22.
18. **C** 1 oz equals 30 ml. 3 oz equals 90 ml. Page 386, Chapter 22.
19. **D** Allow time for chewing and swallowing. Fluids are offered during the meal. A teaspoon, rather than a fork, is used for feeding. Sit and talk with the person. Page 392, Chapter 22.
20. **D** Support the part being exercised. Do not force a joint beyond its present ROM. Move the joint slowly, smoothly, and gently. Do not force the joint to the point of pain. Page 415, Chapter 24.
21. **B** A cane is held on the strong side of the body. If the left leg is weak, the cane is held in the right hand. Page 423, Chapter 24.
22. **B** Position the person in good alignment. Bed linens are kept tight and wrinkle-free. Talk softly and gently. Avoid sudden and jarring movements of the bed or chair. Page 432, Chapter 25.
23. **C** Check behind the ears and under the nose for signs of irritation. Never remove an oxygen device. Do not adjust the oxygen flow rate. Do not fill the humidifier. Page 449, Chapter 26.
24. **A** Tell the nurse at once. Mercury is a hazardous substance. Do not touch the mercury. Follow special procedures for handling hazardous materials. Page 472, Chapter 28.
25. **C** Report and record a pulse rate less than 60 or more than 100 beats per minute at once. The radial pulse is used for routine vital signs. If the pulse is irregular, count it for 1 minute. Do not use your thumb to take a pulse. Page 481, Chapter 28.
26. **B** Count the respirations for 1 minute if an abnormal breathing pattern is noted. People change their breathing patterns when they know respirations are being counted. Therefore the person should not know that you are counting respirations. The healthy adult has 12 to 20 respirations per minute. Page 484, Chapter 28.
27. **A** Report any systolic pressure above 140 mm Hg and any diastolic pressure above 80 mm Hg at once. Then continue to take blood pressures on other persons. Retake the BP in 30 minutes if the nurse asks you to. It is your responsibility to tell the nurse, not the unit secretary's. Page 485, Chapter 28.
28. **C** Rectal temperatures are not taken if a person has diarrhea, is confused, or is agitated. Page 471, Chapter 28.
29. **C** When a person is first admitted to a nursing center, he or she may feel lonely. Therefore introduce the person to other residents. Encourage the person to

participate in activities. Explain procedures, and answer his or her questions. Repeat information as needed. Page 518, Chapter 31.

30. **B** Have the person void before being weighed. A full bladder adds weight. No footwear is worn. Footwear adds to the weight and height measurement. Weigh the person at the same time of day, usually before breakfast. Balance the scale before weighing the person. Page 520, Chapter 31.

31. **D** Keep the skin free of moisture from urine, stools, or perspiration. Reposition the person at least every 2 hours. Do not massage reddened areas. Keep the heels and ankles off the bed. Page 533, Chapter 32.

32. **C** Face the person when speaking. Reduce or eliminate background noise. Speak in a normal voice tone. Speak clearly, distinctly, and slowly. Page 566, Chapter 34.

33. **C** Explain the location of food and beverages. Keep furniture and equipment out of areas where the person walks. Provide lighting as the person prefers. Do not rearrange furniture and equipment. Page 572, Chapter 34.

34. **C** The person with confusion and dementia has the right to privacy and confidentiality. Information about the person's care and condition is shared only with those involved in providing the care. Protect the person from exposure. Page 632, Chapter 37.

35. **C** Ask clear, simple questions. Explain what you are going to do and why. Call the person by name every time you are in contact with him or her. Keep calendars and clocks in the person's room. Page 622, Chapter 37.

36. **D** Exercise the person as ordered. Adequate exercise often reduces wandering. Do not keep the person in his or her room. Involve the person in activities. Do not restrain the person or argue with the person who wants to leave. Page 628, Chapter 37.

37. **B** Restorative nursing programs promote self-care measures. They help maintain the person's highest level of function. The programs focus on the whole person. The care helps the person regain health, strength, and independence. Page 643, Chapter 39.

38. **C** Remind the person of his or her progress in the rehabilitation program. Focus on the person's abilities and strengths. Progress may be slow. Do not deny the disability. Page 647, Chapter 39.

39. **D** Respect the person's right to privacy. Do not expose the person's body unnecessarily. Only those involved in the person's care need to know the person's diagnosis. The final moments of death are kept confidential. So are family reactions. Page 675, Chapter 41.

40. **A** Remember the word RACE. Your first action is to **R**escue the person in immediate danger. Then sound the **A**larm, **C**onfine the fire, and **E**xtinguish the fire. Page 139, Chapter 10.

41. **B** Failure to provide a person with the goods or services needed to avoid physical harm or mental anguish is neglect. Page 29, Chapter 2.

42. **C** You have not been trained to give drugs or to perform sterile procedures. Do not perform tasks that are not in your job description. Page 20, Chapter 2.

43. **C** Report any changes from normal or changes in the person's condition to the nurse at once. Then record your observation. Page 56, Chapter 4.

44. **D** A good attitude is needed at work. People rely on you to give good care. You are expected to be pleasant and respectful. Always be willing to help others. Page 44, Chapter 3.

45. **B** Unnecessary restraint is false imprisonment. Observe the person for complications every 15 minutes. The least restrictive type of restraint is ordered by the doctor. Restraints can increase confusion and agitation. Page 165, Chapter 12.

46. **C** The supine position is the back-lying position. For good alignment, the bed is flat and the head and shoulders are supported on a pillow. Place arms and hands at the sides. Page 208, Chapter 14.

47. **A** Hand washing is the most important way to prevent or avoid spreading infection. Page 181, Chapter 13.

48. **B** To gossip means to spread rumors or talk about the private matters of others. Gossiping is unprofessional and hurtful. If others are gossiping, you need to remove yourself from the group. Do not make or repeat any comment that can hurt another person. Page 45, Chapter 3.

49. **D** Ask a co-worker to help you. The head of the bed is lowered. The person flexes both knees. Friction and shearing cause skin tears and need to be prevented. Page 221, Chapter 15.

50. **A** On a sodium-controlled diet, high-sodium foods such as ham and canned vegetables are omitted. Salt is not added to food at the table. The amount of salt used in cooking is limited. Page 382, Chapter 22.

51. **B** Elastic stockings should not have wrinkles or creases after being applied. Wrinkles and creases can cause skin breakdown. Apply stockings before the person gets out of bed. Apply the correct size. Page 538, Chapter 32.

52. **C** When a person begins to fall, ease him or her to the floor. Also protect the person's head. Page 158, Chapter 11.

53. **A** Before bathing, allow the person to use the bathroom, bedpan, or urinal. Page 286, Chapter 18.

54. **A** Insert a rectal thermometer 1 inch into the rectum. Page 475, Chapter 28.

55. **A** Touch is a form of nonverbal communication. It conveys comfort and caring. Touch means different things to different people. Some people do not like to be touched. Page 83, Chapter 6.

56. **A** A person's information is confidential. The information is shared only among health team members involved in the person's care. Page 45, Chapter 3.

57. **A** Report and record complaints of urgency, burning, dysuria, or other urinary problems. Page 330, Chapter 20.

58. **C** Respect and accept a person's culture and religion. Learn about his or her beliefs and practices. This helps you understand the person and give better care. Page 79, Chapter 6.

59. **C** Wear gloves when giving perineal care. Gloves are needed whenever contact with blood, body fluids,

secretions, excretions, mucous membranes, and non-intact skin is likely. Page 186, Chapter 13.

60. **D** Report any changes from normal or changes in the person's condition to the nurse at once. Then record your observation. Page 56, Chapter 4.

61. **A** If a person is standing, have him or her sit before fainting occurs. Page 664, Chapter 40.

62. **A** The person drinks an increased amount of fluid. Keep fluids within the person's reach. Offer fluids regularly. Page 386, Chapter 22.

63. **B** Communication fails when you talk too much and fail to listen. Page 86, Chapter 6.

64. **A** During bathing, a person has the right to privacy and the right to personal choice. Page 286, Chapter 18.

65. **C** People in late adulthood need to develop new friends and relationships. They need to adjust to retirement and reduced income, decreased strength and loss of health. They need to cope with a partner's death and prepare for their own death. Page 110, Chapter 8.

66. **C** One myth about aging is that mental function declines with age. The other statements are facts about aging. Page 111, Chapter 8.

67. **C** Never put clean or dirty linen on the floor. The floor is dirty. You cannot use the linen. Page 261, Chapter 17.

68. **B** To prevent aspiration, position the unconscious person on one side when you do mouth care. Use a small amount of fluid to clean the mouth. Tell the person what you are doing. Dentures are not worn when the person is unconscious. Page 281, Chapter 18.

69. **B** Encourage people to do their own hair care. Do not cut matted or tangled hair. The person chooses his or her hair style. Brushing and combing are done with morning care and whenever needed. Page 308, Chapter 19.

70. **D** Check between the toes for cracks and sores. These areas are often overlooked. If left untreated, a serious infection could occur. Fingernails are cut with nail clipper, not scissors. You do not trim or cut toenails if a person is diabetic or has poor circulation. Page 316, Chapter 19.

71. **B** If an indwelling catheter becomes disconnected from the drainage system, you tell the nurse at once. Page 343, Chapter 20.

72. **B** Urinary drainage bags are emptied and the contents measured at the end of each shift. Drainage bags must not touch the floor. The bag is always kept lower than the person's bladder. Page 344, Chapter 20.

73. **C** Use elastic tape to secure a condom catheter. Elastic tape expands when the penis changes size, and adhesive tape does not. Do not apply a condom catheter if the penis is red and irritated. Always act in a professional manner. Page 347, Chapter 20.

74. **D** For comfort during bowel elimination, leave the person alone if possible. Provide for privacy. Help the person to the toilet or commode if possible. Page 355, Chapter 21.

75. **A** Help the person from the wheelchair to the bed on his or her strong side. In transferring, the strong side moves first. It pulls the weaker side along. Page 236, Chapter 15.